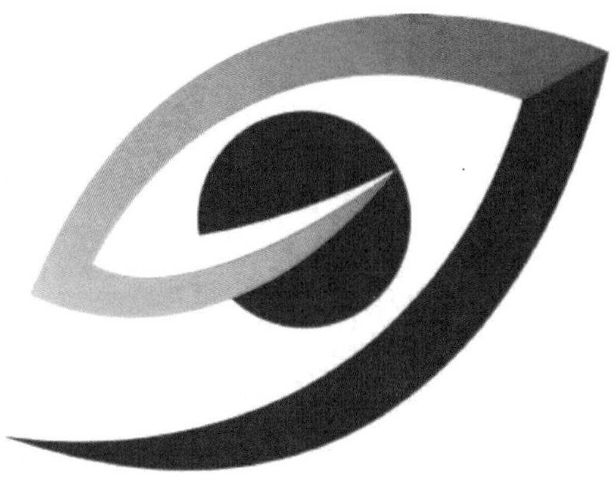

Cure AMD Foundation™

Ancestral Dietary Strategy to Prevent and Treat Macular Degeneration

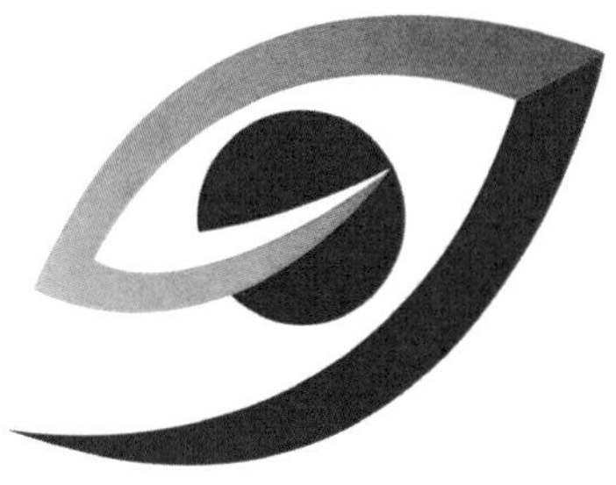

Ancestral Dietary Strategy to Prevent and Treat Macular Degeneration

CHRIS A. KNOBBE, M.D.
Ophthalmologist & Associate Clinical Professor Emeritus

Profound, Revolutionary, and Dramatic Discoveries
Made by Dr. Knobbe, support the hypothesis that AMD may be prevented and successfully treated, through ancestral dietary strategy and "sacred" foods

Cover Design by Derek Murphy, *CreativINDIECovers.com*
Ophthalmic Illustrations by Mark Erickson, *JirehDesign.com*
Book Formatting by Benard Owuondo, *BookGrinds.com*
& Jennifer Woodhead, *gaiadesignstudio.co.uk*

Printed in the United States of America
Published by Cure AMD Foundation™
Boulder, Colorado, USA

First eBook and Print Editions, 2016

For Lisa and Kyla.

And now these three remain: faith, hope, and love.

But the greatest of these is love.

Praise for Chris A. Knobbe, MD, and *Ancestral Dietary Strategy to Prevent & Treat Macular Degeneration*

"In our opinion, Dr. Knobbe has uncovered an important connection between diet and age-related macular degeneration that has the potential to prevent hundreds of thousands, if not millions, of people from progressing to the advanced stages of this disease."

— Editorial Board, Price-Pottenger Nutrition Foundation
Price-Pottenger Journal of Health and Healing, Summer - 2017

"I have found Dr Knobbe's theory well researched and presented in his book. Although no one can accurately say exactly what the incidence of AMD was in the early 1900's, he presents a compelling argument, based in fact, that not only is AMD on the rise and reaching epidemic proportions, but it's coincident with the introduction of processed, nutrient deficient, foods. Perhaps most compelling is, after reading his book, I now find myself taking extra chair time to discuss dietary issues with my patients. I would say this is a must read for any eyecare provider, but particularly those practicing primary eyecare with the goal of preventing AMD."

— Micah W. Rothstein, MD
Ophthalmologist
Eye Care Center of Northern Colorado

"Dr. Knobbe's thesis that macular degeneration is due to dietary causes is well-supported by his research. Drawing on the observations of Dr. Weston A. Price, who studied traditional cultures living on unrefined and unprocessed foods, the author makes his point quite clearly: Our present-day diet is a major culprit in the proliferation of not only AMD, but most likely for many other degenerative diseases of civilization as well. Here is where so many current studies are woefully behind; the answers are right in front of us if we dare to look. Dr. Knobbe has done just that, and he deserves great credit for bringing this topic to the public with this very readable book."

— Ed Bennett, President
Price-Pottenger Nutrition Foundation

"As Founder and President of the Macular Degeneration Association, a 501 (c)(3) tax exempt non-profit organization, whose purpose it is to educate and help prevent vision loss from age-related macular degeneration (AMD), I read and studied Dr. Knobbe's book, *Ancestral Dietary Strategy to Prevent & Treat Macular Degeneration*. I must say, I was surprised – somewhat shocked – by his hypothesis and referenced supportive research. Dr. Knobbe has relied partly on the fact that AMD was once a rare disorder – in fact – it was rare just about 85 years ago, prior to 1930. Today, AMD has reached epidemic proportions – worldwide. Knobbe's hypothesis concludes that AMD develops because of the ingredients of processed, man-made, nutrient-deficient foods.

His research and book also lay out plausible biological mechanisms whereby processed food consumption, which is associated with vitamin and mineral deficiencies and certain toxicities (e.g., from sugar and vegetable oils), ultimately causes this disease. In his book, Knobbe also provides a fundamental nutrition plan to reduce the risk of getting AMD and avoiding its progression.

For these reasons, I have invited Dr. Knobbe to be a speaker at each and every one of the Macular Degeneration Association's patient education conferences in 13 cities across the U.S., annually. I highly recommend his book to anyone who desires to prevent and/or treat this dreadful disease. Finally, we are finding that attendees at our conferences are generally impressed and convinced, that Dr. Knobbe's hypothesis and research, just makes good sense. I am convinced that his message is of critical importance to all of us, but especially for those who desire to preserve their precious gift of sight."

— Larry Hoffheimer, JD Founder & Chairman
Macular Degeneration Association

"It is fairly infrequent that I am asked to review a book for Price-Pottenger as I am simply too busy. A while back, Joan Grinzi, Executive Director of the Price-Pottenger Nutrition Foundation, gave me the Review Copy of *Ancestral Dietary Strategy to Prevent & Treat Macular Degeneration*, by ophthalmologist and author, Chris A. Knobbe, MD. She asked me to take a brief look at it and give my opinion of whether we should think of recommending it. It quickly captivated me so that it received far more than any brief glance.

AMD, or age related macular degeneration, is a misnamed eye condition, which is rapidly increasing in frequency in the U.S. I say misnamed, due to the fact that it is not age related any more than cancer and heart disease are age related. There are millions of people at advanced ages who have none of these conditions. I would re-name it D&LMD for Diet and Lifestyle Related Macular Degeneration, to be more accurate.

As I read through Dr. Knobbe's book, I was pleasantly surprised and then even astonished to find an MD Professor of Ophthalmology with both such an open mind as well as such a good grasp on nutrition and reality even when it directly contradicted his medical school training. Yes, this is likely the best book ever written on AMD, but saying that is doing it a disservice since this book should be read be everyone who cares about their current and future health or the health of their loved ones. Knobbe does such a grand job of exposing frauds and lies regarding diet and disease, that his book could just as easily be re-named ***Everything You Need to Know About Diet and By the Way It Will also Help Your Eyesight***. This book has my highest recommendation for anyone interested in protecting their eyesight (and their health) as they get older."

— David J. Getoff, CCN, CTN, FAAIM (Naturopathic Physician)
Vice President, Price-Pottenger Nutrition Foundation

"I just finished reading *Ancestral Dietary Strategy to Prevent & Treat Macular Degeneration*. Following extensive research, this book is, without doubt, the most comprehensive and useful study on macular degeneration I have found. As a physician and author, may I commend you, Dr. Knobbe, on an excellent book, superbly researched and written. Congratulations!"

— Dr. Felicity Dale, MD, MBBS

"I was introduced to Chris's work at the Ancestral Health Symposium, held at the University of Colorado Boulder, in 2016. I was already well informed about the effects of modern diet/lifestyle on many major chronic diseases such as diabetes, many cancers, cardiovascular events and dementia. As I listened, I realized that it was blindingly obvious (excuse the pun) that the retina was no different to any other complex vascular structure - of course, it would be adversely affected by the same factors identified in other chronic diseases. How, as a doctor myself, did I not realize this before?

But a hypothesis must be backed up by data. Chris presents a compelling review of data from 25 nations, showing that the incidence of AMD, very rare prior to 1930, has risen in parallel with the displacement of traditional diets by processed 'Western foods." This mirrors the same data for other chronic diseases as mentioned above and is robustly backed up by known biochemical mechanisms beyond the scope of this review.

I am convinced on the basis of Chris's evidence review - and saddened by traditional Western medicine's delay in not making consideration of lifestyle factors an immediate first step in preventing and managing all chronic diseases, of which AMD is hugely important. Hopefully the tide is turning, and this work deserves to take credit for being a powerful force towards reducing the incidence of lives affected by AMD."

— Dr. Andrea Steinberg
Family Medicine Physician
Ellerslie Medical Center
Auckland, New Zealand

Acknowledgments

After developing a hypothesis for the cause of macular degeneration, it would be nearly a year-and-a-half of far greater than full-time work to bring this book to a conclusion. When I began, I never imagined that I would need the help of numerous ophthalmologists, scores of vision scientists, reference librarians, the National Institutes of Health (NIH), the USDA Economic Research Service (ERS), and not to mention that I would ultimately rely on the research of many thousands of investigators. So many brilliantly intelligent, dedicated, kind, and caring people, from professors to manufacturers, gave freely of themselves in the name of science. After having given my name, university affiliation, my goal of "investigating the nutritional basis of AMD," and a question or request, these people gave of themselves that it might, one day, help those with macular degeneration.

Among those who provided much assistance, I would first like to acknowledge Pamela "Pam" Sieving, MA, MS, AHIP, reference librarian formerly of the NIH. Pam gave tirelessly to help me uncover studies and relics from the 19th century, even translating one German paper in it's entirety. I would also like to thank Jenny Benjamin, reference librarian at the American Academy of Ophthalmology (AAO), and Mary Ann Huslig, MLS, librarian at the University of Texas Southwestern Medical Center, where I am on the volunteer faculty, both of whom assisted me in tracking down historical research.

I would like to extend a huge debt of gratitude to Professor Ron Klein, MD, at the University of Wisconsin, not only for his own studies, but for helping me with this research nearly from its inception. Secondly, I cannot thank Professor Paulus T.V.M. de Jong, MD, of Erasmus University, Rotterdam, The Netherlands, enough, as he assisted me multiple times and even provided his brilliant historical research on AMD, which I otherwise had never uncovered. Professor Daniel M. Albert, MD, of the University of Wisconsin, also graciously assisted me in researching the history of AMD. For all of their brilliant investigations on AMD, particularly the epidemiologic research, I would like to extend my gratitude to Professor Troels Vinding, MD, of National University Hospital (Rigshospitalet), Copenhagen, Denmark, Professor Johannes Vingerling, MD, of Erasmus University, Rotterdam, The Netherlands, Professor Paul Mitchell, MBBS, MD, PhD, of the University of Sydney, Australia, and Emeritus Professor Alan Bird, MD, of London University.

Professor Johanna Seddon, MD, of Tufts University, has really been iconic in ophthalmology, having paved the way to link macular degeneration with certain dietary elements, when our own colleagues once thought the concept was laughable. I owe to her a huge debt of gratitude, for persevering in so many studies to tie diet to AMD.

I would like to extend a thank you to Professor Ronald Wormald, MD, Moorfields Eye Hospital, London, England, and Jennifer Evans, MSc, PhD, for both helping me in regards to their research of blindness in the U.K. secondary to AMD. Sergio Pagliarini, MD, University Hospital Coventry and Warwickshire, West Midlands, U.K., and Professor Antonietta Moramarco, MD, of the University of Rome, Italy, both were exceptionally kind, gracious, and helpful regarding their research on AMD in Saladra, Italy, where AMD is quite rare. Special thanks to Dr. Moramarco, whose native tongue is Italian, for communicating with me in English, since I can only write and speak one language. The same is true of many other doctors around the world who've helped me.

I must thank Professor Jill Keeffe, PhD, the former director of the Center for Eye Research Australia (CERA), as she helped me reach so many ophthalmologists in the South Pacific Islands. Along that same vein, a huge thank you to the ophthalmologists from Fiji, including Dr Ana Cama, Prevention of Blindness Coordinator, Dr Biu Sikivou, Director of the Pacific Eye Institute, Dr Tarai Rakabu Hicks, and Dr Varanisese Naviri. I owe a great debt of gratitude to Dr. Claude Posala, MBBS, DO, MMED/Ophthalmology, of the Solomon Islands, Dr. Lucilla Ah Ching, of Samoa, and Dr. Rabebe Tekeraoi, of Kiribati. The assistance of these many generous ophthalmologists is of incalculable value, as AMD is exceedingly rare in these island nations.

I owe such an enormous debt of gratitude to so many investigators and authors in various areas of nutrition research. In the area of general nutrition, I owe much to Stephan Guyenet, PhD, of the University of Washington, for his brilliant articles and education through WholeHealthSource.org, as well as his generous donation of various graphs. And if it weren't for the research and books of Loren Cordain, PhD, of Colorado State University, I may have never begun to investigate nutrition myself. I would like to thank Professor Chris Masterjohn, PhD, of Brooklyn College, for directly helping me and providing guidance on categorizing vegetable oils and his brilliant studies on lipid research, Robert Lustig, MD, of the University of California, San Francisco, for assisting me with sugar research, Kris Gunnars, BSc, of Authority Nutrition, for his assistance on vegetable oils, Denise Minger, for her generous support and brilliant analysis of white wheat flour, Chris Kresser, Lac, for broadly sharing his general nutrition knowledge, and Staffan Lindeberg, MD, for helping me with nutrition as it relates to myopia.

Thanks goes to Wanjiku "Ciku" Mathenge, MD, of Kenya, Africa, for assisting me regarding her prevalence study and the diets of Kenyans; to Amar Agarwal, MD, Chandran Abraham, MD, Anusha Venkataraman, MD, and R. Kim, MD, all of India, for assistance in validating the history of AMD in India; and for my friends and colleagues in Texas, Bill Plauche, MD and Andrew Bossen, MD, of Sherman, Texas, and Rajiv Anand, MD, of Dallas, Texas, for giving us perspective on AMD prevalence at home. Also, a great thanks to Bob Wang, MD, vitreo-retinal specialist of Dallas, Texas, for his guidance in preparing a manuscript for scientific publication of this work.

Thank you to Jinan Saadine, MD, MPH at the Centers for Disease Control (CDC) and Jeanine Bentley, of the USDA Economic Research Service, who helped with tables, graphs, and my annoying emails.

I owe a debt of gratitude to Gert Mulvad, MD, member of the Circumpolar Inuit Health Committee, Greenland Center for Health Research, University of Greenland, for his great assistance in locating and sharing research on the changing food consumption patterns in Greenland. Dr. Mulvad is an expert in this area and his assistance was invaluable.

I owe a great thank you to Sally Fallon, Founder and President of the Weston A. Price Foundation, for her assistance, book, lectures, and advice. Personally, I hold Mrs. Fallon in the highest of regards, and I have a deep and reverent respect for her extraordinary knowledge. I would also like to extend a great thanks to Joan Grinzi, RN, Executive Director of the Price-Pottenger Nutrition Foundation, for allowing me to review Weston A. Price's book, *Nutrition and Physical Degeneration*, and also for providing photos from Dr. Price's invaluable research.

Thank you to my extraordinary and amazing friend of many years, Mark Erickson, of JirehDesign.com, for providing the brilliant eye illustrations found in this book. These images help anyone make sense of the pathology of AMD.

I cannot possibly extend enough thanks to the brilliant Marija Stojanoska, MSc, of Skopje, Macedonia, my colleague in this research. She has worked tirelessly with me for months on end – first mining vegetable oil and sugar data in 25 countries, with as much dedication to integrity and accuracy as my own, and secondly, for graphing that data to paint scientifically accurate results. She brought data to the hypothesis proferred herein, which was stunning. I couldn't have done what she did, if I had been given years. I am deeply indebted to her and I hope we can collaborate further for many years to come.

The person I would like to thank the most is the late Weston A. Price (1870 – 1948). If it weren't for Dr. Price's extraordinary dedication and decades of research, published in 1939, I don't believe I would have ever even considered the hypothesis for AMD proffered in this book. We should all learn from this great giant in the field of nutrition, for his research was brilliant, revolutionary, vast, timeless, and beyond compare. Once a person fully understands Price's research, everything in nutrition suddenly becomes clear.

Table of Contents

Part I

Unveiling the Hypothesis

1 CAN ANCESTRAL DIETS ACTUALLY PREVENT AND TREAT MACULAR DEGENERATION?

"Let food be thy medicine and medicine be thy food."
~ *Hippocrates (460 – 370 B.C.)* ~

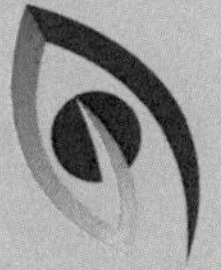

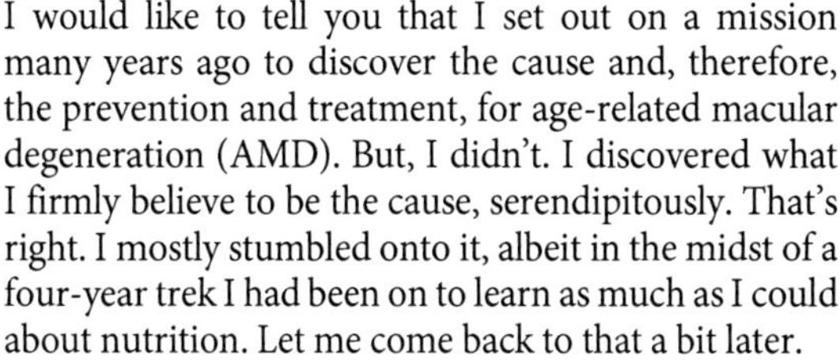

I would like to tell you that I set out on a mission many years ago to discover the cause and, therefore, the prevention and treatment, for age-related macular degeneration (AMD). But, I didn't. I discovered what I firmly believe to be the cause, serendipitously. That's right. I mostly stumbled onto it, albeit in the midst of a four-year trek I had been on to learn as much as I could about nutrition. Let me come back to that a bit later.

As I know you're anxious to hear it, let me immediately unveil the hypothesis that I will proffer in this book, as it leads us not only to a logical and rational strategy for prevention of AMD, but to its treatment as well. Submitted for your consideration, an alternative hypothesis for the cause of macular degeneration:

Hypothesis: The 'displacing foods of modern commerce' are the Primary and Proximate Cause of Age-Related Macular Degeneration.

Corollary: Ancestral Diets Prevent AMD (and may reverse early AMD).

In this book, I will argue that the condition of AMD is, first and foremost, entirely preventable, through any variety of ancestral diets. The term "ancestral diets" refers to the traditional diets of our ancestors – and there are numerous examples that are extremely varied, but they all share certain commonalities when it comes to nutrient density – and none of them contained man-made, processed foods.

Secondly, I will argue that, even once begun, the earliest stages of AMD are often fully or partially reversible, while moderate stages of disease may be stabilized, with proper diet and lifestyle changes. When AMD is not reversible, I will submit to you that preventing progression may be common for those who will alter their diet and lifestyle according to those of our ancestors. I will also review exactly what that means, leaving few if any questions in your mind about how and what to eat in order to save your sight.

Thirdly, I will argue that this condition we now call "*age-related* macular degeneration," is really

diet-related macular degeneration. Just about eighty-five years ago and prior, the condition we call age-related macular degeneration either did not exist, or was extraordinarily rare. An abundance of evidence will support this claim and I will review that in significant detail. So the obvious question becomes: If AMD did not exist just eighty-five to one hundred years ago, how can we possibly draw the conclusion that it is "age-related"? It is therefore, axiomatic, that we draw the conclusion that something in our environment has caused the condition. That something – I intend to show – is our diet.

Fourth, I will demonstrate that there is a dose-response relationship between the consumption of the 'displacing foods of modern commerce', which equate to man-made, processed, nutrient-deficient foods, and the incidence and prevalence of AMD. The evidence shows that, although certain ethnic groups have a lower prevalence of AMD, their prevalence of disease rises rapidly and exponentially once they begin to consume the 'displacing foods of modern commerce'. Furthermore, it is evident that the greater the consumption of these nutrient-deficient, processed, displacing foods, the greater the risk of AMD and its progression.

Fifth, I will conclusively and very carefully review and demonstrate all of the major elements of the "perfect storm," that have resulted not only in AMD, but a plethora of other conditions often referred to as the "diseases of Western influence." This perfect storm, orchestrated through numerous insults to old and even ancient dietary traditions that had sustained us in exuberant and abundant health for thousands of years, has caused suffering, disease, and death in colossal proportions. AMD is one of these diseases.

Sixth, I will show that, at both the individual and population level, it is impossible to have exuberant and abundant health without plenty of whole, natural, unprocessed foods, preferably organic. Alternatively stated, the 'displacing foods of modern commerce' – sooner or later - rob us of our once vibrant health and may also result in numerous catastrophic diseases, including AMD.

Seventh, I will review the fact that it is virtually never the healthiest approach to micro-manage diets that are substantially insufficient in proper whole foods, with man-made, synthetically derived nutrients, such as multi-vitamin/multi mineral supplements. The research conclusively shows that this practice is generally not only *not* beneficial, but it is detrimental to our health. I will review this in some detail, but suffice it to say that taking multivitamin/multi-mineral supplements, may possibly help a minority of patients with AMD, while hurting all the rest. Furthermore, I will show that everyone will benefit to a much greater degree by avoiding supplements, and enriching their diet with naturally produced foods.

Eighth, I will spell out exactly what foods we should consume to prevent macular degeneration, as well as specifically which ones *not* to consume. Both are critical to our health – and an abundance of tradition and science supports this concept.

Ninth, I will review the "sacred foods," which may very well be absolutely critical in helping to prevent and treat AMD; possibly helping to reverse the earliest stages of disease. These sacred foods are the ones that definitely helped to maintain so called "primitive" societies in exuberant health, while preventing diseases like macular degeneration.

Finally, whole food nutrition, with all its associated *natural* vitamins, minerals, phytonutrients, polyphenols, amino acids, fatty acids, etc., is unquestionably the key to vibrant health and immunity to a vast array of disease. Densely nutritious diets that do not include the 'displacing foods of modern commerce' not only prevent AMD, but they prevent and treat a plethora of other diseases as well, including heart disease, stroke, diabetes, hypertension, blood lipid disorders, metabolic syndrome, numerous cancers, Alzheimer's disease, dementia, gout, ulcerative colitis, Crohn's disease, irritable bowel syndrome, Autism, ADHD, depression, osteoarthritis, inflammatory arthritis, numerous inflammatory disorders and autoimmune disorders, including multiple sclerosis, rheumatoid arthritis, and many, many more.

From this introduction, let me follow-up by stating that AMD:

- Is a multifactorial disease, not unlike heart disease, stroke, or diabetes mellitus
- Generally follows a linear progression, based on the gestalt of a person's nutrition and lifestyle, over a lifetime or at least several decades of time
- Is the end-result of numerous, highly complex interactions of highly intricate metabolic pathways, which cannot be reduced to simple terms or treatments (e.g., "we need more synthetic vitamins, zinc, etc.")
- Requires an integrated hypothesis that connects broad-based nutrition (i.e., entire diets, over decades of time) with end results (i.e., development of AMD or lack thereof)
- Must be treated with a multi-pronged therapeutic approach, which includes removal of the 'displacing foods of modern commerce', supplanted with the consumption of nutrient-dense foods.

In follow-up to these points, let me also submit that, in this book, I will proffer biologically plausible mechanisms whereby processed food consumption may produce the pathophysiologic processes leading to macular degeneration.

LET'S DIVE IN…

Since this chapter is both introduction and eye-opener, no pun intended, I'd like to begin by addressing the myth of this reductionist thinking about nutrition. What I am referring to is our widely held belief system, present only for the last few decades, that we can reliably enhance or repair our diet with multivitamin/multi-mineral supplements and/or isolated synthetic nutrients. This is seldom true. In 2003,

David Jacobs, PhD, and Lyn Steffen, PhD, at the University of Minnesota, Institute for Nutrition Research, published a paper reviewing 58 studies providing evidence that real, whole, natural food positively influences health through complex, synergistic mechanisms that are truly beyond our reductionist thinking. In their own words, "There is considerable evidence for the existence of food synergy, the additive or more than additive influences of foods and food constituents on health."[1] In essence, biological systems are generally far too complex for us to reduce into simpler terms.

To continue with the concept of reductionist nutrition versus food synergy, there's also no such thing as "eye vitamins," no more than there are "heart vitamins," "liver vitamins," "brain vitamins," or any other organ specific vitamins. There is also no good substitute for consuming vitamins as they are found in nature. Natural, organic, unprocessed foods are "packaged" with innumerable cofactors, enzymes, minerals, phytonutrients, etc, the way Nature intended them. Every single cell of our bodies, essentially, depends on virtually all the vitamins, minerals, essential amino acids, fatty acids, cholesterol, and hundreds and even thousands of other nutrients and components – all of which are either found in, have their basis in, or are supported by, none other than... you guessed it, *whole food.*

What this means is that it really is an exercise in futility to assert that we need "vitamins that are good for" our heart, liver, eyes, etc. Sure, we do, and I will even review this concept regarding the eye later in the book. But the fact is, most every cell of our bodies requires virtually every single one of those nutrients, and by far and away the best way to get those nutrients is by consuming whole, natural, unprocessed foods. These foods literally supply thousands of nutritional components in perfect combinations, wrapped up in perfectly bio-available "packages." Man-made, synthetic substitutions do not. Hence, their potential danger.

Here's the beauty of what I have just reviewed. **By eating right to save your sight, you're simultaneously going to reduce your risk of a multitude of other diseases and you're going to become tremendously more healthy.** If you need to, you will lose undesirable weight. You will feel better and you will have more energy. Within 72 hours, you will have a reduced risk of heart disease and stroke, type 2 diabetes will begin to reverse, blood pressure will naturally begin to correct itself, blood lipid profiles will normalize (this doesn't mean cholesterol will be lower), arthritis may improve or disappear, inflammatory conditions such as colitis and irritable bowel syndrome will improve or resolve, autoimmune disorders such as lupus, rheumatoid arthritis, and multiple sclerosis may improve or stabilize, and numerous other conditions will likely begin to abate.[2]

So just forget the notion that you're eating right – just for your eyes, or for any other condition for that matter. You're either eating right for everything, or you're eating wrong for – pretty much - everything. That's the beauty of this plan. It's virtually impossible to consume a food that is good for one thing, and bad for another (with very rare exceptions, primarily genetic ones). It is true, but nevertheless, ridiculous, to say, "Oh, I shouldn't have eaten that candy bar, because it's bad for my hips." Sure, the statement is true. But, the candy bar is not only bad for your hips, but it's also bad for your heart, brain, liver, eyes, kidneys, pancreas, teeth, joints, etc., etc. Likewise, when you eat wild-caught sushi and salmon roe (eggs) for dinner, it's not just good for your heart and eyes, it's good for every single cell of every single organ in your entire body. Alright - so sushi is not your cup of tea, you say? No problem. There are plenty of other options.

CHALLENGING THE PREVAILING DOGMA FOR THE CAUSE OF AMD

The prevailing sentiment regarding the elusive etiology (cause) of AMD is repeated over and over in almost every publication that deals with the condition. The typical verbiage is well represented by the following examples, the first of which is taken from Albert & Jakobiec's 1994 edition of Principles and Practice of Ophthalmology. In the chapter entitled "Age-Related Macular Degeneration: Epidemiology," written by Kathleen Egan, MPH and Johanna Seddon, MD. Their candid statement reads, "Since the cause or causes of AMD are unknown, we lack the means for its prevention."[3] This honest and forthright statement, made in 1994, remains true today.

If we go online for the latest reviews regarding AMD, the Mayo Clinic's website (*MayoClinic.org*), written by "Mayo Clinic Staff." Under "Causes" (for AMD) the publication reads as follows: "The exact cause of dry macular degeneration is unknown, but the condition *develops as the eye ages.*" The article continues, "Dry macular degeneration affects the macula – an area located in the center of your retina that is responsible for clear vision in your direct line of sight." Next, under risk factors, the article reads as follows: "Factors that may increase your risk of macular degeneration include: Age, family history of macular degeneration, race, smoking, obesity, unhealthy diet, cardiovascular disease, and elevated cholesterol."[4]

WebMD, in their review states, "age-related macular degeneration is more common in older adults... may be hereditary," and lists "smoking, high blood pressure, high cholesterol, obesity, and being light skinned, female, and having a light eye color" as *risk factors* for AMD.[5]

Little has changed in regard to the theories and hypotheses regarding the cause(s) of AMD for many decades. To illustrate by example, let me review the writings of the historically prominent ophthalmologist and author, Sir W. Stewart Duke-Elder, MD. From 1927 through the 1960's, Duke-Elder was a dominant force in both British and international ophthalmology. As editor-in-chief for the *Duke-Elder Textbook of Ophthalmology* series, which served most English speaking ophthalmologists around the globe during those decades, his writings and editing were both profound and prolific. In his 1941 edition of the series, *Volume III, Diseases of the Inner Eye,* some four pages is dedicated to the review of what was then referred to as "Senile Macular Chorio-Retinal Degeneration (Senile

Macular Degeneration of Haab)." Duke-Elder, with regard to the cause(s) of this condition, states "While the sclerotic origin of senile macular degeneration is generally accepted, van der Hoeve (1918 – 20) considered that the action of light might be a contributing cause."[6] By "sclerotic origin," Duke-Elder was referring to atherosclerosis or "hardening of the arteries" that takes place specifically in the choroid, which is a layer of supportive vasculature beneath the retina (to be reviewed later).

In 1994, the same year I finished my ophthalmology residency training at the University of Colorado Health Sciences Center, in Denver, I purchased the latest definitive treatise on ophthalmology, which was Albert & Jakobiec's *Principles and Practice of Ophthalmology*. This six volume, 5,200+ page, 400 pound gorilla, which requires a wheelbarrow to move (sorry, I digress – and the weight is embellished, but not the page count), has answers for most of the fundamental questions in ophthalmology. In the Basic Sciences volume of the set, in Chapter 109, "Age-Related Macular Degeneration: Epidemiology," the introduction reads as follows:

> "Age-related macular degeneration (AMD) is the leading cause of irreversible blindness in the United States among persons over age 50. **As many as 15 million persons in this age group may be affected by AMD. Little is currently known concerning the cause or causes of this vision-threatening disease.** Among current hypotheses are that ambient light and nutritional and cardiovascular factors are related to the onset and progression of AMD." [7]

In the same series of Albert & Jakobiec's ophthalmology textbooks, volume 2 of the series presents the chapter on the dry form of AMD. The subtitle of "Conclusions and Future Research," reads as follows:

> "Although fairly uniform descriptions of the nonneovascular features of AMD [dry AMD] have been presented, there still is little information on the cause or progression of these changes. Hopefully, current and future epidemiological studies will lead to better understanding of the pathogenesis [fundamental biological cause] of these changes. Interventional trials may allow us to understand what can be done to prevent the development of these changes in the first place or prevent progression to the visually disabling stage of atrophy or choroidal neovascularization [Wet AMD]."[8]

My impression is that the prevailing hypotheses regarding the causes of AMD, are that AMD is caused by aging – hence the term 'age related macular degeneration' – and also a result of "bad genetics," primarily. The fact that genetics is deemed so important is underscored by the fact that much research has centered about genes associated with AMD and many epidemiological studies have assessed race or ethnic background as it relates to the prevalence of AMD. In this book, I will submit that neither age - nor race (genetics) – is a primary cause of this dreadful condition.

To my knowledge, in contrast to all previously held hypotheses regarding the cause or risk factors for AMD, I will proffer the hypothesis that there is really just **one primary cause** for AMD:

> ***Unhealthy, Processed Food Laden, Diet - which is a diet that includes significant proportions of the 'displacing foods of modern commerce', namely processed, nutrient-deficient foods, including vegetable oils, artificially created trans-fats, refined flour and sugar, and invented foods, all of which displace nutrient-rich, natural, organically raised animal and plant foods.***

I will also argue that – even smoking – would likely not contribute to the development of macular degeneration, if the diet were correct, i.e., abundant in natural vitamins, particularly the fat-soluble vitamins, and entirely lacking in truly toxic foods, such as vegetable oils and artificially created trans fats. Disclaimer: I am wholly and entirely opposed to smoking for innumerable reasons, and it can definitely contribute to both the onset and progression of AMD, but it is *not a primary cause* of AMD. I will assert that smoking is a secondary cause of AMD, when the diet is already incorrect and insufficient.

The other "risk factors" listed by the Mayo Clinic and WebMD websites, which are consistent with all recent research and general conclusions, are not actually causes of AMD, in my opinion, but are conditions that "run with" AMD. **Cardiovascular disease, high blood pressure, and obesity, as examples, are not actually risk factors or *causes* of AMD, but rather they are also *effects* of an unhealthy diet and lifestyle, just as the AMD is.**

This type of analogy is the same as author, Gary Taubes (*Good Calories, Bad Calories*, and *Why We Get Fat*), used to explain growth and weight gain as being driven by hormones. In his classic example he writes:

> "...it is absurd to think about obesity as *caused* by overeating, because anything that makes people grow – whether in height or in weight, in muscle or in fat – will make them overeat. Children, for example, don't grow taller because they eat voraciously and consume more calories than they expend. They eat so much – overeat – because they're growing. They *need* to take in more calories than they expend. The reason children grow is that they're secreting hormones that make them do so – in this case, growth hormone."[9]

In like fashion, we do not develop AMD *because* we have cardiovascular disease, high blood pressure, metabolic syndrome, blood lipid disorders, and/or because we're overweight – we have all of those conditions because, in this case, the same mechanism that results in those disorders – a faulty, nutrient-deficient, processed-food laden diet – is also the cause of macular degeneration. In essence here, we just reassign cause and effect.

In all fairness, the term "risk factor" doesn't necessarily imply causation, but I want to be certain that this point is very clear, because practitioners sometimes advise their AMD patients to "lose weight" for example, because that "will help the progression of the AMD." The point is, both being overweight and having AMD are caused by the same thing – and the patient with AMD doesn't likely know how or why he or she is overweight in the first place, if indeed they are overweight. After all, if they understood why they were, they probably would have resolved the problem. It's not that simple – not in today's world.

As such, in order to understand the cause of macular degeneration and, therefore, prevention and appropriate treatment, we absolutely must begin to think about our overall health – our global health, if you will. Our eyes don't live in a vacuum. They're just another organ, just like our heart, liver, kidneys, or brain. So, in order to understand AMD, we must absolutely understand our health and exactly what's wrong – or right – with it.

Incidentally and parenthetically, by the conclusion of this book, you will also understand why, at least here in the U.S. (with numerous nations following suit), we do "overeat." It is true that, in order to gain weight, one must consume more calories than one expends. The question is, why are men and women in the U.S. consuming about 252 more calories per day (we actually do), on average, than we did forty years ago?[10] By the conclusion of this book, you will not only understand why we are consuming more calories, but you will also see that the answer to that question has ties that are strongly related to the cause of macular degeneration. And it's not the calories themselves that are the issue – I assure you.

With that said, get ready to learn a lot more about your body and health than you ever thought you might learn from a book on macular degeneration. We absolutely *must not* attempt to consider macular disease in isolation. Reductionist thinking is why and how we've missed the true cause of AMD. We must consider the gestalt of our health – exactly why, how, and where we went wrong – for if we don't understand the cause, we'll never know the cure. So, as we discuss nutrition as it relates to heart disease, cancer, type 2 diabetes, and even our weight, just remember – every last bit of that is related to our eyes – as well as to macular degeneration.

CURE AMD FOUNDATION™ GOALS...

As Founder and President of Cure AMD Foundation™, our team's mission is to prevent and treat macular degeneration, through ancestral dietary strategy, advocacy, and scientific research. Collectively and without question, we believe that AMD is fully preventable and, therefore, our aim is to "Cure" this disease through prevention. However, this will require a remarkable paradigm shift in global nutrition – certainly, a colossal and formidable task. Nevertheless, it is our goal to reach as many people and populations as possible, with the message contained in this book.

We also collectively believe that, if you should clearly understand the dietary elements responsible for causing AMD (and the myriad of related diseases and conditions that tend to "run with" this disease), you will not only agree – but you will spread this message as well. That said, it is not our assertion that changing your diet today can reverse any pre-existing damage to your maculae and, therefore, restore sight that has already been lost. That, we hope you clearly understand, would be tantamount to advising a smoker that we have a cure for his COPD (emphysema) and metastatic lung cancer (spread to other organs), after he's smoked a pack a day for the last 57 years.

A LIFETIME OF POOR DIET...

Continuing the thought from above, the point here is simple: As much as I am loathe to tell you, many of you have been consuming the wrong foods, and not nearly enough of the right ones, for the past half-century and, quite possibly, your entire lives. Unfortunately, I made many of the same mistakes, until just a few years ago. We made these mistakes, you and I, because we trusted the collective advice of the media, government agencies, our doctors, nutritionists, and even the healthcare profession at large.

That advice went something like this: "Follow a low-fat diet and avoid saturated fat (like the plague), eggs, and butter. Eat heart-healthy, low-fat, butter substitutes. Eat low-fat skinless chicken and turkey, and possibly eat red meat just two or three times a month. Eat plenty of healthy whole grains, fruits, and vegetables."

Most of that advice – I am sorry to say - is deeply and tragically flawed. I'll do my best to make sense of exactly why throughout this book, but remember, this is a book about preventing and treating AMD. Because of that, there won't be quite the detail on heart disease, diabetes, and obesity, however, the dietetic principles are exactly the same! I have directly addressed these other conditions in significant detail, in my last book – *Ancestral Diet Rx*, which is pending publication. In any case, the bottom line here is that – there are limits to the damage control that can be accomplished this late in the game for some of you. Nevertheless, I hope you agree that, if changing your diet could potentially prevent progression of the disease you currently have, wouldn't that be a great accomplishment? Wouldn't that be far better than the potentially inexorable progression of the disease you might appropriately fear, because of "genetics and aging"?

THE FAULT OF OUR HEALTHCARE SYSTEM AND GOVERNMENT

There is a lot of fault here that lies squarely with the medical orthodoxy. We've collectively abdicated our responsibility to educate ourselves and apply fundamental concepts about nutrition to our lives and the lives of our patients. We've shirked this responsibility, in favor of prescription pads, medicines, radiation, chemotherapy, and surgery. As one surgeon once said, "If we can't eradicate it, burn it, freeze it, irradiate it, or cut it out, then what good are we?"

This question is both humorous - and tragic. Because - it's largely the truth. This is a fundamental mistake - and it should give us all pause for concern. As allopathic physicians (traditional medical doctors, of which I am one), we've spent an extraordinary amount of time learning how to diagnose and treat disease. *But, we have virtually no training in nutrition and prevention of disease.* This is an oversight of colossal magnitude - because - if you hadn't noticed - we're pathetic at curing most disease. How many of you out there, with your prescription drugs for diabetes, high blood pressure, arthritis, "cholesterol disorders," heart disease, ulcerative colitis, arthritis, fibromyalgia, depression, etc., took your medicine for a period of time - and were cured of the ailment?

I assure you - that prescription medication is virtually never going to cure your chronic condition. And, of course, you're not being told that it is. Most all medicine is a band-aid. You're being told that your condition has no cure - only a prescription remedy that you will need to take indefinitely. In the eyes of allopathic medicine, this is true. It's true, because the underlying cause of the disease is not known - and not addressed.

We've been led to believe that the components of our diet don't really matter all that much. That, when it comes to diet, it's really mostly a calories in - calories out equation. Yes, that dogma - which I will address as well. We've ignored the fact that whole, unprocessed organic foods, without fabricated, man-made foods such as vegetable oils and trans fats, and without pesticides, herbicides, and GMOs (genetically modified organisms), sustained us in brilliant and exuberant health for thousands of years.

For decades, there has been much ado in the lay press and even in medical research regarding total caloric consumption along with nearly an obsession regarding macronutrient (protein, carbohydrate, and fat) ratios. However, what you will learn is that neither of these generally needs any specific attention - if one chooses to consume a whole foods diet. To gain optimum nutrition, the focus must be on the quality of foods consumed - and not quantity. If the quality is correct, the quantity will virtually always take care of itself, even in a free-feeding situation and with unlimited access.

But your doctor doesn't likely know any of this - because he's never had any formal education in nutrition. He doesn't know because our educational systems have ignored nutrition as a fundamental science. One-hundred-thirty-five years ago and prior, that is, in 1880, physicians really didn't need much education in nutrition. They didn't need it to be good practitioners because, nutritionally, it was a much simpler world. All food was essentially whole, unprocessed, and organic. It was almost impossible to eat an unhealthy diet. Sure, some people didn't get enough food and there certainly were many cases where monotonous diets, such as nothing but corn and pork, caused disease. But, there were no such things as edible vegetable oils, artificially produced partially hydrogenated trans-fat containing vegetable oils (like Crisco), sugars in abundance (generally), high-fructose corn syrups, highly-refined wheat flours, genetically modified corn, soy, sugar beets, and cotton, and grocery stores filled with literally hundreds of thousands of processed, man-made foods that are almost completely devoid of natural vitamins and minerals.

With the onslaught of a degenerative decline in our nutrition, we've become sick as a nation, and we're literally spreading the "disease" not only through exports to the rest of the world, but by the example that we've set. Moreover, our people are generally overweight, ill, and suffering - and the healthcare industry, food industry, and our government have all failed them. The backlash, appropriately, is that these people have become wary of the statements of physicians, the government, and even scientists - and for good reason. They've been led astray, with ill-founded advice that is inconsistent not only with historically proven and time-tested principles, but often with science itself. In essence, the medical field, Big Pharma, and Big Food are now seen to value individual and institutional self-promotion above truth and the common good of our people.

ALLOPATHIC MEDICAL EDUCATION

As a graduate of the University of Colorado School of Medicine in Denver, I received little or no formal education in nutrition. The last time I checked, Harvard Medical School had no required course in nutrition for their medical students either, though they purportedly review relevant nutrition throughout their curriculum. These medical schools are not outliers. They're both par for the course. Patients think that their medical doctors must know about nutrition. The reality is - overall, most of us don't have a clue.

In 2004, researchers from the University of North Carolina, Chapel Hill, surveyed all 126 U.S. medical schools asking the schools to determine the characteristics of the nutrition education that their MD candidates received in medical school. One hundred and six (84%) medical schools responded to the query. The researchers found that 99 of the 106 required "some form of nutrition education; however, only 32 schools (30%) required a separate nutrition course." [11] On average, the students received only 23.9 contact hours of nutrition instruction during medical school, with the range being anywhere from 2 to 70 hours. The researchers also cite "only 40 schools required the minimum 25 h recommended by the National Academy of Sciences." The researchers conclude with, "The amount of nutrition education in medical schools remains inadequate."[12]

I would say that the "nutrition education in medical schools remains inadequate" is an enormous understatement, but in such study publications, statements must remain very pragmatic. So, in short - I agree. Just 23.9 formal education hours in nutrition, on average, huh? About three days worth of classroom time at 8 hours a day... Would you expect your physician to be knowledgeable about nutrition?

I spend a fair amount of time going to the gym. Over the years, I've had the pleasure of knowing and visiting with many friends who might be considered everything from fitness enthusiasts, to personal trainers, to bodybuilders. Quite frankly, I can honestly say that I would trust most of their nutritional advice over that given to me by most any physician I know. It's sad, but true. Fitness enthusiasts learn about nutrition out of necessity. They can't perform at their best or be in their best shape, without at least some body of knowledge. For physicians, that knowledge – or lack thereof – has virtually no impact on their practice at all.

In 2010, Pauline Chen, MD, wrote an article for *The New York Times* entitled "Teaching Doctors About Nutrition and Diet." She reviewed that, once accepted to medical school, she kept getting all sorts of questions about vitamins and diet. Her response was, "Each and every time someone posed such a query, I became immediately cognizant of one thing: the big blank space in my brain." [13] She then relates that, "...what my friends and acquaintances really wanted to know was just what they should or should not eat."

She continues, "Years later, as a newly minted doctor on the wards seeing real patients, I found myself in the same position. I was still getting a lot of questions about food and diet. And I was still hesitating when answering. I wasn't sure I knew that much more after medical school than I did before."

Dr. Chen wraps up this classic encounter with, "One day I mentioned this uncomfortable situation to another young doctor. 'Just consult the dietitians if you have a problem,' she said after listening to my confession. 'They'll take care of it.' She paused for a moment, looked suspiciously around the nursing station, then leaned over and whispered, 'I know we're supposed to know about nutrition and diet, but none of us really does.'"[14]

Let's face it. Medical school curricula have almost no place for nutrition. It's not about prevention. It's all about diagnosis and management once you have disease. It's also not about managing health and reversing disease through dietary and nutritional alteration. To illustrate the point, one day a couple of years ago, I was walking from the hospital back to my clinic, when I encountered one of the family medicine residents (post-graduate doctors in training). I asked him, "So, how's it going?" "Pretty good, " he said. "After a while you start to figure this out - it's just a matter of – they've got this, you give 'em that."

I believe his statement is really a perfect illustration of our current practice of allopathic medicine. It's all about making the diagnosis, at which we are brilliant, followed by the reaching for the prescription pad – unless, of course, a procedure is planned. Which is exactly why today we have over 10,000 medications available to prescribe. Case in point: on a quick review, I counted 77 medications that could be prescribed for hypertension (high blood pressure) alone. I assure you, not one of these will "cure" or permanently reverse the problem. Why? Because none of them corrects the *cause* of hypertension. However, proper diet and lifestyle will very commonly correct hypertension, and it will do it virtually every time for younger healthier patients. On the other hand, nearly all medicines are just a "band-aid." They'll help to manage the problem, but seldom do they actually permanently solve the problem (antibiotics excluded).

Over and over, in my 24 years of practice, I reviewed lists of my patients' medications. As a general ophthalmologist and cataract surgeon, our clinic prepared a lot of patients for surgery. So we definitely were dealing with the older population most of the time. In any case, I would estimate that most patients were on an average of about ten medications, chronically. Many were on 15 to 20 medicines and, in some cases, we would count medication lists that were up to 25 to 30 medicines.

For many years, I observed that the more medications a patient was on, the sicker they usually were. This probably seems like I'm stating the obvious. Those people virtually never come in the office looking vibrant, healthy, and happy. That kind of patient is usually reserved to those who are on little or no medicines at all! But, here's the point. **For years I have discussed diets with my patients – and I learned that there was a very clear pattern. The more that patients subscribed to and followed diets with the 'displacing foods of modern commerce', the more illness and disease they had, including – macular degeneration.** Alternatively, the more that patients followed diets that were more 'ancestral,' the greater their health and lack of disease, including macular degeneration. It is an uncanny correlation. Not to worry – we'll get to the scientific correlative data – and you will be shocked.

DOES MORE MEDICINE TRANSLATE TO WORSE HEALTH?

Now, I'm not asserting that we don't need medicines. We do. Some of them are definitely good. But, over 10,000 medicines? The reality is that the U.S. spends more money on healthcare than any nation in the world. We spent $2.6 trillion dollars on health-care in 2010, which works out to be $8,402 per person, per year.[15] As reviewed elsewhere, if you stack 2.6 trillion dollar bills one upon another, they would reach 170,000 miles into the atmosphere. That is nearly three-quarters of the distance to the moon! Yet, we are one of the least healthy nations in the world. Think a brilliant healthcare system is going to make you healthy? Think again.

Let's take a look at some evidence that we need drastic reform, not only to our healthcare system, but to our food supply. The World Health Report 2000, Health Systems: Improving Performance, ranked our U.S. health care system as 37th in the world.[16] And it's getting worse every year. In fact, according to the report, in 2006 the U.S. "ranked 39th for infant mortality, 43rd for adult female mortality, 42nd for adult male mortality, and 36th for life expectancy." Of the developed nations, we're one of the sickest there is.

In an *American Medical News* article, published in January, 2013, the headline reads, "U.S. found to be unhealthiest among 17 affluent countries."[17] The article cites the results of a study completed by the National Research Council and the Institute of Medicine "to examine why the U.S. has a poorer health status and lower life expectancy than other countries, despite spending the most money on health care." Their findings? "Americans die sooner and experience higher rates of disease and injury than the populations of 16 other high-income countries," including Australia, Austria, Canada, Denmark, Finland, France, Germany, Italy, Japan, Netherlands, Norway, Portugal, Spain, Sweden, Switzerland, and the United Kingdom.

In the same study, areas where Americans ranked poorly included prevalence of cardiovascular disease, diabetes, and obesity. The U.S had the highest rate of obesity in the list of countries studied, the highest rate of childhood overweight and obesity, and one of the highest rates of diabetes. However, that's just the tip of the iceberg. If you were to look at a whole plethora of diseases, including heart disease, stroke, peripheral arterial disease, hypertension, blood lipid ("cholesterol") disorders, osteoarthritis, rheumatoid arthritis, gout, fibromyalgia, irritable bowel syndrome, Crohn's disease, ulcerative colitis, Alzheimer's disease, dementia, autism, autism spectrum disorders, ADHD, depression, anxiety, bipolar disorder, and hypothyroidism - just to name a few – the U.S. likely ranks at the very top. Here, I am just speculating that we do. Otherwise, why else would we spending far more healthcare dollars per capita than any other nation in the world?

But there is a unifying answer to why we're amongst the most ill and spend the most money on healthcare. The answer is because most of our disease and ailments are driven by the same mechanism, namely, a nutrient-depleted, processed food-laden diet, which is chock-full of the 'displacing foods of modern commerce'.

Consuming the 'displacing foods of modern commerce' is also the primary reason that, of 196 nations in the world, we're currently ranked number one for being "most obese."[18] Almost exactly one of every three adult Americans is obese, and approximately 67 percent are overweight. Nevertheless, obesity itself is not the cause of the other conditions, despite what you've probably been led to believe. Obesity is just another condition that runs along with the "diseases of Western civilization."

As an example, let's take a quick look at metabolic syndrome. This is the term physicians use to describe a cluster of six chronic and related conditions, as identified by the National Cholesterol Education Program's Adult Treatment Panel III report:[19]

- **Abdominal obesity**
- **Atherogenic dyslipidemia** (abnormal blood lipid profiles, such as elevated triglycerides, elevated small dense LDL cholesterol, and low HDL)
- **Elevated blood pressure**
- **Insulin resistance with or without glucose intolerance** (pre-diabetes or diabetes)
- **Pro-inflammatory state** (*May play a role in AMD)
- **Pro-thrombotic state** (tendency for clotting – as in heart attack, for example)

Metabolic syndrome is a strong predictor of developing both heart disease and type 2 diabetes. And while components of the metabolic syndrome are present in 80% of those who are obese, we also see some of these metabolic derangements in up to 40% of the U.S. adult population who are normal weight.[20] A study published in the Journal of the American College of Cardiology, in 2013, showed that full-blown metabolic syndrome currently affects about 20% of the U.S. population.[21]

Recall from previous discussion the "risk factors" for macular degeneration? Research concludes that obesity,[22,23,24] high blood pressure,[25,26] and cardiovascular disease.[27,28] are all associated with AMD. Type 2 diabetes[29,30,31,32,33] and diseases of inflammation, or markers of inflammation,[34] are also associated with AMD. And all of these aforementioned conditions are associated with metabolic syndrome – and metabolic syndrome itself is conclusively associated with AMD.[35] Once again, I will assert that these conditions in and of themselves do not cause us to develop AMD. They simply *occur alongside* AMD because they all have the same basis in origin – and that basis is a faulty diet.

THE MAGNITUDE OF THE EPIDEMIC OF AMD

Over and over, I've witnessed the heartache of seeing patients lose so much vision that, they could no longer read, watch television, or drive, and not infrequently, they lost their independence. In some cases, I would sit and listen to my patients lament how they could no longer see their children and grandchildren's faces. In short, the "golden years" became, "not so golden."

Simple and expected daily visual tasks, such as reading a book or seeing one's grandchild, are just a few of the things that we were obviously meant to enjoy in our later years. For most of us, we take it for granted, but for many, the *new* sneak thief of sight – AMD - gradually steals our precious gift of sight – and robs us of some of life's greatest pleasures.

AMD is the leading cause of irreversible vision loss in the U.S. and other developed nations in people over the age of 65.[36]

This ugly and devastating disease is threatening to visually cripple and even blind tens of millions of people across the globe – needlessly. Researcher Dr. Donatella Pascolini, at the World Health Organization (WHO), in Switzerland, estimates that about 5 percent of global blindness is the result of AMD.[37] This translates into about two million people. But this is not just impaired vision – this is blindness. In eyecare terms, that means *best-corrected* visual acuity (with best glasses or contact lenses) of 20/200 or less in the U.S., or 20/400 (3/60) throughout much of the remainder of the world according to the World Health Organization definition.[38]

In 2002, the World Health Organization survey identified AMD as the leading cause of blindness in high-income countries.[39] These studies showed that 14 million people, or 8.7% of the world's blindness and severe vision loss, was secondary to AMD. **In the U.S., by 2004, 54% of blindness in whites was attributable to AMD.**[40] In 2010, the WHO found AMD to be the third most common cause of blindness worldwide, ranking behind cataracts and glaucoma.[41] As of 2010, macular degeneration had replaced cataract as the most common cause of blindness in high-income regions.[42]

Albert & Jakobiec's Principles and Practice of Ophthalmology asserts that as many as 15 million people in the U.S. were thought to have AMD, as of 1994. By my calculations, that number could be as high as 22 million as of 2015. However, the U.S. only represents about 4.5 percent of the world's population, so the number of people with AMD worldwide is staggering (see below). **Ron Klein, MD and colleagues at the University of Wisconsin, determined that AMD affects about one in three adults over the age of 75 in the United States, as of 1992.**[43]

In 2014, researchers from the Singapore Eye Research Institute comprehensively evaluated the world's AMD prevalence data, and estimated that some 196 million people worldwide will be afflicted with macular degeneration by year 2020, with that number projected to rise to 288 million people by 2040. For people between the ages of 45 and 85 years of age, this translates to 8.01% with early AMD, 0.37% with late AMD, and 8.69% with any degree of AMD.[44] Globally, this means that for those over age 50 years, about one person in every 11 has some degree of AMD.

Estimates of AMD prevalence aside, if you take into account the heartache, suffering, and vision loss that I've witnessed, and multiply it by 200,000, which is the approximate number of ophthalmologists (EyeMD's) worldwide,[45] you get some sense of the colossal magnitude of this problem. Yet, this number doesn't even take into account all of the patients that are being managed by optometrists. According to *Primary Care Optometry News*, there are more than 300,000 optometrists worldwide,[46] thereby totaling more than half a million total eye care providers globally, many of whom are literally overrun with AMD patients.

As practitioners, we're also seeing the progression to advanced AMD at an alarming rate and, although wet AMD only represents about 10 to 20% of late AMD cases, if it is untreated it has a devastating visual prognosis. Untreated patients lose about 1 line of visual acuity (on the eye chart) at 3 months, nearly 3 lines at 12 months and 4 lines by 2 years. Those who develop severe vision loss (more than 6 lines lost on the eye chart) increase from 21.3% at 6 months to 41.9% at 3 years. Finally, those with vision 20/200 or worse (legally blind in the U.S.) at the initial exam increased from 19.7% to some 75.7% by 3 years. And for those who already have wet AMD in one eye, the fellow eye develops wet AMD in 12.2% of patients by 12 months and in 26.8% by 4 years.[47] One study showed that once advanced AMD developed in one eye, 43% developed advanced AMD in the other eye within five years.[48] And finally, for an individual with wet AMD in one eye, the risk of legal blindness in both eyes may be approximately 12% over a period of 5 years.[49]

Translation into real world vision terms: If you are affected by AMD and it degrades into the wet variety, without treatment your visual acuity is likely to be reduced by half (what ophthalmologists call a 'doubling of the visual angle') within the first year. In other words, if you start out at 20/40, you will be expected to be about 2/80 within a year, or if you start out at 20/100, you will be expected to be 20/200 within a year. Again, this is without treatment, but millions of people in the world have no access to treatment for this condition.

Human suffering aside, the financial costs to society are staggering. In his assessment of the problem based on statistics from Australia, Gregory S. Hageman, PhD, Professor of Ophthalmology and Visual Sciences at the University of Iowa Carver College of Medicine, states the following:

> "A recent analysis of AMD in Australia predicts that the disease costs $2.6 Billion per year. This is projected to grow to $6.5 billion by 2025, a total cost of $59 billion over the next 20 years. A treatment that reduced the progression by only 10% would save Australia $5.7 billion over that same period of time. Similar analyses for the United States are lacking, but given the demographics and higher cost of medical care in the US, the costs would be projected to as much as twenty-fold higher."[50]

IT'S EITHER OVER-SIMPLIFIED, OR OVERLY COMPLEX

This book is written for everyone. And while I've tried my best to make it readable to those of you who have no medical or nutrition background at all, ophthalmologists, optometrists, and vision scientists may find that it's lacking the detail they desire. My daughter, Kyla, currently seventeen and heading off to college next summer, once said to me, "Dumb it down, Dad." With that said, I've tried to keep her advice and strike a happy medium. I hope you agree and can accept the limitations on either end of the spectrum.

CHALLENGES TO MY HYPOTHESIS...

I have no doubt that my position on AMD and its relationship to diet will be challenged. However, I will not be discredited for being non-scientific, as every major aspect of my entire hypothesis will be supported by fundamental scientific research. Every piece of data comes from third-party reliable and trusted sources. To be sure, I will be very clear as to when and where I draw any of my own conclusions. Finally, just so you're aware - none of this book is based on opinion. Not mine. Not anyone's. It is based on scientific fact, reason, and logic. Every single reference will be provided, right in the text. If you so desire, I invite you to do just as I have done. Go to each and every book, study, and reference, and review them for yourself. Then, see if you don't arrive at the same conclusions that I have.

CHAPTER SUMMARY

I have proffered the hypothesis that the 'displacing foods of modern commerce' are the primary and proximate cause of 'age-related macular degeneration.' The corollary to this is that any variety of ancestral diets, that is, diets that do not contain significant amounts of processed, nutrient-deficient, displacing foods – will not only prevent AMD, but may treat it as well.

I have witnessed the full reversal of early AMD in my own patients, in at least nine patients. However, those virtually all occurred without any advice from me. These were simply people that rather dramatically altered their diet in a healthful way, of their own volition. The key, though, is to begin as early as possible – and to be diligent.

If anything in this chapter seems complex, trust me, to put these plans into action is *deceptively simple.* Once we boil it all down and you practice putting these concepts into action for even a few days or weeks, making healthy food choices to virtually eliminate your risk of macular degeneration or to treat your existing macular degeneration, as well as a whole slew of other degenerative and inflammatory diseases, will very quickly become second nature.

THE GENESIS OF A NOVEL HYPOTHESIS FOR AMD...

The only relevant test of the validity of a hypothesis is comparison of prediction with experience.
~ *Milton Friedman* ~

MY STORY...

I finished my ophthalmology residency in 1994. About a year later, I encountered a 37 year-old young lady by the name of Cheryl, who had the beginning of AMD. She had drusen in both eyes, which are a characteristic early finding in the macula in those with macular degeneration. She was very concerned, as was I, particularly given her young age. Just about a year prior to that, a landmark study in the potential cause of AMD was completed by Johanna Seddon, MD, Walter Willett, MD, and colleagues, at the Massachusetts Eye and Ear Infirmary, in Boston. That study, published November 1994, in the Journal of the American Medical Association, showed that those people who consumed the most dark leafy-green vegetables, like spinach and collard greens, had a 43% lower risk of developing AMD than did those who consumed the least.[51]

Armed with that study and that study alone, I decided to ask Cheryl about her diet. "So do you eat much in the way of fruits or vegetables, Cheryl?" I asked. "No, " she said, "I almost never eat any." "Do you eat any salads at all?" I questioned her a bit further. "No," she said again, "we never eat salad." With that, I told Cheryl about the study published by Dr. Seddon and colleagues, and I advised her she might ought to start eating more leafy greens, like spinach, kale, and collard greens. We made an appointment for Cheryl for six months.

In six months she returned. To my amazement, the early signs of macular degeneration were gone. Not a single drusen anywhere in her maculae (plural for macula). I followed her for the next three years and the early macular degenerative signs never resurfaced. She was "cured," at least of these mild but beginning signs of AMD.

That study and that memory stuck in my head. It shaped the way that I would advise patients who had dry AMD from that point forward. At that point, I was all but clueless when it came to nutrition. As further studies came along (I'll review subsequently), I would advise my patients accordingly, as probably most ophthalmologists would: don't smoke, eat dark leafy greens, take the multivitamin/multimineral (AREDS) supplements, and get some fish oil.

Around the turn of the millennium, I had spear-headed the development of a large on-line database of eyecare and eye conditions, known as *EyeMDLink.com*. That site was eventually acquired from me, in 2008, by Access Media Group (owner of *AllAboutVision.com*). With my background and credentials, the *AllAboutVision.com* team invited me to become a member of their Editorial Advisory Board, which I gladly did.

That same year, I was asked to write an article for AllAboutVision that regarded the prevention and "treatment" of dry AMD. I gladly accepted. As I worked on the literature search for the article, one thing continually struck me. **Over and over, it seemed that every single condition or marker that appeared to be a risk factor for AMD - obesity, hypertension, high triglycerides, high levels of small, dense LDL cholesterol, etc. - *was also a risk factor for heart disease.*** Indeed, research would eventually show an association between AMD and coronary artery disease.[52]

Also, everything that seemed to reduce the risk of heart disease – not smoking, consuming plenty of leafy greens, plus plenty of fruits, vegetables, nuts, and fish in the diet, as well as exercise and a reduction of refined carbs (sugar and white flour, for example), also reduced the risk of AMD. There seemed to be almost no exceptions - right down to the last nitty-gritty detail. I was perplexed. And I was continuously bothered by the myriad of apparent coincidences. Were they both caused by the same thing?

MY OWN CONDITION LEADS ME HERE

Some three years later, in February of 2011, I had had enough. The story takes an odd turn here, so hold on. I had considered myself fairly athletic my entire life. Well, except for a couple years of college when socializing and parties were more important – but that was 30 some odd years ago – and I digress.

What I had had enough of was the arthritis that had plagued me since I was 35 years old. I was now 50. Most days, I would take Aleve and get by, and on my "leg-day" at the gym, I would prepare by taking Celebrex, Aleve, and an aspirin. Then, I would warm up my painful knees (and other joints) for about 15 minutes, and then I could begin to do my squats, leg presses, and so on. Just a few years prior, I regularly did sprints as part of my fitness regimen to stay in shape. But now, my arthritis was too severe. I walked into the gym one day, and I decided to try to do some jogging across the basketball court to warm up. I couldn't do it. The pain was too severe. I hurt everywhere - my knees, ankles, toes, fingers, elbows, and my neck. Luckily, my hips and back seemed to be spared. I literally walked out of the gym that day and went home - without working out – which is something I had never done.

I decided to call a rheumatologist. Even as I made the appointment though, my hopes were fading. Over the previous ten years, I had already seen one rheumatologist, three orthopedic surgeons, three internal medicine docs, and I had consulted every traditional mode of treatment for arthritis I could think of. None could help me, except with short lasting steroid injections and drugs like Celebrex. I got the appointment with the rheumatologist – and it was for Friday, March 4, 2011. I couldn't wait to get in. My hopes were back up again, as my optimism usually wins. At my appointment, the rheumatologist, who was also a friend of mine, gave me a thorough work-over – physical exam of my joints, x-rays, blood work - everything. In conclusion, he said, "Chris, you've got inflammatory arthritis (osteoarthritis)." He showed me the films of my knees, elbows, and my neck. "Your knees look like you're a 400 pound man," he said. I was about 215 pounds and around 13% body fat. Not the six percent I once was, but it was getting harder and harder to move – and my diet was wrong. He went on, "But your arthritis in your elbows and your neck is pretty severe too – and your neck is not really weight-bearing." In the end, he gave me a prescription for an immunosuppressant, called colchicine. I took the prescription and literally raced to the pharmacy to get it that afternoon. The rheumatologist told me the medicine he was prescribing would take two to three weeks to produce noticeable results, so I wanted to start it as soon as possible.

I took the colchicine that day and again the next morning, on Saturday. Later that morning, I had a phone chat with my next older brother, Kyle. Kyle is a steel-mill supervisor in Colorado. He's one of the busiest people I've ever known. A typical work week is 70 hours, sometimes more.

In any case, I told Kyle about my arthritis and the medicine that my rheumatologist had prescribed. Without knowing anything about it, he said, "You need to get off that crap." I was taken aback. In fact, I was almost defensive. But somewhere in the back of my mind, I wondered if he might be right. I wondered, "Could this medicine ultimately cause me to have even more problems?" I knew, after all, that we're still not getting at the root of the problem.

As fate would have it, in the same conversation with Kyle, I asked about the diet that he and his wife had started just about two months prior. I knew something about their "diet" because his wife had sent out a blanket email to the family regarding their results. She and Kyle had collectively lost 55 pounds in the previous ten weeks by following this diet that their doctor prescribed. Kyle told me he had lost about 25 pounds in ten weeks and his blood pressure, which had previously required two medicines and was still high, was now down to 120/70, naturally. He was off both medicines.

"What is this diet, exactly?" I asked. "It's the Paleo Diet –" he said, "You just don't eat grains and dairy, mostly. No breads, cereals, pasta, and no milk or milk products. No beans or white potatoes either." That was it. His version of the entire diet spelled out for me in 12 seconds. Next came the usual conclusion from my 70-hour work-week brother, "Look Chris, I gotta get back to work here." We said our good-byes. But, I was intrigued, especially because I already thought I knew something about nutrition. And I did – I knew what mainstream nutrition had told us, and I knew that pretty well. I knew an upscale version of what the public pretty much knew. I knew nothing else.

So I immediately Googled "Paleo Diet." Lots of sites popped up, but I was attracted to a few key phrases that were most interesting to me, given my own personal condition. The Paleo Diet was, among other things, "anti-inflammatory." Now my antennae were standing straight up. I spent a couple of hours reading about it and after that much research that Saturday morning, I decided, half-heartedly, that I would give it a try. Being a physician, I knew that for any reasonable "experiment," I would need to manipulate only one variable at a time. It was either take the colchicine medicine, or try the diet. I decided to try the diet.

I wasn't convinced at all though, in fact, I was pretty lukewarm about the whole thing. I had experienced so much disappointment in dealing with my arthritis for 15 years, could you blame me? In any case, from my research, I could see that grains, particularly wheat, seemed to be most associated with inflammation. So, I decided, beginning the next day on Sunday morning, that I would completely stop eating wheat. I avoided anything with wheat – like the plague. Without the usual wheat in my diet, I was eating a ton of vegetables – I mean, I was eating my usual hefty meat portions and salads made and eaten right out of a mixing bowl.

By Wednesday morning, three days later, my arthritis was 50 percent better. I was absolutely shocked. My joints hadn't felt that good in probably six years, even with three medicines. I was so amazed, I decided to take it a step further and I quit dairy. No milk, cheese, yogurt, or sour cream. By about day 9 on the diet, I was 80% better. Now, I am about 90 percent better than where I was before the Paleo diet transition. I also don't take any medicines for arthritis, and though my joints still bother me mildly, remember that I had a lot of damage before I started the Paleo Diet. This was truly one of the most transforming events in my life.

Please don't jump to conclusions too fast, here. My recommendations are not just for a Paleo Diet, and you're good to go. Though that would certainly be a good start. As you will see, even the dietary exclusions I made are not always necessary to achieve the same and even better results. Now, I eat grains and I also eat dairy, but it's all in the details, which you will soon understand. So, just hold on… At this point, we're still 4000 feet from Base Camp 1 of our Mt. Everest.

That spring, I bought Loren Cordain's book, *The Paleo Answer*. I read it cover to cover – and I was ten times as shocked as I was about my arthritis. I read the book again. Could all of that be true? Could almost all of the usual ailments that we're facing simply be a result of our diet? It was mind-boggling. Physicians don't think that way. We weren't trained that way – and that's not how I thought.

ORTHODOX MEDICINE'S VIEWS ON NUTRITION – DEBUNKED

I was always fascinated by nutrition. But after reading Dr. Cordain's book, I was stunned. I launched into a journey of my own to discover everything I could. I read everything I could find. I bought book after book – and studied. Being a Clinical Associate Professor of ophthalmology, I had access to our university library. That helped immensely. I downloaded study after study and continued to read and review. I had so much energy from being on the Paleo Diet, I could go to bed at 9:30, get up at 4:00 am, and I would read, study, and write – usually for about two hours, then go to the gym, and then have breakfast and rush off to work. I took my lunch from the hospital back to the office and continued to read. At night, if the family was all busy, I stopped watching television and I continued on my quest.

About a year-and-a-half later after investigating everything I could, I was immensely better informed, but I was still deeply frustrated. The world of nutrition is inconceivably and deeply complex. I still didn't even know the real cause for being overweight. It was deeply disturbing. There are so many theories and hypotheses – sometimes I just wanted to throw up my hands and say, "I can't figure it out." But, I couldn't. I was too deep into it. Plus, I just wasn't raised that way - our parents never let us quit anything. I always felt like, somewhere around the corner, it would all begin to make sense.

About two-and-a-half years into my studies, I was finally seeing the light. I was starting to have a firm grasp on some of the fundamental concepts – and they differed from traditional medicine's orthodox views – vastly. The evidence was there – and I couldn't ignore it.

For example, just for starters, the research conclusively shows that a moderate or high percentage of *natural* fat in the diet is very healthy in every regard and generally causes the most weight loss (Robert Atkins was right all along),[53,54,55,56,57] that our health is benefitted by plenty of saturated animal fats in the diet (from pastured, grass-fed cattle, e.g.),[58,59,60,61,62,63,64] that more than 20 studies show that people who have the highest blood cholesterol live the longest,[65] that sugar in significant quantities is extremely dangerous in terms of weight gain and diabetes development,[66] and that 68 studies conclusively demonstrate that multivitamins/multi-minerals supplements are dangerous and result in higher death rates from all causes, including cancer and heart disease.[67] These, and a myriad of other nutrition and health findings, literally turn the medical orthodoxy on its head.

Just so we don't get off on the wrong foot here, I am not admonishing you to necessarily eat a high fat diet, although that would be fine. What you will understand, by the conclusion of this book, is that macronutrient ratios (ratios of proteins, carbohydrates, and fat) don't make much difference – as long as you're eating whole, natural foods. In the final analysis, you'll see that you can eat 60% of your diet as fat, or 10% as fat. What matters, primarily, is not the ratios of macronutrients, but the *quality of those macronutrients*. All fat and all carbohydrates are not the same!

ANOTHER JOURNEY – BUT NOW ABOUT AMD

It was late in 2013 that the murmurings in my mind led me to begin to consider AMD as possibly "just another" of the many diseases of Western influence. As I had mentioned, it had never left my mind after I wrote the article for AllAboutVision that AMD seemed to have a strong correlation with cardiovascular disease. And those with cardiovascular disease are the same ones with hypertension, blood lipid disorders, pre-diabetes or diabetes, abdominal obesity or overweight, and so on. Once I began to connect the dots that most of these diseases are a result of our Westernized diet, I hypothesized that AMD might be just one more disease that was squarely sighted in the cross hairs of a toxic, highly-processed, nutrient-deficient diet.

To determine if I my hypothesis had any validity, not that it was true necessarily, but if it had any validity, I would first have to answer several critically important questions: First, did macular degeneration always exist, and if so, did it have the prevalence in the population that it does today? If it did not always exist, or at least not to the prevalence that it does today, that would be evidence strongly in favor of a non-genetic basis. Second, if AMD varies between populations, particularly populations of the same ethnic descent, is the variation tied to diet? Third, if AMD had increasing prevalence over time, as I suspected, could this be tied to dietary patterns? If the answer to the latter question was a resounding "yes," then the next question is: What exactly are those dietary patterns? Finally, if the answers to all of the previous questions returned in support of my hypothesis, I would need to ask the most difficult question of all: What has changed about our diets, collectively around the world, that is tied to the increasing incidence and prevalence of AMD? Of utmost importance, that last question needs to be answered regarding both food elements and nutrients that are not only new to our diet, but those that have been diminished or removed from our diet as well, because both may be causal.

The answers to those four questions would lead me on an investigation that would take more than a year – and a review that would include thousands of scientific studies, more books – old and new - than a good mule could carry, plus many more thousands of Google windows opened and closed, sometimes only after my internet browser would freeze because I had dozens of windows all open simultaneously. But maybe this search wasn't in vain, after all.

ONE PATIENT'S ANECDOTE...

In 1998, I met a patient by the name of Jean. She was a 57 year-old white female who presented for a routine eye exam. After dilation, I noted that she had some soft drusen and pigmentary disturbance of her maculae (plural for macula). These are both hallmark signs of early, dry AMD. I discussed with her what we knew about dry AMD at that time, which was mostly that a diet rich in dark, leafy-green vegetables would help to prevent progression of the disease, and that she might want to consider taking multivitamins.

But Jean knew much more about nutrition than I did, even though she hadn't been following her own knowledge. She did not take vitamins. She began what she felt was best: eating a diet filled with whole, natural, unprocessed foods. And living on a farm, she began to eat the vegetables she raised in her own garden, at least part of the year. The next year when I saw Jean, her drusen and pigmentary disturbance was better. I congratulated her on a job well done. That fueled her fire to continue eating a natural diet. Two years after I saw her the first time, she returned again. This time the drusen and pigmentary disturbances were both gone. No evidence. Not a trace.

Today, some 17 years after I first saw her, she has no signs of AMD and, at the age of 75, she remains in vibrant health and has no disease other than some mild arthritis. I learned something valuable from Jean. I also learned from thousands of others – both what worked, and what didn't. I might not have ever learned from all of these patients, both healthy and diseased, but I often took the time to ask - and then – I listened.

WARNING: DEEP SCIENCE AHEAD

At times in this book, you may find yourself feeling a little lost when you read some of the quotes from the many scientific journals which I will reference. If you do, don't worry. Just trudge on through and get to the other side because none of that will affect the take-home messages. I promise. I won't let it. I've put the exact quotes there for the sake of those who are ophthalmologists, optometrists, physicians, scientists, researchers, and even the more erudite – who just want the nitty-gritty detail. So even if some of those are a little above your comfort zone – don't despair - in the end, you will get the main points – because they're plain and simple.

In my opinion, we're all equals here. Some people may not have had the opportunity for higher education, like I did. I was fortunate. My Dad, who passed away in 2011, worked as an automotive machinist his entire life. He supported my mother and us five "kids" through hard-work, dedication, and six-day work weeks. He grew up on a farm in Western Kansas. His father made him leave school in the middle of tenth grade so that he could work on the family farm. He certainly never had the opportunity for higher education. Yet, he provided that opportunity to me and my siblings. We were very fortunate. We might not have been in other circumstances. Maybe my Dad didn't read or write so well, but he was still one of the smartest guys I've ever known – and he wanted more for his children than he ever had himself. He accomplished that goal.

So, maybe your situation is similar to my Dad's. Or maybe you've never had education beyond the 5th grade. Doesn't matter. We're all equals here - and I'm writing to you too. This book is about helping people – all people. Young or old, well or sick, educated or not.

Still, keep in mind, this book is not just "light reading." It just cannot be – and still do justice to something so incredibly important, which is your health – and your vision. The eye itself is at least as complicated as the brain, if not more so. No superficial review of a matter this complex would be suitable. Keep that in mind and, just remember, you will only get out of this what you put into it. I'm going to ask you to work at this, because in the end, it will be worth it. There's an old saying that 'Nothing great ever comes without hard work.' I believe in that principle. And I'm asking you to believe in it too.

CHAPTER SUMMARY & A PROMISE TO DELIVER...

There's an awful lot riding on whether or not I lead you in the right direction regarding your macular degeneration, or your risk for the condition if your eyes are currently healthy. My vow to you is that I will present the evidence in as fair and honest a fashion as possible, I will interpret the data only where I feel it may be needed, and I will make every attempt to clearly spell out the nutritional advice that I believe may truly save your vision. This advice, born out of years of intensive investigative research, combined with 24 years of medical and surgical ophthalmology practice, is entirely driven by my motivation to prevent needless vision loss. Personally, I have witnessed this vision loss countless times in my practice and that, of course, is representative of the devastation that is affecting millions of people all around the world.

In this light, I must point out that the conception of the hypothesis postulated in this text did not dictate the evidence for it – in fact, it was collective evidence that dictated the conception. And as I believe you will see, no matter where we look, the evidence is in support.

In the concluding pages of this book, I will ask you if you believe that there is adequate support for my hypothesis. More importantly, I will ask you to make the changes to your diet (and possibly lifestyle) that I have recommended, and see what this accomplishes for you. I suspect that you will be amazed.

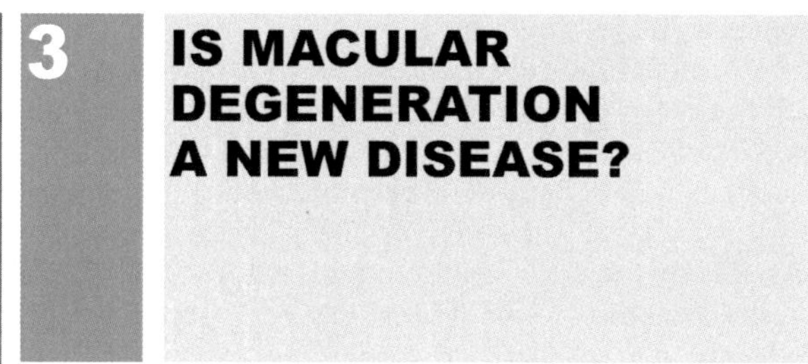

3 IS MACULAR DEGENERATION A NEW DISEASE?

"Those who do not remember the past are condemned to repeat it."
~ George Santayana ~

The fact that we physicians have almost no formal education in the history of disease plays an enormous role in our present view of macular degeneration. As previously shown, most textbooks begin the discussion of AMD with a description of the disease itself, which is common in medical practice. In many book chapters and studies presented in journals, there is a one-sentence description regarding the fact that the disease was described at some point historically. **I firmly believe that this has led ophthalmologists and optometrists to make three inchoate – and erroneous – assumptions:**

1. Macular Degeneration has always existed.
2. The prevalence of AMD always existed to the degree that it does today, and
3. AMD is the inevitable consequence of aging and/or genetics.

All three assumptions are false.

If macular degeneration essentially did not exist, or rarely existed, before about 1930, how can we possibly account for that? Is AMD actually a relatively new disease? If so, then what has changed in our food consumption, environment, or lifestyle to produce this pandemic of disease that we see today?

To answer these questions would require an extensive review of the history of ophthalmology. Thanks be to Google Books search, I was able to find a whole slew of rather ancient books for sale, and purchase I did. Book after book came to my office, and then home to my study. Eventually, I couldn't even find a place in my study to keep them all. They've since been relegated to a new bookshelf, which serves as a second mini-library. But, in these books we find powerful keys to our understanding of the genesis of macular degeneration.

Perhaps the most shocking discovery I made while reviewing these books, many of which hold very prominent positions in the history of ophthalmology, isn't what's in them.

It's what isn't in them.

Curiously missing from almost all of these textbooks before about 1933 is any mention of macular degeneration. "How could that be?" I asked myself. If this is a disease of aging, or a genetic disease, how is that possible? Is it just that ophthalmologists of previous eras couldn't see the macula? Or did AMD just plainly not exist? Let's dig in to this.

Despite the fact that, after medical school and internship, we ophthalmologists complete another three years of residency training, and perhaps another year or two of fellowship training for those who further sub-specialize, most of us have little or no knowledge of the history of our profession. Like nutrition, the history of medicine and/or the history of our specialty generally is not part of the curriculum. There's enough to learn, obviously, and delving into the history of our specialties is not generally deemed to be educational time well-spent. But should it be?

Just before the American Academy of Ophthalmology was founded, in 1896, Rudolph Virchow made the following statement:

> "It is one of the worst aspects of our present developmental stage of medicine that the historical knowledge of things diminishes with each generation of students. Even independent young researchers can normally be assumed to have a historical knowledge of no more than three to five years at a maximum. Anything published more than five years ago does not exist."[68]

In response to this statement, distinguished professor Daniel M. Albert, MD, of the University of Wisconsin School of Medicine, remarked as follows:

> "This unfortunately remains true today. Yet at times of crisis or great change, such as ophthalmology now faces, it behooves us to pause and examine our past and renew our understanding of where we came from, so we may better decide on where we are going." [69]

I agree. And we're in a crisis situation. Tens of millions of people around the world are losing vision to macular degeneration – and at least two to three million are already blind in both eyes – and yet, we don't seem to know what's causing this horrific disease.

This is a long chapter, ladies and gentleman, and sometimes pretty tough reading because there's some science here and there. But I feel that it is absolutely crucial that we take a very close look at the history of this disease – and subsequently our diets - because in those two pursuits we will see the evidence for how and why this disease came about. Armed with that information – we'll know exactly how to prevent it – as well as how to treat it. Once we get through this chapter, everything else in the entire book is less challenging, so just hang in here with me…

1850 – HELMHOLTZ INVENTS THE OPHTHALMOSCOPE

If you're wondering whether 19th century ophthalmologists could see the macula as well as what ophthalmologists call the fundus (macula, optic nerve, retinal vessels, and peripheral retina), the answer is that - after 1851 - they could. They could because of the genius of **Herman von-Helmholtz (1821 – 1894)** - a German born physicist and physician, who invented the direct ophthalmoscope in 1851.[70] This quickly became the instrument known to ophthalmologists as the only way to visualize the "living" posterior segment, or fundus of the eye. Up until that time, no one had ever visualized these anatomical structures in a living eye.

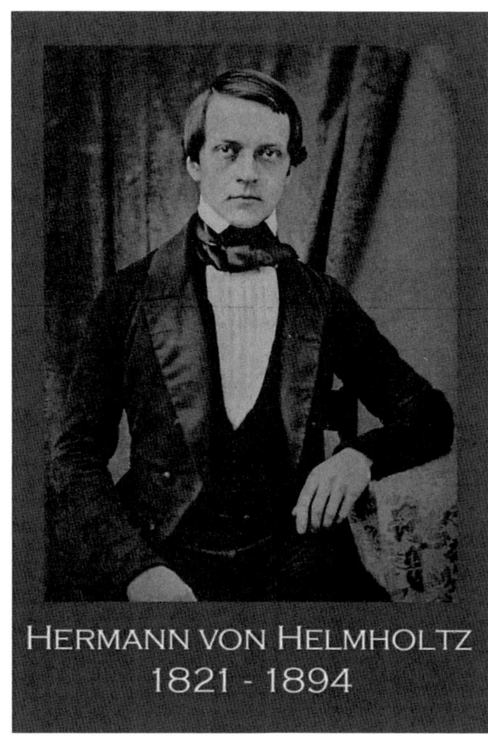

Helmholtz at age 29.
Image courtesy of Richard Keeler, Honorary Curator, The Royal College of Ophthalmologists.

According to Professor Daniel Albert, MD, at the University of Wisconsin, "Helmholtz discovered the ophthalmoscope in 1851, and within ten years, improved models were in use throughout the world… In the case of the ophthalmoscope, machinists were available to construct the basic frame of the instrument. The simple lenses required could be supplied by grinders of spectacle lenses, and the necessary curved and flat mirrors were readily available. The major obstacle was illumination and here a candle, kerosene lamp, gas lamp, or daylight had to suffice." [71]

Helmholtz' ophthalmoscope unquestionably marked the beginning of modern ophthalmology. No other invention has had a greater impact on the advancement of our knowledge in the field of ophthalmology than did the direct ophthalmoscope. As a result, news of Helmholtz' invention spread rather quickly through Europe and subsequently, to the Soviet Union, Asia, the United States, and the rest of the world.

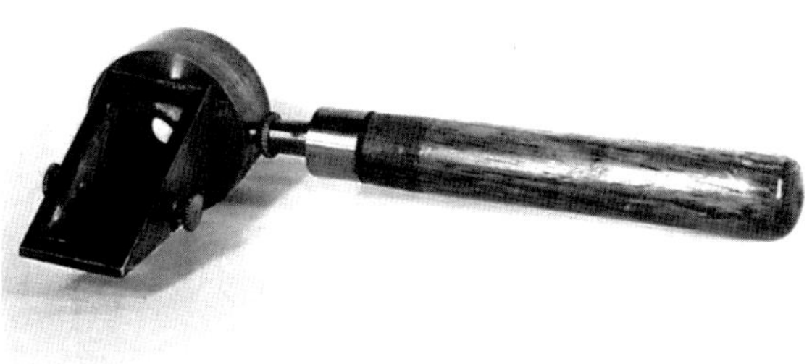

Helmholtz Ophthalmoscope, 1850.
Image courtesy of Richard Keeler, Honorary Curator, The Royal College of Ophthalmologists.

Collaborators would develop numerous iterations of the ophthalmoscope device, which actually continue to this day. With Thomas Edison's invention of the light bulb in 1879 (patented 1880), there would soon be the addition of incandescent light added to the ophthalmoscope - rather than the light of a naked candle, oil lamp, or gas-burning lamp - the light of any of which was harnessed and directed into the eye via a mirror system. By 1885, the first handheld electric ophthalmoscope was developed, marking a dramatic improvement in both design and functionality.

In 1861, a binocular indirect ophthalmoscope was designed to examine the eye, allowing depth perception and a broader field of view.[72] However, like the direct ophthalmoscope, there would be hundreds of iterations developed, with successive improvements in the illumination, functionality, optics, and hence, quality of view.

With the advent of the ophthalmoscope, ophthalmologists began to make numerous observations and discoveries that had, of course, never previously been made. One of the earliest journal articles published was written by Greek ophthalmologist, Andreas Anagnostakis (1826 - 1897). Anagnostakis' publication, in 1853, was entitled, "Attempt to explore the retina of the living eye by means of a new ophthalmoscope."[73]

According to Daniel M. Albert, MD, professor and chair of the Department of Ophthalmology and Visual Sciences, University of Wisconsin, in his textbook *The History of Ophthalmology* (1996), a great many astute observations of the fundus of the eye would be made within just ten to twelve years of Helmholtz' invention.. Albert wrote, for example:

> Elkanah Williams (1822 – 1888) of Cincinnati published two articles in 1854 describing the use of the ophthalmoscope and stating that examination of the living fundus oculi was "by far the most important improvement made in ophthalmology in modern time, and destined to form an interesting epoch in the history of science." In addition to describing the findings in the normal eye, he described retinal detachment, dropsy, varicose vessels as well as brown and grayish patches in the retina."[74]

Dr. Albert reviewed the observations and inventions of other ophthalmologists who collaborated in producing illustrations of the normal and diseased eye, as early as the mid-1850's to early 1860's. He wrote, "Eduard Jaeger in 1854...painted pictures of normal and diseased fundi that required 20 to 40 sittings of two to three hours each. These were initially published in his *Beiträge zur Pathologie des Auges* in 1855 and subsequently in enlarged editions entitled *Ophthalmoscopisher Hand-Atlas* that appeared from 1869 to 1894 in German, French, and English editions." Albert also reported that ophthalmologist, Richard L. Liebreich (1830 - 1917), "published his *Atlas der Ophthalmoscopie*," which "was the first atlas of ophthalmoscopy and a model for all later atlases. The text was in French and German and the illustrations were comprehensive and expressive, reflecting Leibreich's artistic gifts."[75]

Clearly, as early as the 1850's, ophthalmologists were viewing and eloquently describing the macula and other structures of the fundus of the eye. By the late 1880's, they could even visualize the fundus with electric ophthalmoscopes. According to C.R. Keeler, "In 1880, {ophthalmologists} Landolt and Snellen had collected 86 types of ophthalmoscope and by the time Hermann von Helmholtz died in 1894, a great number more had appeared, many designed by the best-known ophthalmologists of the day. On the occasion of the 50th anniversary of the ophthalmoscope, an exhibition was put on in Atlantic City, USA, where no less than 140 different designs were shown. By 1913, Edward Landolt reported that 200 models had been produced."[76]

HISTORY OF MACULAR DEGENERATION IN THE SCIENTIFIC LITERATURE...

In general, I believe there is a rather direct correlation to the prevalence of a condition and the amount of published research on the condition. Let's begin on a brief journey through the literature. *What you are about to see is an incredible paucity of references to macular degeneration up until about the 1930's, which has seemed to grow almost exponentially since then.* I will review the literature as it relates to documented cases of macular degeneration, in chronological fashion, documented by the year and always in relation to Helmholtz' design of the ophthalmoscope in 1851.

In reviewing this seemingly ancient literature, from the 1800s and early 1900s, one thing continually struck me. These physicians and ophthalmologists had exceptional skills and magnificent powers of observation. Their attention to detail and descriptions of the eye are generally far beyond present day ophthalmologists, as we've grown greatly dependent on technology. It is abundantly clear these early ophthalmologists would have rarely missed a detail, let alone something as obvious as the signs of macular degeneration.

Sir Duke-Elder's System of Ophthalmology (1967) reviews the fact that ophthalmogists had discovered drusen, as early as the 1850's – within just a few years of Helmholtz' discovery of the ophthalmoscope. Drusen are the tiny deposits that lie in Bruch's membrane in the macula (or retina, in general) of the eye, which frequently accompany macular degeneration, In fact, Duke-Elder wrote, "The deposition of masses of hyaline material as varicosities, called COLLOID BODIES in Anglo-Saxon literature and DRUSEN in German, occurring in association with the cuticular layers of Bruch's membrane is a common and well known phenomenon which was noted histologically by Wedl (1854) and was first elaborately studied by Donders (1855) and H. Müller (1856)."[77]

Though these ophthalmologists had noted drusen, they apparently hadn't noted macular degeneration of any sort. In general, these drusen were more a sign of aging and perhaps mostly outside of the macula, as degeneration of the macula nor associated vision loss was mentioned.

UNITED KINGDOM STUDY: "SYMMETRICAL CENTRAL CHOROIDO-RETINAL DISEASE OCCURRING IN SENILE PERSONS," BY JONATHAN HUTCHINSON – PUBLISHED 1874

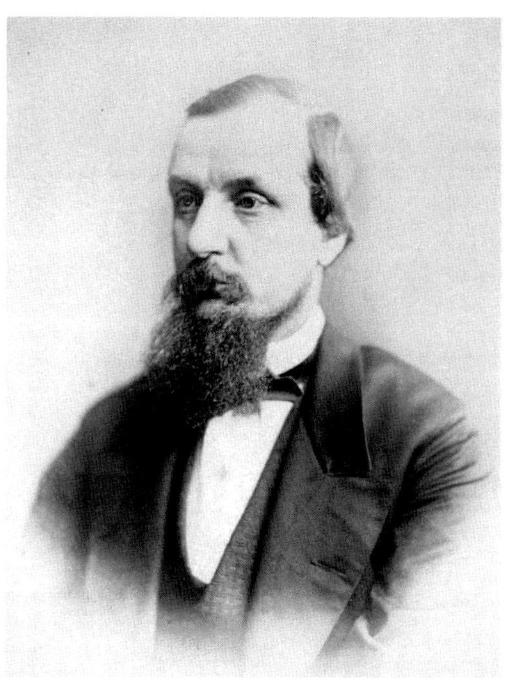

Jonathan Hutchinson

In fact, it would be 23 years after Helmholtz' invention that the presumed equivalent of macular degeneration would be described for the first time. British ophthalmologist, Jonathan Hutchinson, in 1874, had discovered a total of four cases in his career at that point. Though he presented ten cases of macular disease in total, only four appear to be quite consistent with AMD, in my opinion. Let me provide a quick review and just bear with me on this detail, which is presented primarily for the sake of my colleagues.

Of the ten total cases presented in Hutchinson's scientific paper, the first three cases were discovered in three sisters, ages 40, 48, and 60.[78] The three sisters did not appear to have "garden variety" macular degeneration, though they did have macular disease. Sir Stewart Duke-Elder suggested that these sisters likely suffered from Doyne's honecomb retinal dystrophy, a dominantly inherited form of macular disease, rather than AMD.[79] Each of the sisters also had rather severe systemic disease resulting in everything from paralysis to dementia. Dr. Hutchinson notes, "Cases I, II, and III of the following occurred in three sisters, in each of whom a symmetrical disease of the choroid around the disc {optic nerve} and yellow spot {macula} occurred after middle life. The extent and character of the disease were almost precisely alike in the three patients. Two of them had at former times suffered from weakness of one or more limbs apparently amounting for a time to paralysis, slowly passing off, and leaving some permanent weakness." Professor Paulus T.V.M. de Jong, MD agrees with the assertion that these three sisters' cases are consistent with Doyne's honecomb retinal dystrophy, and not AMD.[80]

Dr. Hutchinson described seven more cases. I will briefly review each of these because, as you will eventually come to see, the associated conditions are suggestive that nutrition played a role in these cases – even then.

Case IV was a 60 year-old gentleman with doubtful AMD, as Hutchinson's assistant, Mr. Tay, described the patient as having "a number of very small white spots" that were "in a circle around the disc, passing between it and the yellow spot." He wrote, "There was no trace of haemorrhage anywhere, nor any change at the yellow spot {macula} in either eye."

Hutchinson's case V was a former drinker and smoker, who had "a number of small spots"... "chiefly situated above and below the disc." He stated that the spots did not involve the "yellow spot" in the right eye and in the left eye he wrote "there were a few at the yellow spot." My take is possible early AMD in this case.

Case VI is a 62 year-old woman seen at Moorfields Eye Hospital, who also had cataracts and deafness. Her case notes include the following: "a number of very small white spots were found to be scattered widely over the central part of the fundus, being especially numerous in the yellow-spot region." This one sounds like AMD to me.

Case VII was a "Man of 74" with deafness, cataracts, and failure of sight for several years. He was described as having had "a number of well-defined white spots in the fundus of each eye at the yellow-spot region." This case appears consistent with AMD, in my opinion.

Case VIII was a 64 year old man with albuminuria (indicates kidney disease) whose "complexion was pale and sallow, and his face somewhat puffy; he said that his legs swelled, and were more swelled in the morning than later in the day." On eye exam, he had "small white spots found in the fundus on the nasal side of the disc (none on the yellow-spot side)." In my opinion, this case does not appear consistent with AMD, given that the spots did not affect the macula, that is, the "yellow-spot" side.

Case IX was a 48 year-old man "in bad health" with "failure of sight" for two months, as well as deafness and albuminuria. His right eye had "numerous minute very white dots in the fundus between the disc and the yellow spot, and involving the yellow spot region to some extent." This case appears consistent with AMD.

Case X was a 38 year-old woman with "slight failure of sight" with notes as follows: "a large area in the central part of the fundus was occupied by numerous, small, round, yellowish-white spots" which "occupied each yellow-spot region." This woman's husband had passed away one year prior with complications of syphilis. The woman herself had had four children, the first died at age 18 months, the second died at 2 months, the third was stillborn, and the fourth died at 10 months of age. This case, including the macular changes, is entirely suspicious for syphilis, which can definitely cause infection in the macula and these characteristics.

Hutchinson recognized the initial involvement of the choroid vascular layer supporting the retina as an initial insult, as he wrote, "There is no doubt that the disease is confined to the choroid in the first instance, while the great defect of sight which accompanies it points to implication of the retina secondarily." He described three stages of disease: (1) "scattered very minute yellow-white spots" in the macula and around the disc {optic nerve}, (2) "coalescence of these minute spots and the formation of patches with irregular borders," and (3) "hemorrhage at the yellow spot" {fovea} and "absorption of the blood."

In all, it appears to me that Hutchinson did find four cases out of the ten, which were consistent with non-hereditary AMD - as we are concerned with here (hereditary, or dominant AMD, is exceedingly rare). In the last paragraph of Hutchinson's study he states, "I have failed to find in our standard works and atlases any description of similar cases."

Between 1874 and until the late 1930's, reports of macular degeneration were rare. Duke-Elder (1940) would report that, "The pathology of the condition has been investigated by several authors (Nagel, 1875; Harms, 1904; Friedenwald, 1930; Rones, 1938; and others)."[81]

Let's look at each of these studies in chronological order, with the exception of Harms (1904) as it is in German and I could not get an accurate translation. Of course, we'll review virtually all salient textbooks and papers published during this era and beyond as they related to macular degeneration.

NAGEL, 1875

German ophthalmologist, Albrecht Nagel, presented a very odd case of a 64 year old woman with possible wet AMD, in 1868,[82] who had a dark red net and brilliant white flecks in both maculae, which he called "krystalldrusen." The patient complained of poor vision, metamorphopsia (wavy or distorted vision), and a quivering image. In follow-up on this case, in 1875, the patient had died and a post-mortem exam of her eyes showed very large, hard grains in her maculae that crunched under the tip of a knife. Nagel's conclusion was that these crystalline deposits consisted of carbonic acid lime.[83] Research from 1958 on retinal crystals shows that they may occur in the systemic conditions of cystinosis and oxalosis, that the crystals are highly refractile (as they were in this case), and that they tend to deposit in the macula.[84] Perhaps his 1868 case is more consistent with one of these conditions, rather than AMD. Nagel did report on two additional patients in the 1875 paper, which are more consistent with AMD as we know it.

GERMANY, 1875

Hermann Pagenstacher describes the first known case of disciform degeneration of the macula, which may have been a case of wet AMD that had developed a central scar.[85] His descriptive diagnosis is "choroidioretinitis in regione maculae luteae." Translated to today's English this would be "choroido-retinitis (inflammation of the retina and choroid) in the region of the macula-lutea (macula yellow spot)," the latter of which is the center of the macula.

GERMAN PAPER: *LECTURE BY DR. HAAB* - PUBLISHED 1885

Sir Stewart Duke-Elder (1940) would credit Swiss ophthalmologist, Otto Haab, with the first discovery of macular degeneration, in 1885, dubbing it "Senile Macular Chorioretinal Degeneration, or Senile Macular Degeneration of Haab."[86]

Haab's original paper (1885) is written only in German. I couldn't possibly have read it, however, Pamela "Pam" Sieving, MA, MS, AHIP, reference librarian at the National Institutes of Health and member of the Vision Science Librarians, not only found the article for me, but translated it as well. This article represents a lecture by Dr. Haab, as it reads, "Vortrag, gehalten von Dr. Haab," that is, "Lecture by Dr. Haab." It isn't exactly clear exactly when or where the lecture was presented. The article reads somewhat choppy, apparently, because it is taken directly from the lecture. Here is Pam Sieving's translation of the only aspect of Haab's lecture that deals with 'age-related' macular degeneration:

> ***Sometimes the macular region of otherwise completely normal eyes of older people occurs spontaneously and bilaterally. The changes are often slight, but the impact on vision is great, and the prognosis poor. In the course of this disease strongly pigmented or also light [colored] spots occur in the macular region, finally atrophy of the pigment epithelium. This category of macular disease. This second category of macular disease can well be designated 'senile.'***[87]

In a separate paper and atlas published in 1895, Haab presented several images which indicate that he believed drusen weren't necessarily associated with macular degeneration, as he wrote, "These drusen, also a change in old age, have nothing to do with the macular disorder depicted here (fig. 1a) and should be distinctly separated from this." [88] Even today, though we clearly recognize the strong association of the presence of drusen with AMD, the presence of "small hard" drusen alone are not consistent with a diagnosis of macular degeneration. Other elements are required to make the diagnosis, typically including larger soft drusen and pigmentary disturbances (to be reviewed in Chapter 13).

Perhaps the most important piece of data from the 19th century came from Haab. *From his analysis of some 50,000 patient files, he concluded that "Senile Makulaerkrankung," (translates to 'senile macular disease') affected only about as many people as did traumatic macular disease and myopic (nearsighted) macular disease, both of which are exceedingly rare conditions.*[89],[90]

AUSTRIA - ERNST FUCHS: *TEXTBOOK OF OPHTHALMOLOGY* (PUBLISHED 1892)

One of the most respected names in the history of ophthalmology is Ernst Fuchs (1851 – 1930). Dr. Fuchs was professor of ophthalmology at the University of Vienna, Austria, and besides being a physician, ophthalmologist, and professor, he was a relentless researcher. He published more than 250 scientific publications, creating international recognition for himself. His name is recognized by all ophthalmologists today, if for no other reason than the fact that his name is still used eponymously for multiple conditions of the eye, including Fuchs' corneal dystrophy, Fuchs' heterochromic iridocycltis, and Fuchs' heterochromic uveitis.

In 1889, Dr. Fuch's published his *Lehrbuch der Augenheilkunde* (Textbook of s Ophthalmology), in German. The text was translated into English in 1892. For about five decades, Fuchs' textbook of ophthalmology was considered not only the most authoritative, but also the most widely published reference for ophthalmologists worldwide.[91] It was also translated into Japanese, Chinese, Spanish, French, Russian, and Italian.

I was able to purchase an original copy of Fuchs' Textbook of Ophthalmology, copyright 1892, through a used book re-seller. This book looks awfully ragged, with a mangled spine, torn cover, and yellowed pages, naturally – at 123 years of age - but it reads perfectly. The inside of the front and back covers are marked "Discarded." Little did they know, I would have paid dearly for this historic treasure.

In any case, Fuchs' textbook is just under 800 pages and the content is superb. Most of the descriptions of disease would serve us perfectly well today. Primarily, what has changed is the incidence and prevalence of disease and, of course, the treatment. But for diagnostic purposes regarding innumerable major conditions, this book could still serve us quite well today.

Chapter 10 of Fuchs' textbook is "Diseases of the Retina." It spans 19 pages of the book, but – curiously absent from this chapter is any mention of macular degeneration, or any term even remotely related. Fuchs covers six retinal conditions, including "retinitis, embolism of the central retinal artery, thrombosis of the central retinal vein, anemia of the retina, detachment of the retina, glioma {tumors} of the retina, and injuries of the retina."[92] He even dedicates two full pages of the book to retinitis pigmentosa, a rare degenerative condition of the retina affecting about one in every 4000 people in the United States. I must add, Fuchs review of this condition would rival virtually any account of the disease given today.

In a chapter on "Diseases of the Choroid," Fuchs' references what would be consistent with macular degeneration, and dedicates *one sentence* in the entire book to the condition:

> "Choroiditis centralis is characterized by the deposition of a mass of exudate directly in the region of the macula lutea {central macula}, and thus causes a central scotoma {blind spot}. The most frequent course of it is myopia {nearsightedness}, which, if of high degree, leads late in life, almost without exception, to changes in the yellow spot, which are mainly of an atrophic nature. Inflammatory changes at this spot are often found in syphilis, and also after injuries – especially contusions – of the eyeball. *Finally, a disease of the macula is observed in old people, which usually affects both eyes about equally, and is referable to senile changes.*" [93]

Some 39 years after Helmholtz' invention of the ophthalmoscope, and Fuchs made no mention or reference to the findings of Hutchinson, nor of Haab, and dedicates one sentence to the presumed condition of macular degeneration in this all encompassing textbook. I would submit that this is a very strong indication of the obscurity and rarity of the macular degeneration condition that they had described. Recall additionally, that by 1880, Landolt and Snellen had already collected 86 types of ophthalmoscope, which is pretty strong evidence that the ophthalmoscope was in fairly broad use by 1889 when Fuchs' textbook was published. Therefore, we cannot attribute any lack of diagnosis of macular degeneration to these ophthalmologists lack of ability to visualize it. Any time they would have gazed into the back of the eye with an ophthalmoscope, they would have seen the macula – it's in the dead center of view.

U.S.A.: *A TEXTBOOK OF OPHTHALMOLOGY – PRIMARY SOURCE EDITION* - BY CHARLES AUGUSTUS OLIVER, MD AND WILLIAM FISHER NORRIS, MD (PUBLISHED 1893)

Drs. Oliver and Norris, distinguished professors of ophthalmology at the prestigious Wills Eye Hospital, in Philadelphia, Pennsylvania, wrote an extremely comprehensive and detailed textbook of ophthalmology, for that time. I was able to get a re-print of this text. This textbook is greater than 650 pages in length, has 29 chapters, and includes chapters on diseases of the retina, diseases of the choroid, and even an entire chapter devoted to ophthalmoscopy (examination of the fundus), the latter obviously indicating that virtually all ophthalmologists were utilizing this now standard technology devised by von Helmholtz some 43 years previously. The content of this book is tremendously detailed and, again, could serve us well in terms of diagnosis today.

In the chapter entitled "Diseases of the Retina," there is no discussion of macular degeneration nor anything resembling it. In the chapter entitled, "Diseases of the Choroid," the text begins with "Primary disease of the choroid is generally due to degenerative changes taking place in some part of its vascular network, or to some constitutional affection, such as syphilis. At times, such degeneration is either senile or is the result of *impaired general nutrition* (italics added)." [94]

There is, however, one paragraph on "choroiditis centralis." The described condition, however, does not appear consistent with age-related macular degeneration, in my opinion. I am going to provide the text, which may be a bit deep for non-ophthalmologists and non-optometrists, but nevertheless, here it is for your consideration:

> "Choroiditis centralis (choroiditis circumscripta) is that variety of the disease which localizes itself in the macular region. The patient complains of a gray cloud situated immediately in front of every object looked at. Vision is so reduced that there is an inability to read even course print, except when the book is held close and the head to one side. The ophthalmoscope shows one or more yellowish prominences in the macular region. These are covered by a grayish layer of retina. The rest of the eyeground presents nearly its usual appearance. Later, complete atrophy, which is marked by a sharply-cut white spot that is due to the sclera showing through, appears in the affected area." [95]

This condition appears more consistent with infectious etiology (in that era, likely tuberculous retinitis), vascular insult (e.g., branch retinal artery occlusion), or inflammatory, but does not, in my opinion, appear consistent with macular degeneration. There's never any mention nor any description of the hallmark features of AMD: namely, drusen and/or retinal pigmentary disturbances, such as clumping or loss and, finally, there is no mention of hemorrhage as might occur with wet AMD.

Outside of these two previously captioned phrases, there is no other reference to macular degeneration in this textbook.

U.S. STUDY: *ANOMALIES OF THE RETINAL PIGMENT EPITHELIUM AND THEIR CLINICAL SIGNIFICANCE* - BY HENRY GRADLE (PUBLISHED 1913)

In 1913, Henry Gradle wrote a journal article entitled "Anomalies of the Retinal Pigment Epithelium and their Clinical Significance," which was published in the Transactions of the American Academy of Ophthalmology and Otolaryngology. In this article, he wrote **"According to Rosa Kirschbaumer, anomalies are formed in the pigment epithelium in three-fourths of all eyes of persons over 50 years of age, but are confined mostly to the anterior (ciliary region) and extend only exceptionally toward the posterior pole."** [96] The "anterior" region of the retina is toward the front of the eye and, as far as the eye goes, is located a country-mile from the macula. His reference relates to the work of Rosa Kirschbaumer-Putjata, MD (1851-1923), and his statement that the pigmentary changes "extend only exceptionally toward the posterior pole" indicates that the macula was rarely involved.

GERMANY: *JULIUS HIRSCHBERG'S TEXTBOOK, THE HISTORY OF OPHTHALMOLOGY, Vol. 10 - THE FIRST AND SECOND HALF OF THE NINETEENTH CENTURY* (PUBLISHED 1914-1915)

Another of the most famous and respected ophthalmologists of all time is the German born Julius Hirschberg (1843 -1925). Hirschberg developed the tangent screen test, still used today, which is a measurement of the field of vision using a flat screen.[97] In 1879, he became the first ophthalmologist to use an electromagnet to remove metallic foreign bodies from the eye. Among modern-day ophthalmologists, he is best known for the "Hirschberg test," which is a simple and effective test to determine the presence and degree of strabismus (misalignment of the eyes). He produced ten volumes of his series *Geschichte der Augenheilkunde* (*History of Ophthalmology*) between the years 1899 and 1915.

I was able to get the English version of the Tenth Volume of his *History of Ophthalmology*, published in 1914-1915. This is not a textbook of ophthalmology in the traditional sense, that is, one that reviews all or many of the conditions and treatments that affects the eyes, but rather is really a compendium of "Who's Who" in ophthalmology and the studies and achievements of numerous ophthalmologists. This book, in fact, reviews the practices and research papers written by more than 900 international ophthalmologists, truly from all parts of the world. How Hirschberg ever accomplished actually knowing that many ophthalmologists, as well as their works, I'll never know.

In any case, the book is about 350 pages and has no subject index – only an index of the ophthalmologists names whom he references. As such, the only way I could review this book for any references of macular degeneration was – to read it – which I did. It was an arduous task, because it's chock full of what was trivia, at least to me. Nevertheless, despite the fact that the sub-title of the book is *THE FIRST AND SECOND HALF OF THE NINETEENTH CENTURY*, Hirschberg reviews some detail right up until 1914, which is the first publication date of the 10th volume. A whole slew of diagnoses are considered throughout the book, including for example, "the ophthalmoscopic diagnosis of sclerosis of the retinal vessels, retinal arteriosclerosis, the pathology of papilledema {swelling of the optic nerve} and its changes after trephination, inflammation of the retina and optic nerve, choroiditis disseminata, retinitis haemorrhagica albuminurica, traumatic retinal degeneration, the curability of retinal detachment," and a host of other retinal disorders, indicating that ophthalmologists were constantly evaluating the retina, macula, and optic nerves in that era.

Missing from the entire textbook, however, is any mention of macular degeneration, central choroiditis, or any other term or description of what might be considered age-related macular degeneration. In fact, the macula was apparently so rarely the subject of disease, there is only one mention of the macula in the entire text: "Ein Fall von doppelseitigem Colobom der Macula lutea (Arch. F. Augenheilk. 36:58, 1898,"[98] which translates to "A Case of Double Coloboma of the Macula Lutea." (A coloboma is a congenital defect of the eye, analogous to a cleft lip or palate) I even confirmed from his index of ophthalmologists reviewed that there was no mention of Hutchinson or Haab – the two ophthalmologists that had published perhaps the most prominent papers reviewing what we believe was AMD by that time.

In a few places in the book, Hirschberg reviews causes of blindness, as reviewed by ophthalmologists' studies. One example is that of a report by Carreras y Arago, regarding blindness in Spain, in 1881. He finds 11.09 blind persons per 10,000 inhabitants in Spain. Carreras reported the cause of blindness in 1000 cases from his records: 56 with ophthalmia neonatorum (infectious), 91 with trachoma (infectious), 43 with smallpox, 96 with glaucoma, and 241 with optic nerve disease.[99] He makes no mention as to the cause in the remainder. Nevertheless, there is no reference to blindness from anything affecting the macula.

With Hirschberg's work, we're now up to 1914 – almost exactly a century ago - and there's scant evidence of macular degeneration in an abundance of ophthalmic literature. The prevalence of AMD was, unquestionably, extremely rare.

THE AMERICAN ENCYCLOPEDIA AND DICTIONARY OF OPHTHALMOLOGY – EDITED BY CASEY A. WOOD (PUBLISHED 1914)

Casey A. Wood, MD (1856-1942), was a professor of ophthalmology and Head of the Department at the College of Medicine – University of Illinois. Dr. Wood completed his doctor of medicine in 1877 and his ophthalmology residency at the New York Eye and Ear Infirmary in 1886. According to JAMA Ophthalmology, "He served as president of the American Academy of Ophthalmology and Otolaryngology and of the Chicago Ophthalmological Society and as chairman of the Section on Ophthalmology of the American Medical Association. He was a founding fellow of the American College of Surgeons and of the Institute of Medicine of Chicago." His career achievements and accolades are too numerous to review.

Just three years before he retired from practice, in 1917, he published The *American Encyclopedia and Dictionary of Ophthalmology*. In his text, Dr. Wood describes what may be a *single case of macular degeneration*, in his illustrious 31-year career, as a practicing ophthalmologist and professor of ophthalmology. His description follows:

> "A rare condition of the macular region, which is symmetric and which may be mistaken for central choroiditis, is the occurrence of colloid formations {drusen} resembling those found in the nerve head {optic nerve}. In a case observed by the author both maculae were occupied by rounded, yellowish bodies lying beneath the retinal vessels, and presenting a mulberry-like appearance. The patches were oval and equal in length to two disc diameters. The patient was a man, aged 41 years, and vision was normal. Three similar cases have been seen by de Schweinitz. Nettleship has described a similar case as central, guttate choroiditis with normal vision. His patient showed 'a number of small, perfectly circular, pale grayish-yellow spots thickly congregated at the yellow spot {macular} region, and more thinly scattered all around that part, reaching on the nasal side as far as the disc {optic nerve}.'... The condition does not call for treatment. Choroiditis can be excluded by the fact that vision is normal."

In this reference, Dr. Wood reports what appears to be one case of early macular degeneration, in a 41 year-old man, and his colleagues, Schweinitz and Nettleship, purportedly have seen three cases and one case, respectively.

1920 – NEARLY 5 MILLION PEOPLE OVER 65, YET VIRTUALLY NO AMD

In 1920, the U.S. Census Bureau shows that there were 4.9 million people over the age of 65, as compared to 35 million over 65 by year 2000.[100] As we've witnessed, there were almost no reports of AMD in any U.S. literature. Jumping ahead a bit, by 1990, Professor Ron Klein, MD, and colleagues, found that, "In persons 43 to 86 years of age, the overall prevalence of any ARM (age related maculopathy, translates to dry AMD), was 20.9% and of late ARM it was 1.9%."[101] If the same prevalence rates existed in 1920, even if only considering the population over age 65 in the U.S., there should have been over 1.1 million people affected with AMD. The literature and textbooks would have literally been flooded with studies or reports on macular degeneration, yet there was near complete silence on the subject.

GERMANY: JUNIUS AND KUHNT PUBLISH CLASSIC PAPER ON DISCIFORM MACULAR DEGENERATION (MACULAR SCARRING) – 1926

What is known as "disciform macular degeneration," which is generally considered to be the end-result of wet AMD with a macular scar, was presented in a classic paper by

German ophthalmologists, Paul Junius and his predecessor, Hermann Kuhnt.[102] They described 10 cases, ranging in age from 36 to 76 years of age. Their paper held that "circinate retinitis," a term that might be used for AMD in that era, and disciform degeneration, belonged to a cluster of diseases, not necessarily all AMD. Professor Paulus T.V.M. de Jong, MD, PhD, Director of the Netherlands Ophthalmic Research Institute in Amsterdam and former Chair of the Department of Ophthalmology at the Erasmus University Rotterdam, reviewed this German study (in German language) and confirmed that only one of the ten cases had "increasing drusen-like spots" as well as the fact that drusen "did not otherwise appear in any description of their cases."[103] Professor de Jong continued:

> The word 'senile' appeared once in case II with 'senile vessel diseases.' The causes suggested for the disciform disorders varied from alcoholism and lues {syphilis} to hypertension and atherosclerosis... So what I always considered to be a monograph on end-stage AMD was actually a monograph on discoid macular degeneration caused by different retinal disorders, including a few cases with late AMD! Junius and Kuhnt could not help the fact that for many years their names were coupled to AMD. This was partly because Verhoeff, and later Duke-Elder, added to the original title of their monograph the word 'senile' or started a sub-chapter with: 'Senile disciform degeneration of the macula (*of Junius and Kuhnt*).' [104]

UNITED KINGDOM: DUKE-ELDER'S TEXTBOOK – *RECENT ADVANCES IN OPHTHALMOLOGY* (PUBLISHED 1927)

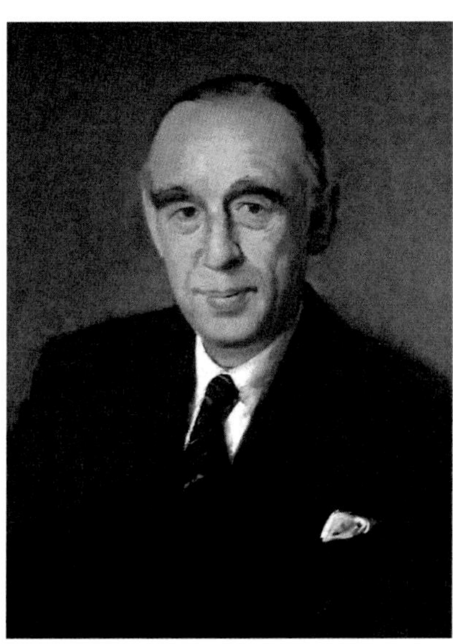

Sir Stewart Duke-Elder.
Image courtesy of the Moorfields Collection.

Sir Stewart Duke-Elder's first textbook, *Recent Advances in Ophthalmology* (1927), was purported by Duke-Elder himself to have been written to "present in a readily accessible form the research work which has been done within the last few years in ophthalmology and its associated sciences." In the introduction of the book, Duke-Elder asserts the following: "The two 'major' diseases of ophthalmology, cataract and glaucoma,..." obviously, no mention of macular degeneration as would most definitely be the case today.[105] In this 340-page book, Duke-Elder makes no mention of anything that could be considered macular degeneration, nor of central choroiditis, an alternate term that might describe AMD.

U.S.A. TEXTBOOK: *DISEASES OF THE EYE* – CHARLES HENRY MAY, MD, (PUBLISHED 1930)

Dr. Charles May (1861-1943) was founding director, professor, and visiting surgeon for the Eye Department at Bellevue Hospital in New York City. He is best known for his *Manual of Diseases of the Eye*, which was a classic textbook and atlas of ophthalmology. The book was published in 23 American editions between the years 1900 and 1963, and it was translated into ten different languages.

I was able to get May's 13th edition of Diseases of the Eye, published in 1930. In this 450 plus page book, Dr. May presents most of the fundamental diseases and conditions of the eye. The book also displays some 20 full-color fundus images, all of which include the macula, and every single color drawing was completed by Dr. May himself. Notably, there wasn't a single drawing of macular degeneration or any condition resembling it.

Under the condition of "Central Choroiditis," which is the term used by Hutchinson and Tay (1874), Dr. May writes:

> **Central Choroiditis** includes a number of degenerative and atrophic changes located at the macula, resulting in a gray, white or red spot, with more or less pigment deposit within the area or surrounding it. It occurs most frequently in *high myopia*, but also in syphilis and after contusions of the eyeball. It results in serious interference with vision and causes central scotoma [blind spot]. *It also occurs as a result of senile changes (central senile choroiditis).*" [106] (Last italics added)

Dr. May reports that high myopia (nearsightedness) is the most common cause of macular degeneration (central choroiditis) at that time, followed by syphilis and contusions of the eyeball. Personally, in my 24 years of clinical practice, I can count the number of cases of significant myopic maculopathy (nearsightedness associated macular degeneration) that I have diagnosed on one hand. In comparison, hardly a day goes by in the clinic that I don't see that many patients with AMD. In fact, I would estimate that in most days of my clinic, every fifth patient or so has some degree of AMD.

U.S. STUDY, 1930: *PATHOLOGICAL CHANGES IN THE RETINAL BLOOD VESSELS IN ARTERIO-SCLEROSIS AND HYPERTENSION* – BY HARRY FRIEDENWALD, MD

In 1930, Harry Friedenwald, MD, ophthalmologist from Baltimore, presented what was known as "The Doyne Memorial Lecture: Pathological changes in the retinal-blood vessels in arterio-sclerosis and hypertension." [107] This was a very lengthy lecture, completely transcribed, that was delivered to the Oxford Ophthalmological Congress at the University of Oxford, in England. This extensive lecture reviewed in every detail the fact that the eye may suffer from vascular disease too. Similar to other organs, there may be "hardening of the arteries" in the form of arteriosclerosis (thickening and "hardening" of the arteries) and arteriolosclerosis (thickening and "hardening" of the very small arteries/arterioles) in the eye. These effects may ultimately involve the retinal arteries and the choriocapillaris (choroidal sclerosis), which means that the inner retina can suffer from loss of good blood flow due to retinal arterial disease and the outer retinal layers (rods and cones and retinal pigment epithelium) can suffer due to vascular disease in the choriocapillaris. **We see here that the eye is no different than the heart or any other organ – that is, the vascular supply can be diminished due to vascular disease. The consequences, as you will see, are frequently devastating.**

Dr. Friedenwald did not specifically discuss macular degeneration, however, but Duke-Elder referenced him and this paper due to the connections he had drawn between vascular disease and AMD.

U.S.A. STUDY, 1937: 84 PATIENTS WITH DISCOID MACULAR DEGENERATION (POSSIBLE WET AMD) IN THE WORLD'S LITERATURE

In 1937, ophthalmologists F.H. Verhoeff, MD, and Herman P. Grossman, MD, published a study in which they reviewed all of the world's literature to that point. Their paper, entitled "The Pathogenesis of Disciform Degeneration of the Macula," discussed the fact that some 84 patients with a total of 129 affected eyes, had been diagnosed and reported with what was most likely some sort of wet AMD, ultimately, with a scarred macula, since 1875. The enormous majority of those appear to have been documented after 1923. Of their reference list, three were before 1900, 10 were between 1904 and 1919, and 20 between 1923 and 1935, strongly indicating an increasing prevalence of disease.[108] Already, the research conclusively illustrates the association with systemic diseases, as the authors report, regarding these 84 patients,

> Many of the reports contained little more than a description of the ocular lesion. Nineteen of the patients were recorded as having general hypertension. Fifteen had general arteriosclerosis. Eight cases were cardiac and four were nephritic [kidney disease]. Four were diabetic. Only three were luetic [syphilis related]... Eight patients died from coronary disease.[109]

Perhaps only a minority of all of the cases of discoid macular degeneration reviewed in this study would be cases of late or end-stage AMD, just as Professor de Jong concluded regarding the Junius and Kuhnt study of 1926, previously reviewed.

U.S. STUDY, 1938: *SENILE CHANGES AND DEGENERATIONS OF THE HUMAN EYE* – BY BENJAMIN RONES, MD

By 1938, macular degeneration was obviously becoming slightly more familiar to ophthalmologists. Ophthalmologist, Benjamin Rones, MD, of Washington, D.C., in his article entitled "Senile Changes and Degenerations of the Human Eye," addressed macular degeneration with much greater detail. He wrote:

> "Greater clinical importance is attached to the so-called senile macular degenerations. The chief complaint of these patients is impaired central vision, and though they are able to get around and carry on their activities, the ability to read and perform the finer visual tasks is considerably diminished. Ophthalmoscopically one sees in the macular regions an irregularity and heaping-up of pigment, with minute and conglomerate whitish patches of drusen and connective tissue. Histologically [examination of the tissue microscopically post mortem] it is evident in these cases that the obliteration of the choriocapillaris [nourishing vascular layer beneath the macula/retina] is of primary importance in producing the retinal changes, for the deeper layers show considerable disorganization and atrophy. There are also present adjacent areas of atrophy and of proliferation of the pigment epithelium, together with drusen on the lamina vitrea [Bruch's membrane]." [110]

Dr. Rones did not address the number or frequency with which he saw macular degeneration in his practice. However, he did state, **"Some individuals have advanced senile changes in their tissues at 40 years of age, while in others there is singularly little evidence of this at 80."**[111] He referred to the affected ocular structures as 'tissues' because his article addressed all of the structures of the eye that were affected by 'senile changes.' In any case, it certainly appears that macular degeneration was much more familiar to Dr. Rones than it was to those that came before him, as he thoroughly addressed the 'senile changes' of the eye in this 17-page study.

UNITED KINGDOM: *DUKE-ELDER'S TEXTBOOK OF OPHTHALMOLOGY* (PUBLISHED 1940)

In great contradistinction to all previous textbook references and journal publications, **Duke-Elder's Textbook**

of 1940 dedicates some 13 pages to both the dry and wet forms of AMD, including some 17 images, six of which are in full-color – and **he refers to macular degeneration as "a common cause" of vision loss in the elderly.**[112] This is a dramatic turn of events. Recall that, just 13 years previously, Duke-Elder's very own *Recent Advances in Ophthalmology* (1927) made absolutely no reference to the macular degeneration condition. **Let's look at the text of his 1940 textbook, beginning with the dry form of AMD:**

> "SENILE MACULAR DEGENERATION, first described as a clinical entity by Haab (1885), is a *common cause of failure in central vision in old people* (italics added). It is characterized by the presence of degenerative changes, usually punctate in nature, occurring bilaterally, limited to the region of the macula, and due to sclerosis and obliteration of the chorio-capillaris in the central area...
>
> The pathology of the condition has been investigated by several authors (Nagel, 1875; Harms, 1904; Friedenwald, 1930; Rones, 1938; and others). The primary changes are found in the choroidal circulation, which shows marked sclerotic changes and hyaline degeneration. The whole thickness of the choroid is affected, but the most advanced changes are in the chorio-capillaris where most of the channels disappear. Colloid bodies {drusen} are frequently seen on Bruch's membrane, and the pigmentary epithelium overlying may be raised by exudative material; the pigment cells show atrophy or proliferation with a dispersal or a heaping up of pigment." [113]

If you're not an ophthalmologist, let me simplify this passage. Duke-Elder gives a very accurate description of the dry form of macular degeneration, the same as we see it today, but he goes on to describe what is seen pathologically when these eyes (and maculae) are later examined post-mortem, under a microscope. In essence, he describes the fact that the choroidal circulation, which is the layer of vasculature beneath the macula (retina) and which nourishes the macula, is subject to "sclerotic changes." The latter simply means the vessels are occluding – obstructing – just as they do in the heart, kidney, or elsewhere in what we call ischemic (oxygen starved) disease. This is really a form of "hardening of the arteries."

Next, in Duke-Elder's textbook, is his view of management of the disease:

> "The treatment of sclerotic lesions of the choroidal vessels, as of all processes of this nature, is extremely unsatisfactory. The condition is due essentially to processes outside medical control – the gradual attrition of age and the stresses of living, the influence of hereditary and constitutional factors, and the accumulated effects of low-grade pathological processes acting over a long time. Moreover, in all such cases we are dealing with tissues of low vitality which are in no condition to respond to therapeutic or stimulatory measures. In view of the fact that toxic influences of a chronic nature do predispose to such changes, the elimination of any septic focus is advisable; and it is significant that a very large number of such cases suffer from a chronic and long-standing streptococcal toxaemia, originating, for example, from the teeth, the throat and the bowel. For the rest, a suitable mode of life and diet, with perhaps mild cardio-vascular stimulants and the administration of iodine and small doses of thyroid is the most that can be done.
>
> Optical appliances [glasses] in cases of macular degeneration may, it is true, tide the patient over for a little time—strong convex lenses [reading glasses], telescopic glasses, and so on—but slowly and irrevocably the central vision diminishes, all fine work and reading become more and more difficult and then impossible, and although field vision [peripheral vision], and with it the ability to get about the world, remains, such people can only be helped in so far as every effort should be made to assist them to accommodate their interests with philosophy and resignation to their limited visual efficiency." [114]

In this section of the book, there are six full-color images devoted to AMD, ranging from the earliest stages where there is mild pigment stippling to the full-blown stage of a large area of central atrophic degeneration of the macula (loss of retinal tissue).

I would like to ask you to highlight, in your mind, Duke-Elder's comment that "a very large number" of these individuals are also afflicted by infections involving the teeth, the throat, and the bowel. This has very significant meaning, and I will elucidate later as to why.

Next in Duke-Elder's 1940 edition of the text, he addresses wet AMD, which is the more threatening and disabling form of the disease. In this text, Duke-Elder refers to the condition as "disciform degeneration of the macula" and/or "senile macular exudative choroiditis." Here are selected portions of the text:

> "DISCIFORM DEGENERATION OF THE MACULA is a condition, frequently bilateral, characterized ultimately by the development of a localized mass of organized tissue situated under the retina. Such a picture may have a composite aetiology; but one proved cause is the occurrence of a haemorrhage from the chorio-capillaris extravasating between Bruch's membrane and the pigment epithelium. In general terms the cases may be divided into two classes, senile and juvenile; in the first the haemorrhage is usually due to sclerotic changes in the choroid; in the second its aetiology is obscure...
>
> The typical case develops in a patient over middle life with arterial disease; it commences with a

haemorrhage at the macula and terminates with the presence of a tumour-like mass of organized tissue at the macular region which abolishes central vision.

While senile disciform degeneration of the macula is not a common condition, it is commoner than would be supposed from the fact that only some 130 cases have been reported in the literature; Kahler and O'Brien (1935), for example, met 12 cases in their clinic in one year, and Davenport (1926) gathered a series of 17. It is definitely associated with age, occurring most commonly in the sixth decade; the youngest recorded case was 39 (Neame, 1923) and the oldest 83 (Kahler and O'Brien, 1935). Males are affected more frequently than females (10: 7), most of the patients have arterial disease, while hypertension, nephritis [kidney disease], diabetes and occasionally syphilis (3 cases) may be accompaniments. In rather more than half the cases the condition is bilateral, and in a few the second eye has been involved after the first has been observed." [115]

In this last paragraph of the text, I would again like you to observe that, in this presentation, all of the worst cases of macular degeneration (wet AMD) are found since approximately the year 1926, as noted above. As we get further in the book, you will see the dietary and nutritional significance of this and why I am pointing it out now.

UNITED KINGDOM: *SYSTEMIC OPHTHALMOLOGY, 2ND EDITION* – BY ARNOLD SORSBY (PUBLISHED 1958)

British ophthalmologist, Arnold Sorsby, was a Research Professor of Ophthalmology at the London University. According to the famed Dutch ophthalmologist, Petrus Johannes Waardenburg, MD, Dr. Sorsby completed invaluable research, published numerous books in the field of ophthalmology, including three volumes of Modern Trends in Ophthalmology, which was published in 1940, 1948, and 1955, and "his work culminated in his attempt to classify the choroidal and retinal dystrophies." [116] This final work would include analysis of macular degeneration.

In Sorsby's Systemic Ophthalmology (1958), he writes:

> "Senile macular degeneration" – It is often difficult to assess the significance of macular changes in elderly people. Bilateral lesions with atrophy, pigmentary disturbance and colloid [drusen] formation, especially if they affect vision, are often labeled senile macular degeneration. The histological changes reported are not incompatible with this idea consisting essentially of sclerosis of the choriocapillaris in the central area. ***Yet it is far from certain that these are cases of simple senile change. They are not nearly so frequent as would be expected*** and some of them are definitely hereditary, progressing to cause extensive retinal and choroidal damage, such as the cases of dominant fundus dystrophy of late onset described by Sorsby, Mason and Gardner (1949). It seems probable that in many cases of "senile macular degeneration, ***factors other than simple senile change are at work***, some of them possibly genetic." [117]

In this paragraph, the eminent Professor Sorsby made it clear that macular degeneration is not just a "simple senile change," meaning that it's not just about aging. He followed this statement with "They are not nearly so frequent as would be expected," which, I believe was his assertion that the frequency would be dramatically higher (than it was at that time) if this were simply an aging ("senile") change. His final statement, "factors other than simple senile change are at work..." obviously alluded to the fact that something more ominous was involved.

U.S.A. STUDY: *DISEASES OF THE MACULA IN THE AGED* – BY ABRAHAM KORNZWEIG, MD (PUBLISHED 1965)

One-third of an Elderly Nursing Home Population Now Afflicted with AMD

In 1965, U.S. ophthalmologist Dr. Kornzweig, presented his paper regarding the pathologic (post-mortem) study of 194 eyes "obtained at consecutive postmortems at The Jewish Home and Hospital for Aged in New York City. The residents range in age from 65 to over 90 years, mostly in the 75 to 85 decade." The results? **A staggering 33.5% of all eyes had evidence of "senile macular degeneration."** [118] Another 2.1 percent had "Kuhnt-Junius Disciform Macular Degeneration," which is the term used then for the end-result of what we call "Wet AMD."

Out of the 194 eyes examined by Dr. Kornzweig, he reviews the following findings:

> **"Sixty-five eyes, 33 per cent, showed the changes associated with senile macular degeneration, in varying stages of severity from mild to very advanced. The pathologic changes" include "atrophy of the cone cells, depigmentation of the pigment epithelial layer [retinal pigment epithelium], and drusen,"[119] among other findings.**

In Kornzweig's series of cases, he pointed out that the nourishing layer of vessels beneath the retina – the choriocapillaris – was relatively unaffected. He wrote, "The choriocapillaris appears to be unaffected. Similarly, the retina adjacent to the macula also appears to be relatively normal. It seems as if this portion of the retina acts as a separate organ, subject to influences that do not affect the other parts of the retina." [120]

This next one is a deep passage for non-ophthalmologists, but let me state this for all of our sake, because this is a critical turning point in understanding the AMD disease process, and then I'll simplify! Kornzweig's astute observations continue, as he wrote:

"Several authors, Parsons,[121] Friedenwald,[122] Rones,[123] Woods,[124] Duke-Elder,[125] and others, have attributed the cause of senile macular degeneration to sclerosis of the choroidal vessels in the region of the macula and especially of the choriocapillaris. There is thickening and hyalinization [thickening of the vessel walls] of the choriocapillaris and obliteration of many vascular channels. The sclerotic changes in the choroid may be widespread, but the limitation of the retinal changes to the macula indicates the greater vulnerability of this region.

The eyes that have been examined in this study do not bear out this conclusion. The choroid and choriocapillaris appear to be fairly normal under the light microscope. There is sclerosis of the larger choroidal arteries in many of these eyes, but this is a fairly common finding in many aged eyes. Other authors who have had an opportunity to examine, pathologically, eyes with a clinical history of senile macular degeneration have reported the same observations. Nagel,[126] Harms,[127] Behr,[128] and Klien[129] state that the choroid and the capillary layer appear relatively normal in such eyes. Klien[130] has helped to clarify this situation by pointing out a difference between ordinary senile macular degeneration and degeneration of the macula due to sclerosis of the choroidal vessels primarily and uniquely in the region of the macula. In the latter condition the pigment layer and the choriocapillaris are markedly atrophic and there is advanced sclerosis of choroidal arteries. The cones and rods in this area are also atrophied so that the external limiting membrane rests on the lamina vitrea. In ordinary senile macular degeneration, the choroid and choriocapillaris show little involvement." [131]

At this point, we're beginning to see two distinctly separate processes that seem to be leading to AMD:

1. **Sclerosis of the Choriocapillaris**: First, we see that the choriocapillaris, which is the nourishing vascular layer beneath the macula, may undergo sclerotic changes whereby the vessels occlude, thus eliminating or severely reducing blood supply to the overlying macula and leading to macular degeneration.
2. **Degeneration of the Retinal Pigment Epithelium (RPE)**: A distinctly separate process may occur as well, one in which the retinal pigment epithelial cells, which are also required to support the macular rods and cones (photoreceptors), may also undergo degeneration and even disintegration, leaving behind their pigment in clumps. This, in turn, may also result in loss of the overlying photoreceptors – and thus, AMD.

Clearly, two separate pathological processes seem to be at play. Could this mean two separate causes, both related? Let's move on…

U.K.: *DUKE-ELDER'S SYSTEM OF OPHTHALMOLOGY* (PUBLISHED 1966)

In 1966, in Sir Stewart Duke-Elder's textbook series, *System of Ophthalmology*, we see a dramatic and stunning change in the prevalence of macular degeneration. Let me quote the introduction to Duke-Elder's section of the book subtitled "Senile Macular Chorioretinal Degeneration (Senile Macular Degeneration of Haab)":

> **SENILE MACULAR DEGENERATION, first described as a clinical entity by Otto Haab (1885), is a common cause of failure in central vision in old age, occurring in some 25% of people between 65 and 80, and 30 to 40% over the age of 80 years** (Kornzweig et al., 1957; J.-P. Bailliart, 1961). It is characterized by the presence of *degenerative changes, usually punctate in nature, occurring bilaterally, limited to the region of the macula, and in most cases due to sclerosis and obliteration of the choriocapillaris in the central area.*
>
> The view that infective or toxic influences of a chronic nature predispose to such changes is difficult to refute but equally difficult to prove; but the advice of the previous generation to remove foci of infection cannot be substantiated unless in the interests of the general health. For the rest, a suitable mode of life and diet with perhaps mild vasodilators is the most that can be done in the early stages. Perhaps the most useful – and innocuous – method of therapy is an abundance of vitamins associated with nicotinic acid {vitamin B3} for its vasodilatory properties. In all these cases, however, the results of treatment are difficult to assess… [132]

It is tremendously interesting to note, once again, that Duke-Elder refers to the possibility of "infective or toxic influences" in relation to AMD. Please recall that, in his 1940 *Textbook of Ophthalmology*, he wrote that "a very large number of such cases suffer from a chronic and long-standing streptococcal toxaemia, originating, for example, from the teeth, the throat and the bowel."

Also in this passage, I believe this is the first time that multivitamins are recommended for macular degeneration, as Dr. Duke-Elder asserts, "Perhaps the most useful – and innocuous – method of therapy is an abundance of vitamins associated with nicotinic acid…"

Recent evidence clearly shows, however, that the widespread use of multivitamins certainly hasn't reduced the incidence or prevalence of macular degeneration. Nevertheless, Duke-Elder considered multivitamins to be "innocuous", as have most other physicians to date, but the evidence may surprise you. We'll tackle the risks and benefits of consuming synthetic vitamins in Chapter 18.

Finally, I would like to mention that Duke-Elder's recommendation for multivitamins was obviously made without the backing of any research. This is by no means meant to undermine the eminence of Dr. Duke-Elder. He remains one of the most esteemed ophthalmologists of the past century and his recommendation was obviously made in good faith. But, with the knowledge of current research, this recommendation as well as the assertion that multivitamins are innocuous will be challenged.

U.S.: *FRAMINGHAM EYE STUDY* (1973 TO 1975)

Next, let me note that the diagnosis of AMD starts to get messy at this point, because each study had different criteria for the diagnosis, for example, some required that vision be reduced, others did not. When vision is not a criterion that has to be met, then the prevalence numbers go way up. If vision is not a criterion, then obviously, anyone with any characteristic drusen or pigmentary disturbance in the macula will be included, and prevalence goes up.

In the Framingham Eye Study, investigators looked at the prevalence of AMD with and without vision loss. This was a survey of the surviving members of the Framingham Heart Study, which was begun in 1947 in Framingham, Massachusetts. A total of 2477 members of the Framingham study were examined for AMD. **If vision loss to 20/30 or worse and drusen were both considered to be requirements of the definitive diagnosis, 1.6% of those between 52 and 64 had AMD, 11.0 percent of those between 65 and 74, and 27.9% of those between 75 and 85**. If visual criteria were not considered, then those numbers went up to 35, 47, and 50 percent of the same age brackets, respectively. **Overall, 8.8% of subjects between 52 and 85 years of age were diagnosed with AMD.** [133,134,135]

COPENHAGEN CITY STUDY, DENMARK (1985 TO 1986)

In Copenhagen, Denmark, the prevalence of AMD was determined for the years 1985 to '86. For those with vision loss and retinal findings of AMD, for the age brackets of 60 - 64, AMD affected 2.3%, ages 65 - 69, 5.9%, ages 70 - 74, 12.1%, and between ages 75 - 80, the prevalence of AMD was 27.3 percent. For those with retinal findings and no visual criteria, the numbers increased to 14.6, 23.8, 29.0, and 45 percent, respectively.[136]

THE BEAVER DAM EYE STUDY, U.S. - 1988 TO 2005 (ONGOING)

In Beaver Dam, Wisconsin, the prevalence of AMD was assessed over a period of some 17 years. This study began with a baseline examination of some 4926 people age 43 to 86 years, followed by repeat examinations every five years for those still in the area and still living. There were 1913 still available for exam by 2008 to 2010. In the following age brackets: Ages 43 to 54, AMD affected 8.4%, ages 55 to 64. 13.8%, ages 65 to 74, 18.0% and at ages 75 plus, the prevalence of early AMD was a whopping 29.7 percent. For each category, the prevalence of late (advanced) AMD was 0.1, 0.6, 1.4, and 7.1 percent, respectively.[137] It might be worth reiterating that nearly one-third of those 75 and older had early AMD in this study.

THE BLUE MOUNTAINS EYE STUDY, AUSTRALIA (1992 – 1993)

A total of 3582 people, aged 49 to 90+, residing in two adjoining communities located in the Blue Mountains area west of Sydney, Australia, underwent examinations to evaluate for the presence of AMD. For those with the presence of "soft drusen" (mild to moderate AMD), the prevalence was 3.6% for those 49 to 54, 6.5% for those 55 to 64, 15.9% for those 65 to 74, 26% for those 75 to 84, and 40.2% for those 85 years of age and older. The prevalence of advanced AMD, defined as either wet AMD or geographic atrophy in this study, was 0.0% for those aged 49 to 54, 0.2% for those 55 to 64, 0.7% for those 65 to 74, 5.4% for those 75 to 84, and 18.5% for those over 85 years of age.[138]

U.S.: ALBERT & JAKOBIEC'S *PRINCIPLES AND PRACTICE OF OPHTHALMOLOGY* (PUBLISHED 1994)

Recall that Albert & Jakobiec's 1994 *Principles and Practice of Ophthalmology* made the statement, **"As many as 15 million persons in this age group [over 50] may be affected by AMD,"**[139] and this is in the U.S alone. At that time, the U.S. population was around 250 million,[140] which means that somewhere in the neighborhood of six percent of the entire population was affected by AMD.

The prevalence of AMD was reviewed in Albert & Jakobiec's textbooks via research that I have presented directly from the studies themselves, e.g., the Framingham Eye Study, the Copenhagen City Study, and others.

U.K. STUDY: *IS THE INCIDENCE OF REGISTRABLE AGE-RELATED MACULAR DEGENERATION INCREASING?* – BY RICHARD WORMALD, MD, AND JENNIFER EVANS, MSC, PHD (1996)

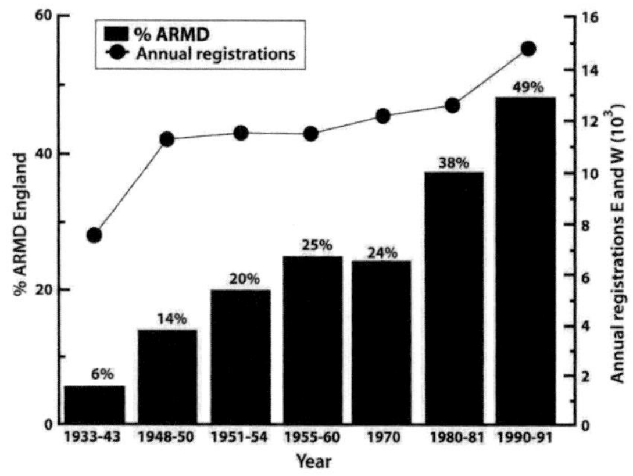

FIGURE 3.1 Annual new registrations for blindness in England and Wales 1933-90 and proportion of registrations attributed to age-related macular degeneration (ARMD) in England.

This is the only study of its kind, that is, one in which the incidence of AMD (as related to blindness) was projected over time. This study, however, was aimed at testing the hypothesis that the age specific incidence of blinding AMD has increased in Britain over the past 60 years or so. The researchers extracted data from the government registration system whereby social services for the blind are coordinated in England and Wales.

In the author's own words regarding their results, "After controlling for changes in the age structure of the population, registration rates for all causes, cataract, glaucoma, and optic atrophy have decreased while registrations attributed to ARMD [Age-Related Macular Degeneration] have increased in the order of 30—40%." Their conclusion? "These findings are compatible with the hypothesis that the incidence of ARMD is increasing in Britain." [141] They further state, **"In the 1930s only 6% of the certificates analyzed were attributed to ARMD; in 1990 nearly 50% of registrations were attributed to ARMD."** [142] **By 2014, a separate study showed that AMD either fully accounted for or was a contributor to blindness in 56% of those registered as blind in the U.K.**[143]

There is little or no question that this is some of the most powerful evidence indicating that the prevalence of AMD is markedly increasing. Though this study is indicative of the worst kind of AMD ("wet" AMD or severe geographic atrophic AMD), it is still a strong reflection of the degree of AMD overall. As of the date of this study (1996), the authors purport that AMD was already responsible for blinding some 17,500 people in Britain each year (recent years). Again, keep in mind that this is *blindness*, which in Great Britain, requires that best-corrected visual acuity is less than 20/400 in both eyes (Blindness in the U.S. is best-corrected visual acuity 20/200 or less in both eyes). The numbers of people whose vision loss was negatively affected, but not blinding, in Britain, would likely be at least a couple-hundred fold higher, as late AMD only occurred in 1.6% of the population in the Beaver Dam Eye Study, but that wouldn't necessarily be in both eyes in the same person.[144]

Alan C. Bird, MD, distinguished Emeritus Professor of Ophthalmology and honorary consultant at Moorfields Eye Hospital, London, United Kingdom, in a study published in The Journal of Clinical Investigation, in 2010, wrote that **"AMD is recognized as causing more than 50% of blind registration in Western society and is now designated as one of the major blinding diseases of the world. In contrast to the current high prevalence of AMD, in the 19th century, it was considered a rare disorder and described as "chorioretinal disease in senile persons"**, the latter of which is referenced to Dr. Hutchinson's 1874 study, which I've reviewed previously in this chapter.

Dr. Bird continues, "There is evidence that the current increased prevalence of AMD cannot be fully explained by increased life expectancy. Furthermore, the disease is now recognized as a burden in societies in which it was considered rare 30 years ago. Low prevalence of AMD in some populations not of European descent has been well documented in the past. However, the disorder has become common in the last 2 decades in urban communities in Japan, and in the last 3 years, the rate of hospital referrals has doubled (M. Uyama, personal communication). Publications imply that a similar change in prevalence may be occurring elsewhere in east Asia. There is also a strikingly high prevalence of macular disease in elderly Inuit in Greenland." [145]

Some four years later in 2014, in a *Distinctive Voices* lecture given at the Beckman Center in Irvine, California, Professor Bird made the following update and statement:

> "...Because it's {AMD} undoubtedly relatively rare 50 years ago and it's now very common.... Age-related macular disease accounts for 57 percent of blind registration in the United Kingdom. Huge! It's exactly the same in North America. It's exactly the same in the rest of Western Europe. It's an enormous burden on society." [146]

A REVIEW OF THE AMERICAN ACADEMY OF OPHTHALMOLOGY'S JOURNAL - *OPHTHALMOLOGY*

I searched the American Academy of Ophthalmology's (AAO) official journal, *Ophthalmology*, for articles/studies that included the term "macular degeneration" anywhere in their content, as far back as their on-line database shows (1965). In the 1960's, there were no studies presented on macular degeneration in this journal, in the 1970's, five studies mentioning macular degeneration, in the 1980's, 84 studies, in the 1990's, 238 studies, from 2000 through 2009, there were 1344 studies, and from 2010 to April of 2015, already 1444 studies presented.[147] At the current rate, there will be more than 3000 studies published dealing with AMD during the decade from 2010 to 2020, in this single journal alone. I believe this is consistent with the pandemic of AMD that we see as well as the frenzy of scientific research directed at cause, prevention, treatment, and cure.

CHAPTER SUMMARY

As we've seen in this chapter, following the invention of the ophthalmoscope in 1850, ophthalmologists were clearly observing and detailing the macula, retina, and optic nerves – and by the early 1860's, there were already multiple significant atlases of the fundus of the eye. It was some 23 years, however, after Helmholtz' invention, before Jonathan Hutchinson would describe the first four cases of macular degeneration, in 1874. In 1885, Otto Haab gave a lecture detailing some of the characteristics of macular degeneration and, in 1895, Haab presented several cases with associated images. In 1892, Ernst Fuchs' *Textbook of Ophthalmology* devoted one brief sentence to the condition, which did not address frequency, nor did he mention the findings of Hutchinson or Haab. Oliver and Norris' *Textbook of Ophthalmology*, in 1893, appears to have no references to macular degeneration at all. By the end of the 19th Century, despite numerous iterations of the ophthalmoscope, retinal atlases, and extraordinarily detailed descriptions of the retina, we see only a very small number of cases of macular degeneration in the span of 50 years of potential discovery.

Julius Hirschberg's *The History of Ophthalmology*, written in 1914 – 1915, which is a summary of ophthalmology in the 19th century and up to 1914, failed to mention macular degeneration at all. And again, In Duke-Elder's *Recent Advances in Ophthalmology* textbook, published in 1927, no mention is made of macular degeneration whatsoever. In 1930, Charles Henry May's textbook, *Diseases of the Eye*, devotes only one sentence to the condition of macular degeneration. There is no notation of its frequency, once again, which appears to be indicative of the rarity of the condition. Furthermore, Dr. May reports that myopic (nearsighted) macular degeneration, a rare condition, is the primary cause of macular degeneration. In total, by 1931, we have 80 years of ophthalmic history following the invention of the ophthalmoscope, and all we have are scattered and rare reports of macular degeneration.

In 1930, Harry Friedenwald's study showed that "choroidal sclerosis," the vascular phenomenon of obliteration of the retina's nourishing vascular layer, was well observed in pathological studies. This condition could clearly lead to loss of photoreceptors – the rods and cones. In 1937, Verhoeff and Grossman reviewed some 84 patients with 'disciform degeneration of the macula' that had been documented in the world's literature, between 1875 and 1937. Many or most of those cases may not have been late AMD, but rather, other causes of macular scarring. In 1938, Benjamin Rones corroborated Friedenwald's study and, in fact, he correlated clinical loss of central vision with signs of macular degeneration and, at post-mortem exam, findings of obliteration of the choriocapillaris. At this point, we begin to see that researchers showed that macular degeneration found its roots in vascular disease, at least in part.

In 1940, in the U.K., we suddenly see that Duke-Elder, in his *Text-Book of Ophthalmology*, reported that macular degeneration was "a common cause" of vision loss in the elderly. This was a profound and entirely new statement at the time – something that had never been documented. He still did not address frequency, however. But he reviewed both the dry and wet forms of macular degeneration and, in great contradistinction to his 1927 textbook, which didn't even mention macular degeneration, we now see 13 pages of text and 17 images devoted to AMD. He drew connections with streptococcal toxemia from the teeth, throat, and bowel, and recommended a "suitable mode of life and diet" as the primary treatment of choice.

In 1958, Sorsby's *Systemic Ophthalmology* textbook addressed the etiology (cause) of macular degeneration. Sorsby surmised that "*factors other than simple senile change are at work*..." In 1965, Kornzweig completed post-mortem studies on the eyes of residents who died in a nursing home with average ages of about 75 to 85, showing that a staggering 33.5% had evidence of AMD. Though not exactly a population representative of the public (these were nursing home residents), at this point we can clearly see that an epidemic of macular degeneration may have been developing in the elderly of our nation. We also begin to see two separate pathological processes at work: 1) Sclerosis of the choriocapillaris vessels, and 2) Diminution and disintegration of the retinal pigment epithelium.

By 1966, Duke-Elder's Textbook of Ophthalmology reported that "some 25% of people between 65 and 80, and 30 to 40% over the age of 80 years" had some degree of AMD. Duke-Elder considered that "infective or toxic influences of a chronic nature" may be at fault, and recommended "an abundance of vitamins associated with nicotinic acid {vitamin B3}."

After 1966, there are many studies that corroborate the epidemic of macular degeneration. These include the Framingham Study (U.S.), the Copenhagen City Study (Denmark), the Beaver Dam Eye Study (U.S.), the Blue Mountains Eye Study (Australia) and others, all of which found AMD to approach or even exceed 30% of the population in those 75 years of age and above.

Wormald and Evans showed that AMD accounted for only 6% of blind registrations in England and Wales between 1933 to 1943, and that by 1990 to '91, AMD accounted for 49% of blind registrations, indicating a dramatically higher prevalence and/or severity of the disease, even after accounting for other blinding diseases.

In summation, we see that documented cases of AMD were very rare between 1850 and 1900, with a few more sporadic cases up until 1930, and then an obvious surge of clearly documented AMD cases in the 1930s. Prevalence of AMD rose to epidemic proportions by the 1960s and 1970s, at least in the U.S. and U.K. Incidence and prevalence appears to remain approximately at or above those levels today.

The question is: Why?

ONE GIANT LEAP FORWARD

In the first chapter, I briefly reviewed the dogma surrounding the cause of AMD. Perhaps the term "dogma" here is a little strong, because if anything, there are also abundant references stating the cause of macular degeneration "is unknown," just as you have read from the Mayo Clinic's website and Albert & Jakobiec's *Principles and Practice of Ophthalmology.* If there is a dogma regarding the cause of AMD, it is that it has generally been blamed on two primary risk factors – namely, advancing age and genetics.

The definition of dogmatism is "the tendency to lay down principles as incontrovertibly true, without consideration of evidence or the opinions of others." At this point, I would like to pose two questions for you to ponder:

- First, if AMD is truly an "age-related disease," shouldn't it have affected the elderly the same just 50 years ago? A century ago? One-hundred-and-fifty years ago? As you've now seen, AMD was practically non-existent just a century ago. How can this possibly be considered "age-related"?
- Second, if AMD is a genetic condition, shouldn't AMD have been as prevalent a century or more ago, as it is today? Are we to believe our genetics have changed this drastically, in 85 years?

These are the pivotal, and fundamental, questions that I want you to consider- and re-consider - as we progress through this book.

To my knowledge, no one previously has ever stated that macular degeneration is caused almost exclusively by diet. However, ophthalmologists have had an inkling about nutrition and its link to AMD for over a century. Utilizing nutrients from food to treat the eye dates back to the era of Hippocrates. In ancient Greece, the home of Hippocrates, vitamin A deficiency was treated by squeezing the juice of liver onto the surface of the eye.[148]

Quite frankly, the association of eye disease and nutrition is anything but new. Let's just very briefly touch on this concept now, as we'll be reviewing the concept of nutrition and AMD throughout this book.

DISTURBANCE OF THE RETINAL PIGMENT EPITHELIUM (RPE) AND DIET

As early as 1913, ophthalmologist Henry Gradle, MD, of Chicago, noted that retinal pigment epithelium (RPE) disturbances were associated with a faulty diet and that a peculiar "stippling or granular condition" of the macula was sometimes associated, even in children and young adults. In addition, Dr. Gradle found that the primary symptoms these patients presented with were "asthenopia," which is the medical term for eyestrain, but these youngsters often had neurotic tendencies as well. An excerpt from Dr. Gradle's study below:

> "All of these patients complained of ocular discomfort, described sometimes as a burning or, rather oftener, as an ache, and usually accompanied by more or less headache. While reading intensified the discomfort, most patients complained more or less even while resting the eyes, and indeed very commonly much discomfort was noticed at once on rising in the morning. Perhaps this was due to the effect of daylight on the eye sensitized by darkness; for as a rule, these patients were annoyed by strong light of any kind." [149]

Dr. Gradle's young patients referenced in this passage present with classical symptoms that were likely associated with vitamin A deficiency, which includes dry eyes as evidenced by the discomfort, burning, and uncomfortable eyes, photophobia (sensitivity to bright light), and perhaps even vitamins B or D deficiencies, which might play a role in the neurotic tendencies. Dr. Gradle recognized the nutritional deficiencies, however, as his recommendations for treatment were as follows:

> "In some instances the temporary relief from the use of smoked {tinted} glasses was very striking, more so than I have ever seen in any other form of functional disturbance of the eyes… For ultimate success, however, I trusted to measures directed against the neurotic condition – liberal outdoor exercise, sojourn in the country, bathing, correction of habits and diet, iron if required, and sometimes strychnia. About one third of the patients lost their eye complaints and headaches under this treatment; another third were improved to a variable extent, while the balance could not be watched a sufficiently long time to be recorded regarding the final outcome."

In 1936, in a study published in the Transactions of the American Academy of Ophthalmology and Otolaryngology, Arthur Bedell, MD, wrote, "In certain conditions, *such as disturbed nutrition*, the chromatophores [retinal pigment epithelial cells] which normally have branched processes lose their processes and have the appearance of clump cells."[150] (Italics added) In this passage, we see that Dr. Bedell had tied "disturbed nutrition" to abnormalities in the RPE. When the RPE is severely disturbed, altered, or in the worst case scenario – undergoes atrophy - we then lose the rods and cones (photoreceptors) that were supported by the lost RPE cells. This is the hallmark of macular degeneration.

FAULTY CIRCULATION AND AMD

As early as 1893, Doctors Oliver and Norris noted that "impaired general nutrition" could play a role in disease of the vascular choroid, which nourishes the retina (macula). They wrote, **"Primary disease of the choroid is generally due to degenerative changes taking place in some part of its vascular network... At times, such degeneration is either senile or is the result of impaired general nutrition. Secondary disease of the choroid is exceedingly frequent."** [151] They also noted that hemorrhages in the macula could be related to a deficient diet, as they wrote, "Where degenerative changes have occurred in the cerebral blood vessels, hemorrhages in the retina are not infrequently the forerunners of apoplexy [stroke with severe symptoms]. They are also common accompaniments of albuminuric retinitis [retinal disease associated with kidney failure], and may be very frequent in many diseases of malnutrition where the character and composition of the blood have undergone marked changes."[152]

Ophthalmologist Benjamin Rones, MD, whom we've discussed previously, author of the scientific study "Senile Changes and Degenerations of the Human Eye," published in the American Journal of Ophthalmology (1938), wrote the following summary of his article, taken in its totality:

> Analyzing the factors contributing to the diversity of senile changes in the ocular tissues leads to the conclusion that the vascular changes are of fundamental importance. *Impaired nutrition* resulting from this will explain the deposition of fat globules in the various structures. It is also well known that initial proliferative changes leading to subsequent degenerations are attributable to faulty circulation. The old adage that 'a man is as old as his arteries' can thus be also applicable to the changes that occur in the eye during advancing years.[153]

In the substance of the same article, Rones draws connections to the circulation of the choroid, which is the vascular layer beneath the macula that supports the health of the macula itself. He wrote:

> **The role played by the choriocapillaris in the nutrition of the retina is of the utmost importance, and consequently any great impairment of its function must necessarily exercise a deleterious influence upon its dependent tissues.** The pigment epithelium [retinal pigment epithelium, which lies immediately beneath the macula] is an early sufferer from this diminished circulation, and its changes are partly of a proliferative and partly of a degenerative nature.[154]

This connection, as relevant today as the day it was written, may explain exactly why cardiovascular disease and its risk factors are virtually the same risk factors for AMD.

As previously reviewed, recall that in 1940, Sir Stewart Duke-Elder recommended "a suitable mode of life and diet" for "senile macular degeneration," and he repeated this same recommendation again in 1966. In 1966, as you may recall, he also recommended "an abundance of vitamins."

In their book, *Macular Degeneration,* published in 2004, Philip Penfold, PhD, and Jan Provis, PhD, wrote, "A rigorous test of a nutrient-deficiency hypothesis of AMD-associated photoreceptor death awaits more information about normal nutrient delivery mechanisms across the RPE/Bruch's membrane complex, intra-retinal contributions to photoreceptor nutrition, changes in these mechanisms with age and pathology, and differential effects on rods and cones." [155]

Penfold and Provis went on to review the fact that Don Gass, MD (1973) suggested that the dry, atrophic form of macular degeneration and the wet form of the disease may both be manifestations of the same disease process. They wrote:

> It would appear, therefore, that in the adult macula there is a critical relationship between limited blood supply and high metabolic demand. Even minor perturbations of circulation, for example in incipient vascular disease, may lead to metabolic stress in foveal neurons and/or glia. Such perturbations and the resultant stress may generate signals that induce the neovascular changes associated with wet AMD. Chronic failure of choroidal vascular supply at the macula may result in atrophy or dry AMD usually considered to be the natural end-stage of the disease.[156]

Johanna M. Seddon, MD, ScM, Professor of Ophthalmology at Tufts University School of Medicine and Director of Tufts Medical Center Ophthalmic Epidemiology and Genetics Service, and her colleagues have completed numerous studies that have enhanced our understanding of nutrition and AMD. In her book, *Eat Right for Your Sight,* which is primarily a cookbook, she wrote the following in the introduction:

> When I began my career as an ophthalmologist and retina specialist, a large percentage of my patients were elderly with macular degeneration. I, like every other eye doctor in the world, didn't have answers to questions from patients or their families as to why they developed the disease. We'd say, "It occurs with aging." The only treatment we had to recommend (laser surgery, now rarely used) left behind damaging scar tissue.
>
> Many eye doctors were skeptical when I began my research on nutrition, lifestyle, and macular degeneration. At scientific meetings, my talks were scheduled near lunchtime, and moderators would joke about the study of diet and eye disease. Then, from 1994 to 1996, we reported that the antioxidant nutrients lutein and zeaxanthin, which are also called carotenoids (abundant in spinach and kale), along with the anti-inflammatory nutrients called omega-3 long-chain polyunsaturated fatty acids (found in salmon, sardines, herring, and mackerel), could reduce the risk of macular degeneration, the leading cause of vision loss among the

elderly. We discovered that 6,000 μg of lutein and 2,000 μg of zeaxanthin per day from food sources like spinach and summer squash could reduce the risk of macular degeneration by 43 percent and 2 or more servings per week of fish (rich in omega-3 fatty acids) could reduce the risk by 40 percent.[157]

CHAPTER SUMMARY

Researchers have tied the cause of macular degeneration, repeatedly, to vascular disease (in the choroid), an altered and thickened Bruch's membrane, degeneration of the RPE, and loss of the photoreceptors (all to be reviewed in Chapter 6). The question is: What happened to our diet, beginning about the turn of the 20th century, to potentially cause AMD – and why have we seen a true epidemic of the disease in the past 50 years or so? To answer that, we need to look at our culinary history – and that is coming up in a couple of chapters.

As you can see, ophthalmologists have been entertaining the hypothesis of faulty nutrition as a cause of macular degeneration for more than a century. In fact, there's been quite an explosion of research in the past 25 years regarding nutrition and AMD. However, I believe most of this research misses the most crucial points, because a thorough analysis of the history of nutrition has never been examined in parallel with the epidemiology of AMD. Once we complete a thorough analysis of our dietary history, and then tie that to available research that supports biologically plausible mechanisms, I believe you will agree that we can take one giant leap forward – and we can indict a faulty diet as the villain in this long and tragic story.

5 DID OUR GENETICS CHANGE?

I feel it is a compulsory that I include a chapter on this question, since there is a near constant repetition that genetics plays a major role in AMD. So, did our genetics change over the past century – or century-and-a-half? The short answer? No. Now, can we move on to the next chapter?

Alright, I'll explore this question briefly, for all of our sake. In brief, as most of you probably already understand, if our genetics haven't changed in the past century or so, we can't blame our genetics for our current epidemic of AMD, right? And we've already seen that AMD was exceedingly rare at the turn of the 20th century, right?

To date, more than 30 different "genetic polymorphisms" (think genetic variations) have been characterized that are believed to play a role in AMD.[158] This research has certainly required an immense amount of dedication and a staggering sum of money. Yet, clinician scientists, Lucia Sobrin, MD, MPH, and Samaneh Davoudi, MD, of Massachusetts Eye and Ear Infirmary, in an article in Ophthalmology Management, wrote, "While there has been extensive genetic discovery and excellent risk prediction models developed thus far in AMD, no prospective studies to date have proven that predicting increased disease risk will make a difference in AMD patient outcomes."[159] That's correct. Not a single study has shown that all of this genetic profiling will benefit any patient in any way, as it has never led to any methodology to treat the condition. And the short answer is that it's not going to.

As previously reviewed, I believe it is this unfounded belief system and our collective failure to examine the history of AMD that has led us to believe that AMD has always been so prevalent and that it, therefore, has a genetic basis. It obviously has no such prevalence in history and, consequently, no such genetic basis.

Recall Dr. Kornzweig's research, published in 1965, in which he studied nursing home patients, most of which were 75 to 85 years old? Repeating the findings: "Sixty-five eyes, 33 per cent, showed the changes associated with senile macular degeneration, in varying stages of severity from mild to very advanced." Since this was 1965, most of these patients were born around 1880 to 1890. If we go back just 20 to 40 or 50 years, we're now roughly in the era in which their parents and grandparents were born. Obviously, virtually none of their grandparents had AMD, as we know that by 1930, reports of AMD were scarce. Possibly some of their parents developed AMD, as they may have lived into the 1940's or so, but probably very few of them developed the condition.

So, if their parents and/or grandparents didn't have AMD, and our assertion is that it might be genetics, is that even plausible? Is it reasonable at all? My answer – possibly, but very unlikely. Why? Enter: Epigenetics.

If you're not familiar with epigenetics, let me give a very brief review. This will be so short and dirty that it is truly an injustice, which might very well be the case with every single chapter of this book since each one is very capable of being a book in itself. But since no one wants this book to be the length of *War and Peace*, it is a necessity.

The definition of epigenetics is "the study of changes in organisms caused by modification of gene expression rather than alteration of the genetic code itself." In short, this means that our genes can be turned "on," "off," or perhaps somewhere in-between, based on "environmental influences." These environmental influences are legion – and according to epigenetics expert, Jill Escher, MA, JD, may include exposure to such things as drugs and pharmaceuticals, industrial chemicals, pesticides, cigarette smoke, exogenous hormones, endocrine disruptors (such as BPA and phthalates in water bottles), plasticizers, radiation, acute stress, exercise, and nutrition,[160] or lack thereof, the latter of which would include vitamins, minerals, phytonutrients, fatty acids, amino acids, and all the macronutrients in general (proteins, fats, and carbs).

I think we understand some of this intuitively, but this science is very new having only begun in the '90s. Let me give an example. Our DNA is like the architectural blueprint for a beautiful brick and stone home with a pool. The blueprint itself is generally thought to be immutable. It serves as the master-plan for constructing the home. To build the home though, requires all sorts of "sub-contractors" to fulfill the plan. We would need foundation "subs," framers, carpenters, masons, electricians, plumbers, insulators, concrete, deck, and pool sub-contractors, maybe more. Each sub-contractor not only needs his training and experience, but he also needs equipment, tools, and raw materials. The raw materials would include lumber, bricks, stone, dry-wall, paint, electrical wiring, plumbing, and so on.

Once the home is finished, let's say that we now own this home for 80 years. In that duration, the home will sometimes need maintenance and repair. Perhaps in those 80 years, there are hailstorms that damage the roof, hurricane-force winds that knock a tree into the picture window, foundation settling that results in cracks in the wall, and pipes that break under a winter freeze. In both the building and the restorative phases, we need sub-contractors, tools, and raw materials, once again.

Our bodies are like that. Just think of our blueprint as being the DNA. **In order for the DNA to build the body, it needs sub-contractors, which would include hormones and enzymes. Those in turn need "tools," such as all vitamins and minerals, and "raw materials," such as proteins, fats, and carbohydrates, but also includes all nine essential amino acids, essential fatty acids, phytonutrients, etc., all in innumerable combinations.**

If you don't give the body what it needs, you come up short in terms of either development or repair. Let's say a gale-force wind blows a tree down that smashes through the front window. If you call a glass repair guy in, but you cannot provide a new window as a replacement, he might cover the window with plastic or a board. It's not what you want, but you didn't provide the most desirable "raw" materials. Or, lets say you buy the window, but you don't have anyone to install it. This is analogous to missing vitamins or minerals. The raw material is there, but you're missing the enzymes and tools. In this case, you're still coming up short – and your house begins to "degenerate." The hail that damages the roof, the gale-force winds that knock out the window, and the frozen and busted pipes are all analogous to oxidized particles – also known as free radicals. They cause damage and we need the correct hormones, enzymes, vitamins, minerals and so on to effect repair.

This is exactly how I want you to think of your body – and your eyes. You absolutely must give them the raw materials, vitamins, minerals, and appropriate environment in which to thrive and properly repair.

In our bodies, including our eyes, if we're missing critical nutrients, the effects can be devastating. Personally, I think we are overlooking these nutritional deficiencies – and I think we're overlooking them in a very big way.

In the realm of epigenetics, it might be stated that our environment can dysregulate our genes. It's not that the blueprint is changed, but environmental influences affect the regulations of our genes. It's a built-in mechanism whereby the genes modify their action based on environmental availabilities, such as nutrients, but also may be effected by the presence of toxins and poisons, such as pesticides and herbicides. In one sense, this is a fail-safe mechanism designed to modify the body in accordance with the nutrients that are provided.

Physicians, especially our pediatric and obstetric colleagues, are well aware of the deleterious effects of missing nutrients. For example, spina bifida, a condition in which the spinal cord and meninges (the protective sheath around the brain and spinal cord) incompletely develops in the unborn baby due to insufficient intake of folic acid – a common B-vitamin. Vitamin K deficiency in newborns causes uncontrolled bleeding and underdeveloped faces and bones in newborns. Rickets, a vitamin D deficiency, is characterized by soft, weak, and disfigured bones and muscles, which will often become permanent. Scurvy, first noted in sailors who spent months at sea, is a deficiency of vitamin C that is characterized by lethargy, bleeding gums, loss of teeth, and eventually, death. Pellagra, a disease originally discovered in early settlers, was found to occur in people consuming mostly corn. Corn lacks vitamin B3 (niacin) and the deficiency leads to diarrhea, dermatitis, dementia, and death. Beriberi, a disease originally endemic in Asia, occurred almost exclusively in the more elite of society while the poor were spared. This disease is secondary to a vitamin B1 (thiamine) deficiency, which is found consistently in cereal grain husks and bran. The rich had washed and polished their rice consistently – to a degree that would remove the husks and bran – thereby removing vitamin B1. The poor did not. The signs and symptoms of Beriberi included severe weight loss, muscular weakness, central nervous system disease, cardiac arrhythmias, heart failure, and death for those untreated. Vitamin B12 deficiency (hypocobalaminemia) is associated with deterioration of the brain and spinal cord, usually beginning with fatigue, irritability, depression, and memory loss. Mania and psychosis may eventually ensue, which may become irreversible. B12 is found only in animal products, so strict vegans will all get this disease without proper supplementation. These are just a few examples of diseases and conditions that occur as a result of nutritional deficiencies, all of which fall into the epigenetics category.

After the next chapter, I will introduce you to the work of Weston A Price, who completed a stunning volume of real-life work in the field of epigenetics, and presented his work some 50-plus years before the term epigenetics was even coined.

COMPLEMENT FACTOR H VARIANTS AND OTHER GENES – LINKED TO AMD

The complement pathway is a critical component of the innate immune system and the alternative pathway of complement functions through an ancient pathway to defend us against infectious organisms. There is an entire cluster of genes that is associated with regulation of the complement system and, as it turns out, there are polymorphisms (variants) of the complement factor H (CFH Y402H) gene that are associated not only with macular degeneration, but also with certain renal (kidney) diseases.[161] CFH actually plays an anti-inflammatory role.[162] As such, the proposed mechanism that this CFH variant may play is that it fails to properly inhibit the complement system, thereby increasing inflammation.

Some studies have shown that certain variants of the CFH gene confer greater risk of macular degeneration in some populations.[163] In fact, Australian researchers Ammarin Thakkinstian and colleagues completed a meta-analysis in 2006, and according to these authors, "the CFH polymorphism is involved in (or in other words, the CFH allele contributes to) over half of all AMD, slightly higher than previous estimates."[164]

In addition to CFH, other complement factor genes, including ARMS2 A69S,[165] CFB, complement component 2 (C2), C3, the age-related maculopathy susceptibility 2/HtrA serine peptidase 1 gene, and finally, the LOC387715 gene, all confer greater risk for AMD.[166,167]

Let's get some perspective here on these genetic risk factors and their relationship to AMD, because even these are not nearly as powerful as one might think. According to Dr. B. Jeroen Klevering from the Netherlands, "The CFH Y402H and ARMS2 A69S gene polymorphisms [variants] are the two most important genetic risk variants associated with AMD."[168] People can have one, two, or no copies of these alleles (genes). For those that are homozygous for the CFH gene, that is, they have the worst case scenario, which is two copies of the gene, they develop wet AMD 2.8 years earlier than those that have no copies of the gene. For those people that are homozygous for the ARMS2 gene, again with two copies, they develop wet AMD 5.2 years earlier than those with no ARMS2 genes. Obviously, even for those with the most risk in terms of heredity, the development of AMD is not tremendously different. It's not as if people with the worst genetic risk profiles develop AMD 20 or 30 years sooner than those without.

I am not at all surprised that certain genes, such as these variants of the CFH and the ARMS2 genes, most definitely place individuals at higher risk for AMD. At this point, it might be a good reminder to recall that, in many industrialized populations that have been studied, rates of AMD run up to 30% and 40% or more of the population by age 75 to 80, depending on the criteria used. If the criteria for the presence of drusen and/or pigmentary disturbance in the macula are used in the definition of AMD, many more than that would qualify to have AMD. Is it any wonder that some genes would be associated with AMD in more than half of the population? In fact, I would assert that if the diet of a population is severely deficient in micronutrients and replete with processed foods – and every individual consumes it, virtually 100% of those who live long enough will have some form of AMD.

FAMILY AND TWIN STUDIES OF AMD PATIENTS

Hyman and colleagues, in 1983, found that AMD patients were three times as likely to report a positive family history for AMD than their age-matched controls. At that time and in that particular study, 21.6% of 228 AMD patients gave a positive family history for AMD.[169]

In 1997, Dr. Johanna Seddon and colleagues examined 119 AMD patients and found a prevalence of AMD in 23.7% of the first degree relatives compared with only 11.6% in the first degree relatives of 72 control patients without AMD. Their conclusions state, "Results suggest that macular degeneration has a familial component and that genetic or shared environmental factors, or both, contribute to its development."[170]

Twin studies should prove the genetic basis of AMD, if there is one. Monozygotic twins (MZ, or "identical twins") share 100% of their DNA while dizygotic twins (DZ, or "non-identical twins") share approximately 50% of their DNA. That is, dizygotic twins are no more alike than siblings.

Ophthalmologists Sanford Meyers, MD and Froncie Gutman, MD, from the Division of Ophthalmology at The Cleveland Clinic Foundation, completed an excellent study of twins between the years 1986 and 1994. They examined some 98 pairs of MZ twins and some 38 pairs of DZ twins. They found that of the 98 pairs of MZ twins, who ranged in age from 44 to 86 years, with an average of 65 years, some 25 pairs both had macular degeneration and of the remaining 73 pairs, neither had AMD. In the 38 pairs of DZ twins, 5 pairs both had AMD, 26 pairs both did not, and the remaining 7 pairs were discordant, that is, one had AMD and the other did not.[171]

In this study, the concordance in the MZ twins was 100 percent, whereas concordance was only 42 percent in the DZ twins. Obviously, this is strong evidence that there is a genetic component to the development of AMD. However, this study did not address dietary consumption in any meaningful way, likely because the authors didn't believe it was all that significant, as is generally the belief.

In this study, the authors state, "The dietary history included questions on the type and frequency of vegetables, fruits, or vitamins; we did not perform serum levels of micronutrients or calculate semiquantitative micronutrient levels based on diet." And their results state, "We did not identify any environmental or nongenetic risk factors for age-related macular degeneration from the occupational, residential, dietary, or medical histories of the twins." But the results section of the study makes no other mention of their dietary histories at all. That is, these two statements quoted are the only statements made relating to diet in the entire study.

In this case, we don't know if the monozygotic twins were both consuming similar diets their entire lives or not. I would submit that, more than likely, they were. The question is, were the 25 pairs of MZ twins that both had AMD both consuming vegetable oils, artificially created trans-fats, white flour, sugar, and other processed foods, throughout their lifetime, to a greater degree than the 73 pairs who both did not have AMD? This question was never addressed and, therefore, we'll never know.

Another twin study completed by ophthalmologists Christopher Hammond, MD, and colleagues at the St. Thomas' Hospital, London, United Kingdom, was presented in the journal *Ophthalmology*, in 2002. This was a much larger, population based study, which evaluated 506 twin pairs, 226 of which were MZ twins and 280 of which were DZ twins. They averaged 62 years of age. In this case, the heritability of age-related maculopathy (ARM) was estimated as 45%, which was obviously a much lower concordance rate than the previous twins study reviewed.[172]

I'll wrap up this brief chapter with a quote from S. Boyd Eaton, MD, who might be considered the original founder of the Paleo diet, when he wrote, "Our genetic makeup, especially that regarding our core metabolic and physiologic characteristics, has changed very little between the emergence of agriculture, roughly 10,000 years ago, and the present."[173] As you can see, even for hard-core evolutionary biologists, the belief is that our core genetic profiles have changed little in 10 millennia. Should we believe they've changed in just a century?

CHAPTER SUMMARY

There is little or no evidence that our core genetic makeup has changed in the past 150 years or so. Even the hard-core geneticists and evolutionists would generally agree with that. The studies of the Complement Factor H and ARMS2 genes, family studies, and particularly twin studies do suggest that there are genetic characteristics that put some people at greater risk for AMD than others. I think that is quite clear.

However, it certainly doesn't indicate that any of those people who are at greater risk genetically would have developed AMD had their diets been consistent with ancestral dietary principles. **I would submit that the genes that put people at higher risk are nothing more than "susceptibility genes," that is, genes that increase the likelihood of developing AMD.** Those probably exist for most every single pathologic condition there is. People with light-colored skin are more likely to sunburn – but only if over-exposed to the sun. Women smokers are more likely to develop lung cancer than men.[174] And when it comes to AMD, whites have a greater risk of developing AMD than African-Americans. But, neither race developed AMD, except in exceedingly rare circumstances, before about 1930.

We currently have an epidemic of AMD. In the words of British physician and researcher, David Grimes, MD, of the Blackburn Royal Infirmary, "...it is obvious that an epidemic cannot be due to faulty genes, which have a stable prevalence over a long period of time. However, genes can have an influence on susceptibility..." [175] This is exactly the case with AMD.

In the United States, Great Britain, Australia, and many other nations that have followed suit, enormous percentages of the populations are consuming severely nutrient deficient, processed food diets that result in a vast array of disease conditions. Studying the genetics of these disastrous conditions is tantamount to studying the genetics of holocaust victims, who were placed on diets of instant coffee for breakfast, watery soup that might contain a piece of turnip or potato peel for lunch, and a 300 gram slice of black bread with less than an ounce of sausage, cheese or margarine for dinner[176] – and then trying to predict who would get disease, malnourishment, and emaciation – based on their genetics. It's an exercise in futility. You already know the answer.

Our genetics are not what have changed to result in an epidemic of AMD, obviously. What has changed – and changed drastically in the past 135 years – is our environment, particularly our food supply. It is staggering what has happened to it since the year 1880. This changes our epigenetics – and what we will see is that that the consequences are pathological changes, which may be devastating.

Next, we'll take a brief review of what AMD is – at the microscopic level. Glad you're still with me. We're nearing Base Camp One of our Mount Everest.

6 A PRIMER ON AMD

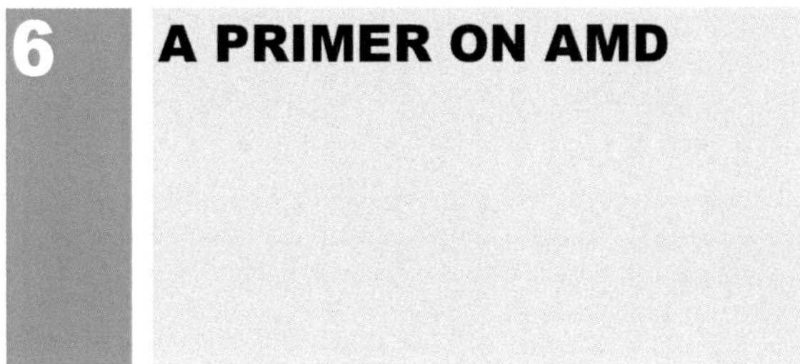

Age-related Macular Degeneration (AMD) is the leading cause of worldwide blindness in the elderly and has been the leading cause of irreversible vision loss and blindness in the developed world for a number of decades. The macula, which is the central retina, accounts for only about four percent of the retina, but it is by far the most important part of the retina since it is responsible for central vision. The macula is responsible for one's ability to discern faces, to see stop signs, to read print, and so on. If the macula is destroyed, the impact on vision is devastating. Hence, the importance of discovering the true etiology and treatment for AMD.

I will not give an extensive review of the anatomy and pathology of AMD in this chapter. The fundamentals in these areas are covered in great detail in numerous publications and, as such, I will keep this relatively brief so as to emphasize etiology, prevention, and treatment through nutritional means. This chapter will be a mix of clinical presentation, anatomy, physiology, pathology, and nutrition, all as they relate to AMD. At times, it might get a little deep for those of you who are non-scientists. But once we get through this chapter, the remainder of the book is far less scientific and complex. So just hang in here with me through one additional tough chapter - so that we can understand some of the fundamentals of AMD. Trust me – understanding a little further what is going on with AMD at the microscopic level will really help to make sense of its prevention and treatment as well.

THE INITIAL PRESENTATION

In the early stages of macular degeneration, visual loss is typically mild and usually asymptomatic. However, one may begin to notice blurred vision, blind spots, decreased contrast sensitivity (harder to see in dim illumination), abnormal dark adaptation (difficulty adjusting from bright to dim lighting), and the need for brighter light to accomplish normal visual tasks. With progression, the affected individual will lose more central vision, definite blind spots may develop, and if dry AMD suddenly becomes wet AMD, distortion of the vision (metamorphopsia) and profound central vision loss may occur. Even without wet AMD, however, dry AMD may progress into more advanced AMD known as geographic atrophy, which may also result in rather profound central vision loss, albeit at a more insidious pace.

MACULAR ANATOMY AS IT RELATES TO AMD

The macula is only about 6 millimeters in diameter – that's almost exactly one-fourth of an inch This entire book all comes down to what's going on in that quarter-inch area of retina in the back of your eye. The macula itself comprises only about four percent of the entire retinal area, but yet it is responsible for about 10 degrees of our central vision as well as the enormous majority of our useful vision. The fovea, located at the center of the macula, is the area responsible for the most acute vision. It is only about 2 millimeters (1/13th of an inch) in diameter and yet represents approximately 5 to 6 degrees of our central vision, which is the area of maximal visual acuity. This is arguably the most important 2 millimeters of your entire body, as without it, you would have a rather large central blind spot in your vision. Suddenly, you'd be unable to read or see a person's face.

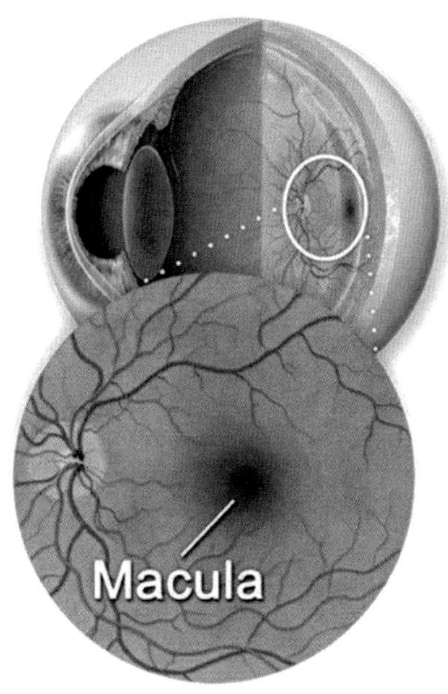

Deep to the neural retina, from the front to the back of the eye, lies the retinal pigment epithelium, followed by Bruch's membrane, the choriocapillaris, and then the sclera, which is the outer white of the eye (see the image below). Most of this chapter will focus on the retina, specifically, the photoreceptors (rods and cones), the retinal pigment epithelium (RPE) located just behind the retina, Bruch's membrane, which separates the retina from the choriocapillaris, and then the choriocapillaris itself, which is the primary blood supply to the macula. Got it? Stay with me. Just one step at a time and we'll build on simple foundations...

THE MACULA

The fovea is so critically important to vision – and yet many researchers say, "paradoxically, it has the least blood supply." This isn't exactly a paradox, in my opinion. Let's examine why.

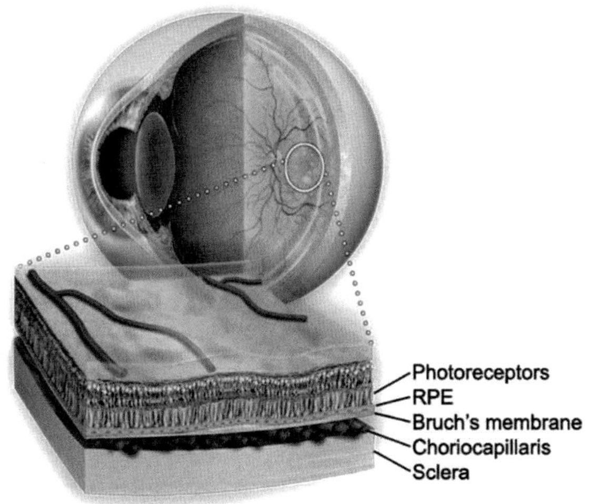

Illustration courtesy of Mark Erickson , JirehDesign.com.

The fovea has a central area known as the foveal avascular zone (FAZ), which is a central area of the fovea approximately 400 to 500 microns (one micron equals one thousandth of a millimeter) across, which has no blood supply on the retinal side. This is thought to be a specialization associated with high visual acuity, as the presence of vessels in this area on the retinal side would compromise vision. This is the reason that the relative lack of vasculature in the fovea is not truly a paradox. It is truly the perfect design, quite frankly, apparently as long as nutrition and blood supply remain adequate.

The choroidal circulation, which is deep to the retina and beneath the retinal pigment epithelium, would therefore be required to play a bigger role in oxygenating and nourishing the fovea. And as we've seen, it is the choroidal circulation that is compromised in AMD.

PHOTORECEPTORS – RODS AND CONES

Photoreceptors, known as rods and cones, are responsible for converting photons of light ("light rays") that are transduced into a biochemical signal (known as phototransduction) that is transferred to the brain, first through bipolar cells, and then to the retinal ganglion cells, the latter of which synapse in the brain (via the optic nerve) to allow us to actually "see." Rods are responsible for light and dark vision, that is, they cannot perceive color, but are highly adapted for low light vision. Cones are responsible for color vision and are highly adapted for acute, high-definition vision.

Outside of the fovea, rods are the predominant photoreceptor, where they outnumber cones 20:1 on average. There are about 120 million rods in each eye. Anatomically, cones become increasingly common toward the center of the fovea. At a distance of 500 microns (1/2 millimeter) from the center of the fovea, rods and cones are equal in presence. Rods become increasingly scarce within 300 microns of the center of the fovea and the central 100 microns of the fovea is made up purely of cones.

There are only about 90,000 cones in the central 2mm of the retina.[177] According to vision researcher, Anita Hendrickson, at the University of Washington Department of Ophthalmology, "Therefore our highest visual acuity depends on the functional integrity of less than 100,000 cones out of almost 5 million, emphasizing how critical optimal health of the fovea is for good vision throughout life."[178]

According to physicist Francois Delori, PhD, Associate Professor of Ophthalmology at Harvard Medical School and Senior Scientist at the Schepens Eye Research Institute, the "photoreceptor cells have the highest metabolic rate of cells in the body." He states that their "activity is very demanding in energy and nutrients" and that this "is possible only through an exquisitely organized support and protection system."[179] His statements are founded and supported by the research and writings of Cohen and Noell, in the textbook *Biochemistry of the Retina,* from as far back as 1965.[180]

RETINAL PIGMENT EPITHELIUM (RPE)

The photoreceptors are dependent on the retinal pigment epithelium (RPE) and the RPE cells are dependent on the photoreceptors. Extraordinarily, it appears that the the vascular layer beneath the RPE, which provides 90% of the oxygen and virtually all of the nutrients to the photoreceptors via the RPE, is dependent on the RPE for its own health! This is one of the most spectacularly mutually supportive roles in the body.[181] In fact, mutations in the genes responsible for RPE functionality often lead to degeneration in the photoreceptors and mutations in the genes controlling photoreceptor functionality may result in degeneration of the RPE.[181] It's as though one can't really live without the other.

The photoreceptors, working harder than any other cells in the body, are also the subjects of intense "oxidative stress," which means that reactive oxygen species (ROS) are developed rapidly. To resolve this problem, the photoreceptors "shed" the outer 10% of their photoreceptor segments (which are closest to the RPE) every night. The RPE must engulf these outer segments, degrade, and re-process them. Since one RPE cell services approximately 30 photoreceptors, the RPE has perhaps the highest burden in the body to break down oxidized debris.[182] More importantly, if an RPE cell goes kaput for any reason, the 30 photoreceptors that it supports will also go "belly-up." If this occurs over a significant area, we get what is called geographic atrophy – and this is devastating to vision.

The roles of the RPE are so numerous, and the research so incredibly detailed and voluminous, I could easily fill the rest of this book just discussing the RPE. In order to keep this brief and on-target to our goals of understanding how nutrition plays such a critical role in our vision, let me just begin by summarizing a few of the crucial functions of the RPE, all of which obviously are critically dependent on nutrients, good blood flow, and of course, plenty of oxygen.

German scientist and researcher, Olaf Strauss, PhD, is Professor of Experimental Ophthalmology, University Hospital, in Regensburg, Germany. He has spent more than 25 years studying the RPE and it's relationship to health and disease of the eye. To summarize the major findings of his research, the RPE:

Stages of Macular Degeneration Progression

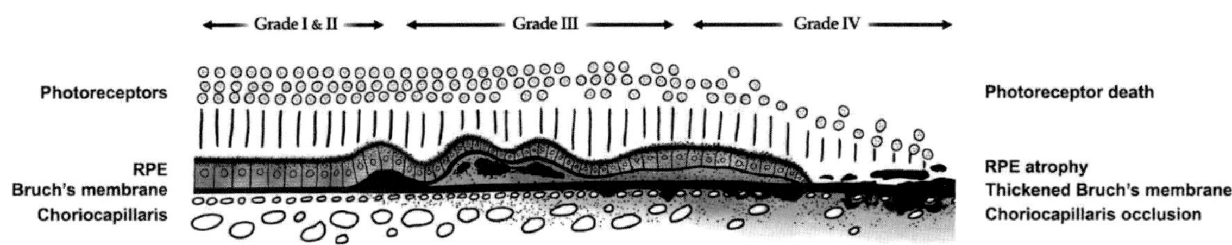

Schematic Illustration Courtesy of Mark Erickson, JirehDesign.com.

- Forms one side of the blood-retinal barrier, which is critical to controlling what substances can get into and out of the retina.
- Takes up nutrients such as glucose, amino acids, fatty acids, minerals, ions, carotenoids (e.g., lutein and zeaxanthin), and vitamin A derivatives, while it must remove and transfer to the choriocapillaris various waste products, including lactic acid, carbon dioxide, and various metabolic end-products.
- Plays the critical role of maintaining the visual cycle (converting all-trans retinal to 11-cis retinal – to be discussed).
- Phagocytocizes (engulfs) the photoreceptor outer segments, which contain the photoreceptor opsin proteins. This is part of the restorative and regenerative process of the photoreceptors.
- Secretes a variety of growth factors that are essential to the functional and structural integrity of the choriocapillaris endothelium (inner lining of the blood vessels) as well as the photoreceptors, which includes vascular endothelial growth factor (VEGF).
- Secretes immunosuppressive factors, which are critical to the immune privilege of the eye.

Dr. Strauss states, "With these complex different functions, the RPE is essential for visual function. A failure of any one of these functions can lead to degeneration of the retina, loss of visual function, and blindness."[181]

The vascular layer that supports the RPE, which also lies immediately below it, while being separated from the vessels by Bruch's membrane, is the choriocapillaris. In the dry and atrophic type of AMD, the choriocapillaris is seen to degenerate, i.e., occlusion occurs.[183] It is not clear whether this is a cause or a consequence of degeneration and atrophy of the RPE. In any case, Dr. McLeod and colleagues found that atrophy (cell death) of the RPE occurs prior to degeneration of the choriocapillaris. This implicates the RPE as the likely starting point for AMD.[184]

Unfortunately for us, when the RPE is destroyed, whether that is secondary to inflammatory, infectious, ischemic (blood flow and oxygen deprivation), toxic, nutritional deprivation or other means, it doesn't grow back. That's right, ***the RPE of the human and virtually all mammals is remarkably non-regenerative.***[185,186,187]

Researchers Brandon-Luke L. Seagle, MD, PhD, at the University of Chicago, Department of Chemistry, and his colleagues at the University of Chicago Department of Ophthalmology and Visual Science and the Institute for Biophysical Dynamics, state that, ***"RPE cells are nonregenerative and must last a lifetime to maintain sight."***[188]

Marco A. Zarbin, MD, PhD, Chair of The Institute of Ophthalmology and Visual Science at the New Jersey Medical School, in Newark, New Jersey, in his review of the pathogenesis of AMD, states, **"In response to decreased oxygen delivery/metabolic "distress", the RPE may elaborate substances leading to CNV [choroidal neovascularization, or "wet AMD"} growth. Perhaps RPE atrophy, followed by choriocapillaris and photoreceptor atrophy, is a response to decreased nutrients/increasing metabolic abnormalities…"**[189]

Chung-Jung Chiu, DDS, PhD, who has done immense investigation involving the study of vision at the Laboratory for Nutrition and Vision Research, Tufts University, puts it like this:

> "…The first indication of AMD is observed in the outer retina, primarily involving the retinal pigment epithelium (RPE) and associated tissues. The RPE lays on a basal lamina, known as Bruch's membrane, and together they form the outer blood retinal barrier (oBRB). The oBRB separates the

retina from the choroid plexus. The choroidal circulation receives 65 – 85% of the blood that flows to the retina through choroidal arteries and is vital for the maintenance of the outer retina (particularly the photoreceptors). A very high density of mitochondria and lysosomes in RPE also indicates a high metabolic activity. The RPE serves as a headquarters in outer retinal metabolism; it oxygenates and nurtures the outer retina and is also responsible for processing metabolic waste generated from visual cycle. The high energy requirements of the RPE stem from requirements for metabolism including proteolytic burden, because every night each RPE must digest the outer 10% of the photoreceptor discs that are shed by 30 photoreceptors. In fact, the RPE has the highest proteolytic burden in the body." [190]

It's getting pretty deep, I know. The simplified version is this: the retina (rods and cones, primarily) depends greatly on the RPE. The RPE, in turn, depends on the blood supply of the choroidal circulation. Amazingly, the choroidal circulation itself depends on growth factors secreted by the RPE – in an amazingly mutually beneficial relationship. The RPE gets oxygen and nutrients from the choroidal circulation. If the choroid is compromised, the RPE suffers and, if the RPE suffers, the choroid and the retina suffer. *We must strongly consider that, lack of proper nutrients, i.e., vitamins and minerals, may cause the RPE to suffer first. This is followed by failure (degeneration) of the vascular layer, which is the choroid/choriocapillaris.* In turn, the RPE atrophies (undergoes cell death) followed by photoreceptor (rods and cones) cell death. This is the dumbed-down version of a critical concept we'll need for the rest of the book. Okay? Got it? Let's move on.

attempting to understand and explain the physiology of vision. It will never be fully understood. I assure you. The complexities are far beyond us. I will only just briefly touch on this physiology. In fact, to even call this entire chapter a thumbnail sketch is definitely a stretch.

Nevertheless, let's begin with the fact that processing visual information begins with the detection of light by the photoreceptor cells (rods and cones). In order to detect light, the photoreceptors must utilize a derivative of vitamin A, known as 11-cis retinal. When 11-cis retinal is bound to an opsin signaling protein, a visual pigment molecule is formed. In the rod cell, this is known as rhodopsin, and in the cone cell, as iodopsin. When photons of light hit this molecule, the 11-cis retinal is isomerized to all-trans retinal, which is associated with the straightening of the molecule as seen below. This induces an electrical signal that is conducted from the photoreceptor to the bipolar cell, ganglion cell, and eventually the ganglion cell processes synapse with neurons in the visual cortex of the brain to create an image.

The all-trans retinal, located in the photoreceptor, must be transported out of the photoreceptor to the retinal pigment epithelial cell, where it is converted back to 11-cis retinal in three enzymatic steps. The latter is transported back to the photoreceptor to complete the visual cycle. It is believed that interphotoreceptor retinoid-binding protein (IRBP) is responsible for transporting the 11-cis retinal back to the photoreceptor, though the mechanism of transport is not clearly understood. The process of regenerating 11-cis retinal from all-trans retinal is thought to take place exclusively in the RPE cells as it relates to rod function. However, it appears that the cones are able to regenerate 11-cis retinal in a separate cycle that takes place in the Müller cells, the latter of which are supportive cells that stretch from the photoreceptor layer to the ganglion cell layer.[191] According to Cynthia Owsley and colleagues at the University of Alabama at Birmingham, "Unlike rods that derive vitamin A preferentially from the RPE and choroidal vasculature, cones have alternative sources of vitamin A through the retinal vasculature, Mueller cells, and retinoid-targeting mechanisms that are selective for cones."

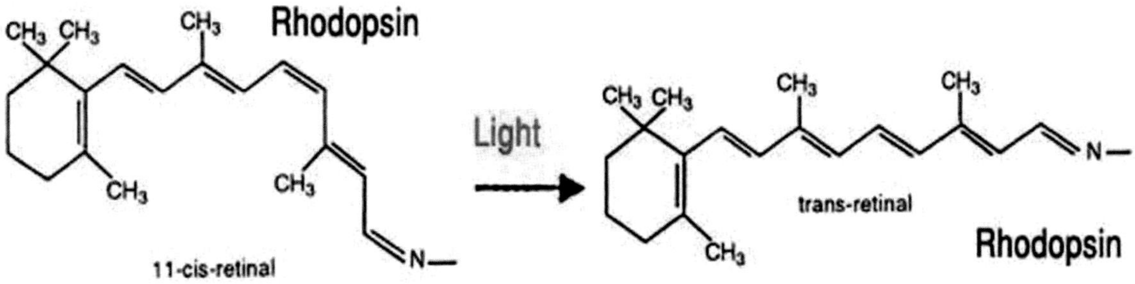

THE VISUAL CYCLE – VITAMIN A IS THE ESSENTIAL INGREDIENT

To process vision, a number of metabolites of vitamin A, known as retinoids, are required. These include retinyl esters, retinol, retinoic acid, and oxidized and conjugated metabolites of both retinol and retinoic acid. In fact, to produce vision requires numerous carrier proteins, enzymes, vitamins, minerals, ions, carotenoids, and cofactors involved in what is truly a dizzying array of metabolism that has perplexed thousands of scientists all around the globe for decades. Many of these researchers have spent their entire lives and careers studying, researching and

BRUCH'S MEMBRANE

Bruch's membrane lies between the RPE and choriocapillaris. It is in this layer that significant degenerative changes occur that apparently play yet another role in the development of AMD. Bruch's membrane contains the basement membranes of both the RPE and the choriocapillaris and sandwiched between those are two collagenous layers with a middle elastic layer. The middle elastic layer is one-third to one-fifth as thick in the fovea as it is in the peripheral retina, perhaps to allow greater diffusion of molecules both directions in the extremely metabolically active fovea (central macula).[192]

Bruch's membrane generally tends to thicken as we age. In fact, what is known as basal laminar or basal linear deposits cause progressive thickening of Bruch's, which is thought to be a significant precursor to AMD.[193,194] **Dr. Ramrattan and colleagues found that Bruch's membrane generally tends to double in thickness between childhood and approximately 90 years of age.**[195] **It is believed that this thickening and basal laminar deposits may serve as barriers to the diffusion of oxygen and perhaps other nutrients to the photoreceptors.**[196] In response to this, the RPE and outer retinal layers may increase production of vascular endothelial growth factor (VEGF) and other growth factors that cause the growth of new vessels (ultimately, wet AMD).

Christoph Spraul, MD, and colleagues at the Emory University School of Medicine, Department of Ophthalmology, Atlanta, Georgia, examined 51 eye bank eyes that had various stages of AMD and compared them to 40 age-matched controls without AMD. They evaluated the degree of basal laminar deposit according to a classification scheme set forth by Sarks and van der Schaft et al. The degree of basal laminar deposit is graded as follows: Grade 0, which is none; Grade 1, which is small solitary patches on the basal side of the RPE; Grade 2, which is a thin, continuous layer, less than half the height of the RPE; and Grade 3, which is a thick layer, greater than or equal to half the height of the RPE. They found that the median (average) score for both the dry AMD and wet AMD groups was a 3 and the median score for the control group was only a 1, which was highly statistically significant.[197] Thirty-five of the 40 eyes with AMD had grade 3 basal laminar deposit whereas only 3 of the 40 control eyes had basal laminar deposit as severe as grade 3.

Dr. Spraul's group also discovered significant differences in the degree of calcification of Bruch's membrane in the wet AMD group versus the control group. A critical difference between non-AMD patients and those with wet AMD is physical breaks in Bruch's membrane, as this allows the vessels of the choroid to break through Bruch's and "grow" beneath the retina, often subsequently leaking fluid and bleeding. **They found that in the wet AMD group the mean degree of graded calcification was 1.6 with a median number of five breaks in Bruch's membrane, whereas in the control group, calcification only averaged 0.8 and there were zero breaks in Bruch's membrane.**[196] In the dry AMD group, calcification averaged 0.8 – the same as the control group – however, those eyes averaged one break in Bruch's membrane.

In a study by Ron Klein, MD, and colleagues at the University of Wisconsin Department of Ophthalmology and Visual Sciences, subjects with higher pulse pressures (difference between the systolic, or upper, and diastolic, or lower blood pressure number) were found to be more likely to have macular findings consistent with early AMD, as well as wet AMD, findings. High pulse pressure is an indication that the arteries have become stiff and less pliable secondary to vascular disease. The authors drew analogies with AMD as they wrote, "These findings indicate relationships between higher pulse pressure (a presumed indicator of age-related elastin and collagen changes in Bruch's membrane)..." [198] This is yet another indication that cardiovascular disease and the thickening and changes in Bruch's membrane share a common cause.

The question is why are the patients with AMD developing thickening (basal laminar deposit and basal linear deposits) of Bruch's membrane to a much greater degree than patients without AMD? Secondly, why are patients with wet AMD developing calcification and breaks of Bruch's membrane to a much greater degree than patients with dry AMD, who fare better, or those without AMD, who fare the best?

I will propose that this may very well be the result of multiple and varied deficiencies of the fat-soluble vitamins, particularly vitamins A, D and K, but particularly K2 (to be reviewed in Chapter 16), combined with the presence of an abundance of polyunsaturated fatty acids (PUFA) in the diet, the latter of which may contribute to deposition of oxidized lipids in Bruch's membrane.

Deficiencies of the fat soluble vitamins play a complex but tremendous role in numerous degenerative disorders and this will be reviewed in some detail. However, at this point, one should understand that at least 17 different vitamin K-dependent proteins have been identified to date that are involved in soft-tissue calcification. For example, osteocalcin, matrix Gla protein (MGP), and possibly Gla-rich protein are all inhibitors of soft-tissue calcification and all are dependent on vitamin K for their activity.[199,200] **A vitamin K2 deficiency might play a significant role in calcification of the soft-tissue of Bruch's membrane, just as it does in the calcification of coronary vessels, aortic valve calcification, and in chronic kidney disease where vascular calcification is extensive.**[201]

Research has shown that there is a progressive increase in the lipid content of Bruch's membrane throughout life.[202] Thus, Bruch's membrane becomes a lipid rich barrier, which has been implicated in AMD development.[203] Assessment of the type of lipids present in Bruch's membrane is imprecise, but evidence suggests that the increased lipids consist of neutral fats with esters of both saturated and unsaturated fatty acids and phospholipids. I have hypothesized that the greatest contribution to this may come from the PUFA vegetable oils that we consume to extreme excess, perhaps through indirect mechanisms – and which will be reviewed in detail.

Further, calcification, lipid deposition with consequent thickening, and basal laminar deposits may collectively serve as barriers to the diffusion of gases, nutrients, and metabolic by-products between the photoreceptors and the choriocapillaris.[204] A decrease in choroidal blood flow, which is the vascular layer that supports the RPE and photoreceptors (to be reviewed below) might reasonably be expected to decrease the clearance of metabolic debris and by-products from the RPE cells, which could then deposit that debris within Bruch's membrane.

Drusen, the yellow-white deposits that are so characteristic of AMD, accumulate in Bruch's membrane exclusively. According to internationally acclaimed ophthalmologist and researcher, Professor Paulus T.V.M. de Jong, MD, PhD, of the Netherlands Ophthalmic Research Institute, "Drusen often have a core of glycoproteins, and their outer domes contain crystallins, chaperone proteins, apolipoprotein E (APOE), vitronectin, and proteins related to inflammation (amyloid P, C5, and C5b-9 complement complex)." [205] We must strongly consider the fact that elements of inflammation occur in drusen, as this may signal a role for a significant inflammatory component to the development of AMD.

THE CHORIOCAPILLARIS

The choriocapillaris has the greatest blood flow by mass of any tissue in the body.[206,207,208] However, it's no wonder there is a relatively tremendous blood flow in the choriocapillaris. The choriocapillaris has the job of bringing oxygen and nutrition to the photoreceptors. The photoreceptors, in turn, do more metabolic work per unit of mass than any other tissue in the body. Metabolically speaking, they're the top-fuel dragsters of the body – and yet incredibly, they cannot stop working - ever. They're performing metabolic functions while we sleep and while we're awake. Processing vision is a phenomenally intensive task.

As such, to properly care for and nourish our photoreceptors and their supportive tissues, which include Bruch's membrane, the RPE and choriocapillaris, we need a tremendously good blood supply – and a supply of blood that is rich in nutrients and oxygen, and scarce in any variety of toxins.

With that said, let's take a look at some studies regarding blood flow in the choroid of patients with AMD.

Dr. Spraul and colleagues found fewer large choroidal vessels in the submacular choroid in eyes with AMD versus eyes without AMD ($P < 0.001$), but with early proliferation and subsequent atrophy (closure) of the capillaries of the choriocapillaris, in those with AMD.[209] This might be interpreted as a proliferative response to hypoxia (poor oxygenation) early on with subsequent degeneration of the capillaries of the choriocapillaris with disease progression.

In fact, multiple studies have demonstrated reduced choroidal blood flow in dry macular degeneration. Juan Grunwald, MD, Professor of Ophthalmology at the University of Pennsylvania, and investigator at the Scheie Eye Institute, is world renowned for his research on blood flow in the retina. In 1998, he and his colleagues compared the choroidal blood flow and volume in AMD patients versus age- and blood pressure-matched control subjects without AMD. **They found that, in subjects with AMD, choroidal blood volume was 33% lower than that of control subjects ($P = 0.005$). They also found that average choroidal blood flow in subjects with AMD was 37% lower than those without AMD ($P = 0.0005$).** [210]

It has been shown, by Doctor Penfold and colleagues and by Dr. Curcio and colleagues that reduced blood flow and loss of patency of the vessels in the choriocapillaris is associated with degeneration of the RPE and cell death of the adjacent photoreceptors and outer retinal layers.[211] [212] Furthermore, Dr. Curcio and colleagues at the Department of Ophthalmology, University of Alabama, found that diminution of the choriocapillaris was associated with adjacent RPE degeneration and that "complete loss of the choriocapillaris was associated with RPE atrophy." [212]

According to John Lovasik, PhD, and Hélène Kergoat, PhD, chapter authors in the book *Ocular Blood Flow,* "A global reduction in choroidal blood flow is not a common clinical occurrence. However, there is increasing evidence that a regional reduction in choroidal blood flow occurs in patients with age-related macular degeneration even before there is any clinical evidence of a significant disruption in the macular anatomy. Thus, a subnormal choroidal perfusion of the macula may be a major risk factor for this age-related macular disease."[213]

Perhaps even more convincing that vascular disease plays a big role in AMD, researchers at the Indiana University Macular Degeneration Clinic and Research Center compared ocular blood flow in 25 patients with AMD versus 25 control subjects without AMD. They performed color Doppler imaging to analyze the blood flow of various vessels that perfuse the eye, such as the posterior ciliary arteries and the central retinal artery. An examiner of the results was masked as to which patient was in which group. **The researchers found that, in the nasal posterior ciliary artery, for example, the mean blood velocity measured 1.45 cm/sec in the AMD group, versus 1.96 cm/sec in the control group. This is an average blood flow decrease of 26% in the AMD group versus the control group, which was highly statistically significant ($P = .0012$). This also held true for the central retinal artery, where the average blood flow was 1.37 cm/sec in the AMD group, versus 1.95 cm/sec in the control group – again, the results being highly statistically significant ($P = .0007$).**[214]

INFLAMMATION AND AMD

A number of studies have suggested that inflammation plays a significant role in the development of AMD.[215,216,217,218] Drusen, the metabolic deposits at the level of Bruch's membrane that are so characteristic of AMD, have been shown to contain proteins that are associated with both acute and chronic forms of inflammation. For those who want the nitty-gritty detail, these proteins include serum amylopid P component, apolipoprotein E, immunogloblulin light chains, Factor X, and complement proteins C5 and C5b-9 complex.[219] What is important here is that all of these proteins are associated with inflammation and, of course, inflammation has been tied to coronary artery disease in thousands of studies (PubMed search linking "coronary heart" or "coronary artery" and "inflammation").

The point here is that, once again, we see a correlation between AMD and heart disease, right down to the molecular level. In fact, Robert F. Mullins, MS, PhD, Professor of Ophthalmology and Visual Sciences at the University of Iowa, in the last study mentioned wrote, "The compositional similarity between drusen and other disease deposits may be significant in view of the recently established correlation between AMD and atherosclerosis." [220]

The brilliant Johanna Seddon, MD, and colleagues at Massachusetts Eye and Ear Infirmary and Harvard Medical School, showed that C-reactive protein (CRP), a marker in the blood for systemic inflammation, is associated with a substantially higher risk of AMD. In fact, she and her colleagues found that for those whose CRP was in the upper 25% were 1.65 times more likely to have AMD than those whose CRP was in the lowest 25%. Their conclusion: "Our results suggest that elevated CRP level is an independent risk factor for AMD and may implicate the role of inflammation in the pathogenesis of AMD." [221]

The connection between inflammation and AMD is being reviewed here not just for the sake of completeness, but like everything in this book, it has a link to diet. What we find is that a diet high in refined sugars and flour, that is, a diet replete with processed foods, is a set-up for disturbed gut health, which leads to inflammation in remote areas of the body such as vessels in the heart and in the eye.[222]

PUTTING THIS ALL TOGETHER...

Allen Taylor, PhD, senior research scientist at Tufts University's Laboratory for Nutrition and Vision Research, and his colleagues, in a recent paper entitled "Diminishing Risk for Age-Related Macular Degeneration with Nutrition: A Current View," summarized most of the concepts reviewed so far as follows: "Since photoreceptors do not have their own blood supply, it is crucial for nutrients from the choroidal blood supply to cross Bruch's membrane and enter the RPE and photoreceptors. Adequate nutritional support to the RPE also facilitates efficient turnover of photoreceptors. The combination of inadequate nutrition and the inability to properly degrade and dispose of cellular debris may contribute to the formation of deposits in the RPE-Bruch's membrane region. Basal laminar deposits accumulate between the RPE basement membrane and the RPE plasma membrane. These are thought to precede the formation of drusen, which are established clinical indicators for early AMD. Drusen are often found between the RPE and the choroid and contain a variety of lipids and proteins, including ubiquitin and advanced glycation end products, as well as inflammatory mediators." [223]

CLINICAL ASPECTS OF AMD

From a clinical standpoint, AMD is classified as either the "dry" form, which is really an atrophic type of disease, or the "wet" form, which is a type of exudative or neovascular (new vessel) disease. The dry form almost always precedes the wet form, though wet AMD does rarely present without a known history of the dry form of the disease. Approximately 10 to 15% of all dry AMD cases will eventually progress into wet AMD.

ATROPHIC "DRY" AMD

From a histologic (study of tissue) standpoint, AMD exists when there is atrophy (tissue loss) of both the RPE and the photoreceptors. If there is neovascularization, which is new vessel growth, then the condition becomes wet AMD at that point.

The characteristic clinical findings of dry AMD begin with the deposition of drusen in the macula and disruption of the retinal pigment epithelium (RPE), the latter of which lies just deep to the retina proper.

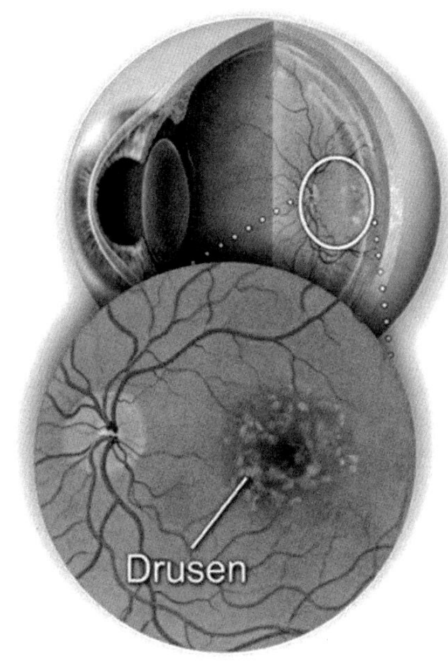

Dry AMD, illustrating characteristic drusen.
Illustration courtesy of Mark Erickson, JirehDesign.com.

As previously reviewed, drusen are small, yellowish deposits that form at the level of Bruch's membrane, which is just deep to the RPE. Drusen are thought to be the end result of certain metabolic insults with resultant inflammation and immune-mediated processes.[224]

"Disruption of the RPE" generally indicates that certain areas of RPE cells undergo cell death, perhaps as a result of injury, infection, or circulatory impairment, with or without an inflammatory response. In any case, loss of RPE cells and the overlying photoreceptors is known as *geographic atrophy (GA)*. When GA becomes marked, vision loss may be severe and this can and does frequently occur without the patient ever developing wet AMD.

Of course, we've already reviewed the fact that there is reduced choroidal blood flow and volume in patients with dry AMD, as well. And when we see complete loss of the choroid, there is loss of the overlying RPE. With loss of the RPE, there is loss of photoreceptors – again, GA. When that occurs, vision is lost. It's just a matter of how many photoreceptors are lost – and where. The more one loses, the worse the vision. In the dreaded scenario that photoreceptors are lost in the central 200 to 400 microns of the macula, that is, in the fovea, there is a rather drastic loss of central vision. This is when the affected person may no longer be able to read or possibly see faces with the affected eye or eyes.

WET AMD

Approximately 10 to 15% of dry AMD patients will have progression to "wet AMD." If wet AMD is left untreated, the natural progression is leakage of fluid, possible bleeding, and subsequent scarring of the macula, which is often referred to as a disciform scar. This natural progression of the disease usually takes place over the first few months or perhaps within the first two to three years. This, of course, leaves the patient with loss of central vision, often down to the "counting fingers" level, meaning that the patient can only count fingers perhaps a few feet away with the affected eye. When one eye develops wet AMD, the risk to the opposite eye of developing wet AMD is about 4 to 12 percent per year.[225]

Next, let's take a look at how wet AMD develops. In wet AMD, typically all the signs of advancing dry AMD already exist. As reviewed previously, the next typical pathologic event is a break in Bruch's membrane, which is then followed by the growth of neovascular (new vessel) tissue arising from the choroid and poking its ugly head up under the retina proper. From there, the neovascular tissues, which are inherently abnormal, tend to leak serous fluid or exudates into the retina. This raises the retina like a microscopic bubble underneath, thereby distorting the retina and, as such, also distorting the vision.

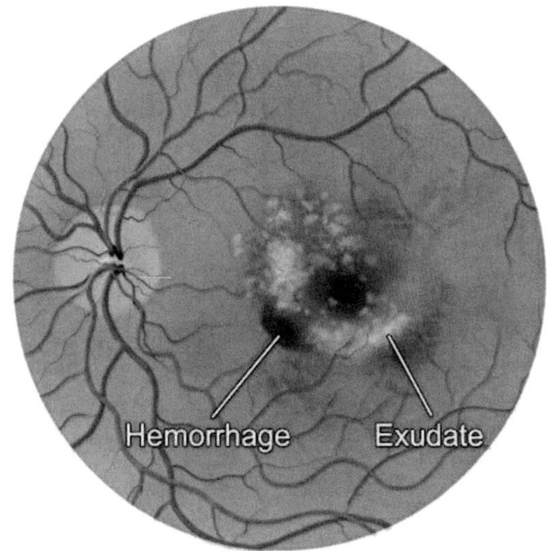

Wet AMD.
Illustration courtesy of Mark Erickson, JirehDesign.com.

Precisely what mechanism is behind the development of wet AMD is not clear, however, it appears that both a break in Bruch's membrane and higher levels of vascular endothelial growth factor (VEGF) are required. Though VEGF is normally secreted by the RPE and other retinal structures, multiple mechanisms have been implicated in the development of neovascularization in the retina, including local hypoxia (low oxygen levels) in the retina, RPE cell death with wound healing responses, and inflammatory processes. In each case, production of VEGF, primarily from the RPE, appears to be the major impetus.[226,227,228,229] Simultaneously, what we see is that in the hypoxic (oxygen starved) retina, there is also reduced secretion of pigment epithelium-derived growth factor (PEDF) by the RPE, and PEDF is a potent anti-angiogenic factor.[230]

The simplified version is this: what happens here is that, in those individuals who develop loss of choriocapillaris circulation due to vascular disease, and perhaps also have thickening of Bruch's membrane, the retina becomes hypoxic – oxygen starved. In this scenario, the pigment epithelial derived growth factor (PEDF), which prevents new vessel growth, diminishes in production, while VEGF, which enhances new vessel growth, may be increased in production or, alternatively, functions unopposed by PEDF. This is obviously a mechanism to attempt to bring greater blood flow to an ischemic (oxygen and perhaps nutrient starved retina), however, the whole situation really goes south when there are concurrent breaks in Bruch's membrane. In this scenario, the new vessels growing in the choriocapillaris can then break through Bruch's membrane and grow under the retina.

TREATMENT OF WET AMD – ANTI-VEGF DRUGS ARE BOTH FRIEND AND FOE

In wet AMD, if the neovascular vessels, known as choroidal neovascularization (CNV), break and bleed into the retina, there is a much greater chance of scarring and severe vision loss. As such, bleeding is a particularly ominous sign. Regardless of whether there is serous fluid, exudate, or bleeding with CNV (wet AMD), today the treatment is generally the injection into the eye of one of the vascular endothelial growth factor (VEGF) inhibitors. These drugs include Avastin, Macugen, Lucentis, and Eylea, and they may require injection as often as once a month if the wet AMD persists.

The VEGF inhibitor drugs have truly made a tremendous advance in the treatment of wet AMD. Patients who once would have lost their central vision due to wet AMD are now maintaining central vision for years, albeit many are required to return for repeated injections on a monthly basis – generally considered a small price to pay for retaining central vision.

However, as great as the anti-VEGF drugs are, they do nothing to prevent the progression of dry AMD and, in fact, they may make dry AMD progress more rapidly. Very briefly, let's look at why.

Vascular endothelial growth factor (VEGF) is exactly what its name calls it. It acts like a local growth factor, or hormone, for endothelium. The RPE secretes VEGF in low concentrations on a continual basis in healthy eyes[231] [232] in order to prevent apoptosis (cell death) of the inner lining (endothelium) of the choriocapillaris and to keep the endothelium intact and highly functioning.[233] Interestingly, VEGF plays a substantial role in the life and integrity of the RPE cells as well,[234] and we've previously reviewed the vast importance of the RPE to the health of the photoreceptors. But, VEGF plays other roles too.

VEGF is expressed both by adult photoreceptor and Müller cells, the latter of which are a type of glial cell that plays a supportive role to the photoreceptors, with numerous metabolic functions important to the function of the photoreceptors.[235],[236]

In a mouse model, after VEGF inhibition for 14 days there was a significant increase in cell death in the inner and outer nuclear layers of the retina. In fact, within one month the neural cell death was severe enough to be associated with reduced thickness of both the inner and outer nuclear layers and a decline in retinal function demonstrated by electroretinogram.[237] This is an indication that photoreceptors and Müller cells may also undergo cell death as a result of VEGF inhibition.

In fact, we now have two more recent studies that show monthly injections of the anti-VEGF drugs are associated with a higher degree of geographic atrophy. In the Comparison of Age-Related Macular Degeneration Treatment Trials (CATT), approximately 20% of patients developed geographic atrophy (GA) within two years of treatment, which generally means a serious decline in vision despite the success in terms of resolution of wet AMD disease.[238] Additionally, patients given ranibizumab (Lucentis) fared worse in this development than did patients given Avastin. Results of the HARBOR Study at Wills Eye Hospital, in Philadelphia, Pennsylvania support the findings that GA is greater in patients given monthly anti-VEGF injections as well.[239]

The bottom line here? **The RPE, choriocapillaris, photoreceptors, and Müller cells are all at risk of atrophy (cell death) with severe and protracted inhibition of VEGF, which most certainly occurs with multiple and repeated anti-VEGF injections for recurrent or persistent wet AMD.** With this knowledge, we should obviously be very cautious with the use of VEGF inhibitors and use them precisely to control wet AMD and only when the benefit appears to clearly outweigh the risk.

DARK ADAPTATION – A MEASURE OF OVERALL NUTRITIONAL STATUS?

A person's ability to adjust from bright light to dim light, known as dark adaptation, may be an excellent marker of the overall nutritional status as it relates to the development of AMD. Let's take a look at why, because I believe this is a critical issue to understand as it relates to AMD.

The human eye can function at the extremes of brightness and darkness. In fact, the brightest and dimmest light signal that the eye can perceive are a factor of roughly one billion apart. However, in any given moment of time, the eye can only sense contrast ratios that are about one thousand orders of magnitude apart. This is because the eye continually adapts its definition of complete darkness, or what is black, and it accomplishes this primarily by altering the sensitivity of the photoreceptors – the rods and cones.

Scotopic sensitivity relates to vision in dim light, which is chiefly based on the function of the rods in the retina. This functionality has been shown to be based on age, however, it is also based on the health of the eye and nutritional status, particularly vitamin A status. The eye takes anywhere from about 30 to nearly 50 minutes to maximally dark adapt, that is, to fully adapt from bright sunlight to complete darkness. Complete dark adaptation takes approximately 30 to 35 minutes in people in their 20's and up to about 50 minutes in the elderly.[240]

Researchers Gregory R. Jackson, PhD, Cynthia Owsley, PhD, and Gerald McGwin Jr, PhD, at the University of Alabama, collectively made ground-breaking research in the field of dark adaptation. They state the following:

> "Scotopic sensitivity loss in older adults is observed in peripheral retinal areas where there is negligible rod loss and is not accentuated in the areas of heightened rod loss (Jackson et al., 1998), suggesting that rod loss cannot account for older adults' sensitivity impairment in the dark. Furthermore, there is little change in the amount of rod photopigment, rhodopsin, throughout adulthood.... An alternative hypothesis to explain older adults' scotopic sensitivity loss is that the visual cycle, the biochemical pathway responsible for rhodopsin regeneration, is perturbed with age... Slowing of the visual cycle results in a prolongation of dark adaptation kinetics." [241]

Let me simplify this a little. The authors are conveying that the loss of dark adaptation is not secondary to the loss of rod photoreceptors in the aging eye, nor is it apparently due to loss of rhodopsin pigment, but rather, the visual cycle itself (conversion of vitamin A from inactive to active forms) is abnormally delayed.

Finally, the tie to AMD: Doctors Owsley, Jackson, and colleagues, in their research, found that patients with early AMD had rod-mediated dark adaptation that was much slower (13 minutes on average) than in age-matched controls without AMD.[242] This was true even for patients with AMD who had no visual loss.

Researchers, Jackson and Owsley, along with researchers Christine A. Curcio, PhD, and Kenneth R. Sloan, PhD, also at the University of Alabama, chapter authors in Penfold & Provis' book, *Macular Degeneration,* wrote the following:

> Dark adaptation is a good candidate for a test of visual function, because dark adaptation relies on retinoid cycle components contained within the same layers where ARM-associated lesions are located… The retinoid cycle provides 11-cis-retinal, a metabolite of vitamin A, to the photoreceptors for photopigment regeneration. Aging and ARM {age-related maculopathy – same as AMD} – related changes may retard dark adaptation by a variety of mechanisms working either independently or in concert to reduce the pool of 11-cis-retinal available to the photoreceptors. Debris in Bruch's membrane may slow the passage of vitamin A from the choroid to the RPE, the RPE may process retinoids less efficiently due to age- or disease-related change… [243]

In a study entitled, "Delayed Rod-Mediated Dark Adaptation Is a Functional Biomarker for Incident Early Age-Related Macular Degeneration," researchers Cynthia Owsley, PhD, and colleagues wrote,

> **We previously showed that the rate of rod-mediated dark adaptation in older adults with normal retinal health or AMD accelerated after a 30-day course of high-dose retinol [vitamin A], whereas cone-mediated dark adaptation was unaffected. These findings support a nutritional barrier/retinoid deficiency hypothesis.** [244]

To review and simplify once again, a 30-day high-dose vitamin A supplementation improved dark adaptation both in normal adults and those with AMD. This suggests that, for one thing, we tend to be vitamin A deficient – most all of us. Otherwise, why would vitamin A supplementation improve dark adaptation? Secondly, the "nutritional barrier" hypothesis refers primarily to the thickening of the Bruch's membrane, which acts as a barrier to transporting nutrients to the photoreceptors.

Dark adaptation is not only an indicator of vitamin A status, but of the general health status of the eye, implicating multiple pathological factors as well as numerous nutritional factors, all of which must simultaneously take place to produce AMD. The point here is that this is a multifactorial problem. A delayed dark adaptation is likely an indicator that numerous conditions typically must exist in order for this condition to occur. Just as authors Jackson, Owsley, Curcio, and Sloan pointed out, there must be multiple mechanisms at play in order for this condition to occur. And obviously, not everyone develops AMD, so what's the difference between those with AMD and their prolonged dark adaptation times and those with healthy eyes and normal dark adaptation times? I will assert that this condition may be due to multiple nutritional deficiencies, combined with the pathological consequences of a diet replete with processed foods, which ultimately may lead to vascular disease at the choroid/choriocapillaris level, thickening and calcification of Bruch's membrane, and dysfunction of the RPE. The end result, of course, is RPE cellular dysfunction and death followed by photoreceptor death.

THE COUP DE GRÂS: DELAYED DARK ADAPTATION PREDICTS AMD

Owsley's group assessed 325 people with dark adaptation at baseline and again three years later, to determine if delayed dark adaptation might predict the development of AMD. Their answer?

> After age adjustment, older adults in normal macular health with abnormal dark adaptation in the tested eye at baseline were approximately 2 times more likely to have AMD in the tested eye by the time of the follow-up visit compared with those who had normal dark adaptation at baseline. They also were approximately 2 times more likely to have AMD in either eye at the follow-up visit.[245]

This indicates one of two things as it relates to those who are destined to develop AMD: This is either a damning indictment of a deficient vitamin A status, or a perturbed pathway to get vitamin A to the RPE and photoreceptors, or both. There are no other conclusions that I can draw from the collective body of this research. I am quite certain these authors agree with that statement. But, one must realize, vitamin A does not act alone. It works in concert with the other fat soluble vitamins, and this too will be reviewed subsequently.

Make note: These apparent nutritional deficiencies, pathological processes, and ultimately, the ramifications of consuming a diet replete with the 'displacing foods of modern commerce,' have not and will not, be solved by consuming vitamins or multivitamins in pill-form. This has been proven repeatedly, for decades, and I will also address this in further detail in coming chapters. The problem can only be addressed with real, whole, unprocessed foods.

CHAPTER SUMMARY

AMD is the leading cause of blindness and irreversible vision loss in developed nations. **It is defined at the tissue level by loss of RPE and photoreceptors (rods and cones).** Clinically, it is diagnosed by the presence of drusen, pigmentary disturbances, and geographic atrophy (GA) in the dry form of the disease. GA is indicative of loss of both RPE and photoreceptors. In the wet form of AMD, choroidal neovascularization (CNV) is indicated by the presence of subretinal fluid, exudate, or hemorrhage.

We've reviewed the fact that the photoreceptors (rods and cones) have the highest metabolic activity of any cells in the body. The retinal pigment epithelium (RPE) is a workhorse as well, perhaps second only to the photoreceptors themselves in terms of metabolic activity. In fact, the RPE must work side-by-side with the photoreceptors at a metabolic pace that rivals or exceeds that of any cells in the body, in order to process the incredibly complex task of vision. The photoreceptors, RPE, and other associated retinal cells are highly dependent on an excellent blood supply, oxygen, and nutrients in the form of vitamins, minerals, carotenoids, lutein, zeaxanthin, DHA, glucose, amino acids, fatty acids, cholesterol, etc (all to be reviewed subsequently).

The choriocapillaris is the vascular bed that supplies blood, enriched with oxygen and nutrients, to the RPE, photoreceptors, and outer retina. **There is a substantially reduced blood volume and blood flow in the choriocapillaris in patients with AMD versus those without the disease.** I will submit that the cause of the vascular occlusive disease in AMD is virtually identical to that which occurs in coronary artery disease (heart disease, heart attacks, and related disease of the heart, such as congestive heart failure). Interestingly, just as I wrapped up this chapter, this week a study was published in the British Journal of Ophthalmology, finding a strong association between coronary artery disease (CAD) and early AMD.[246] I will review this in more detail subsequently as well and I will precisely review the diets and mechanisms behind both conditions, of course, and exactly what to do about it.

Bruch's membrane tends to thicken with age secondary to basal laminar deposit, which is much more severe in patients with both dry and wet AMD than those without. Secondarily, Bruch's membrane tends to calcify with advancing age, and those with wet AMD show a far greater degree of calcification as well as breaks in Bruch's membrane, as compared to those without AMD or those with dry AMD. Thickening of Bruch's membrane may cause diminished transfer and diffusion of nutrients and waste products across the membrane, from the RPE to the choriocapillaris and back. I have proposed that this may specifically be related to multiple fat soluble vitamin deficiencies, and that vitamin K2 deficiency may play a role in this regard.

Research has definitively shown that early AMD is associated with prolonged dark adaptation times. This is strongly indicative of dysfunction of the vitamin A visual cycle, if not a frank vitamin A deficiency. This may also indicate that Bruch's membrane thickening and disease of the choriocapillaris/choroid prevents vitamin A from being properly transported to the RPE and photoreceptors. In short, we might assert that all of this is ultimately secondary to chronic multiple fat-soluble vitamin deficiencies, including vitamins A, D, and K2, and the multiple sequelae that would ensue, including thickening of Bruch's membrane, reduction of the choriocapillaris, deterioration and dysfunction of the RPE, and ultimately, cell death of the RPE and photoreceptors.

Individuals with delayed dark adaptation times were shown to be twice as likely to develop AMD within a three-year period. We can only imagine what this number might be if the study were 10 or 20 years long! But, as reviewed, this is strong evidence of either a frank vitamin A deficiency or a perturbed mechanism to get vitamin A, and perhaps its many cofactors, to the RPE and photoreceptors.

The photoreceptors and their supportive cells, primarily the retinal pigment epithelium (RPE), are the metabolic top-fuel dragsters of the entire human body. **Wouldn't it make sense that the nutritional requirements of the most metabolically active cells in the body would also be the ones that require an abundance of key nutrients, such as natural vitamins, minerals, carotenoids, phytonutrients, DHA, glucose, amino acids, fatty acids, etc., from an abundance of natural and varied whole foods?** Wouldn't that also suggest, that these cells may be the ones most sensitive to minor perturbations of the nutrient profile? What would happen to a top-fuel dragster if you filled the tank with regular gasoline? Should you expect anything different from the most metabolically active cells in your entire body, if they are given substantially inferior nutrients – over a lifetime?

Part II

So the Villain is Modern Food?

7 WESTON A. PRICE – UNEQUIVOCALLY, THE GREATEST NUTRITION RESEARCHER IN HISTORY

"Life in all its fullness is Mother Nature obeyed."
~ Weston A. Price, DDS ~

Weston A. Price, DDS (1870 – 1948), was a scientist, researcher, and a dentist from Cleveland, Ohio who, in the opinion of many nutrition researchers, conducted the single most important body of nutrition research that has ever been produced. It is my opinion that Dr. Price's research is, without question, more important than virtually all other nutrition research combined. The fundamentals of his findings provide a framework and template for understanding nutrition that is beyond compare. If you're not familiar with Dr. Price and his research, in this chapter I will attempt to provide a thumbnail sketch of his studies from which one can draw vast conclusions regarding the numerous "diseases of Western civilization."

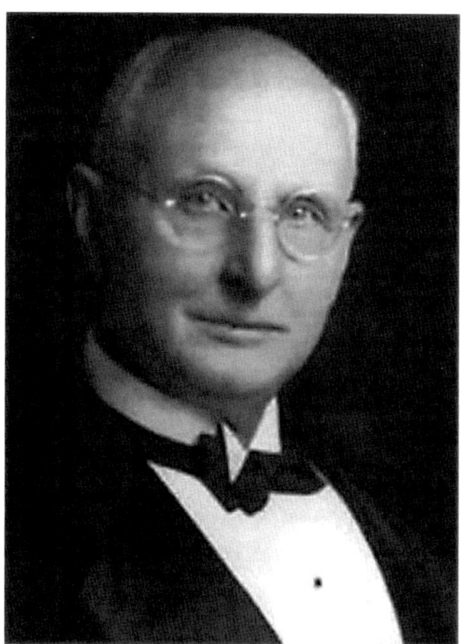

Weston A. Price

Dr. Price was born in Newburgh, Ontario, Canada, in 1870. He graduated from the University of Michigan College of Dentistry in 1893 and began his practice initially in Grand Forks, North Dakota. Later that year, he

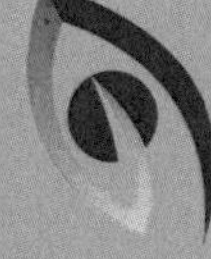

moved and began practice in Cleveland, Ohio. By the end of that century, Price noted minimal decay of teeth in his own patients, yet he had already begun to suspect nutrition as a critical element in the development of tooth decay.

By the early 20th century, Price had become a prolific researcher; he founded the National Dental Association (NDA) in 1914 and held the position of chairman for the NDA from 1914 through 1928. During this time, he conducted numerous studies in his field, the results having been published in the peer-reviewed journals of his day.

By the early part of the 20th century, Price had become disturbed by an ever-increasing incidence of children with crowded, misaligned (crooked) teeth, which seemed to go hand-in-hand with dental caries (cavities), narrowed faces and dental arches (the crescent arrangements of teeth), overbites, pinched nostrils, and other facial deformities. Perhaps even more alarming, Price found that the affected children were more likely to suffer from frequent infections, allergies, asthma, poor vision (refractive errors), behavioral problems, and in the worst scenarios, even reduced intelligence. In adults, he was beginning to see the development of rampant tooth decay, which was frequently accompanied by systemic diseases, including arthritis, osteoporosis, diabetes, irritable bowel, chronic fatigue, and poor overall health. The teeth, he believed, represented a mirror to the health of the body.[247] In fact, Dr. Price had made the observation that burgeoning degenerative disease was prevalent in this country by the end of the 1920's.

Dr. Price believed that the health of the American people was progressively worsening, for reasons that were unclear. He did not believe that such physical degeneration was consistent with God's plan for His people. Furthermore, in his dental practice, patients were asking him what constituted a "healthy diet" – a question to which he did not have an answer.

While seeing rather rampant tooth decay in his practice in Cleveland, Price was simultaneously intrigued when he witnessed the photographs of members from "primitive tribes" from all around the globe who generally appeared to have perfectly straight and beautiful teeth, all while apparently living in primitive conditions and without dentists. In fact, according to Sally Fallon Morell, founder of the Weston A Price Foundation, "One of the most common observations that Westerners had when they discovered these isolated people – was what beautiful teeth they had. Even the first settlers to America described in their diaries – the native Americans as having teeth - broad, and straight, and white – as piano keys. And this intrigued Dr. Price very much because this is not what he was seeing in his practice." [248]

"A comprehensive study of modern degeneration will require the use of controls," Dr. Price wrote in his 1939 text. But, given the dramatic changes that had already occurred with the American people of his day, he explained, "It became necessary to look elsewhere in Nature's great biological laboratory, which has been in operation through the history of life."[249] And thus began his worldwide study.

Price set out on a mission to discover the answers to two fundamental questions:

1) Did these isolated peoples living in primitive conditions not suffer from dental deformities, cavities, and dental disease and, if not, did they also enjoy excellent general health?
2) What were the diets that would lead to such physical perfection?

In short, Dr. Price sought to determine "standards of excellence," a term that describes the general health and physical well-being of the human body under Nature's perfect guidance. These questions and goals would take Dr. Price on a mission that would require an entire decade of his life to complete – from approximately 1929 to 1939. During that time, Price would travel to 14 different countries, on 5 different continents, and he would personally examine tens of thousands of people, including natives from hundreds of different tribes and cultures.

Price specifically sought out populations that were isolated from civilization – or at least isolated from the influencing effects of foods outside of each culture's traditions. He also sought out similar populations, often nearby, that had begun to regularly consume Westernized foods. This was a genius decision that would make his discoveries immeasurably unique and robust, because one could then compare the health implications provided by ancient dietary wisdom against those provided by modernized cuisine – no matter what population was being analyzed. In other words, he was in search of a universal effect on dental and even general health, which was independent of confounding factors, such as race, geographic locale, genetics, etc. This was possible because, in many of these studies, Dr. Price would observe a population in a given geographic locale that was surviving on traditional foods, whereas an otherwise entirely similar population living in a nearby town or village could be studied that had incorporated many of the Westernized foods into their diets. The timing of Price's study would also make this investigation one that could never again be truly replicated, since so few populations now exist that are consuming their native traditional diets without the influence of modernized, processed foods.

Price and his wife, Florence, who assisted him in these endeavors, would travel by steamship, prop planes, automobiles, canoes, and sometimes on foot for great distances, to search out these isolated populations and tribes that were, in some cases, even nomadic in character. When they arrived at the various towns, villages, and nomadic tribe tenements where they hoped to make observations, Dr. Price would carefully explain his research to the elders of the population, often via translators. When and if they agreed, which was virtually always, he would carefully examine the teeth of every individual, making precise and systematic notations, often documenting his findings with thousands of photographs. But his observations didn't end with examination of their teeth. He simultaneously made many astute observations regarding the general health of these peoples and, when occasionally available, had enlightening discussions with their health-care providers as well.

In the next few pages, I'll briefly review the findings of just a few of the populations that Dr. Price studied and provide just a very small sampling from his book, *Nutrition and Physical Degeneration,* published in 1939. This book is a treatise and anthology of nutrition, greater than 500 pages in length, and absolutely chock-full of mind-boggling discoveries and detail.[250]

PEOPLE OF THE LOETSCHENTAL VALLEY, SWITZERLAND

Dr. Price's first population to study was the people of the Loetschental Valley, in Switzerland. This was a population of about 2,000 people, isolated from civilization for nearly 1200 years. Without even a single road with which one could reach them, the long final path to their village could be traversed only on foot. In this high Alpine valley, Dr. Price found both children and adults of extraordinary physical condition, with wide faces and dental arches, in which every single individual naturally had nearly perfectly straight and beautiful teeth. In great contrast to his practice in Cleveland, where tooth decay and misaligned teeth were rampant, Dr. Price had to look in three mouths to find evidence for one cavity, typically. In a study of the teeth of the children examined in this valley, only 0.3 percent showed any current or previous evidence for a cavity. These people were also found to be in extraordinary health, with virtually no signs of disease. Whereas tuberculosis was considered to be the greatest affliction of Switzerland at the time, as it was then in much of the world, government officials confirmed there had never been a case found in the Loetschental Valley. These people had neither physician nor dentist, because there was virtually no need for either.

Curious to know what these completely isolated people in this nearly mile-high valley in the Swiss Alps were consuming for food? The primary staple for numerous meals was a slice of whole rye bread and a thick slice of summer-made cheese, which was typically about as thick as the slice of bread. With that, they drank the fresh whole raw milk of either goats or cows – unpasteurized, of course. In fact, fresh raw milk was their chief source of calories. From the milk, they also made cream and butter. They only had meat to eat about once a week, and that was typically veal, because the climate wouldn't allow them to raise many cattle for slaughter. The rye bread was painstakingly produced – beginning with the whole grain, which was originally thrashed by hand, but eventually, thrashed by water-driven turbines to create the flour. The dense, rye whole grain bread was then raised in sourdough fashion, without yeast, and this took up to several days to complete and about another two weeks to completely cure. This type of fermentation process, used by many cultures practicing traditional culinary methods, tremendously increases the vitamin and mineral availability of the grain. These Swiss villagers had few vegetables due to a very long winter, however, they were able to produce a few vegetables during their short summer.

As in every population in supreme health that Dr. Price ultimately discovered, the Swiss villagers of the Loetschental Valley had a sacred food. In this case, that particular food was the butter made from cows that had grazed on the rapidly-growing green grass of springtime and early summer. This was a deep-orange colored butter, which, as we will see, was a tremendous source of fat-soluble vitamins (A, D, and K) – particularly, vitamins A and K2.

Dr. Price took food samples from most every culture and analyzed those samples in his lab in Ohio. In the case of the people of the Loetschental Valley, he found that the typical and average amount of fat-soluble vitamins (A, D, and K – in this case), as well as the average mineral intake of calcium and phosphorus, would far exceed that of the typical American child.[251]

In great contrast to the people of the Loetschental Valley, modernized Swiss people, who lived virtually anywhere where roads were to be found, had already begun to develop widespread tooth decay, facial and dental arch deformities (with crooked teeth), and extreme susceptibility to disease. **Wherever roads were developed, modern stores quickly followed that sold Westernized foods – white flour and other refined cereal grains, sugar, vegetable oils, sweets, canned goods, jams, jellies, pastries, sweetened fruits, and chocolate. These types of foods were what Dr. Price referred to as the "'displacing foods of modern commerce',"** which is the term that I used in Chapter One of this book and, of course, from where I borrowed the term. Along with consumption of the displacing foods, came a greatly reduced consumption of raw milk products (in this particular population).

GAELIC PEOPLE OF THE OUTER HEBRIDES ISLANDS – SCOTLAND

Dr. Price studied the people in the islands of the Outer Hebrides off the northwest coast of Scotland. These Gaelic people lived in cottages that were heated with fireplaces that often had no chimneys, which left the smoke to pour into their homes and out through the thatched roofs. This eventually made the roof black, giving rise to the term "black houses," as their homes were often called. Like the Swiss villagers of the Loetschental Valley, these Gaelic people were tremendously healthy, with straight teeth, stalwart physiques, and were unquestionably of noble character.

The breathing of smoke in these "black houses," often day and night when the weather was cold, was not associated with development of tuberculosis, however. Incredibly, Dr. Price found that their tremendously healthy diet, with plenty of fat-soluble vitamins and minerals, completely protected them against not only tuberculosis, but numerous other afflictions as well.

The soil on the Isle of Lewis in the Outer Hebrides is very rocky and not conducive to vegetation. Hence, very few vegetables could ever be grown. Fruit was practically unheard of. Likewise, lack of grass meant that almost no livestock could be raised and, therefore, they had virtually no dairy products. However, they could raise oats on the island and a small crop of barley. As such, these people survived primarily on oat products, a meager amount of vegetables, but a tremendous variety of seafood, including fish, lobsters, crabs, oysters, and clams. Unlike us, however, these Gaelic people ate the entire fish – including the heads, the organs, and the fish liver. The sacred food of these people was baked cod's head stuffed with oats and chopped cod's liver! This was a typical breakfast food for their growing children. As will be reviewed in detail later, the organs of the fish and the associated oils are excellent sources of the fat-soluble vitamins A, D, and K2.

The smoke laden thatch from their rooftops was removed once a year and placed in their fields to provide fertilizer. Dr. Price tested the island thatch against commercial fertilizers and found that only the island thatch could produce mature crops of oats. These people knew exactly what they were doing with their fertilizer plan – and it worked exceedingly well to produce mature and nutritious oats.

On the nearby Isle of Lewis, Dr. Price found that only 1.3 out of every 100 teeth of the children had ever been attacked by dental caries (cavities) and these people also had wide dental arches with straight teeth and virtually no need for dentists.

Also on the Isle of Lewis, but in great contrast, were the people of the seaport town of Stornoway. Here, there were plenty of options for the 'displacing foods of modern commerce', including white bread, angel food cake, many other white flour products, canned marmalades, canned vegetables, sweetened fruit juice, jams, and confections of every sort.

Dr. Price found a tremendous degree of tooth decay in Stornoway. He assessed 100 people there between the ages of approximately twenty and forty years of age, and found that 25 of them already were wearing artificial teeth, and that approximately that many more would have benefitted from them had they been able to afford them. He provided a photo of two brothers, side-by-side, both raised together consuming the foods of their traditions. The young man who continued to consume the traditional foods of oats and seafood remained in extraordinary health, with excellent teeth. His brother, who had been consuming the modernized foods, including white bread, jam, sweetened coffee, and sweet chocolates, had extensive tooth decay and was missing a number of teeth, including two of his upper front teeth. The boy's father lamented his concerns for this son, as he had a great deal of trouble in arising to go to work, due to his fatigue.

INDIAN AND ESKIMO POPULATIONS IN CANADA AND ALASKA

Dr. Price studied some 39 Indian and Eskimo populations located in Canada and Alaska. In the natives consuming their traditional diets, he found supremely healthy people with almost no evidence of tooth decay. The Eskimos ate a densely nutritious diet, though they had few food choices. They consumed mainly fresh fish, caribou, the organs of large sea animals, kelp, some berries, and seal oil. According to Sally Fallon Morell, when Dr. Price spoke to a doctor who lived among the Eskimos for 30 years, "He learned that there had never been observed by this doctor a case of cancer, heart disease, tuberculosis, or any condition requiring an operation among those who ate their ancestral foods. Among the Eskimos who were eating the 'displacing foods of modern commerce', he found all of the diseases of the Western world." [252]

In general, the "coming of the white man" and the "white man's food" meant a predictable and fateful plight of deterioration in physical health and a multitude of diseases.

Bethel is a Canadian settlement on the Kuskokwim River where a number of Eskimos were to be found. Some lived on native foods and some were consuming the displacing foods. Dr. Price found twenty-seven Eskimos living on natural and native foods and, of their 796 teeth examined, only one tooth was found to have caries. This was a rate of 0.1 percent. In contrast, he examined 40 individuals who had been living on modernized foods that had been shipped in by government supply boats. In this group, of some 1,094 teeth, 252, or 21.1 percent, had already been attacked by decay. This is the situation that will be found, over and over – and over again – in Dr. Price's studies.

The Eskimos would wear their teeth down tremendously by utilizing their teeth constantly in the process of making clothes and tanning leather. In any individual consuming a typical Western modernized diet, this would have frequently exposed the pulp of the teeth (with decay and abscess), but in these healthy Eskimos consuming their traditional diets, the teeth still had secondary dentin, which kept the teeth from decay.

Dr. Price also noted that he virtually never heard an Eskimo infant or child cry, except when they were either hungry or frightened. This was a theme that he would also find to be common among numerous populations who were feeding their young the healthy, native diets that were traditional. These infants and children were alert, happy, and rarely cried.

In the adult population who began to consume significant quantities of the 'displacing foods of modern commerce', there was rampant tooth decay, rotting teeth, loss of teeth, abscesses, and so much pain that the affected Eskimos often became suicidal – citing the pain and agony of dental disease as the only reason for their circumstance. In most of the areas a dentist was not available.

In the very first generation of children born to families who had begun to consume the displacing foods, there was narrowing of the dental arch and mid-face, with consequently misaligned teeth, crowding of teeth, narrowing of the nostrils and over time, dental caries.

The majority of Eskimos living in their traditional culture and consuming traditional foods chose to reside near deep waters, where Dr. Price found that they were experts at spearing salmon from their kayaks. Fish was common in their diet. They would also spear seals, from which they would harvest "seal oil." The seal oil is the fat of the animal and is densely nutritious. They often dried their salmon, and then would break off pieces of it, dipping it in the seal oil as they ate it. Dr. Price took samples of the seal oil back to his lab and found that it was one of the richest sources of vitamin A that he had ever analyzed.

The Eskimos also saved all of the salmon eggs (roe) and they typically spread them out to allow them to dry, for later consumption. Along with the seal oil, the salmon eggs would likely have been considered their other sacred food. Dr. Price found that fish eggs were considered a sacred food for a number of cultures – as they are, once again, densely nutritious, containing multiple vitamins, minerals, omega-3 fatty acids, and many of the ingredients necessary to begin life, all in significant proportions.

THE MASAI TRIBE OF KENYA AND TANZANIA - AFRICA

Dr. Price studied the Masai people of Eastern Africa. They are a semi-nomadic and Nilotic people that primarily inhabit southern Kenya and northern Tanzania. Price described the Nilotic tribes, which are those from the Nile Valley, as having been "chiefly herders of cattle and goats" that "have lived primarily on dairy products, including milk, and blood, with some meat, and with a varying percentage of vegetable foods." [253] He wrote that they were "characterized by superb physical development, great bravery and a mental acumen that made it possible for them to dominate because of their superior intelligence." He also described them as "tall and strong," and in reference to these Nilotic tribes, stated, "It is of great significance that we studied six tribes in which there appeared to be not a single tooth attacked by dental caries nor a single malformed dental arch. Several other tribes were found with nearly complete immunity to dental caries. In thirteen tribes we did not meet a single individual with irregular teeth." Contrast that with what he says next: "Where the members of these same tribes had adopted modern civilization many cases of tooth decay were found. In the next generation following the adoption of the European dietaries dental arch deformities frequently developed." [254]

"Where the members of African tribes had attached themselves to coffee plantations," Price wrote, "and were provided with the imported foods of white flour, sugar, polished rice and canned goods, tooth decay became rampant." [255]

Dr. Price studied 88 Masai tribe members and examined some 2,516 teeth in these individuals. Of all of these, only four members had dental caries with a total of 10 caries (cavities), which translates to only 0.4% of their teeth having ever been attacked by tooth decay.[256] In Kenya, a physician by the name of Dr. Anderson, who was in charge of a government run hospital there, advised Dr. Price that he had "observed that they did not suffer from appendicitis, gall bladder trouble, cystitis {urinary bladder infection}, and duodenal ulcer. Malignancy was also very rare among the primitives." [257]

Part II So the Villain is Modern Food?

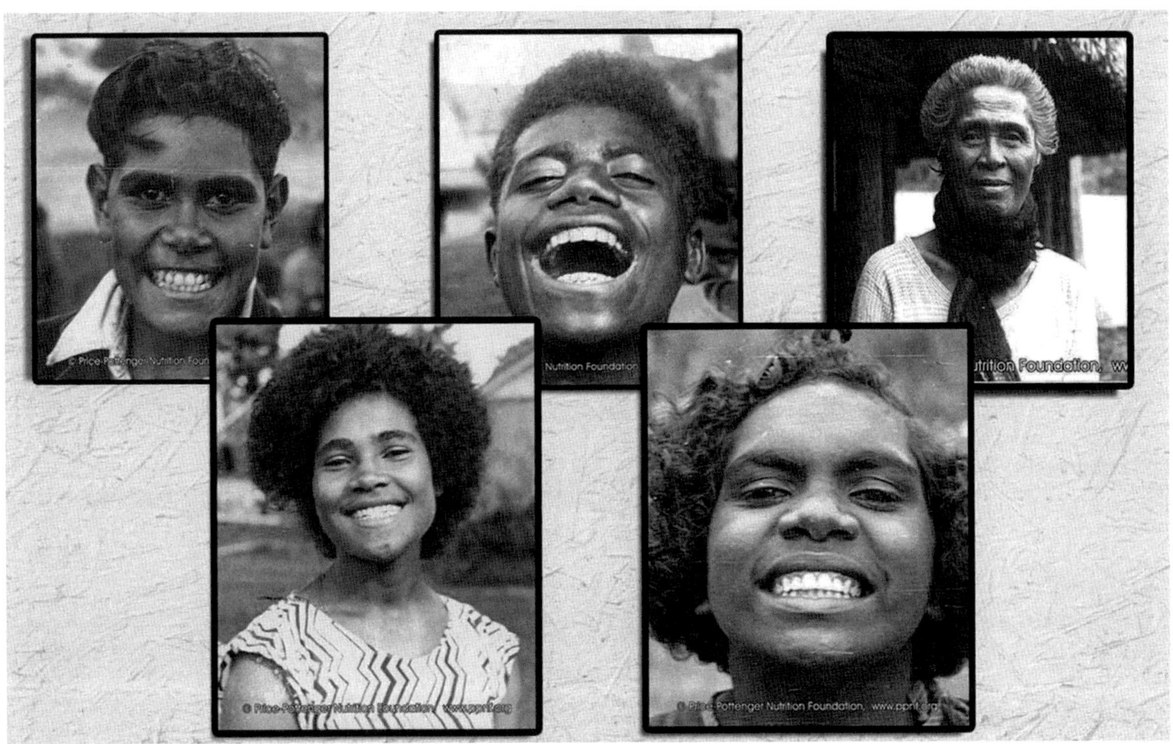

Images of Tribal Members In Various Populations That Continued Their Ancestral Diets.

NUMEROUS OTHER POPULATIONS STUDIED

Dr. Price would study numerous additional populations, including North American Indians, Polynesians and Melanesians in the South Pacific Islands, various other African tribes, the Australian Aborigines, the New Zealand Maori, ancient civilizations of Peru, and Peruvian Indians. In every case, what he found, time and time again, were people in superb health – so long as they adhered to the primitive diets of their ancestors – and rapidly failing health, infectious disease, and degenerative diseases, all combined with tooth decay, in those who opted for the modernized foods.

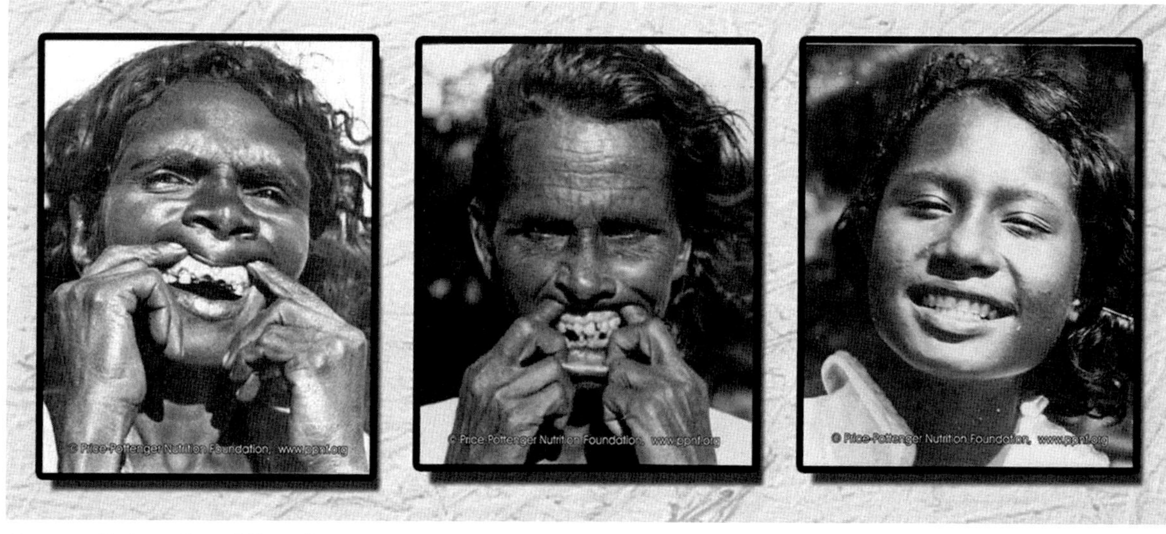

Images (left and middle) of primitive Australian Aborigines who had been placed on reservations and fed white man's foods of commerce. The Aboriginal woman on the far right continued her primitive diet.

In the majority of populations, Dr. Price found that for those who adhered to their traditional diets, less than one percent of their teeth had ever been affected by caries. However, in those who consumed significant proportions of the displacing foods, as many as 20 to 40 percent or more of the teeth were affected by caries.[258]

KEEN EYESIGHT IN NATIVES ADHERING TO TRADITIONAL DIETS

Sally Fallon Morell, who is Founder and President of the Weston A. Price Foundation, author of the brilliant book (with combined cookbook), *Nourishing Traditions,* and not to mention also a brilliant orator, has given numerous presentations regarding Dr Price's work and the incalculable benefits of following a traditional diet contrasted against the colossally destructive effects of a Westernized, processed food-laden diet. In her presentation, "Nourishing Traditional Diets – The Key to Vibrant Health," which is available on YouTube, Sally states, "The native people had very keen eyesight and hearing. One of the first things that goes when we start eating processed foods is that keen eyesight and hearing – and suddenly, everyone needs corrective lenses." [259]

Sally's statement is fully backed by the findings of Dr. Price as well as by recent research. In fact, researchers Loren Cordain, PhD, S. Boyd Eaton, MD, Jennie Brand Miller, PhD, Staffan Lindeberg, MD, PhD, and Clark Jensen, OD showed that consumption of a Westernized, hormone-altering diet, reliably produces "juvenile-onset myopia" (nearsightedness). They also reference the fact that "a number of human studies have shown that myopes {the nearsighted} have more dental caries than non-myopes." [260]

In the March 10, 2016 issue of *Ocular Surgery News,* the cover story headline reads "Concern for myopia progression increases with alarming rise in global prevalence." [261] The article, written by associate editor Kristie L. Kahl, states, "Globally, high myopia is ranked second behind cataracts as the leading cause of visual impairment, with 10% of all myopes having 6 D of refractive error or more, according to a review published by Liu and colleagues. Myopia has nearly doubled in the last 30 years in the U.S., going from a 25% prevalence rate in 12 to 54-year olds in 1971 – 1972 to a 42% prevalence rate in 1999 – 2004. In East Asia, nearly 50% of urban populations are myopic, while its prevalence in university student populations is approximately 90%." [262]

Curiously, the prevalence of obesity in U.S. adults was about 13% in 1960 and remained at that level until about 1980. Obesity then climbed to 23% by 1988, 30.5% by 1999, 34.3% by 2005, and a dramatic 35.7% by 2011.[263] Obesity more than doubled in the U.S. between 1980 and 1999 – in the span of just 19 years – and precisely during the same era that myopia nearly doubled. Besides obesity (BMI greater than 30), an additional 34% of Americans were considered overweight (BMI of 25 – 30) by 2008. The rate of obesity in children ages 6 to 19 was under 5% in 1963, rising to about 10% by 1988, and was at 17% by 2008.[264] And along with the obesity and overweight came skyrocketing rates of metabolic syndrome,heart disease, diabetes, hypertension, and as we'll review in detail later, a worldwide epidemic of AMD. Do you suppose these are all mere coincidences? Do you suppose our diet might stake a claim in all of these?

The *Ocular Surgery News* article also raises the more concerning issue – that myopia is not just about greater need for glasses. "Higher degrees of myopia," Kahl continues, "are associated with an increased rate of glaucoma, retinal detachment, macular choroidal degeneration, myopic choroidal neovascularization and myopic retinoschisis, as well as early onset cataract, amblyopia and strabismus." [265]

Kahl also quotes Susan Vitale, PhD, MHS, of the National Institutes of Health, who said, "I think that [researchers] are learning more and more all the time about the different mechanisms of myopia, but they still don't completely understand what the cause is. They particularly don't understand the cause of this increased prevalence seen over the last 10 to 20 years in a lot of different countries." [266] And, of course, Vitale's statement is correct. Most researchers don't know the cause. However, Loren Cordain's group obviously hit the nail on the head – and over the next four chapters – you will clearly understand exactly what it is about a processed food-laden diet that holds the underpinnings for not only myopia, but AMD as well.

THE TEETH TELL THE TALE!	
STRAIGHT TEETH	**CROOKED, CROWDED TEETH**
Plenty of room in head for pituitar, pineal, hypothalamus	Compromised space for master glands in the head
Good skeletal development, good muscles	Poor development, poor posture, easily injured
KEEN EYESIGHT AND HEARING	**POOR EYESIGHT AND HEARING**
Optimal function of all organs	Compromised function of all organs
Optimistic outlook, learns easily	Depression, behavior problems, learning problems
Round pelvic opening, easy childbirth	Oval pelvis opening, difficult childbirth

Table courtesy of Sally Fallon Morell, Weston A. Price Foundation.

Returning our attention to macular degeneration, this is obviously much more concerning than myopia, because it is much more threatening to vision and is also affecting the masses. Interestingly, Dr. Price made no mention of vision loss in any of the people of the primitive tribes that he studied. He did, however, confirm that many had vision far better than the white man. For example, he wrote,

> "I have been impressed many times in my studies with the superior physical development and acuteness of the senses of the primitive races. This is strikingly illustrated in the visual acuity of the Maori of New Zealand, the Aborigines of Australia and some African tribes." He continued, "I was advised that the Australian Aborigine could see a mile away animals that the white man could not see." [267]

Price also referenced the fact that archeologists discovered a prehistoric cave wall painting of the Pleiades star group, known as "Severn Sisters." The ancient artist had painted ten stars in the constellation, however, current day astronomers can only see six stars in the constellation with the naked eye, requiring a telescope to see the other four. Without a doubt, our pre-historic ancestors had amazingly acute eyesight, quite similar to modern day natives who consume the traditional foods of their culture.[268]

Price referenced the fact that modern-day Maori of New Zealand could see satellites of Jupiter, which could only be visualized by the white man with the aid of a telescope. The confirmation that their vision was this acute came when they could reliably notify the viewer through the telescope as to when an eclipse of one of the stars would occur.[269]

DR. PRICE ON VITAMIN A IN THE RETINA AND VITAMIN A IN EYE DEVELOPMENT

Price wrote, "Now modern science knows that one of the richest sources of vitamin A in the entire animal body is that of the tissues back of the eyes including the retina of the eye." He continues, "In Chapter 18 I refer to the work of Wald on studies of vitamin A tissues. He states that extracts of eye tissue (retina, pigment, epithelium, and choroid) show the characteristic vitamin A absorption band and that they are potent in curing vitamin A deficient rats. He shows also that the concentration of vitamin A is constant for different mammals."[270] Dr. Price even referenced the fact that many natives of the island countries consumed the eyes of fish, which were shown to be a rich source of vitamin A.

Vitamin A is not only critical to the normal development of the eye, but to vision itself, as we've reviewed. Vitamin A was once referred to as the "xerophthalmic vitamin," which literally translates, "dry eye vitamin." We seemed to have forgotten this connection.

Finally, Dr. Price referenced the work of Fred Hale and his studies with vitamin A deprivation and re-introduction, in pigs:

> One of the most important contributions in this field has been made by Professor Fred Hale, of the Texas Agricultural Experiment Station, at College Station, Texas. He has shown that many physical

deformities are readily produced by curtailing the amount of vitamin A in the ration of pigs. He produced 59 pigs that were born blind, every pig in each of six litters – where the mothers were deprived of vitamin A for several months before mating and for thirty days thereafter. In pigs, the eyeballs are formed in the first thirty days. He found, as have several others, that depriving pigs of vitamin A for a sufficient period produced severe nerve involvements including paralysis and spasms, so that the animals could not rise to their feet. He reported that one of these vitamin A deficient pigs that had previously farrowed a litter of ten pigs, all born without eyeballs, was given a single dose of cod liver oil two weeks before mating. She farrowed fourteen pigs which showed various combinations of eye defects, some had no eyes, some had one eye, and some had one large eye and one small eye, but all were blind.[271]

In this passage, it is clear that the single dose of cod liver oil was beneficial to a degree, but after months of vitamin A deprivation, just one dose was not enough to produce fully anatomically correct and functional eyes. Dr. Price continued,

> One of the very important results of Professor Hale's investigations has been the production of pigs with normal eyes, born to parents both of whom had no eyeballs due to lack of vitamin A in their mother's diet. The problem clearly was not heredity. Two litters, one containing nine pigs and the other eight, which were born to mothers that had been deprived of vitamin A before mating and for thirty days thereafter, produced the following lesions: All had complete absence of eyeballs; some lacked development of the opening of the external ear; others had cleft palate, harelip, displaced kidneys, displaced ovaries, or displaced testes.[272]

Dr. Price goes on to review anecdotal reports from farms in Texas, where in one case, pigs were born blind to a mother sow when there was no green grass available for consumption for some 14 months during the years 1934 to 1935 due to drought conditions. In a similar situation, in 1935, pigs borne blind due to deficiency of vitamin A in the mother, subsequently mated after being fed foods with significant vitamin A. All of their offspring were not only normal, but healthy and with normally sighted eyes.[273] If this had been considered a form of hereditary congenital blindness, then how would the blind pigs produce normally sighted offspring?

DR. PRICE ON VEGANISM

For those of you not aware, vegans are those who eat only from plant foods, i.e., they avoid any foods from animal sources, including eggs and dairy. So called 'lacto-ovo vegetarians,' consume eggs and dairy, but no other animal products. Dr. Price was disappointed that he did not find a supremely healthy culture existing exclusively on plant sources for food. At the conclusion of his studies, he lamented,

> "As yet I have not found a single group of primitive racial stock which was building and maintaining excellent bodies by living entirely on plant foods. I have found in many parts of the world most devout representatives of modern ethical systems advocating the restriction of foods to the vegetable products. In every instance where the groups involved had been long under this teaching, I found evidence of degeneration in the form of dental caries, and in the new generation in the form of abnormal dental arches to an extent very much higher than in the primitive groups who were not under this influence." [274]

DISEASES ASSOCIATED WITH THE "NUTRITION OF COMMERCE"

Dr. Price consistently found that people living on their traditional diets not only had excellent dental health, as well as straight and aligned teeth, most of them had never heard of or seen a toothbrush. Furthermore, they were supremely healthy, with "stalwart physiques," absence of disease, great immunity to infection, and of "noble character." In one passage, Price described this as follows:

> Associated with a fine physical condition the isolated primitive groups have a high level of immunity to many of our modern degenerative processes, including tuberculosis, arthritis, heart disease, and affections of the internal organs."[275]

Back home in America, Price also confirmed that, for those suffering tooth decay, not only were the diets insufficient in phosphorus, but he stated, "Fat-soluble vitamins have been deficient in practically every case of active tooth decay." Yet, he showed that tooth decay could be halted and even reversed by the addition of these vitamins and, of course, through natural foods. Price wrote, "The program that I have found most efficient has been one which includes the use of small quantities of very high-vitamin butter mixed in equal parts with a very high vitamin cod liver oil." These exact food sources (these are whole *foods* and not supplements) are commercially available and I will review in Chapter 21. "High-vitamin butter is simply that which comes from cows grazing on rapidly growing green grass and "high-vitamin cod liver oil" is a whole food that comes from the soaking of cod liver in brine (salt solution), ultimately skimming off the oil that accumulates at the top, which is fantastically abundant in the fat soluble vitamins.

FAT-SOLUBLE VITAMINS, WATER-SOLUBLE VITAMINS, AND MINERALS IN TRADITIONAL DIETS

The single most important element of Dr. Price's studies was his analysis of the vitamins and minerals in native diets as compared to the typical American diet of his day. Price obtained samples of foods from every tribe and culture that he studied and he very systematically sent the foods back to U.S. laboratories for vitamin and mineral analyses. Literally tens of thousands of these studies were performed. In conclusion, **Dr. Price found that traditional native diets contained, at least ten times more fat-soluble vitamins – A, D, and K - and four times more water-soluble vitamins – which is the entire B-complex and vitamin C – than did American diets of the 1930s.**[276] Furthermore, he found that the native traditional diets contained dramatically more minerals than did American diets, ranging from 1.5 times as much to up to nearly 60 times more for some minerals, including calcium, phosphorus, magnesium, copper, iron, zinc, and iodine.[277]

For example, Price wrote, "It is of interest that the diets of the primitive groups which have shown a very high immunity to dental caries and freedom from other degenerative processes have all provided a nutrition containing at least four times these minimum requirements; **whereas the displacing nutrition of commerce, consisting largely of white-flour products, sugar, polished rice, jams, canned goods, and vegetable fats [vegetable oils] have invariably failed to provide even the minimum requirements.** In other words the foods of the native Eskimos, for example, contained 5.4 times as much calcium as the displacing foods of the white man, five times as much phosphorus, 1.5 times as much iron, 7.9 times as much magnesium, 1.8 times as much copper, 49.0 times as much iodine, and at least ten times that number of fat-soluble vitamins." [278] In general, the native diets supplied anywhere from approximately two to eight times the minimum daily requirements of calcium and phosphorus and up to 28 times more magnesium.[279]

Dr. Price often referred to vitamins as "catalysts" or "activators." Without them, he made it abundantly clear that we are not able to assimilate minerals in our diets, no matter how abundantly we might consume them. Perhaps this should give us pause as we consider the enormous doses of calcium supplements consumed with ever increasing and progressive osteoporosis, just as one example. Vitamins A and D are critically important to the proper development *and maintenance* of the health of the brain, nervous system, *eyes*, bones, and sexual development, but virtually every cell of our bodies is dependent upon these vitamins. Again, I don't want to revert too much to reductionist thinking – and start naming biological processes dependent on these vitamins, as if they're the only ones. They're clearly not. The cellular dependency on these vitamins is ubiquitous. And with regard to the minerals, you can take these in pill form, but without adequate quantities of the natural vitamins, you won't properly absorb or utilize them.

SACRED FOODS – SUPPLY FAT-SOLUBLE VITAMINS IN GREAT QUANTITIES

The fat-soluble vitamins, A, D, and K, like all the vitamins, are absolutely critical to health. They work together in a synergistic fashion with each other as well as the water-soluble vitamins, minerals, and cofactors, the complexity of which cannot be understood or appreciated by today's science. Each of the native populations that Price studied that continued to consume their traditional diets had a food that was generally considered to be sacred. These were foods, known to be critically essential to health and vitality, to prevent disease and degeneration, and in many cultures, known to provide for healthy pregnancies, easy delivery, strong and sturdy babies, and healthy, robust children. The knowledge of such sacred foods was passed down from their ancestors through generation after generation.

For many societies, such as the Swiss villagers of the Loetschental Valley, the sacred food was the butter made from cattle grazing on rapidly growing green grass. This butter is extremely high in the fat-soluble vitamins, including vitamin K2 – the latter of which is a vitamin recently discovered to play a major role in cardiovascular disease when deficiency is present.[280] **Other sacred foods included, for example, cod liver for the Gaelic people of the Outer Hebrides, organ meats and whale blubber for the Eskimos, and fish eggs (roe) for the Indians of South America living in the Andes mountains.** Dr. Price stated, for example, "The Indians of the high Andes were willing to go hundreds of miles to the sea to get kelp and fish eggs for the use of their people." [281] Analysis of each of these foods shows that they are tremendous sources of fat-soluble vitamins.

"ACCUMULATED WISDOM"

To quote Dr. Price from his 1939 *Nutrition and Physical Degeneration,* "In my studies of these several racial stocks I find that it is not accident but accumulated wisdom regarding food that lies behind their physical excellence and freedom from our modern degenerative processes, and, further, that on various sides of our world the primitive people know many of the things that are essential for life—things that our modern civilizations apparently do not know. These are the fundamental truths of life that have put them in harmony with Nature through obeying her nutritional laws." [282]

MORE FROM WESTON A. PRICE – "THE CHARLES DARWIN OF NUTRITION"

It is my suggestion that, if you only read one more book in your lifetime, it should be Weston A. Price's *Nutrition and Physical Degeneration,* published by the Price-Pottenger Nutrition Foundation (*PPNF.org*). I believe this text should be required reading for every single health care provider on the planet – and perhaps every single parent or parent-to-be, and anyone who desires to maintain or improve their health. Not only do our lives and our own health depend on this knowledge, so does that of our children and their children. *PPNF.org*, with free resources as well as membership availability, is a tremendous resource for ordering and further information. They also display a brilliantly conceived summary chart of the 14 "tribes" that Dr. Price studied, their particular foods, and their percentage of cavities, both on their traditional diets and with modernized diets where applicable. To view the chart, just go to *PPNF.org*, and search for "Dr. Price's Tribal Food and Cavity Chart." Finally, though I've given a thumbnail sketch of *Nutrition and Physical Degeneration* in this chapter, to call this even a "brief review" is like comparing an 8-foot dinghy to the Titanic.

My first-runner-up category for additional reading belongs to Sally Fallon's *Nourishing Traditions.* This book is not only brilliant, it is yet another stroke of genius. Mrs. Fallon simplifies the complicated web of eating in today's world using Weston A. Price principles – and she does it magnificently. *Nourishing Traditions* also includes a large cookbook that espouses the principles of traditional food preparation and has loads of excellent recipes. Sally Fallon is one of the most knowledgeable people in the nutrition industry – and if it weren't for her and the Weston A. Price Foundation, of which she is the founder, I may have never known about Weston A. Price. My hat is off to Mrs. Fallon. The Weston A. Price Foundation (*WestonAPrice.org*) is also a tremendous free resource, with even greater benefits for those who choose membership status.

CHAPTER SUMMARY

According to Dr. Price, the "'displacing foods of modern commerce'" included white sugar, white flour, white rice, canned goods, syrups, jams, confectionary, and vegetable oils.[283] According to a documentary film (available at the Weston A. Price foundation's website) regarding Price's work, the narrator states, "He labeled refined carbohydrates as the 'white plague,' and included in this group all sugar and white flour products." [284]

Dr. Price's ingenious studies showed that physical degeneration occurred independently of an individual's race, ethnicity, genetic heritage, or for that matter, his or her geographic locale, stress level, lifestyle, etc. Physical degeneration occurred in culture after culture, for those who consumed the 'displacing foods of modern commerce' instead of their traditional diets. The implications are profound – and indeed apply directly to the development of numerous diseases and degenerative conditions. This includes heart disease, cardiovascular disease, diabetes, metabolic syndrome, hypertension, arthritic diseases, Alzheimer's disease, cancers, autoimmune diseases, depressive and anxiety disorders, attention deficit disorders, autism, and more. It is my assertion that 'age-related macular degeneration' - a degenerative disorder – is among these diseases of Western civilization and is yet another disease produced by a faulty, processed food-laden diet.

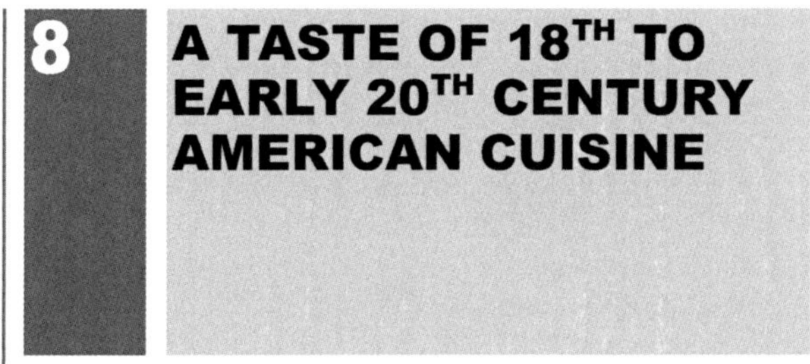

8 A TASTE OF 18TH TO EARLY 20TH CENTURY AMERICAN CUISINE

"A sufficiency of wholesome and well-prepared food is absolutely necessary to the preservation of health and strength, both of body and mind."
~ Eliza Leslie ~
(Author, Miss Leslie's Directions for Cookery, 1851)

Now that we've reviewed the epic work of the great Weston A Price, I believe it's only appropriate to take a look at American cuisine – and what has happened to it. If we can agree that there is an abundance of evidence that macular degeneration was exceedingly rare before 1930, wouldn't it be compelling to know what kinds of foods we were consuming before, around, and after that time frame, and examine the temporal relationship of such food consumption to the development of AMD? Perhaps more importantly, wouldn't it be equally compelling to know what kinds of foods *we weren't consuming*?

With that said, I will devote this entire but brief chapter to the review of this exceedingly important topic.

AMERICAN COOKERY: AMERICA'S FIRST COOKBOOK, 1796 – by Amelia Simmons

In fact, we're going to begin with *American Cookery*, which is the first American-authored cookbook, written and published in the United States, in the year 1796. This book is not only germane to our subject matter, but is truly a historic document. The re-published edition is entitled, *The First American Cookbook: A Facsimile of "American Cookery," 1796*, by Amelia Simmons, which is published with a prologue by Mary Tolford Wilson.[285] This short book is a rich source for Colonial American cuisine – and of course, a great source of evidence as to the kinds of foods our ancestors were consuming.

In this book, Simmons begins by advising how to choose good quality meats, poultry, fish, and vegetables, and then reviews general matters in their preparation. The very first page of the book, entitled "DIRECTIONS for CATERING, or the procuring the best VIANDS, FISH, &c," ("viand" translates literally, "an item of food") begins with how to select meats. For example, she wrote, "Cow Beef is less boned, and generally more tender and juicy than the ox, in America, which is used to labor." She advised how to select mutton, lamb, veal, pork, salmon, shad, lobster, oysters, and numerous other seafood selections, chicken and numerous other kinds of poultry, including peacock, turkey, goose, duck, and many others.

In the "Receipts" (the term used for recipe in that era) of her book, she begins with roast beef, roast mutton, roast veal, and roast lamb. There are "receipts" for "To smother a Fowl in Oysters," "To Stuff a Leg of Veal," and even "To Dress a Turtle."

Butter is used for what seems like every recipe, and not infrequently in very large amounts. Her "Stew Pie" used a half pound of butter, "Sea pie" was made with four pounds of flour, one and a half pounds of butter, and her "Chicken Pie" (chicken-pot pie) was made with one and a half pounds of butter plus gravy.

There were numerous recipes for desserts, which used butter, eggs, and sugar liberally. Her "Plumb Cake" included 21 eggs and 3 pints of cream. Her "Plain Cake" was made with 3 pounds of sugar, 3 pounds of butter (12 sticks in today's terms), one quart of milk, and 9 eggs. Simmons' "Rich Cake" was made with 2 pounds of butter, 15 eggs, and a half pound of sugar.

Very occasionally, she used the term "shortning," in some recipes, which Mary Tolford Wilson confirms that in later editions of the book, was "corrected to 'shortening' – to denote fats, specifying that the proportions she used were 'half butter and half lard.'" Wilson goes on to review that the term "shortning," or later, "shortening," was a term that was obviously familiar to Americans in the late 1700's. In fact, she points out that the term was included in Webster's American Dictionary of the English Language in the year 1828.[286]

It's very interesting that the term "shortening," in that era, refers to a half butter – half lard mix, both of which I will show throughout this book, are incredibly healthy. In fact, those are the fats that helped sustain us in tremendous health for thousands of years. However, until I read this cookbook, along with Mary Tolford Wilson's explanation, "shortening" in my mind had always meant Crisco, which if you're not familiar, is the dreaded man-made concoction of trans-fats that was the invention of Proctor & Gamble, back in 1911. I will come back to this nightmarish substitute for butter and lard later in this book – and it isn't pretty.

One term that I never found in this book, is "oil." There was no such thing as any type of "vegetable oil" mentioned – not even olive oil. This is a critical piece of information that will resurface repeatedly throughout this book, because that, along with trans-fats (e.g., Crisco), will have vast implications for our health, or lack thereof. I believe this is critical to the development of AMD as well.

AMERICAN CUISINE IN THE ANTEBELLUM ERA (1781 TO 1860) – THE ANTEBELLUM PERIOD

by James and Dorothy Volo

Next, we will review the American cuisine in what is commonly known as the Antebellum Era – the era beginning in 1781, when the U.S. Articles of Confederation were ratified, and ending at the beginning of the civil war in 1860.

James and Dorothy Volo wrote *The Antebellum Period*, a historical book regarding this period of time. It this book the authors review food consumption during this era - and they do so with authority. In the book, they write:

> "Modern issues of vitamins, salt, fiber, and fat content were virtually nonexistent for most people during the antebellum period. A few groups emerged during this time urging people to refrain from eating meat or to increase grain consumption, but generally their followers were thought to be eccentric by most Americans. Some women's magazines and receipt [recipe] books did urge balance and moderation in diet… Most meals at this time contained meat, which was likely to be high in fat content, and bread in one form or another. Frances Trollope, a visitor to the United States in the 1830s, was shocked by the American diet. She remarked on the extraordinary amount of bacon and other meats eaten in American homes. 'Ham and beef steaks appear morning noon and night.' Equally astonishing to her was the way eggs and oysters, ham and apple sauce, beefsteak and stewed peaches, salt fish and onion were eaten in combination." [287]

The authors go on to review that pork was the most common meat to be consumed, particularly for Southerners. In fact, pork might commonly be served three meals a day without raising an eyebrow. Due to lack of refrigeration, this pork wasn't necessarily even fresh – it might be salt pork or smoked pork. The method of salting and drying preserved the meats for much longer periods. The farmers' and planters' wives often sold their cured hams and any excess lard, butter, or eggs, all of which were staples in the diet.

Beef was quite popular in the North. In fact, beef cuts might be stored in barrels packed with snow. The beef was even aged by hanging it to dry for a period up to several weeks before preparing it to be served. Lamb was less popular then, however, it was available many times in spring and early summer.

Chicken was a common meat for early Americans – and was generally eaten fresh. In addition, chickens had the general appeal of being egg producers – and eggs were eaten in abundance when available.

The Volo authors continue:

> "In the South and rural areas, hunters would supplement the cuisine by bringing home such victuals as geese, rabbits, squirrels, wild turkeys, partridges, pheasants, deer, and reed birds. The meat supplied in this manner was particularly important for poorer families.
>
> "Fish and seafood were eaten in abundance in shore communities… Freshwater fish included bass, cod, sturgeon, pickerel, perch, pike, whitefish, and catfish. Fish could be salted or smoked but much of

it was eaten fresh or made into chowder or stews. Oysters were extremely popular. They were eaten fresh but were also pickled and canned." [288]

MISS LESLIE'S DIRECTIONS FOR COOKERY (1851) – by Eliza Leslie

I am including a review of this cookbook, from 1851, because the author, Eliza Leslie (1787 – 1858), was unquestionably the 19th century's most popular, prolific, and successful American cookbook author. *Miss Leslie's Directions for Cookery* was first published in 1837, with her 37th edition in 1851 later becoming an unabridged reprint by Dover Publications, Inc., with an introduction by Jan Longone.[289] Miss Leslie's 60th and last edition was printed in 1870, some 12 years after her death. In her introduction to the 37th edition of the book (from 1851), Longone writes, "Every writer on America's gastronomic history has lauded Miss Leslie." Obviously, Miss Leslie's writings not only shaped American cuisine in the 19th century, but reflected typical cooking styles and ingredients as well.

Miss Leslie's cookbook is truly a vast compilation, not only of recipes, but of general gastronomical knowledge. This book is packed with over 500 pages of recipes and general instructions for the cook.

First, she wrote an entire chapter each on soups, fish, shellfish, beef, veal, mutton and lamb, pork, venison, poultry and game, gravy and sauces, vegetables, eggs, pastry and puddings, cakes, preparations for the sick, and more.

Just like Amelia Simmons' *American Cookery*, when a fat needed to be added to the dish, it was almost always butter. Once again, butter was used in liberal amounts. Practically every vegetable was either cooked in butter or served with melted butter. In the chapter on "Gravy and Sauces," there is a section devoted to melted butter, in which she wrote, "Melted butter is the foundation of most of the common sauces." Her "Plain Omelet" was made with six eggs, leaving out whites of two, and cooked in "a quarter of a pound of butter in a frying-pan."[290]

Lard was used in various dishes, but far less commonly than butter. She recommended frying calves' liver in lard, for example. Oysters, which were much more commonly consumed in that era than currently, were frequently on the menu. Miss Leslie's "Minced Oysters" recipe began with "fifty nine large oysters" to be fried in up to one pound of lard.

I only found the term oil used once in this book – and that was under "To Dress Lettuce As Salad." The directions for preparing this salad include the term "sweet oil," which I had to investigate. Sweet oil is actually a derivative of olive oil, which was perhaps used occasionally, but definitely appears to be a rarity for that era.

Her concepts and recommendations are in keeping with the traditions of our forefathers, obviously, as she frequently recommends that the organ meats be included with the meal. This was particularly evident with most of the poultry dishes, where she recommended that these typically be mixed into the gravy. For roast fowl, for example, she wrote, "Leave out the livers, gizzards and hearts, to be chopped and put into the gravy." For her roasted duck, she recommended that one "Reserve the livers, gizzards, and hearts to put in the gravy." For roast goose, her recommendation again was, "Having parboiled the liver and heart, chop them and put them into the gravy."[291] This is in keeping with what might be considered sacred, or at least traditional, foods for early Americans.

Her recipe for "Liver Puddings" states, "The best liver puddings are made of boiled pigs-feet and livers, mixed together in equal portions." With regard to the pigs livers, she states, "Boil some pigs' livers. When cold, mince them and season them with pepper, salt, and some sage and sweet marjoram rubbed fine."[292]

I'd like to finish this segment with dessert, just like a fine meal, but there's too many of them and I cannot choose. So let's just review the fact that Miss Leslie's menu even included a recipe for "dough nuts" (donuts) – which were also fried in lard![293]

FOOD ON THE FRONTIER – MINNESOTA COOKING FROM 1850 TO 1900 by Marjorie Kreidberg

I've selected this next book, *Food On The Frontier – Minnesota Cooking from 1850 to 1900 With Selected Recipes*, by Marjorie Kreidberg, because chronologically, it is in the time frame that is appropriate to consider next, but also because it is a very thorough review that should be quite representative of American cuisine during that era.

Approximately two-thirds of this book is dedicated to a review of the general knowledge required for cooking and there is tremendous review and devotion to the tasks of canning, drying, pickling, and the difficult, laborious, and even complex task of attempting to preserve meats in an era when electronic refrigeration was not available.

When it comes to the actual foods and recipes, author Marjorie Kreidberg states, "Although the principal item in pre-Civil War American diets was meat (especially beef), the food available from 1850 to 1900 was unexpectedly varied, considering the transportation and distribution systems of that time. There were some surprises in the lists of foods Minnesotans ate at mid-century, too; chief among them was oysters. Another surprisingly long-lived food choice was salted codfish, which was sent upriver by steamboat to Minnesota in the 1850s and shipped by rail after the late 1860s. Codfish seems to have been a staple food in many Minnesota homes at least until 1900. A wide variety of vegetables were consumed by Minnesotans in the late 19th century, but only a few were eaten raw in salads. The exception was the popular cabbage made into coleslaw... Much more to Minnesotans' liking were salads made of potatoes, meat, fish, poultry, and eggs. Without a doubt, desserts made up the largest single category of recipes contributed to Minnesota church-sponsored cookbooks." [294] And just as in the previously reviewed cuisine, the desserts were made with plenty of butter, eggs, and yes, even sugar.

According to Kreidberg, the recipes for this book are drawn from 19th century cookbooks and manuscripts that were the collections of the Minnesota Historical Society – obviously, adding tremendously to their authenticity. Kreidberg wrote, "Like their 20th century descendents, the pioneers seem to have preferred beef to other meats, although pork, veal, liver, heart, tongue, brains, and sweetbreads (thymus and pancreas, also known as offal or organ meats) were also popular." In addition to common recipes which won't be reviewed, the book included recipes for "Larded Liver," which is calf's liver wrapped in bacon or ham served with gravy; "Fritot of Chicken," which is the only meat I found that included "two spoons of olive oil,' but which is fried in lard; and "Fried Potatoes," which are fried in "plenty of fresh butter, or butter and lard mixed."

The terms "salad oil" or "olive oil" were used just several times in this book, including "3 teaspoons salad oil" in "Sweet Potato Salad," "three teaspoons salad oil or melted butter" in "Chicken Salad," "oil and vinegar" in the "Herring Salad," and "One egg-yolk, add oil drop by drop, by drop, beating rapidly," for the "Oil Dressing (Mayonnaise)."

My "take" is that there is slightly more use of "oil" in this recipe book than from the recipes given by Simmons prior to 1851. Nevertheless, the use of olive oil is still very, very minimal in the latter half of the 19th century and its use is almost exclusively in salads and not in cooked items.

One of the critical elements of our dietary history also took place during the timeframe of the subject matter of this book (1850 – 1900), and that was the "revolutionary advancement of grain milling" which was the design and development of roller mills that would, in general, replace traditional millstones. This took place in the 1880s and was a two-part invention, the first requiring the use of a "middlings purifier," which removes the husks from grains of wheat, but which was subsequently used to separate the outer "bran" of the wheat grain from the endosperm – the latter of which becomes flour. It did this by passing the partially ground "middlings" over a screen with a stream of air blowing across that literally would blow the lighter bran away. The second part of this innovative process was the development of the roller mill, which was far more efficient at breaking up hard wheat varieties and separating the bran from the endosperm, thereby giving a purer form of flour which also was considered to result in better bread.[295]

Kriedberg references this in her book, as she states, "Shortly after installing middlings purifiers, flour mills in Minnesota were able to replace millstones with rollers, and by 1880 Minneapolis became the flour-milling capital of the nation. The impact of this revolution was manifest in a variety of ways. To the local housewife, however, it meant a more accessible supply of an excellent, white flour made from Minnesota-grown, hard spring wheat." [296]

However, this new roller mill technology appears to have been a double-edged sword, as the more efficient milling technique could therefore remove both the bran and the germ of the wheat grains efficiently, thus creating a flour that was almost pure endosperm and perhaps more appealing to the palate, at the expense of a significant loss in nutrients.[297] [298] This may explain, at least to some extent, that when Weston A Price repeatedly found cultures developing degenerative conditions after adopting Westernized diets, they were typically consuming "*white flour*, white sugar, canned goods, ..." vegetable oils, etc. Hence, our eventual return to at least some understanding that the consumption of "whole grains" is more beneficial, because then we retain the nutritional benefits of both the bran and the germ of the wheat. Today though, unfortunately, there are other potentially negative considerations to the consumption of wheat, and this will be covered in the chapter on grains.

1905 COOKBOOK – FOOD FOR BODY AND SOUL

by Judy Steiger Howard

This treasure of a book was written by Judy Steiger Howard, published in 2011, and is based on numerous heartwarming stories of pioneers in the Oklahoma region, even before Oklahoma was a state (1907). The book was obviously the result of much painstaking research through the files of multiple Oklahoma libraries, newspaper archives, and the donations by numerous individuals of historic photos from the era, which is centered from late 19th century to approximately 1905. According to Howard, "*1905 Cookbook – Food for Body and Soul* combines unpretentious, delectable recipes with a glimpse into the lives of those courageous, God-fearing pioneer women who left family, friends and the comforts of first homes to homestead a hostile and barren landscape before Oklahoma became a state."[299] These anecdotes are combined with a fascinating weave of photos, biblical scripture, and over 300 recipes – with all of the latter documented to have been written by these peoples.

These pioneers had to live off the land, yet they somehow survived and appear to have remained well-nourished and in good health. Howard states, "If the pioneers were lucky in hunting, they might feast on a roasted prairie chicken, squirrel, duck, Jackrabbit, prairie dog, pheasant or catfish. Women and children collected twigs, branches and animal chips for fuel for the campfires. They dug a trench, erected poles to hang the cooking pots, and started the fire with friction matches called lucifers." [300]

A "Grocery List for Surviving the First 3 Months" of this life read as follows:

> "100 pounds of flour for each adult, 37 pounds of bacon, 15 pounds of pilot bread (hardtack), 3 pounds of coffee, 1 pound of tea, 13 pounds of sugar, 1/3 bushel of dried beans, 5 pounds of rice, ½ bushel of dried fruit (mostly dried apples), 1 pound of saleratus (baking soda), 5 pounds of salt, ¼ bushel of cornmeal, dry yeast, 8 pounds of parched or ground corn, ½ keg of vinegar for cooking and drinking

to cure your ills from drinking tainted water, cinnamon sticks and a few spices and lemon extract, your best laying chicken for eggs. Tie on the back of the wagon the family cow for milk and butter." [301]

Virtually identical to the "receipts" of the previous century, around 99 percent of the recipes that called for a fat (that wasn't already in the food, such as animal meats and eggs) was in the form of butter, lard, or both combined. For example, bread called for "1/2 teacup lard," "Rusks" (hard, dry biscuits) called for "2/3 cup lard or butter," "molasses drop cake" called for "1/2 cup lard or butter," "delicious chicken pie" called for "1/1/2 teacups lard," roast turkey was fried in butter and lard, and doughnuts called for "4 tablespoons melted butter" and were fried in "hot lard."[302]

Out of more than 300 recipes in this book, I could only find four that called for olive oil, but two of those called for either melted butter or olive oil. When olive oil was called for, it was used very sparingly. "Chicken Salad" called for 1 tablespoon olive oil; "Salad Dressing" called for ½ cup melted butter, 3 tablespoons olive oil, and 1 pint whipped cream; but "Good Salad Dressing" called for eggs, vinegar, mustard, salt, pepper, sugar, and sour cream, but no olive oil! "Bean Salad called for 1 tablespoon melted butter or salad oil" (olive oil) and "Potato Salad" called for "olive oil or melted butter."[303]

The vegetables, sweet potatoes, corn, salad dressing, fried tomatoes, "potato loaf," lima beans, and asparagus recipes all called for butter. Desserts were probably just an occasional treat for these homesteaders, but those recipes frequently called for sugar, butter, and eggs, of course.

My favorite recipe of all is the "Recipe for a Happy Home":

> "6 cups of love, 3 cups of forgiveness, 1 cup of friendship, 5 spoons of hope, 3 spoons of tenderness, 4 quarts of faith, 1 50 gallon barrel of laughter, (and) 2 cups of loyalty. Mix love and loyalty thoroughly with faith. Blend it with forgiveness and tenderness. Add friendship and hope. Sprinkle uproariously with laughter. Bake it with sunshine. Serve daily with generous helpings to everyone you meet." [304]

CHAPTER SUMMARY

In this chapter, we've reviewed four highly representative cookbooks that span a period from colonial times, in 1796, to 1905. In this era, virtually ninety-nine percent of the fats consumed – and probably more – were of animal origin. These consisted of animal fats directly from beef, pork, chicken, mutton or lamb, any variety of wild animals, plus large amounts of eggs, butter and lard, the latter of which is rendered pork fat. We see that the majority of homes probably didn't even have olive oil, which was generally the only edible oil available at that time, though a few had coconut oil. When "salad oil" (olive oil) was called for, it was used very sparingly and they virtually never cooked with it.

As you can see, our ancestors consumed very high amounts of saturated animal fats, and extremely low amounts of polyunsaturated fats, the latter of which are present in very large amounts in "vegetable oils," such as corn, soybean, canola, sunflower, safflower, cottonseed, and a few others. Our requirements for polyunsaturated oils is very small and this, along with multiple other reasons to be reviewed, may impose substantially increased risks for AMD.

Prior to the early 1900s, the consumption of offal, such as liver, heart, brain, pancreas, kidneys, and other organ meats was commonplace – and many early Americans considered this fare routine and typical. Many meals were prepared either with the organ meats, or with the organ meats cooked and thrown into the gravy.

Finally, we see that, at least prior to the 1880s, wheat would have been considered "whole grain," given that it was ground using millstones, instead of roller technology, the latter of which certainly makes a purer form of white flour, but at the expense of nutrient loss. There are other issues with the differences in wheat during this era as compared to current forms of wheat, such as changes in proteins due to intense hybridization and the common use of herbicides, all of which will be reviewed subsequently.

Rates of heart disease, cancer, diabetes, and apparently, many degenerative disorders, were all extremely rare during the period from the late 1700s until just after the turn of the 20th century. Recall that AMD was virtually non-existent during this era as well. History tells us that most Americans that met an early demise usually succumbed to any number of infectious causes, for which there was no treatment.

Wouldn't it make sense that all of this absence of disease might be related to a diet naturally high in vitamins, particularly fat-soluble vitamins, and virtually absent in processed foods - particularly white flour, refined sugar, canned goods, vegetable oils, and artificially created trans fats? This begs the question: Were early Americans, consuming their traditional diets, just as the cultures that Weston A. Price discovered who were also consuming their traditional diets? I believe the answer is a resounding yes. In other words, they were consuming the diets that their ancestors had followed, probably for hundreds of years, and they were generally in supreme health – as long as they could get enough food as well as a variety of food.

In the next chapter, we will consider what happened to our diets in the 20th century – and the perils that have followed.

Part III

"Displacing Foods" are the Culprits

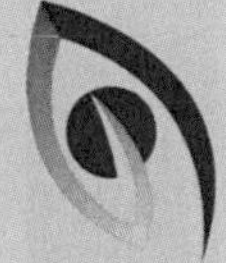

9 THE 20TH CENTURY AND THE NEW "STANDARD AMERICAN DIET"

"If man made it, don't eat it."
~ Jack LaLanne ~

For those of you who don't know Francois Henri "Jack" LaLanne (1914 – 2011), he was an American icon for fitness, nutrition, and exercise. He was often referred to as "the Godfather of fitness" and the "first fitness superhero."[305] I remember him from his television show, *The Jack LaLanne Show*, which I recall watching from the time I was just five or six years old back in the mid 1960's. This show ran for some 34 years – longer than any television program regarding fitness.

LaLanne, who had become a very successful natural bodybuilder, wasn't always that way though. As a teenager, in the late 1920's, Jack said he was addicted to sugars and sweets. "As a kid, I was a 'sugarholic' and a junk food junkie," he said. "It made me weak and it made me mean. I had boils, pimples, and suffered from nearsightedness. Little girls used to beat me up."[306]

At the age of 15, Jack's life began to undergo a transformation after he and his mother attended a lecture by a nationally recognized nutritionist, Paul Bragg, who advised Jack to give up the sugars, sweets, and junk food. Jack began to exercise daily and he rapidly became fit. By the age of 21, he opened the nation's first health and fitness club in Oakland, California, where he also offered exercise and nutrition advice with the primary goal being to help people improve their overall health. Many doctors advised their patients against using LaLanne's health club. They even warned their patients that "LaLanne was an exercise 'nut,' whose programs would make them 'muscle-bound' and cause severe medical problems," including heart attacks and loss of sex drive.[307] LaLanne, at the age of 80, remained brilliantly healthy and fit, and he continued to workout daily until the age of 96, when he passed away secondary to a bout of pneumonia for which he refused to see a doctor.[308]

My favorite quote of LaLanne's, "If man made it, don't eat it," is a mantra that I try to live by. I believe this is a mantra that would serve us all extremely well, because when followed, it eliminates any possibility of consuming processed food. If you're not aware, processed food might be defined as "the transformation of raw ingredients, by physical or chemical means into food, or of food into other forms. Food processing combines raw ingredients to produce marketable food products that can be easily prepared and served by the consumer."[309]

The consumption of processed food, as you're going to see, is quite literally the downfall of Western society and, unfortunately, most of the world is following suit. For numerous reasons, which I will try to convey throughout this book, the consumption of processed foods has caused us to develop heart disease, cancer, arthritis, dementia, numerous other afflictions as well as great suffering and, of course, I believe, to develop AMD.

THE STANDARD AMERICAN DIET (SAD) – BEGINS TO TAKE SHAPE IN THE EARLY 20TH CENTURY

There were four major changes to the American diet that began to occur primarily following the turn of the 20th century, which impacted our health dramatically, and which I believe also play a central role in the development of AMD:

1. **Refined Flour production using roller milling technology, beginning 1880**
2. **Vegetable oil (Cottonseed oil) production and consumption – beginning 1880 and spreading rapidly post 1900**
3. **Proctor & Gamble's Crisco (hydrogenated vegetable oil, or trans fats) invention, production, and mass distribution – beginning 1911**
4. **Increasing consumption of sugar from 1822 through 1999**

In the next chapter, we'll review each of the above in detail. For now, I just want to introduce the major historic changes to our diet and begin to lay the foundation for what is to come. What we will see is that the introduction of these new "foods" (with vegetable oils and hydrogenated vegetable oils, the term "foods" is used loosely here) to our diet, combined with the alteration of other foods (e.g. refining of grains) results in at least two major effects.

First, refined wheat flour, takes the place of whole wheat flour. This came about as the result of stone mill technology being replaced by roller mill technology. The result was our first ever processed, nutrient deficient food – white flour.

Second, the introduction of vegetable oils, which severely displaced the consumption of animal fats. Animal fats had previously been the major and primary source of the fat-soluble vitamins A, D, E, and K.[310, 311] With the development of vegetable oils, manufacturers would produce – and a global market of people would ultimately consume – billions of pounds of vegetable oils, with devastating effects. This began in the late 19th century with the production of cottonseed oil, but eventually numerous other vegetable oils would be produced. The U.S. has been the market leader in the production and distribution of soybeans, which are primarily used for soybean oil, since prior to 1975.[312]

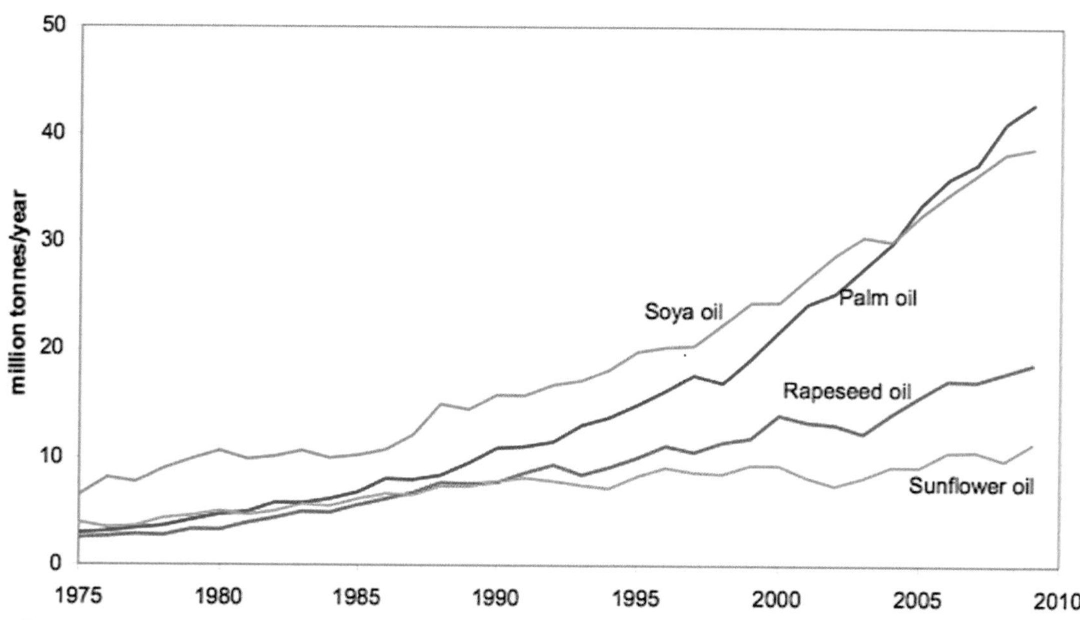

FIGURE 9.1 Annual growth of major edible oils production (palm, rapeseed, soy and sunflower oils).
Source of the data: www.fas.usda.gov/psdonline

Third, in 1911, Procter & Gamble formulated and introduced Crisco - the first hydrogenated vegetable oil. If there was ever a quintessential imitation food, this was it. As we'll review in the next chapter in detail, Crisco was developed by artificially hydrogenating liquid cottonseed oil. The oil is placed in huge steel containers, heated and placed under high pressure while bubbling hydrogen gas through the oil in the presence of a metal catalyst. The result is a solid substance that has an appearance similar to lard, but which could be made inexpensively given the fact that cottonseeds otherwise had little or no use.[313] **Proctor & Gamble marketed Crisco as the "healthier alternative to cooking with animal fats and... more economical than butter."[314]** With a deft marketing plan that included that one sentence, a large marketing budget, and free cookbooks targeted at housewives with 615 recipes all requiring Crisco, Procter and Gamble took on lard and butter as market competitors. Crisco would soon gain and control enormous market share, while lard and butter sales began their decline. In the coming decades, despite a myriad of disastrous health effects (to be reviewed), P & G would sell trillions of pounds of Crisco to unsuspecting customers who "bought" their marketing campaign and their completely unsubstantiated health claims.

Fourth, increasing consumption of sugar, in various forms, further displaced the consumption of even more nutrient-dense foods (such as whole grains, fruits, and vegetables) that would have otherwise been in the diet.

If I may continue the list of major developments in the American (Western) diet, which have played major negative and destructive roles in our health in the latter half of the 20th century, they would include:

5. **The indictment of saturated fat and cholesterol as causative factors in the development of heart disease – 1950s**
6. **The recommendation for a low-fat diet – late 1970s**
7. **The mass consumption of processed foods**
8. **The genetic modification of foods (genetically modified organisms – GMOs) and their mass production and consumption**

Let's take a look at each of these developments briefly...

If the displacement of animal fats, including butter and lard, by vegetable oils and hydrogenated vegetable oils (Crisco) weren't bad enough, we then had the ominous development of the indictment of saturated fat and cholesterol as causative factors in heart disease. This development began in the 1950s and, as most of us are probably aware, spawned a fear that animal fats, including eggs, butter and lard, were the evil culprits behind heart disease. As you recall from Weston A. Price's research, the meats, butter, lard, and whole milk from grass-fed animals are all collectively tremendous sources of natural vitamins A, D, and K.

With regard to organ meats such as liver, which were still staples to many American homes in the 1960s, an end came to their consumption as well – courtesy of the government having vilified saturated fat and cholesterol for playing causative roles in heart disease.

For those of you not aware, the so-called "diet-heart hypothesis" – which claims that saturated fats raise cholesterol, and elevated cholesterol causes heart disease, has been debunked repeatedly.[315] If you're not aware of this, I will review this in further detail in subsequent chapters.

To add insult to injury, in 1977 a U.S. Senate Select committee, led by George McGovern, published its "Dietary Goals for the United States," which was our government's stance that a low-fat diet would help to reduce "killer diseases" that were truly already in epidemic proportions. These recommendations made to the people of the United States, included the blanket recommendation to reduce dietary fat to no more than 30 percent of calories, to reduce saturated fat to no more than 10 percent of calories, and to decrease cholesterol intake to 300 mg per day (a medium sized egg contains about 186 mg of cholesterol).[316]

The Big Food manufacturers, including Nestle, Nabisco, Pillsbury, Coca-Cola, General Mills, Kellog's, Mars, Unilever, Tyson Foods, and others, in order to maintain profits in the billions, responded to the recommendation for low-fat foods and they did so in a big way. Fat in food tastes great, but in order to make sales, they needed foods pleasing to the palate, which were also low in fat. The substitute? Sugar.

In fact, this opened up a whole new market for Big Food manufacturers: the low-fat market. In response to this, literally thousands of newly manufactured food options would come on the market, mainly in the form of packaged, processed, ready-to-eat foods. Not surprisingly, most of these foods would be made from some combination of white flour, sugar in the form of HFCS, vegetable oil, partially hydrogenated vegetable oils (trans-fats) and usually, soy lecithin (an emulsifier) to hold the food together. So, whether it was a cookie, a pop-tart, or a frozen pizza, it generally was found to have a mixture of these ingredients.

Incredibly, these manufactured foods could be made dirt cheap and pleasing to the palate. Plus, since the U.S. Farm Bill had already underwritten the cost of corn and soy, farmers could sell corn and soybeans at a small profit, even when these crops cost more to grow and harvest than the market price would bear. Manufacturers took advantage of these government subsidies to spawn a new type of sugar, known as high-fructose corn syrup (HFCS) and, of course, to produce soybean oil. The HFCS was a cheaper alternative to cane sugar. With that availability, soft drinks and processed foods, old and new, suddenly became loaded with sugars that were mostly of the HFCS variety. By the late 1990's, HFCS had become the most common sweetener for foods and soft drinks in the United States.[317] And, as we've reviewed, soybean oil became the number one vegetable oil in the U.S while we simultaneously became the global leader in soybean oil exports.

All of this set the stage for the mass production of processed foods – commodity agriculture, if you will – which became increasingly prominent after about 1950.

Commodity agriculture is the term that describes the belief that the primary objective of farming is to produce as much food and/or fiber as possible for the least cost. It isn't about quality of food. And it's not about your health. In fact, most processed food, most fast food, and most convenience foods – are not produced to provide you with good nutrition and to benefit your health. They're produced with one primary goal in mind: profits to the manufacturers.

Quite frankly, these are foods that most of our great grandparents wouldn't have even recognized as food and currently includes items like breakfast cereals, pop-tarts, pastries, frozen pizza, frozen dinners, potato chips, pretzels, wheat thins, salad dressings, barbecue sauce, candies, candy bars, confectionary, soft drinks, energy drinks and so on. Incredibly, literally thousands of these nutritionally deficient items would ultimately be sold as "healthy snacks," typically because they were either low in fat, had added synthetic vitamins, or both.

In her book *Nourishing Traditions*, Sally Fallon of the Weston A. Price Foundation draws on the research of the brilliant Mary G. Enig, PhD (1931 – 2014) when she wrote, "During the sixty-year period from 1910 to 1970, the proportion of traditional animal fat in the American diet declined from 83 percent to 62 percent, and butter consumption plummeted from 18 pounds per person per year to four. During the past eighty years {~1920 – 2000}, dietary cholesterol intake has increased only 1 percent. During the same period the percentage of dietary vegetable oils in the form of margarine, shortening and refined oils increased about 400 percent while the consumption of sugar and processed foods increased about 60 percent." [318]

Alright. We've made it to Base Camp One of our Mount Everest. We're making good progress!

CHAPTER SUMMARY

Heart disease,[319] cancer,[320] diabetes, and macular degeneration (previously reviewed in Chapter 3) were all exceedingly rare at and before the turn of the 20th century. At that time, there were practically no food choices that could be considered to be processed foods. People had no choice but to consume whole, organic, and unprocessed foods. The only fats in the diet came almost exclusively from animal fats, which included plenty of animal meats, whole raw milk, butter, and eggs, with just a smidgen of olive oil (and for some, coconut oil) here and there. And because cows grazed on grass, and particularly green grass anytime it was available, they produced milk (and butter) that was high in the fat-soluble vitamins A, D, and K.

With the introduction of both vegetable oils as well as hydrogenated and partially-hydrogenated vegetable oils (trans fats) into our diets at the turn of the 20th century, there was a gradual displacement of the healthy, vitamin-rich animal fats, which had sustained man in supreme health for thousands of years. This displacement, particularly of lard and butter, led to a severe reduction in the consumption of the fat-soluble vitamins A, D, and K.

With the advent of roller mill technology and the consequent replacement of millstones for the grinding of wheat (and other grains), there was the introduction of refined flours, which are associated with the displacement of B vitamins and minerals that are present in whole grains. This is particularly important for wheat, which plays a pivotal role in the Western diet. Simultaneously, increasing consumption of sugar further displaced nutrient-dense foods, of any and all varieties.

The indictment of saturated fat and cholesterol, as causative factors in heart disease, combined and exacerbated by a low-fat diet recommendation, further displaced the consumption of the healthy saturated animal fats, such as butter, lard, and eggs.

The untoward health effect of all of these factors combined cannot even begin to be calculated. However, the net effect appears to be consistent with a dramatic increase in heart disease, cancer, degenerative diseases, inflammatory diseases, and... macular degeneration. In the next chapter, we'll explore these details further – and perhaps we'll begin to understand a little more deeply, just exactly how and why modern diets have wreaked such havoc in our lives.

10 THE PERILS OF "DISPLACING FOODS" *PART I: VEGETABLE OILS & TRANS FATS*

"The introduction of industrial food processing has without a doubt had the most detrimental effect on our health of any other factor in the last few hundred years - and possibly in the entire history of humankind."

~ Chris Kresser ~

In 2011, a gentleman by the name of Mr. Squires came into my office. At the age of 94, he presented for his "first eye exam in 30 years." He just wanted a checkup to "be sure there was nothing wrong." Mr. Squires was about 6'4", maybe 210 pounds, absolutely one of the fittest, most alert, composed, energetic, and supremely kind people I have ever met. He had absolutely no diseases at all – no heart trouble, high-blood pressure, cancer… nothing - not even arthritis. I could swear to you he didn't look a day over 70 – and fitter than most anyone I'd ever seen over age 60. He was still running his own farm.

I completed a dilated eye examination. Incredibly, he had absolutely no cataracts (I've witnessed this twice in 24 years of ophthalmology practice, i.e., a patient older than 90 without cataracts). His maculae were as pristine as most 40 year-olds – not the slightest macular degeneration – not even one detectable druse (drusen is plural), even with ocular coherence tomography (OCT), which is the ophthalmologists version of an MRI of the retina.

I asked Mr. Squires what and how he had eaten throughout his life. He said, "Well, I grew up on a farm and then I started my own farm. We've always raised our own beef and chickens – and collected their eggs - and mostly eaten from our own gardens. We drink the (raw) milk and make butter from one of our cows. My neighbor raises his own grass-fed cattle and chickens too. So we just swap animals, 'cause neither one of us wants to eat our own!"

Contrast that anecdote with this one: Just days after Mr. Squires came in, Mr. Don H. presented to me, at the age of 51. He was about 6'2", but 340 pounds – morbidly obese, with high-blood pressure, congestive heart-failure, two previous heart attacks, renal (kidney) disease, osteoarthritis, irritable bowel disease, and he was on 16 medications. He was "disabled due to heart failure." An examination of his eyes showed he had early cataracts and moderate AMD (2+ soft drusen) both eyes, with best-corrected vision of 20/25 in each eye.

I asked Mr. H. what he ate. In summary, he said, "Cereal and milk for breakfast, ham and cheese sandwiches on white bread or maybe peanut butter and jelly for lunch, quite a few frozen burritos, and… well, a fair amount of fast food for dinners." I asked what he drank and if he ate snacks, to which he replied, "I like to drink some Dr. Peppers here and there, and a 24 ounce Gatorade [made with sugar, of course] at night. I snack on some potato chips and – maybe a candy bar here and there, but not too often."

Now, let me ask you: Do you think that diet has anything to do with the drastic differences in the health of these two gentlemen? Perhaps the presence of AMD? Let me tell you, anecdotally, I have briefly interviewed thousands of patients regarding their diets over the years. Similar scenarios played out in my exam rooms, over and over – and over.

If it's not clear to you, please notice that Mr. Squires consumed virtually nothing but pasture raised (free-range) beef, chickens, and their eggs, along with organic fruits and vegetables from his own garden, primarily. He and his family drank raw (unpasteurized) milk and made butter from the same. There was virtually nothing in his diet that could be considered processed.

Mr. Don H., on the other hand, consumed a diet that was virtually entirely processed. Cereal (processed grains) and pasteurized (processed) milk for breakfast, sandwiches made with processed meats, or peanut butter and jelly, all on white bread (all man-made, processed foods), factory-produced burritos, and fast-foods frequently at night. He drank a large amount of sugar in his drinks. None of the meats he consumed were pasture-raised and, in fact, most all of his meats were processed, as was virtually everything else in his diet. Mr H's diet was atrocious. It was an absolute metabolic and nutritional disaster, severely nutrient-deficient, lacking in vitamins and minerals, and chock-full of man-made, processed, high omega-6 vegetable oils, refined sugars, and refined flour. If there were ever a quintessential diet – a poster-child diet – if you will, for what Weston A. Price referred to as a diet containing the "'displacing foods of modern commerce,'" this was it. And Mr. Don H. was paying the price for it I am very sorry to say. I could fill this book with similar examples.

VEGETABLE OILS

As far as most of the world was concerned, at the beginning of the 20th century, the only edible oil-producing crop present anywhere on the planet would have been olive trees, which were grown primarily in Europe with much smaller crops in California.[321],[322] Most of the world relied almost exclusively on animal fats, such as lard, butter, and beef tallow, for cooking purposes.[323]

In the year 1900, U.S. inventor and manufacturer Mr. Valerius D. Anderson, successfully produced the first continuously operated Expellar® press, which would dramatically increase the efficiency of extracting oils from seeds as well as initiate the beginning of what would become an entire industry surrounding the production and sale of "vegetable oils." This technology would eventually lead to the development of the so called Edible Oil Industry.[324] Incidentally, I sometimes put the term vegetable oils in quotes, because these oils don't actually come from vegetables at all. These oils mostly come from seeds and would be better termed "seed oils," with the exception of corn oil (a grain) and soybean oil (a legume).

The first seed oil produced, however, was actually cottonseed oil and early on – it was far from being considered a potential food item. Cottonseed oil was first produced in the late 18th century on a very small scale. A Professor Olmstead, at the University of North Carolina, had "ascertained that a fine illuminating gas may be obtained from cottonseed." [325] Indeed, the purpose at that time was to illuminate homes and businesses with gas lamps running on the oil. It was used for a time as a lubricant for machinery but for most of the 19th century it was utilized as lamp oil. By many accounts, it was said to compare favorably with whale oil.[326]

In the 1850s, cottonseed oil was demonstrated to be edible. After the American Civil War (1861 - 1865) – the demand for edible oil began to increase and by 1880, the Southern U.S. had produced some forty-one cottonseed oil mills. According to author H.C. Nixon, "There was French complaint in 1880 that refined cottonseed oil was reaching France under the name of olive oil from Spain and Italy. With New Orleans shipping 73,782 barrels to Europe, including 40,000 barrels to Italy, in the year ending August 31, 1879, there might be a question as to spurious olive oil, concerning which 'the world must draw its own conclusions.'" "The new product," Nixon continued, "was destined to circle the globe in competition with olive oil and eventually under correct labels." [327] Cottonseed oil, from it's beginnings as lamp oil and machine oil, had become edible oil by 1880 and a competitor of olive oil in some markets. Eventually, it would become a major competitor of butter and lard. The first "vegetable oil" had been introduced to the world and was gaining much ground by the end of that century.

Today, the so-called vegetable oils are extracted not only from cottonseed, but from soybeans (soybean oil), corn, rapeseed (canola oil), sunflower, safflower, cottonseed, grapeseed, peanut, and a few others. The edible oil industry, capitalizing on the marketing and sale of oils that were less expensive than lard, butter, or olive oil, would become a mega-industry. Ultimately, this industry would sell hundreds of millions of tons of vegetable oils, every year, to global markets – all from these highly processed, heated and chemically treated oils that simply did not exist in our food supply until nearly the turn of the 20th century. In the last few decades, the typical American grocery store has an entire section of the store that is devoted to vegetable oils.

According to the research of Loren Cordain, PhD, and his colleagues at Colorado State University, **"In the United States, during the 90-year period from 1909 to 1999, a**

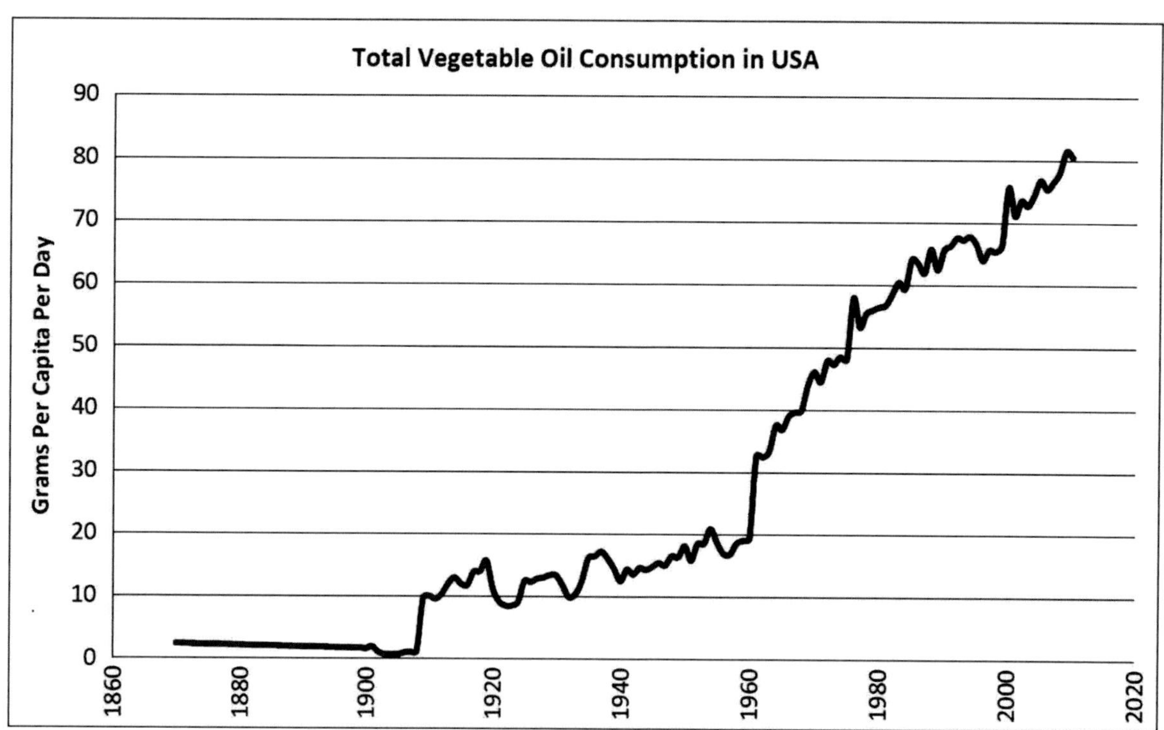

FIGURE 10.1 **Per capita consumption of vegetable oils in the United States, 1880 to 2011.**

References: For data of 1870 – 1899: Calculation of vegetable oils (linseed, cotton, castor, poppy seed and rape seed) produced per capita, Census 1870 and Population 1790-1990.

For data from 1899 – 1908: Margarine, presented as Apparent Civilian Per *Capita Consumption of Foods: 1849-1970, Historiical Statistic* of the U.S. Colonial Times to 1970, U.S. Dept. of Commerce, p. 331, *https://www.census.gov/history/pdf/histstats-colonial-1970.pdf*

For data from 1909 – 1960: Vegetable margarine and shortening, Added fats and oils (fat-content basis): Total and per capita food availability, USDA Economic Research Service.

For data from 1961 – 2011: SUM of vegetable oils FAOSTAT, Food Balances, *http://faostat3.fao.org/download/FB/FBS/E*

striking increase in the use of vegetable oils occurred. Specifically, per capita consumption of salad and cooking oils increased 130%, shortening consumption increased 136%, and margarine consumption increased 410%." [328] These are tremendously large increases in consumption, however, had the comparisons begun just 30 years earlier, that is, in 1879 rather than 1909 – the result would have been infinitely greater in the consumption of cooking oil, shortening, and margarine. This is true because cottonseed oil, i.e., "cooking oil," didn't become available until 1880, "shortening," a term used to refer to cooking fat, is generally made from vegetable oils which are often hydrogenated (trans fats), and "margarine," a term used for butter substitutes, is also generally made from vegetable oils, some of which are hydrogenated and generally mixed with smaller amounts of animal fats.[329]

According to the USDA Economic Research Service, "per capita availability of added fats and oils (unadjusted for waste and spoilage) reached about 86 pounds per person in 2005, up 33 pounds from 1970. Of the 2005 total, nearly 86 percent consisted of vegetable oils and related products, such as margarine, shortening, and cooking and salad oils. Animal fats, such as butter, lard and edible tallow {beef fat}, made up the remaining 14 percent." [330] **This is a staggering statistic, that is, 86% of 86 pounds is 74 pounds of added vegetable oils and related products per person, per year.** Recall that, from the research of Loren Cordain, in the year 1900, the consumption of olive oil (generally, the only available oil at that time) would have been in the range of about 0.5 pounds per year.[331] **Alternatively stated, in the year 1900, approximately 99% of the added fats in cooking would have been in the form of animal fats (i.e, butter, lard, and beef tallow), whereas by 2005, that number had dropped to 14 percent!** And we're supposed to believe that saturated animal fats cause heart disease?

After adjusting for losses, the USDA Economic Research Service showed that in the year 2005, the average per capita food supply in the U.S. provided 59.6 grams a day of vegetable fats and oils (salad and cooking oil, shortening, margarine, and other edible fats and oils).[332] If we convert 59.6 grams of oil (9 calories per gram) into calories, we get 536 calories. **On a 2,200 calorie per day diet, this means that vegetable oils account for about 24% of the caloric total!** Keep this number in mind because we're going to reference this again.

Globally, Barry Popkin, PhD, showed that the "Principal vegetable oils include soybean, sunflower, rapeseed, palm, and groundnut [peanut] oil. With the exception of groundnut oil, global availability of each has approximately tripled between 1961 and 1990." [333] This level of consumption also makes vegetable oils significant proxies – "markers" if you will – for processed food consumption.

How They're Made... In 1971, Organic Merchants representatives Paul Hawken and Fred Rohe, authors of a brief paper, "The Dangers of Vegetable Oil Extraction and Processing", wrote "One very basic difference between our way of looking at vegetable oils and the industrial oil technician's viewpoint should be understood. When he sees dark color, it represents the presence of 'impurities' – material that prevents the oil from being light colored, odorless and bland in taste. From our viewpoint, those 'impurities' look desirable – the things which impart color, odor and flavor are NUTRIENTS. It is both tragic and ironic that removal of nutrients should be equated with 'purity'. Tragic because if those nutrients were present they would contribute to the health of the consumer. Ironic because establishing the desired 'purity' really results in producing poor quality food." [334]

The process of making vegetable oils is so complicated, that I'm just going to give you the extremely condensed version. First, the seeds are harvested. Note: if the beginning product is soybean, canola (rapeseed), or corn, in the U.S. there is a 95 percent chance they're also GMO. The seeds are husked, cleaned, and crushed. Then, they're heated to temperatures varying from 110 to 180 degrees Fahrenheit, usually using steam. The seeds are then run through a high-heat seed press, where they are crushed to begin oil extraction. The resulting pulp and oil is then placed in a petroleum-derived hexane solvent bath and heated again with steam. The product is centrifuged and phosphate is added to help separate oil and seed residue. Next, the hexane is boiled off and further evaporated, as it is otherwise toxic in and of itself. Regardless, the hexane remains in the oil at up to 100 parts per million.[335] The resulting "crude vegetable oil" then undergoes degumming to remove phosphatides ("gums"), followed by the addition of caustic soda or soda ash in a procedure called neutralization, and then the oil is bleached with agents such as fuller's earth, activated carbon, or activated clay. Finally, the oil is deodorized with pressurized steam, at temperatures exceeding 500 degrees Fahrenheit.[336]

An excellent and professionally made video demonstrating the process of making Canola oil is available on *YouTube.com* under the name, "How It's Made – Canola Oil." [337] This process may be fairly well generalized to most all vegetable oils. Ironically, this four-minute video is an attempt to sell the viewer on the healthful benefits of canola oil, because "It has the lowest level of saturated fat – seven percent. It also contains more healthy omega-3 fatty acids and is high in monounsaturated fat, which lowers cholesterol."[338] This kind of advertising, combined with these kinds of products, is exactly why those who have bought into this marketing, these products, and this line of reasoning are often riddled with disease. If this isn't clear to you just yet, I promise it will be by the end of this book.

Every step that requires heat, pressure, and chemicals may produce oxidized products that would smell and taste rancid, except for the deodorizing procedure.[339] These highly oxidized fatty acids are extremely dangerous products when consumed. The vitamin E, chlorophyll, and carotenoid pigments are mostly destroyed in this process. Manufacturers often add BHT and BHA in attempt to replace the vitamin E, however, both of these substances have been suspected of causing cancer and brain damage.[340]

The expeller press is the only other method of oil production for so-called vegetable oils. This method utilizes a screw or continuous press with a constantly rotating worm shaft. The heated or cooked raw material goes into one end and is put under continuous pressure until discharged at the other end, while the oil is squeezed out. With this technology, temperatures usually range between 200 and 250 degrees and this technique cannot, therefore, be considered "cold pressed." This technique should be referred to as "expeller pressed."

Contrast these methods with the gentle method of oil extraction by way of the hydraulic press. This is the only method of oil extraction which literally and truly can be called "cold pressed," and only sesame seeds and olives will yield enough oil to be processed this way. Hence, their superior nature in every respect, particularly in regard to our health. According to Hawken and Rohe, Organic Merchants only use the term "virgin" for olive oil produced via "the first pressing by a hydraulic press without heat" whereas the term "'cold pressed' will refer only to hydraulic pressing without heat." They go on to state, "These oils are the closest possible to the natural state, therefore have the most color, odor and flavor – in a word, the most NUTRITION – but they will often be unavailable because so little is produced this way."[341]

According to Hemi Weingarten of Fooducate (*Fooducate.com*), regarding the term "cold pressed, he states, "Some companies go to great efforts to maintain a temperature below 90 degrees Fahrenheit when pressing the oil. In Europe the term "cold pressed" is regulated and oils cannot exceed that temperature. But in the US, there is no such regulation. Cold pressed could mean anything under 400 degrees…" [342]

Omega-6 to Omega-3 Ratios and Vegetable Oils … I think almost everyone has heard of the omega-3 fatty acids and I presume most everyone has heard of the omega-6 fatty acids too. Most people seem to know that they need more omega-3 fats. That's true, because both the amount of these fats and their ratios play a huge role in inflammation, which seems to play a fundamental role in "diseases of civilization." But *it won't help in the long run to just supplement omega-3 fish oils*, for example, without changing your diet. Let's investigate why.

There are just two essential fatty acids in the human diet. This means we must get these from diet, because we cannot make them. One is the *omega-6 linoleic acid (LA)*, which predominates in vegetable oils. The second, is the *omega-3 alpha linolenic acid (ALA)*, which predominates in fish and is much more prominent in cattle (beef, mutton, etc.) raised on grass. Excellent sources of the omega- 3 ALA include fish, eggs, whole milk, regular cheese, beef, nuts and seeds (particularly walnuts).[343]

It has generally been concluded that the ratios of these two fatty acids are exceedingly important to inflammation – and that inflammation plays a role in numerous Western diseases, including cardiovascular disease, cancer, osteoporosis, and inflammatory and autoimmune diseases.[344]

However, what you will see is that it is not just the ratios that are important. If that were the case, we would have solved this problem with a boatload of omega-3 supplements, like flaxseed oil and fish oil. That obviously is an oversimplification and it hasn't worked. It's more about the "dose" of these oils – particularly the "over-dose" of omega-6 oils as a result of our mega vegetable oil consumption. Let's look at the details…

Omega-3 fatty acids certainly have anti-inflammatory effects, such as the reduction of interleukin 1β, tumor necrosis factor-α (TNF-α), and interleukin-6, whereas the omega-6 fatty acids do not have such properties.[345] The omega-6 linoleic acid (LA) is converted in our bodies to arachidonic acid (AA) – a mediator of inflammation - whereas the omega-3 alpha linolenic-acid (ALA) may be converted to eicosapentaenoic acid (EPA) and the critically important, docosahexaenoic acid (DHA) – both of which have anti-inflammatory effects.[346]

You've probably heard of EPA and DHA, because they're prominent in fish oil. If one is given ALA (18 carbons and 3 double bonds) in the diet, the body can synthesize EPA (20 carbons and 5 double bonds) and DHA (22 carbons and 6 double bonds).[347] However, we still need to realize that the omega-3 ALA and the omega-6 LA are both polyunsaturated fatty acids (PUFA) and that the requirements for PUFAs is very, very small. This is consistent with the consumption of these oils by our healthy 19th century ancestors.

There is tremendous interest in the omega-3 and -6 fatty acids, particularly the long-chain omega-3 fats EPA and DHA and their ratio to the long-chain omega-6 arachidonic acid – and rightly so. The assertion, repeated often, is that the "ratio of omega-6 to omega-3 is too high in Western diets." Artemis Simopoulos, MD, endocrinologist and Founder of the Center for Genetics, Nutrition and Health, in Washington, D.C., has done much research and publication in this area. In 2006, she referenced the fact that our Western diet was deficient in omega-3 with a ratio of omega-6 to omega-3 of somewhere between 15:1 and 16.7:1, instead of the 1:1 ratio that was believed to be the case with wild animals and our distant ancestors.[348] Much research backed her assertion.[349] [350] [351] [352] [353] [354] [355] Simopoulos' earlier study, in 1991, showed that the typical American diet already contained between 11 to 30 times more omega-6 than omega-3 fatty acids, which should likely dramatically contribute to inflammatory disorders.[356]

As a result of this well-confirmed recognition that the ratio of our omega-6 to omega-3 ratio was just too high, we collectively began to treat this primarily with the pouring on of the omega-3 fatty acids. This was accomplished by increasing consumption of flax seed oil and fish oil, primarily. This has had limited, but definite success, even with heart disease.[357] [358]

In 2011, the entire landscape would begin to change, however, regarding this assertion that it's all about the omega-3: omega-6 *ratio*, as bona fide evidence began to emerge regarding the tissue-level consequences of such high consumption of PUFAs, in the form of vegetable oils.

Nutritional neuroscience researchers, Dr. Tanya Blasbalg and colleagues, at the National Institutes of Health in Bethesda, Maryland, systematically quantified the intake of the omega-6 LA and the omega-3 ALA, from the years 1909 to 1999. They modeled expected intake of these fatty acids in 1909 using traditional early 20th century dietary practices as well as the foods that would come from early 1900's farming and breeding techniques. **First of all, this research shows that the estimated consumption of soybean oil increased more than 1000-fold between 1909 to 1999, from 0.006% to 7.38% of energy.**[359] In fact, in 1999, soybean oil was our fourth greatest contributor of calories, only behind sugar, dairy, and grains. **This brilliant research also shows that, from 1909 to 1999, the consumption of the omega-6 LA increased from 2.79% to 7.21% of energy, whereas the omega-3 ALA increased from 0.39% to 0.72% of energy. The ratio of omega-6:3 ratio increased from 5.4:1 in 1909 to 9.6:1 in 1999.**[360]

Blasbalg's research also showed that the consumption of the long-chain omega-6 fats (arachidonic acid – AA) and omega-3 fats (EPA and DHA), both decreased since 1909.[364] These fatty acids decreased because animals in recent decades are primarily fed soy and grains, whereas in the early 20th century cattle were almost exclusively grass fed and, of course, we've largely replaced the consumption of animal fats in our own diets with seed oils.

Dr. Blasbalg and her colleagues did something even more brilliant. They utilized a reliable and proven model to determine the relative presence of omega-3 fats at the tissue level, that is, in cell membranes, based on the 1909 versus 1999 diets.[365] **This showed a decrease of omega-3 fatty acids in cell membranes of 38% from 1909 as compared to 1999. This is a drastic reduction in omega-3 fatty acids and this is also indicative of a decrease in EPA and DHA at the tissue level, which may play a tremendous role in the development of disease.**[366] Previous research conclusively shows that there is competition for the omega-3 and omega-6 fats at the tissue level and that dietary proportions of these fats are critical determinants of the proportions of these fatty acids in cellular membranes.[367] As far as whether its omega-3 or omega-6 fatty acids that end up in cell membranes, research has repeatedly shown that excess omega-6 linoleic acid – as we get with the typical American (Western) diet – ultimately inhibits omega-3's from ending up in cell membranes.[368 369 370 371]

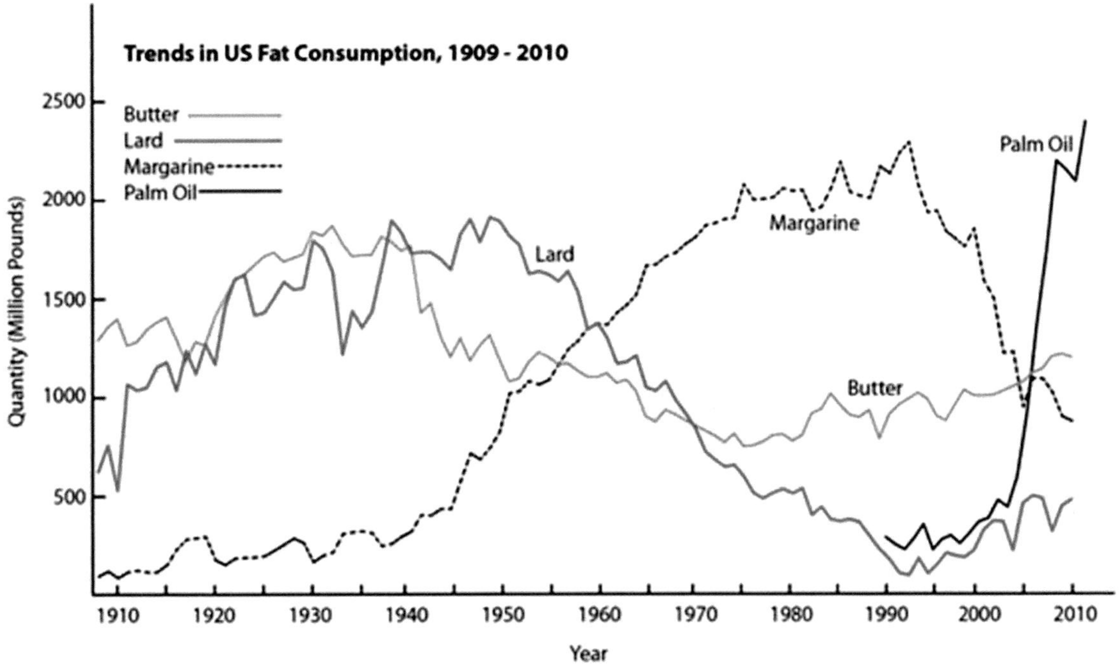

If we assume that early Americans in 1909 consumed the same calories per day that Americans did in 1971, which is approximately 1955 calories per day (NHANES 1971) and we know that Americans were consuming approximately 2250 calories per day in 1999 (NHANES 1999-2000),[361] **this translates to a consumption of just 5.0 grams per day of omega-6 LA and 0.76 grams per day of omega-3 ALA in 1909, whereas those numbers increased to 18 grams omega-6 and 1.8 grams omega-3 in 1999.** Many studies corroborate this typical high level of PUFA intake in industrialized societies.[362 363]

The total consumption of both omega-3 and omega-6 in 1909 was just about 5.76 grams per day, which came mostly from animal fats (e.g., butter, lard, beef tallow) and that increased to a whopping 19.8 grams per day in 1999. In a nutshell, consumption of omega-6 fats tripled and omega-3 fats doubled during this interval of time.

Neurobiologist, obesity researcher, and author, Stephan Guyenet, PhD, at the University of Washington, compiled the data on the accumulation of omega-6 fat, linoleic acid, in the body fat of humans based on six different U.S. studies between the years 1961 and 2008.[372 373 374 375 376 377 378] That data was compiled into a graph by Dr. Guyenet, and is presented below.

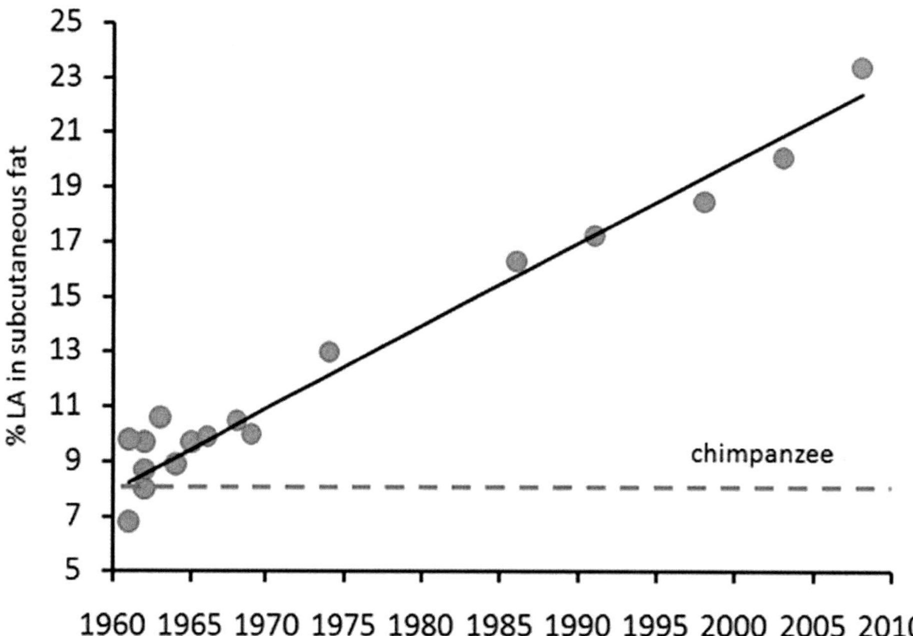

Omega-6 fat, Linoleic Acid, in the fat tissue of U.S. subjects, 1960 – 2010.
Graph courtesy of Stephan Guyenet, PhD (WholeHealthSource.org)

As we can see, many studies confirm that these changes in consumption of omega-3 versus omega-6 fats are directly linked to increasing consumption of these fatty acids, with omega-6 fats steadily increasing in the tissues of our bodies. Many disease conditions have been linked to the proportions of the omega-3 and omega-6 fatty acids in tissues, including everything from sudden cardiac death, to psychiatric conditions, to ulcerative colitis.[379 380 381]

DRASTIC CHANGES IN OMEGA-6 AND OMEGA-3 PUFAS APPEAR TO BE A MAJOR FACTOR IN AMD

Getting back to the eye and to macular degeneration, researchers have conclusively shown that the long-chain omega-3 PUFA's, particularly DHA, are present in abundance in the human retina, and that these fatty acids exert structural, functional, and neuro-protective roles.[382 383] **The highest concentration of DHA in the retina is in – *the photoreceptors* – where it plays a crucial role in their differentiation (during development) as well as their function and survival.**[384] It is critical to understand that the long-chain omega-3 PUFAs, such as EPA and DHA, play critical anti-inflammatory roles[385] and inflammation is thought to potentially play a pivotal role in the development of AMD.[386]

According to French researchers Doctor Marie-Noëlle Delyfer, Dr. Benjamin Buaud, and colleagues, at the University de Bordeaux, "The neuroprotective role of omega-3 LC-PUFAs in AMD has been demonstrated by a number of epidemiologic studies that observed a decreased risk for AMD in subjects with high intakes of omega-3 LC-PUFAs. Among other potential mechanisms supporting neuroprotection, it has been suggested that dietary intake of omega-3 LC-PUFAs may favor the retinal accumulation of lutein and zeaxanthin and thereby increase macular pigment density." [387]

The question is: Could this doubling of consumption of omega-3 and tripling of consumption of omega-6 fats, as a result of enormously increased consumption of vegetable oils (PUFAs), along with an approximate 38% reduction in omega-3 fats in our tissues, also play a role in AMD? To a certain extent, this question was addressed by the Age Related Eye Disease Study (AREDS) group back in 2007. The AREDS group looked at a number of potential causative factors in AMD, and lipids consumption was one "arm" of that study.

The AREDS study was highly structured and complex in design, however, the over-simplified design of the study was such that a total of 4757 participants from 11 different retina clinics, between the ages of 55 and 80, were enrolled and evaluated. They were classified into five different groups based on presence and degree of AMD, with group 1 being free of drusen or with "nonextensive small drusen" (considered the control group), group 2 with intermediate AMD, group 3 with intermediate AMD including large drusen, group 4 with the worse form of AMD called geographic atrophy (GA), and group 5 with either current wet AMD or the presence of signs of previous wet AMD, such as macular scars. The subjects all completed food-frequency questionnaires (FFQ) and then highly complex analyses completed in order to quantify and qualify the various lipids consumed.

In this arm of the AREDS research, the researchers found the following:

1. Subjects consuming higher levels of omega-3 fats and higher omega-3 rich foods had a lower likelihood of developing wet AMD
2. Subjects in the top 20% of omega-3 consumption were 40% less likely to develop AMD during the study
3. There were trends of decreasing likelihood of wet AMD with increasing intake of the long-chain omega-3 PUFA's, such as EPA and DHA, as well as total omega-3's.
4. Subjects who were in the top 20% of consumption of the omega-6 fat, arachidonic acid (AA), which is present in great amounts in vegetable oils, were 1.5 times more likely to be in the wet AMD group than participants in the lowest 20% AA consumption group.
5. Of the long-chain omega-3 PUFAs (EPA and DHA), the greatest protective effects for wet AMD were for those people consuming the most DHA (typically, high fish consumption). [388]

The AREDS study and its findings add a very important element to our understanding of the genesis of AMD. This study underscores the position that AMD (or wet AMD, in this study) is much less prevalent in those who consume higher amounts of omega-3 fats. Secondly, it shows that those consuming the highest amounts of omega-6 fats, such as arachidonic acid (AA), which are abundant in vegetable oils, have the greatest chance of developing wet AMD. The researchers write, "These results and those from other observational analytic investigations suggest that modifying diet to include more foods rich in omega-3 LCPUFAs {long-chain PUFAs} could result in a reduction in the risk of having NV {neovascular, or wet} AMD." [389]

Given the evidence we've seen from Dr. Blasbalg's study and the fact that we now understand that there is competition for the omega-3 and omega-6 PUFA's in cellular membranes, along with the critical roles that the long-chain omega-3 fats exhibit in our retina, I would submit that eliminating the vegetable oils from our diets is a major and critical step in preventing AMD and/or preventing its progression.

Regarding the AREDS group's findings in this study, I would also submit that the results would have been tremendously more dramatic, had a true control group been represented in this study. In this study, the "control group" (group 1) was a group that was defined by either having no drusen or "nonextensive small drusen," that is, these subjects had little or no true AMD, despite many having some early and small drusen. In my opinion, however, *all groups in the study were actually in the "experimental group,"* if you will. In other words, all groups are drawn from American people that were consuming some variation of the standard American diet, presumably virtually all of which already had relatively high consumption of vegetable oils, trans fats, refined flour and sugar, and likely very low in micro-nutrients, particularly fat-soluble vitamins and minerals. This is what Stephan Guyenet, PhD, sometimes refers to as comparing "the sick to the sicker." [390] The perfect control group, on the other hand, would be one that consumed a traditional diet of our ancestors – a diet consistent with pre-year 1880 American traditions and conditions. Yes, I realize that no such groups likely even exist in the U.S.A. and that there are darn few Jack LaLanne types running around. But, as I said, that would make the perfect control group – and had such a control group existed, I firmly believe the results would have been much more dramatic. Nevertheless, the AREDS group did the best they could with what they had – groups of Americans, most all consuming some variation of the Standard American Diet presumably, with the groups having the worst AMD also consuming the most omega-6 fats, that is, consuming the most vegetable oils (among other problems).

VEGETABLE OILS, CARDIOVASCULAR DISEASE, CANCER, AND MORE...

The polyunsaturated oils, that is, the vegetable oils, are highly unstable oils. Because the polyunsaturated oils have unpaired electrons (not paired to hydrogen atoms), they tend to become oxidized when subjected to heat, light, oxygen, and water. As we've seen, they're subjected to all of these conditions to extreme degrees during nearly every phase of their production. According to Sally Fallon, of the Weston A. Price Foundation, these rancid oils and their associated free radicals "...are extremely reactive chemically. They have been characterized as 'marauders' in the body for they attack cell membranes and red blood cells, causing damage in DNA/RNA strands that can trigger mutations in tissue, blood vessels and skin. Free radical damage to the skin causes wrinkles and premature aging, free radical damage to the tissues and organs sets the stage for tumors, and free radical damage in the blood vessels initiates the build-up of plaque. Is it any wonder that tests and studies have repeatedly shown a high correlation between cancer and heart disease with the consumption of polyunsaturates?"[391]

Indeed, the research backs up Fallon's statements, among other things, showing that polyunsaturated fats increase oxidative stress,[392,393] decrease nitric oxide production causing vascular endothelial cell dysfunction[394] (which may associate with high blood pressure), and also cause increased endothelial cell inflammation[395] leading the path to vascular diseases including coronary artery disease.[396]

Again, summarizing a boatload of scientific research that backs up her statements, Sally Fallon writes, **"Excess consumption of polyunsaturated oils has been shown to contribute to a large number of disease conditions including increased cancer and heart disease, immune system dysfunction, damage to the liver, reproductive**

organs and lungs, digestive disorders, depressed learning ability, impaired growth, and weight gain." [397]

VEGETABLE OILS AND BLOOD LIPIDS (LDL, HDL, OXIDIZED LDL)

So we're told that vegetable oils reduce LDL, the supposed "bad" cholesterol carrying molecule, right? Yes, it's true. Vegetable oils do reduce LDL,[398 399 400] however, these same studies show vegetable oil consumption causes reductions in HDL (or subfractions of HDL), the "good" cholesterol carrier. Subsequently, I'll show you that reducing LDL is generally not even beneficial. In any case, high levels of HDL have also been shown to decrease the risk of heart disease.[401 402] So we sure don't want to be decreasing HDL.

Fred Kummerow, PhD, a scientist at the University of Illinois who is lauded by numerous colleagues for his pioneering work, was the first scientist to publish evidence that linked trans fats to heart disease. Simultaneously, he exonerated saturated fat and cholesterol. Incredibly, that was 1957. Today, at 101 years of age, Dr. Kummerow is the oldest living active scientist and he continues to help unravel the supposed mysteries of heart disease, though they really haven't been mysteries to him at all.

Just in the past several years, Dr. Kummerow authored or co-authored two papers in scientific journals in which he indicts an excess of polyunsaturated (vegetable) oils as having major responsibility in the development of atherosclerosis.[403 404] In essence, he reports that LDL, the supposed "bad cholesterol," is not the problem at all. What really matters is whether or not those LDL particles have become oxidized. And this is where things get really interesting.

Dr. Kummerow says, **"Cholesterol has nothing to do with heart disease, except if it's oxidized."**[405] **He goes on to explain that the process of oxidation of LDL particles is particularly severe when consumed vegetable oils are subjected to high temperatures such as in frying. But even without frying, these unstable molecules, once consumed, are highly likely to become destructive and dangerous parts of LDL particles.** As a result of their unstable molecular structure, the polyunsaturated oils simply oxidize easily, which is in great contrast to the stability of the saturated fatty acids, which are found in animal fats, butter, lard, coconut oil, palm and palm kernel oils.

Where the science begins to point its finger at vegetable oils is when we see what these oils are doing to LDL particles. What the research conclusively shows is that these nasty polyunsaturated oils wiggle their way into our LDL particles where they, not surprisingly, make them much more likely to oxidize, just as Dr. Kummerow said.[406,407,408,409,410,411]

These oxidized (again, think rancid) LDL particles are the beginning of a crucial step in heart disease as these particles are the ones that deposit in the vascular endothelial cells and begin the development of plaques in arterial walls.[412] Japanese researchers from the University School of Pharmaceutical Sciences, in Tokyo, state, **"Accumulating evidence indicates that oxidized low-density lipoprotein (OxLDL) is a useful marker for cardiovascular disease. The uptake of OxLDL by scavenger receptors leads to the accumulation of cholesterol within the foam cells of atherosclerotic lesions."** They go on to state, "In the last three decades, a large volume of studies have established that oxidized low-density lipoprotein (OxLDL) is a useful marker for cardiovascular disease (CVDs). The measurement of OxLDL correlates with the presence of CVDs and indicates that OxLDL is a potential prognostic marker for future health events. OxLDL is known to stimulate macrophages to induce foam cell formation and inflammatory responses." [413]

Finnish researcher Pohjantähti and colleagues reviewed and summarized 50 different studies that support the conclusion that atherosclerosis is strongly tied to oxidized LDL and that this is strongly tied to metabolic syndrome (abdominal obesity, high blood pressure, abnormal blood lipids, and insulin resistance with associated pre-diabetes or diabetes).[414]

Thus, we have not only the beginning, but the perpetuation of atherosclerosis as a result largely of oxidized LDL. Chris Masterjohn, PhD, who holds his doctorate degree in Nutritional Sciences and is currently Professor of Health and Nutrition Sciences at Brooklyn College at the City University of New York, has published numerous articles and discussed this hypothesis for heart disease in great detail.[415,416]

In simplified form, what we see is that the concentration of LDL cholesterol in the blood has virtually no relationship to the development of atherosclerosis, rather, it is the duration and presence of oxidized-LDL in the blood that is associated with the development of atherosclerosis. Oxidized-LDL is taken up by the endothelial cells lining our arteries as a means of removing these dangerous particles from the blood. The macrophages of the vascular wall (intima layer) have "scavenger receptors" which ingest and clean up these nasty oxidized-LDL particles, in the process becoming "foam cells." [417] The accumulation of Ox-LDL in the foam cells of atherosclerotic lesions has been demonstrated using monoclonal antibodies, in human coronary and carotid arteries, and in the aortas of rabbits.[418,419,420,421] Eventually, a core of cellular debris, oxidized and crystallized cholesterol, calcium, and dead cells develop in the intima layer, with overlying smooth muscle cells and endothelium – the "fibrous cap." This is the atherosclerotic plaque.[422] Should the plaque rupture, a thrombus (clot) develops at that site and, of course, if it is large enough to occlude the lumen of the vessel, an infarct occurs. If that is in the heart, that's a myocardial infarction – heart attack.

The important thing to realize is that it is oxidized-LDL that appears to accumulate in atherosclerotic plaques – and for most people, the oxidized-LDL comes primarily from the consumption of polyunsatured vegetable oils.

Bringing this back to macular degeneration, it is known that the retinal pigment epithelium (RPE) cells have LDL receptors – and these receptors then are meant to take up LDL.[423] Naturally, they would. Every cell must have lipids and cholesterol. Much research has confirmed that LDL participates in supplying lipids to the retina,[424 425 426] and this is accomplished by way of sending those lipids through the RPE cells.[427 428]

This would lead us to also speculate on the very distinct likelihood that the RPE is taking up these oxidized LDL particles and then they're being deposited into Bruch's membrane, contributing to the lipid deposits found in Bruch's membrane, as well as its thickening, and thereby, decreasing its permeability to nutrients.

In support of this hypothesis, low-density lipoproteins have been found in the retina and the RPE, as they are important to the retina's lipid supply.[429] *If LDL is there, then we also know that oxidized LDL is there, particularly in people consuming polyunsaturated vegetable oils! This was confirmed by Nataliya Gordiyenko, PhD and colleagues, who showed that RPE cells not only take up LDL, but also oxidized LDL, both in great quantities.*[423] *Oxidized LDL levels in the blood have been shown to be higher in AMD patient than in controls.*[430] *And finally, lipid peroxidation products, which are those that come from the oxidation (breakdown) of polyunsaturated fatty acids (PUFAs), among which malondialdehyde (MDA) is the most abundant, have been shown to be dramatically higher in AMD patients ($p < .001$).*[431] *This all makes perfect sense. Perhaps these findings are our strongest evidence indicting oxidized LDL – due to polyunsaturated vegetable oil consumption – in the cause of AMD.*

Not to oversimplify here, as there are unquestionably other factors involved in atherosclerosis, including high blood pressure, smoking, obesity, etc. However, with the exception of smoking, the remaining risk factors (obesity, high blood pressure, diabetes, etc.) are all secondary to our "Westernized diet," that is, the consumption of the 'displacing foods of modern commerce,' meaning that atherosclerosis is directly caused by a processed food-laden diet and, therefore, "runs with" obesity, diabetes, high blood pressure, and, of course, AMD.

In 2001, British researchers from St. Bartholomew's and the Royal London Hospital's School of Medicine reviewed all of the available science and presented a research paper attempting to alert the food industry to the perils of vegetable oils. In the abstract of the paper, the authors wrote:

> "The purpose of this report is to alert the foodservice industry, particularly the fast-food industry, of an emerging health issue. Considerable evidence has accumulated over the past two decades that heated cooking oils, especially polyunsaturated {"vegetable"} oils, may pose several types of health risks to consumers of fried foods and even people working near deep fat fryers. Heat degrades polyunsaturated fatty acids to toxic compounds; saturated {animal} and monounsaturated fatty acids {e.g., oleic acid in olive oil} are resistant to heat-induced degradation. Several types of diseases may be related to the exposure of humans to food- or air-borne breakdown products of heated oils including atherosclerosis, the forerunner to cardiovascular disease; inflammatory joint disease, including rheumatoid arthritis; pathogenic condition of the digestive tract; mutagenicity and genotoxicity, properties that often signal carcinogenesis; and teratogenicity, the property of chemicals that leads to the development of birth defects." [432]

VEGETABLE OILS AND AMD – PERHAPS THE GREATEST SMOKING GUN OF ALL?

If vegetable oil consumption plays a substantial role in atherosclerosis and heart disease via the production of oxidized-LDL, and AMD is characterized by vascular occlusion (atherosclerosis) of the choriocapillaris, which nourishes the outer retina and photoreceptors, shouldn't this be a major risk factor for AMD as well? Many studies suggest this would be true.

A number of researchers have hypothesized that hypertension (high blood pressure) and atherosclerosis, through reduced blood flow in the choroidal vasculature as well as lipid deposition in Bruch's membrane (which reduces permeability), may increase the risk of AMD.[433 434 435 436]

As far back as 1994, a study from Rotterdam, the Netherlands, completed by Johannes Vingerling, MD, Paulus T.V.M. de Jong, MD, and colleagues at the Erasmus University Medical School Rotterdam, entitled "Age-related Macular Degeneration Is Associated with Atherosclerosis" was published in the American Journal of Epidemiology. [437] In this study, the researchers evaluated the carotid arteries of the neck for atherosclerotic disease, as measured by ultrasound, as well as the presence of AMD. In their own words they state, "In subjects younger than age 85 years, plaques in the carotid bifurcation were associated with a 4.7 times increased prevalence odds of macular degeneration; those with plaques in the common carotid artery showed an increased prevalence odds of 2.5."[438] Their research confirmed that lower extremity vascular disease was associated with a 2.5 fold greater chance of having AMD as well. The authors wrote, "These findings suggest that atherosclerosis may be involved in the etiology of age-related macular degeneration."[439]

Researchers from the University of Sydney, in Sydney, Australia, found that patients with stenosis greater than 50% in any coronary artery had nearly a two-fold greater chance of having AMD; they also found that those who had obstructive coronary artery disease in all three main vessels of the heart had a 2.67 fold greater chance of having AMD.[440] Ronald Klein, MD, and colleagues at the University of Wisconsin, studied over 11,500 adults ranging in age from 48 to 72 years of age, and found that carotid artery plaque and focal retinal arteriolar narrowing (a sign of atherosclerosis) were 1.77 and 1.79-fold more likely, respectively, in patients with an early sign of AMD, known as "retinal pigment epithelial depigmentation."[441]

In another study by Dr. Ron Klein and colleagues, subjects with AMD were more likely to have cerebral white matter lesions, which are indicative of small vessel disease (strokes, on a small scale) in the brain, and to have lower total cholesterol (yes, lower).[442] The authors wrote, "The association with small vessel strokes as we report here suggests a possible role of hypertensive small vessel disease, possibly in larger choroidal vessels, in the pathogenesis of ARM [Age-Related Maculopathy - same as AMD}.

In a study presented in 2001 by Johanna Seddon, MD, and colleagues at the Massachusetts Eye and Ear Infirmary, Harvard Medical School, the investigators found that **"higher vegetable fat consumption was associated with an elevated risk for AMD. After adjusting for age, sex, education, cigarette smoking, and other risk factors, the odds ratio (OR) was 2.22 for persons in the highest vs those in the lowest quintiles of intake (P for trend, .007)."** [443] *That is, those in the top 20% of amount of vegetable oils consumed were 2.22 times more likely to have AMD than those in the bottom 20% of vegetable oil consumption.* They also found that the risk was significantly higher for those in the highest 20% versus lowest 20% of intakes of monounsaturated fats (like olive oil and peanut oil) and polyunsaturated fats (generally, most vegetable oils) with odds ratios of 1.71 and 1.86, respectively. Specifically, higher consumption of the omega-6 fat, linoleic acid (again, think vegetable oil), was also associated with a higher risk for AMD (P for trend, .02). Finally, this research group found that higher intakes of omega-3 fatty acids were associated with lower risk for AMD, but only in those consuming diets low in omega-6 fats. For the cherry on top, they found that higher consumption of fish reduced risk of AMD, but again, only when the diet was low in the omega-6 fatty acid, linoleic acid (i.e. vegetable oil).[444]

In a separate, prospective study, with a follow-up period of 4.6 years, **Dr. Seddon and her colleagues found that increasing vegetable fat intake had a strong relationship to AMD progression with a risk ratio of 3.82 (3.82 fold higher risk) for those consuming the highest 20% of vegetable oil intake versus the lowest 20%.** Once again, in this study, higher fish intake was associated with a lower risk of AMD progression for those who consumed lower omega-6 linoleic acid fats. They also found nuts to have a protective effect against AMD progression.[445]

Including the two studies above, at least eight more studies indicate substantially increased risk of AMD with diets containing significant PUFA vegetable oils and/or trans fats (vegetable oils are a major source of trans fats – see below) [446,447,448,449,450,451,452,453]

VEGETABLE OILS ARE A HUGE SOURCE OF TRANS FATS

Though we'll be reviewing trans fats in detail in the next section of this chapter, it's important to realize that vegetable oils are loaded with trans fats, despite the fact that this is not on their labels and the government may not regulate this. **Researchers Sean O'Keefe and colleagues, at the University of Florida, Food Science and Human Nutrition Department, evaluated the United States' most common supermarket vegetable oils, soybean and canola, and found that they contain anywhere between 0.56% and 4.2% trans fatty acids.**[454]

In other research, 19 different commercial samples of vegetable oils being marketed and sold in Belgium, Hungary, and Great Britain were analyzed for their trans-fatty acid content. The vegetable oils were found to have trans fats ranging from 0.0 to 4.6%, with a mean of 1.1%.[455]

These percentages compute to very significant amounts of trans fats – up to several grams per day – given our enormous consumption of vegetable oils. As we'll see in the next section, this alone could result in many devastating consequences, yet the vegetable oil labels still don't show that they even contain trans fats and, obviously, manufacturers won't assess for or publish this data unless mandated by the government.

VEGETABLE OILS DISPLACE ANIMAL FATS & BUTTER WITH ASSOCIATED VITAMIN K2 DISPLACEMENT – ANOTHER MAJOR FACTOR IN AMD?

Perhaps one of the very worst effects of vegetable oils consumption, is that they have displaced the healthy and densely nutritious fats that were once staples in our diets – namely, butter and lard, both of which (combined) are excellent sources of the fat soluble vitamins (A,D, E, and K). *According to the research of Berta Friend, M.A., butter consumption was at 17.7 grams per person, per day, in 1909 – 1913, gradually decreasing to 6.5 grams per day, by 1965.* Lard consumption was 14.9 grams per day in 1909 decreasing to 11.6 grams per day by 1965.[456] Let's briefly assess one critical nutrient that was displaced in this egregious scenario – that of vitamin K2.

According to the USDA Food Facts Sheet, October, 2012, one teaspoon of vegetable oil, defined as "refined canola, corn, cottonseed, olive, safflower, soybean, sesame, sunflower, or any combination of these," contains Vitamin A 0%, Vitamin C 0%, Calcium 0%, and Iron 0%." [457] In fact, according to the USDA National Nutrient Database, soybean oil has 0.37mg vitamin E, 8.35 micrograms of vitamin K1, and no other vitamins at all in a one-teaspoon serving.[458]

In great contrast to soybean oil and all other vegetable oils, pastured butter is a rich source of vitamin K2, just as Weston A. Price had determined back in the 1930s.[459] However, the amount present depends entirely on the degree to which the cow from which the butter came was grazing on rapidly growing green grass. In his book, *Nutrition and Physical Degeneration,* Dr. Price wrote, "It has been shown that dairy products in Hereford vicinity {Texas} may vary through a range of fiftyfold in a few weeks' time in the vitamin A and activator X [later determined to be vitamin K2] content, the range depending directly on the fodder [feed for cattle or livestock]. There is a sharp rise at the time that the green pasturage is added to the ration of the cows." [460]

The critical point that is not to be missed here, is that any vitamin K in any vegetable oil is vitamin K1, whereas it is vitamin K2 that is the one vitamin absolutely critical in preventing atherosclerosis.[461 462] Vitamin K1 is preferentially utilized by the liver to activate various proteins involved in blood clotting. However, it is vitamin K2 that is essential for depositing calcium into bones and teeth, where it belongs, and not into soft tissues such as arteries, where it does not belong.[463]

Could a deficiency of vitamin K2 be a major factor in AMD, via its effect on calcification and thickening of Bruch's membrane? As we've reviewed, calcification of Bruch's membrane, which may ultimately affect the transmission of metabolites to and from the RPE and photoreceptors, might play a significant role in the development of AMD. Could a lack of K2 also play a role in the occlusive vascular disease of the choroid? We'll come back to this again in Chapter 16.

In a brief summary of this section of the chapter, I believe that vegetable oils may play a major role in macular degeneration, through the following mechanisms:

- Inflammation secondary to their high omega-6 content associated with enormous consumption in societies consuming Westernized diets (AMD is associated with inflammation)
- Ability to oxidize LDL, which then deposits into arterial walls beginning the process of atherosclerosis (AMD is characterized by occlusion of the larger choroid vessels and capillaries of the choriocapillaris)
- Displacing animal fats, including butter and lard, which are excellent sources of the fat soluble vitamins, particularly vitamin K2 (lack of K2 may play a role in calcification of Bruch's membrane, which could reduce perfusion of metabolites between the choriocapillaris and the outer retina – that is, the RPE and photoreceptors. The consequent death of RPE and photoreceptors is the sine-qua-non of AMD)

OMEGA-3 FATTY ACIDS AND FISH CONSUMPTION REDUCE AMD

In great contrast to the damaging effects and higher risks of AMD with the omega-6 rich vegetable oils, numerous studies show an association of reduced risk of AMD with increasing consumption of omega-3 fatty acids in foods, particularly the consumption of fish.[464,465,466,467,468,469,470,471] The fish with the highest omega-3 (DHA and EPA) fatty acid content are primarily salmon, herring, mackerel, and sardines.[472] Consuming fish at least two to three times a week definitely reduces the risk of AMD. Make note: consuming omega3 fatty acids as supplements has not been shown to reduce risk of AMD. This is only accomplished by *consuming foods* naturally rich in omega-3 fats, the best example being fish!

TRANS-FATS: SHOULD WE TRUST NATURE, OR CHEMISTS?

As we reviewed in the last chapter, there were no artificially created trans-fats until Procter and Gamble created Crisco, in 1911. William Procter, a candle maker, and his brother-in-law soap maker, James Gamble, teamed up with German chemist, E.C. Kayser in 1908, to "bring to market" the science of hydrogenation, in the form of – food. That's right. Food. At the time, the company Procter & Gamble was competing for market-share with fourteen other candle and soap makers in Cincinnati, Ohio, and electric lighting and kerosene lamps were beginning to hamper candle sales. The brothers had already found good use from cotton seeds in that they had devised a method to substitute hardened cottonseed oil for animal fats (stearic acid, or "stearin"), which were much more expensive, to make candles.

In fact, for centuries, animal fats were used in making candles – and Procter and Gamble's modification of cottonseed oil already closely resembled a paraffin wax. Making this into a "cooking fat" (in their opinion) wasn't a far cry. In fact, to jump ahead momentarily, as recently as 2008, researchers at Iowa State University went back to partially hydrogenated vegetable oils as the basis for a new candle wax. Doctors Tong Wang and Liping Wang, in 2008, wrote, "Fats of animal origin have long been used for making candles, but such candles are typically of lower quality because of the greasy texture, rancid odor, and sooting during burning. Partially hydrogenated vegetable oil (PHVO) may provide a promising replacement of petroleum wax [paraffin] and the traditional tallow [beef fat] wax because of its more desirable environmental and combustible properties." As it turns out, the researchers were successful. They went on to state, "The resulting modified PHVO may either be used by itself for candle-making or other appropriate uses."[473]

Let me reiterate, just by making minor chemical modifications to the PHVO, the researchers have made the trans fats (partially hydrogenated and fully hydrogenated vegetable oils) that are in our current food supply into a better candle wax!

Let's just take a step back and look at the big picture here. Does it make any sense at all that we should take cotton seeds (which we don't eat), grind and crush them to extract oils, add hexane solvent, remove and evaporate the hexane, add an alkaline solution, centrifuge it down, add water and centrifuge again, bleach and deodorize the oil (because the color is dark and the oil is rancid, which smells badly), then take that oil and boil it while bubbling hydrogen gas through it (in the presence of a metal catalyst) until it becomes a solid — and then – eat it?[474] This is supposed to be a replacement for butter and lard? I doubt that anyone who ever watched this process at the factory would even begin to believe that this waxy substance should be in our food supply. Yet, we call this "food" – and it's been in our food supply for over a century! To me, this is truly just mind-boggling.

Because industrially produced trans fats are cheap and they also preserve food, the processed food manufacturers buy them by the trainload and they've pumped them into thousands of food products for many decades. These trans fats (particularly when combined with sugar) are the reason that you can buy a Hostess Fruit Pie that has sat on the shelf or in a vending machine for weeks – and it still tastes fresh. They're a tremendous preservative, allowing pastries to routinely set on shelves for at least four or five weeks before beginning to lose that fresh taste. [475]

As briefly reviewed in the previous chapter, P & G had a brilliant marketing plan for Crisco from its inception, as well as the financial strength to create an enormous campaign. Their target audience was primarily housewives. In addition to calling Crisco "the healthier alternative to lard and… more economical than butter," they touted it as "healthier, more digestible, cleaner, more economical, more enlightened, and more modern than lard" in any variety of marketing campaigns including print, radio, and eventually, television.[476] They portrayed women who cooked with Crisco as good mothers – looking out for the health of their children, even conveying the message that children fed Crisco – instead of lard – grew up with good characters.

This campaign worked, in fact, to the tune of billions of dollars. A substance that, by almost no stretch of the imagination could be considered food, which was more like candle wax, entered our food system – eventually on a global scale – and billions and billions of tons would be sold and consumed by people. Crisco, and eventually, many other hydrogenated and partially hydrogenated vegetable oils, would become commonplace in our food supply. Manufacturers would eventually use partially hydrogenated vegetable oils in tens of thousands of processed foods.

By 1989- 1991, a study representative of the U.S. population found that the mean percentage of energy ingested as trans fatty acids was 2.6%, which translates to 6.4 grams of trans fats per person per day.[477]

NATURALLY OCCURRING TRANS FATS

If anyone ever tells you that there are trans-fats that occur naturally, it's true. Researchers sometimes call these "ruminant trans fatty acids," shortened to rTFAs. In our case, just think of ruminants as beef, though rTFAs would be present in virtually all animals. These types of trans fats typically account for around 2 to 5% of the fat in dairy products and about 3 to 9 percent of the fat in beef and lamb and only about 0.2 to 2 percent in pork and chicken.[478 479] Not to worry about these fats though – because they're good for us!

Suffice it to say that these naturally occurring trans fatty acids, such as vaccenic acid (VA) and conjugated linoleic acid (CLA) have never been shown to have negative health consequences in humans and, in fact, have been shown to have many anti-cancer and anti-prostaglandin (anti-inflammatory) effects.[480,481]

From a cardiovascular standpoint, they've actually been shown to have a beneficial effect on blood pressure and triglyceride levels in the blood. Researchers at the Quebec Research Center in Quebec City, Canada, for example, state, "These data suggest that rTFA may have beneficial effects on cardiometabolic risk factors conversely to their counterpart iTFA [industrial trans fatty acids – man-made trans fats]." [482] In a review article by researchers at the University of Texas Health Science Center, in San Antonio, they found that CLA "has been attributed many beneficial effects in prevention of atherosclerosis, different types of cancer, hypertension, and also to improve immune function."[483]

THE DEVASTATING HEALTH EFFECTS OF ARTIFICIALLY CREATED TRANS-FATS

Heart Disease… Dr. Fred Kummerow's biochemistry, lipid and animal research led him to believe and publish that trans fats were the primary cause of heart disease, in 1957. He pinned the problem on 14 different synthetic compounds found in the trans fats, which were particularly common in margarines, fried foods, and cake mixes. Kummerow pointed his finger at the fact that artificially created trans fats cause the body to produce less prostacyclin, which he shows causes blood to flow smoothly and, without it, may result in blood clotting. He said, "I think the lesson of this whole thing is don't tamper with nature. They were making 14 different fatty acids that had no business being there."[484] With regard to the presence of trans fats in our modern food, Dr. Kummerow said, "The industry is very powerful, and they love to have this stuff in the diet because it has a long shelf life." [485]

Kummerow's most recent book, *Cholesterol Is Not the Culprit*, was released in 2008. Today, at the age of 101, Professor Kummerow holds an emeritus position at the University of Illinois – and he continues to do research and to publish.

Consumption of the industrially produced trans fatty acids (iTFA) have been consistently shown, in observational studies, to be strongly linked to coronary heart disease.[486,487,488] These studies specifically point out greater risk of coronary heart disease (CHD) in people consuming higher amounts of these artificially created industrial trans fats, particularly in those people consuming foods containing significant quantities of them, such as margarine, cakes, and cookies.

These iTFAs are close enough in molecular structure to the normal cis-type TFAs (that would normally be found in milk, beef, cheese, etc.) that the body absorbs them and incorporates them into our cell membranes.[489] From here, these disastrous wax-like molecules apparently disrupt cellular signaling and wreak all sorts of havoc.

Rozenn Lemaitre, PhD, MPH, biochemist and research professor at the University of Washington, Cardiovascular Health Research Unit, along with her colleagues, found that higher total trans fat levels in red blood cell membranes were associated with a modest increase in sudden cardiac arrest. However, higher levels of the omega-6 linoleic acid in the trans fat version were associated with a 3-fold increased risk of sudden cardiac arrest.[490]

One study reports that if people were to replace partially hydrogenated vegetable oils with alternative fats and oils, the risk of coronary heart disease may be reduced by as much as 50%.[491]

Dr. Kummerow and his colleagues found that the piglets of sows fed hydrogenated fats during pregnancy and while nursing, resulted in the uptake of trans fats into their plasma and aortic wall, along with increased deposition of calcium into the aortic wall which, Kummerow states, "could play a role in atherogenesis ('hardening of the arteries')." Once there, the trans fats severely affect essential fatty acid metabolism, causing changes in the vasculature of 7 week-old piglets that mimics the beginning of atherosclerosis.[492] It appears that the trans fats caused a reduction in the quantities of long-chain omega-6 fats in the arterial cells, with a resultant uptake of calcium and beginning of arterial plaques, even in baby piglets receiving trans fats purely via the womb and mother's milk.

In a meta-analysis type study (review of all research) on trans fats, Canadian researchers reported in the British Medical Journal that "Saturated fats are not associated with all cause mortality, cardiovascular disease (CVD), coronary heart disease (CHD), ischemic stroke, or type 2 diabetes" … while they simultaneously reported that, **"Trans fats are associated with all cause mortality, total CHD, and CHD mortality, probably because of higher levels of intake of industrial trans fats than ruminant fats."** [493]

TRANS FATS ASSOCIATED WITH OTHER DISEASES

Trans fats have been associated with many other diseases and conditions, but because these conditions are not particularly germane to the subject matter of AMD, I will not fully review them here. Nevertheless, I want you to be aware that trans fat consumption has been associated with increased risk for diabetes,[494] obesity,[495,496,497] cancer,[498] Alzheimer's disease,[499] depression,[500] and infertility in women.[501]

TRANS FATS AND AMD

If trans fats cause coronary artery disease and confirmed atherosclerosis, and AMD is associated with atherosclerosis, particularly of the choroid and choriocapillaris vascular network, wouldn't it make sense that trans fats could be another molecular mechanism in the etiology (cause) of AMD?

The research in this area is pretty substantial. But, it's very difficult to ferret out the effects of trans fats from vegetable oils (mostly polyunsaturated oils), and monounsaturated oils, because there's just too many variables. Even the most sophisticated statistical analyses, known as regression analyses, cannot truly decipher these confounding variables. With that said, there's some data in all this complexity.

Once again, Johanna Seddon, MD, and colleagues at the Massachusetts Eye and Ear Infirmary, Harvard Medical School, investigated the roles of these various fats on AMD. She and her associates found that trans fats increased the risk of progression of AMD by 2.39 fold (P for trend, .008).[502]

Elaine W. Chong and colleagues, at the University of Melbourne, Centre for Eye Research Australia, found that higher trans fat intake was associated with an increased prevalence of late AMD. The odds ratio for those in the highest 25% of trans fat intake was 1.76 fold greater than those in the lowest 25 percent.[503]

There are a few other studies that link AMD with increased trans fat consumption as well.[504,505,506]

There is even more evidence that indicates trans fats may be another smoking gun in AMD: French researcher, Lionel Bretillon and colleagues, at the Eye and Nutrition Research Group, Dijon cedex, France, showed that trans fatty acids from the diet (these were vegetable oil based trans fats) were found in the RPE and choroid of human eyes.[507] This finding is strongly suggestive that fatty acids in our diet actually reach our retina, rather fully intact. Hence, great concern for what we're eating!

AVOIDING TRANS FATS

You can avoid trans fats completely, but you must be vigilant about selecting your foods. For the most part, avoid fast foods unless you can confirm that no trans fat has been added. Avoid processed foods completely, if at all possible. Remember Jack LaLanne's mantra, "If man made it, don't eat it." If you do purchase any processed food, be absolutely certain the ingredients do not contain either of the terms "hydrogenated vegetable oil" or "partially hydrogenated vegetable oil." Both contain trans fats.

In the U.S. since 2006, package labeling regarding trans fat may be misleading, because the FDA has allowed manufacturers to state "O Grams Trans Fat" on their front label, when the product may contain up to 0.5 grams trans fat per serving. There is absolutely no amount that is safe, so you must read the ingredients list if you're consuming processed foods.

Remember, vegetable oils contain trans fats too, even when the labels don't include this information. This is the case because the extraction of these oils with heat, pressure, and chemicals obviously results in hydrogenation – whether the manufacturers intend it or not.

The last recommendation is to consider buying organic food items. Organic foods cannot contain trans fats and, of course, their presence would certainly go against the grain of any organic producer. To include trans fats in such foods would truly be an abomination of the organic ethic.

In 2013, 102 years after the introduction of trans fats into our food supply and with tens of thousands of processed foods having contained them, the U.S. FDA issued a preliminary statement that trans fats will no longer have a "generally regarded as safe" (GRAS) status. On June 16, 2015, the FDA finalized its determination, removed trans fats from GRAS status, and set a three-year time limit for manufacturers to remove them from all processed foods.[508]

Let me wrap up this segment on trans fats with a quote from Jennifer Swift, medical researcher who wrote an article for *tfX.org*, which is the website for the company known as tfX: The Campaign Against Trans Fats in Food. She wrote, **"As for the fact that trans fats are seriously toxic, causing premature death and misery on a massive scale, much of the worldwide food industry just doesn't care. Only one other industry that treats its customers with the same callous disregard, knowingly selling them products that will lead to unnecessary illness and premature death – the tobacco industry."** [509]

CHAPTER SUMMARY

The acronym for the "Standard American Diet" (SAD) is truly befitting, because the effect of a diet that is replete with nutritionally deficient, processed foods, is devastation to both mind and body – and that includes our eyes. In our current world, if we desire to have good health and to take care of our eyes, we need to really work at avoiding processed foods.

VEGETABLE OILS & AMD...

In summary, with regard to vegetable oils, we have a strong temporal relationship between the introduction of vegetable oils into our food supply and the onset of AMD. The vegetable oils were introduced in 1880, with cottonseed oil first, and production and consumption steadily increased throughout the 20th century with the additions of many other vegetable oils into the market, including the oils of soybean, corn, sunflower, safflower, rapeseed, grapeseed, rice bran, and recently, canola oil. As we've seen, AMD was virtually non-existent in the early 20th century, but became a "common cause of vision loss in the elderly" in the 1930s (Duke-Elder, 1940), increased to epidemic proportions by the 1960s ,and is still increasing in incidence and prevalence globally. Like heart disease, AMD obviously doesn't develop over a few years, which is why we rarely see this condition before the age of about 40 or 45. The condition likely takes several decades to become clinically evident once the dietary onslaught has begun.

We also have a highly biologically plausible mechanism for vegetable oil consumption to be causative for AMD: Polyunsaturated oils, high in omega-6 fatty acids, find their way into cellular membranes and begin a cascade of inflammation. Omega-3 fats, on the other hand, are anti-inflammatory. The AREDS studies show that diets high in omega-6 fats such as vegetable oils are associated with greater risk of AMD, whereas diets high in omega-3 fats, especially long-chain omega 3's, such as EPA and DHA from fish, reduce the risk of AMD.

Polyunsaturated oils deposit themselves into the LDL molecules, which then easily oxidize. These dangerous, reactive molecules are rapidly removed from the circulation by the endothelial cells of our vessels, deposited into the intima layer of the vessel wall, where macrophages ingest them – thereby, beginning an inflammatory and atherosclerotic process. AMD is associated with vascular occlusion in the choriocapillaris and atherosclerosis, in general.

For the coup de grâce, vegetable oils displace vitamins and minerals present in butter and lard, which are the fats that vegetable oils largely replaced. This is particularly true for butter made from cows grazing on green grass, which was previously Americans' primary source of vitamin K2. Lack of vitamin K2 has been shown to play a major role in cardiovascular disease via calcification of arteries. By inference, that same deficiency of vitamin K2 might lead to calcification of Bruch's membrane, which impedes nutrient transfer between the choriocapillaris and the photoreceptors (outer retina).

In order to prevent AMD and limit the progression of existing AMD, we must absolutely minimize our consumption of omega-6 fats, by virtually eliminating vegetable oils from our diets. When we accomplish this, we will almost certainly have enough omega-3 fats in our diets already from meats, eggs, and seafood. This, I believe – and this alone – may have the single greatest impact on preventing and/or stabilizing AMD.

TRANS FATS & AMD...

We reviewed much research that shows how trans fats are associated with vascular disease, even causing the beginning of plaques in the aortas of baby piglets that received trans fats only through the womb and via mother's milk. If this is the case, imagine what a lifetime of consumption of trans fats might do? Furthermore, if the vasculature of baby pigs that are fed trans fats begins to develop disease, is it any stretch to imagine that the choroidal circulation of the eye should be immune?

Remember, if you do consume any processed foods, which essentially means just about anything that is packaged, boxed, canned, labeled, or has an ingredient list of more than three items, you will need to watch out for trans fats. You cannot depend on a label which reads "0 grams trans fats" because the FDA allows the food to contain up to 0.5 grams trans fat and still be labeled as "0 grams trans fat." Any amount is dangerous. If the ingredients list reads "hydrogenated" or "partially hydrogenated" followed by the name of the oil, it has trans fat. Don't buy it. If you already own it, throw it away!

As far as fats in your diet, stick with butter and lard as much as possible, particularly for cooking. The animal fats are the most stable at high temperatures and, just like our 19th century ancestors who did not have heart disease or macular degeneration, these are the fats we should be consuming. They're also the ones that supply significant quantities of the fat soluble vitamins A, D, and K, which are absolutely critical to our health in countless ways. When at all possible, try to get organic butter from pastured cows that graze on green grass, as this will greatly increase the concentration of vitamin K2. This may play an enormous role in preventing cardiovascular disease and, I believe, AMD as well.

In order to avoid vegetable oils and trans fats, you will need to prepare most of your meals at home. I cook virtually everything in pastured, organic butter, because it tastes great and it's very healthy, though lard is great for cooking too. If the recipe calls for olive oil or other oil and cooking/baking is required, just use butter or lard instead. When high temperature cooking is *not* required, you may use unrefined (cold-pressed) coconut oil or virgin olive oil, in relatively small quantities. Palm oil and palm kernel oil, which are also saturated oils like coconut oil, may also be considered for cooking. But again, keep the portions of these small and opt for cooking in animal fats when possible.

When eating out, you're in a danger zone because most restaurants cook with soybean oil, with canola oil and corn oil coming in a distant second and third place in terms of volume.[510] I believe we're a lot safer in finer restaurants where you can actually inquire as to how foods are cooked (e.g., with butter vs. vegetable oil). I actually ask for our foods to be cooked in butter, or no oil at all, depending on the restaurant and the situation. I've found most restaurants will try to comply, because they depend on repeat business. But don't be afraid to ask! If you're told that no butter is available for cooking, which is not unusual, try to opt for something that requires no oils at all. Just be vigilant about this because your life, health, and vision all depend on it!

11 THE PERILS OF "DISPLACING FOODS" *PART II: WHITE FLOUR, WHITE SUGAR, AND PROCESSED FOODS*

"White flour, pretty much wherever it shows up throughout the world, metabolic havoc ensues."

~ Stephan Guyenet, PhD ~

(WholeHealthSource.org)

WHEAT: THE GOOD, THE BAD, AND THE UGLY

One common theme that resurfaces repeatedly throughout this book is this: Whenever and wherever we witness the displacement of nutrient dense foods for non-nutrient dense ones, degeneration and disease are sure to follow. That's the theme of this entire chapter, as you will see. In the end, once again, I will submit that the development of AMD is strongly connected to nutrient deficiencies and that the consumption of white flour, refined sugar, and processed foods greatly contributes to the development of such disease.

When we crack the deceptively simple little grain of wheat, we're truly opening up Pandora's box. Wheat is perhaps one of the most troubling of all foods to draw conclusions from available research. This is because there are two diametrically opposing camps on wheat and its effects on health and, in this case, I think the truth falls squarely somewhere in the middle. As usual, we need to get into the nitty-gritty details to decode the conflicting science and epidemiology.

To lay a brief foundation, I believe there are potentially three major concerns with the consumption of modern-day wheat, as it relates to our health:

- Nutrient deficiencies associated with the consumption of white flour, and
- Leaky gut associated with the consumption of the protein of wheat - gluten - which may lead to inflammation and autoimmune conditions in many people, and
- The spraying of wheat with any number of herbicides, which has been common since the 1940s.

As mentioned, in this chapter, we'll concern ourselves primarily with the nutrient deficiencies associated with consuming white flour.

Today, some authors have implicated wheat as the cause of undesirable weight gain, heart disease, diabetes, and a boatload of other systemic disease.[511,512,513] From the much larger opposing camp, such as the Whole Grains Council, the statement from their "Whole Grains 101" page reads as follows: "The medical evidence is clear that whole grains reduce risks of heart disease, stroke, cancer, diabetes and obesity. Few foods can offer such diverse benefits." [514] As so often occurs in the field of nutrition, we have this dichotomy with two fiercely opposing camps. How can they both evaluate the same research and return with opposing points of view? Are they both wrong? Both right?

After months of reading and frustration, I've decided they're both right. Well, sort of. The problem, in a nutshell, is that the findings from research from wheat consumed as whole grains and wheat consumed from white flour are often conflated. And the two foods are entirely different physically, nutritionally, metabolically, and biochemically. Secondarily, wheat and/or gluten doesn't affect everyone the same. I am living proof. So perhaps we're seeing both sides of the story and the end-result is whatever outcome one chooses to focus upon. As usual, the Deity lies in the details.

The physical and physiologic consequences of consuming whole-grain sourdough bread made from organically grown wheat that is slowly fermented over many hours or days as compared to Wonder Bread, which is made from non-organic, herbicide treated, white flour raised with a huge dose of a single yeast over a period of about an hour, and with synthetic vitamins, sugar, and soybean or canola oil additions, are utterly, completely, and entirely different. The former scenario may present a gut-healthy, nutritious component of a diet, whereas the latter will wreak metabolic havoc in every single human that consumes it. It's too bad that they're both being considered as wheat because the differences for the consumer are drastic. Yet, in the end, the analysis by some researchers and authors is that "they're both wheat – and all wheat is bad."

Consider, for example, consuming a sweet potato baked in the oven with butter and cinnamon added (not only a tremendously healthy side dish, but one of my absolute favorites) versus sweet potato chips made in a factory where the sweet potatoes are peeled, dried, blanched, treated with citric acid, and then fried in soybean, sunflower, or cottonseed oil with sugar, cornstarch (GMO in the U.S.), and tapioca dextrin added for additional flavor.[515] I wouldn't eat those on my death bed. It's tragic, but we could draw similar analogies for every real food item there is. Big Food manufacturers have managed to take nearly every naturally grown food there is and process it into something that can be sold for a greater profit while simultaneously contributing to the demise of our health.

A BRIEF HISTORICAL REVIEW OF WHEAT...

As I've alluded to, wheat is a duplicitous grain, at least from my perspective. There is a long history of wheat consumption that appears positive and has few negative connotations, though there were apparently always at least a small number of cases of celiac disease related to gluten consumption, which date as far back as the 2nd century AD.[516] Wheat has served numerous generations of people and has been consumed in many societies for the past 10,000 years with apparently few health issues. But, by the late 19th to early 20th century, that unmarred history began to change.

It seems clear from a review of the pertinent history that the negative effects of wheat were present on a broad scale in the early 20th century. If you recall, Weston A. Price confirmed that the consumption of white flour was one of the major contributory factors to the demise of the health of many cultures. In review of his 1939 classical book, *Nutrition and Physical Degeneration*, Dr. Price did not find a single healthy tribe, culture, or population that was consuming wheat in the form of white flour. The healthy Swiss villagers from the Loetschental Valley consumed rye bread as a staple, but only whole grain rye which was ground on millstones followed by a lengthy sourdough fermentation process for about two days, followed by a curing process for about two weeks;[517] the Gaelics in the Outer Hebrides consumed oats as a staple; and many of the African tribes consumed corn (maize) and millet, but virtually none of them consumed wheat in the form of white flour. In fact, it was when previously healthy populations introduced wheat (and other processed foods) into their diets in the form of white flour, that a severe and generalized degenerative condition ensued.

I believe we must question the biological effects of wheat in the form of white flour because if this has something to do with macular degeneration (and a host of other diseases and disorders), then I feel compelled to share it with you. I firmly believe there are some very compelling reasons to assert that wheat consumption, *specifically in the form of white flour*, may also be associated with the development of AMD.

In all of my research, most of our chronic disease conditions began to appear within the first few decades after the turn of the 20th century, which I have alluded to previously. **I've also reviewed the fact that stone mills for grinding wheat began to be replaced with roller mill technology, beginning in 1880 and this new technology spread rapidly in the following decades. This appears to be a pivotal turning point in our health.** Of course, as we've also reviewed, vegetable oils and trans fats were introduced just around the turn of the 20th century as well.

Recently, I watched a video of a presentation by highly-acclaimed author, Michael Pollan, who has written several books on nutrition including *In Defense of Food*, which I hope to read soon. In any case, his research led to a similar conclusion, as he made the following remarks in this presentation: "So I was really curious as to determine the turning point, when food processing went bad. And the more I looked at it the more I realized it was the invention of the roller mill in the 1870s and 1880s. The roller mill is what gave us *really* white flour. Before that, you could get whitish flour – it tended to be a little yellowish – uh – because basically you were grinding it on a stone mill and then you were sifting it as finely as you could and you got rid of lots of the bran but you couldn't quite get rid of that smushed germ, which turned out was keeping people healthy to a very large extent… it was a goal [to have white flour] and it was achieved with these [roller] mills that, for the first time, made it possible to break off the bran and the germ immediately and leave that starchy white endosperm as basically all you were going to eat, which is mostly starch and it has some protein as well." [518]

In fact, indicting wheat, per se, as a major cause of heart disease, cancer, diabetes, stroke, Alzheimer's disease, etc., is discordant and irreconcilable with the history of wheat consumption in the United States. The USDA's Economic Research Service confirms, **"From a low starting point in the 1600s, consumption of wheat flour rose to about 225 pounds per capita in 1880, and then fell to about 110 pounds a century later."** [519] The USDA's sub-headline reads, "Flour Consumption Declines for the First Two-Thirds of the 20th Century." Wheat consumption rose modestly to 146.3 pounds per person in 2000 following government recommendations to reduce fats in the diet (~ 1980), dropping back down to 132.5 pounds per person by 2011, as a result of greater adherence to low carbohydrate diets.

ously mentioned conditions rose to epidemic proportions, including macular degeneration.

Now I ask you, how can we possibly blame wheat, per se, in all of these conditions that were medical rarities when we consumed the most wheat? But, take that same healthy, whole-grain wheat, spray it with herbicides as it's growing, and then make white flour and an abundance of processed foods out of it, and we're suddenly dealing with a completely different beast.

With regard to the refining of wheat flour, roller mill technology meant that the bran and germ of wheat could be completely removed. Removal of the germ, which contains B vitamins and omega-3 and omega-6 fats, meant that there was nothing left in the flour to go rancid, which is the process of lipid oxidation. [520] In fact, millers desire is to completely remove the germ (embryo) as this tremendously increases shelf life. This is exactly why flour can be stored in enclosed containers for years and still be "safely" consumed.

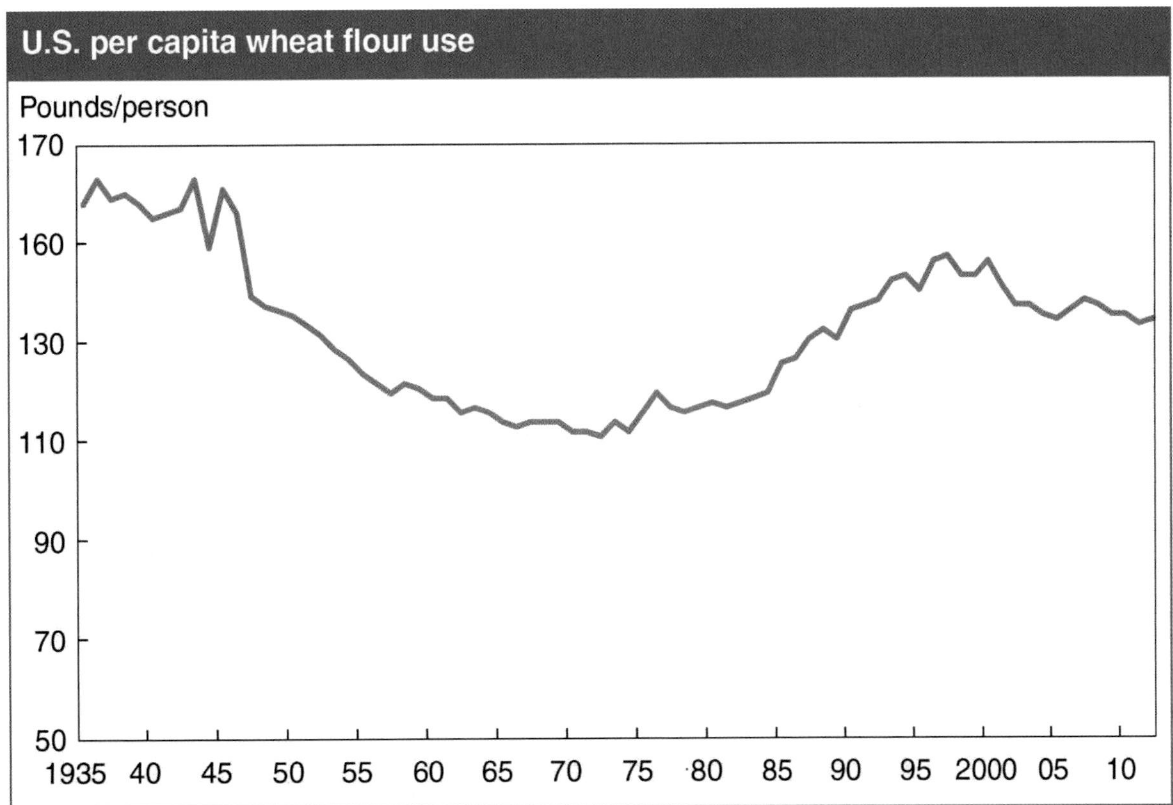

Source: USDA, Economic Research Service calculations based on U.S. Department of Commerce, Census Bureau and Bureau of Economic Analysis data.

The point is, when our wheat consumption was at its highest, in 1880, we had virtually no heart disease, and the conditions of obesity, type 2 diabetes, stroke, cancer, and Alzheimer's disease were medical rarities. Macular degeneration had only been observed and documented by two ophthalmologists. As consumption of wheat began to fall, and fall drastically over the next century, all of the previ-

Meanwhile, complete removal of the bran simultaneously removes additional B vitamins, minerals, and fiber while leaving the miller with an extremely white flour. Before and not long after the turn of the 20th century, white flour was considered highly desirable. Very white bread was considered the most "pure" and was, in fact, the most sought after. Historically, pure white flour was only for the elite, as the intense milling and lengthy sifting process required to produce it also meant very expensive flour, which few could afford.

Ironically, according to roller mill industry expert, Grant Campbell, the skill of the miller is measured "in terms of the amount and purity of white flour that he can produce." [521] This is a travesty, because the "purity" of the flour, in miller's terms, is inversely proportional to the amount and degree of nutrients carried in the flour, as we will witness based on laboratory analysis (to be presented subsequently).

Palmer and Neaverson, in their book, *Industry In The Landscape, 1700 - 1900*, review the fact that, in Great Britain, the baking of bread remained in the home as a domestic responsibility at least until the 1870s. "Bread ovens" were commonplace in the home in that era. Then, with the introduction of steam tube ovens in the mid-nineteenth century combined with the development of mechanical kneading machines, mass production of the baking of bread began by 1900.[522] Obviously, once bread could be mass produced at a low cost combined with the public's desire for white flour, the stage was set for bread to be made of highly refined white flour, with barely a smidgen of nutrition.

According to John Burnett (1925 - 2006), Emeritus Professor of Social History at Brunel University in London, as early as 1847, a physician by the name of Dr. Daniel Carr had promulgated the nutritional advantages of brown bread over white. That year, he published his book *The Necessity of Brown Bread for Digestion, Nourishment and Good Health.* In this book, the first known developed argument for the benefits of 'wholemeal' (whole grain in our terms) was made, evidenced by the following quote:

> "It is for a wise purpose that the Deity has so intimately associated in the grain the several substances which are necessary for the complete nutrition of animal bodies." [523]

In London, "The Bread Reform League was founded in 1880 by May (Mary Anne) Yates, an amateur artist and member of the Ladies' Sanitary Association," Burnett continued. "On a visit to Sicily she had admired the fine physique of the peasants who lived principally on brown bread, and contrasted their vigour with the ill-health she saw in English towns, especially among poor children. Her conclusion that white bread, the staple food of the working classes, was a principal cause of malnutrition, led her to renounce her artistic career, sell her jewelry, and devote the next forty years to changing British tastes from white bread to brown." Burnett continued, "Bread was the largest item in working-class budgets, supplying around half of energy needs. Average consumption was 6.7lb per person, per week, but in poor families it was almost the only food eaten by women and children: men monopolized any meat available, a custom tacitly accepted as the prerogative of the 'breadwinner'. By 1880, British loaves were almost universally made of white wheaten flour." [524]

I find it very intriguing that, up until nearly 1880, a *whole grain wheat bread* was supplying nearly half of energy needs for the "working classes" while many of the poor consumed even more of their energy needs from bread, yet history tells us that they did not have the diseases that currently plague us (again), such as heart disease, cancer, diabetes, and Alzheimer's. Obviously, the whole grain wheat and rye breads that had been consumed for millennia held enough nutrition to prevent most nutritional deficiency diseases, including macular degeneration, even when they accounted for more than half of consumed calories.

Because of the advent of roller mill technology, the once sought after white bread, previously a luxury only for the privileged, was suddenly a staple food for the working class and the poor. May Yates and the Bread Reform League persisted in calling this new flour 'denatured,' and her campaign persisted, mainly through the distribution of pamphlets to physicians, members of parliament, and other influential people. She argued that 'wheatmeal bread' prevented a wide range of ailments ranging from constipation and indigestion to the dreaded tuberculosis, which was often fatal before the advent of antibiotics. Yates insisted that the chief victims of this 'impoverished bread' were the little children, particularly the poor whose diet depended greatly on bread.[525]

It didn't help Yates case, however, that the esteemed British physician and nutritionist, Sir Henry Thompson, had published his 1880 treatise *Food and Feeding,* which conceded that brown bread, containing the germ and bran, might be "richer in nutrients, but the presence of numerous rough, branny fragments so stimulates the action of the intestines, that the material is hurried along the digestive tract without that complete digestion and absorption of its nutritive matters which white bread undergoes." [526]

Yates obviously made astute observations that had gone unnoticed by Sir Henry Thompson, which obviously were also eventually validated repeatedly and in numerous cultures in the 1930s by Weston A. Price. Just as it is today with Big Food and processed, nutrient-deficient foods, Yates' cries fell mostly on deaf ears. In 1900, twenty years after beginning her campaign, 95 percent of the bread consumed in England was still of the nutrient-deficient white variety. Within 20 years of the widespread use of roller mill technology and broad distribution of white bread, even young British males had become so weak and frail that 35 percent of army volunteers for the South African War (1899-1902) were rejected as unfit. Social reformers attributed this to nothing more than 'urban growth' producing weak, stunted 'City Types.'[527]

In fact, the conditions pellagra, a vitamin B3 (niacin) deficiency characterized by dermatitis, diarrhea, dementia, and death, and beriberi, a vitamin B1 (thiamine) deficiency characterized by numerous neurologic, heart, and gastrointestinal symptoms that generally leads to death, were conditions that became worldwide epidemics as a direct result of roller mill technology.[528,529]

According to Katherine Czapp of the Weston A. Price Foundation, "Seventy percent of all bread eaten in the United States was baked at home in 1910, but the percentage had plummeted to 30 by 1924. In 1927, the Continental Baking Company first introduced Wonder Bread, and three years later presented sliced Wonder Bread in a protective wrapper to the national market." [530] Czapp, in her continued review of the history of Wonder Bread, claims that the U.S. Government chose Wonder Bread for an experiment dubbed "the quiet miracle," in which their bread was chosen to be "enriched" with "vitamins and minerals as a way of ameliorating deficiency diseases suffered by the poor." She continues, "what officials never acknowledged was the fact that it was the new foods themselves that were impoverished." [531]

The addition of synthetic vitamins to Wonder Bread and other breads is credited with greatly reducing the incidence of pellagra and Beriberi.[532] However, this also appears to be strong evidence for the lack of nutrition in commercially produced bread in which white flour is the primary ingredient. What we witness with the introduction of synthetic vitamins into bread, as is virtually always the case, is that the addition of synthetic vitamins is a poor substitute for whole food nutrition. We will review this in greater detail in the chapter on vitamins (Chapter 21).

THE SCIENTIFIC EVIDENCE AGAINST WHITE FLOUR...

If the research of Weston A. Price and the deleterious effects that white flour (and processed food) played on culture after culture weren't enough, we now have scientific evidence that documents the loss of nutrients in white flour as compared to whole grain flour.

University of Minnesota nutrition researchers Joanne Slavin, David Jacobs, and Len Marquart, in a paper published in *Critical Reviews in Biotechnology*, state that, "Wheat flours are characterized by the flour extraction, which is defined as the proportion of flour by weight, derived by milling from a known quantity of wheat. **The extraction rate is used to define different types of wheat flour. When the extraction rate is 75% or less, a typical white flour is generated.** If the extraction rate exceeds 80%, the flour will contain non-endosperm particles, and if the flour extraction approaches 100%, a wholemeal flour is generated."[533] At 100% extraction (wholemeal) versus 75% extraction (typical white flour), their research shows that the fat content is reduced from 2.7 to 1.4% and total fiber is reduced from 14.5% to 3.1%. For the same extraction rates, calcium is reduced from 0.44 to 0.25 mg/g, phosphorus from 3.8 to 1.3 mg/g, zinc from 29 to 8 ppm, copper from 4.0 to 1.6 ppm, and iron from 35 to 13 ppm. Finally, and again for the same extraction rates, thiamine (B1) is reduced from 5.8 to 2.2 μg/g, riboflavin (B2) from 0.95 to 0.39 μg/g, vitamin B6 from 7.5 to 1.4 μg/g, folate from 0.57 to 0.11 μg/g, biotin from 116 to 46 μg/g, and niacin (B3) from 25.2 to 5.2 μg/g.

Comparable to most natural foods that provide vitamins in many different isomers, whole-grain wheat contains six of the eight different isomers of vitamin E. In brief, vitamin E comes in 8 different isomers, known as alpha-, beta-, gamma-, and delta-tocopherol, and alpha-, beta-, gamma-, and delta-tocotrienol. Of these eight, wheat germ contains alpha-, beta-, gamma-, and delta tocopherol, and alpha- and gamma-tocotrienol.[534] Contrast that to most any vitamin or multi-vitamin supplement, in which you will find nothing but alpha-tocopherol.

The oil of the germ also contains 6 different plant sterols and 3 different sterylglycosides, again all isolated mostly to the wheat germ oil.[535] Numerous phytochemicals are found in the bran of wheat.[536] Yet, we remove most of these, including the six different isomers of vitamin E, when we shear away the bran and the germ using roller mill technology to produce a "nice white" flour.

If wheat is a considerable portion of the diet (e.g., 20% of calories, as it is today),[537] **the reduction in fats (omega-6, omega-3, saturated and monounsaturated fatty acids), fiber, minerals (including calcium, phosphorus, zinc, copper, and iron), B vitamins (B1, B2, B3, B6, folate or B9, and biotin or B7), E vitamins (tocopherols and tocotrienols), and phytochemicals in white flour as compared to wholemeal flour, is drastic.** This alone appears to have significant deleterious consequences to one's health, particularly for those whose diets include considerable amounts of wheat.

Despite the fact that many people think they're eating a fair amount of "whole grains," they're generally not. The "Whole Grain-Rich Criteria," set forth by the USDA requires that at least 50 percent of the grains in the product be whole grains with the remainder being either whole or "enriched" (added vitamins), in order to meet this standard. If it does, then it is suitable for school meal programs.[538] According to the Whole Grains Council, "The US government has very few actual regulations for whole grain labeling. At this time, the FDA's prohibition of misleading and false labeling is one of the strongest forces in this area... In line with common sense, we advise manufacturers to use the words "whole grain" in the name of a product only if the product contains more whole grain than refined grain." [539]

It's pretty obvious that there's some significant wiggle-room when it comes to labeling and, as such, "whole wheat" and "whole grain" may not truly have nearly as much true whole grain as we would hope. **Indeed, the research shows that the great bulk of grain is actually consumed as white flour.**[540] Hence, the continued epidemics of degenerative diseases that Weston A. Price so eloquently described in 1939.

THE "HEALTHY WHOLE GRAIN" BREAKFAST CEREALS

Thousands of farmers produce wheat, but they're generally not the ones processing it into varieties of white flours and subsequently into extruded breakfast cereals (e.g., Cheerios, Puffed Wheat, Trix, Cinnamon Toast Crunch, Lucky Charms, Special K, etc.), as well as nutritionally deficient breads, pancakes, waffles, Twinkies, Wheat Thins, pretzels, crackers, pastries, rolls, Danish, crescents, donuts, cookies, etc., etc., etc. Most all of these are made with nutrient-deficient, white flour, and they often include vegetable oils such as soybean or canola oil, sugars (e.g., high fructose corn syrup), and an arsenal of additives including synthetic vitamins and preservatives.

Loren Cordain, PhD, S. Boyd Eaton, MD, and colleagues found that 85.3% of the cereals consumed in the U.S. diet are now "highly processed refined grains."[541] Once again, this means that the grains are devoid of the bran and germ, leaving only a nutrient-deficient food to be consumed.

Perhaps even worse than the nutrient deficiency, a typical food manufacturer's breakfast cereal is produced by the process of extrusion. Extruders are machines that force grains that have been mixed into a slurry through a stationary barrel under high temperature and pressure while being cut at the end by a spinning blade. These devices create the various shapes desired, such as Cheerios, Froot Loops, etc. The shaped product is carried on a stream of hot air momentarily while a nozzle sprays a coating of oil and sugar all over it. The latter protects the pieces from becoming soggy when soaked in milk. Some of the issues associated with extruded grains include denatured and fragmented proteins, starch gelatinization, and production of "reactive molecules…not found in nature."[542] According to one industry analyst, the extrusion process destroys "much of the nutrient content of the ingredients," damages vitamins added prior to the extrusion, and is destructive of a critical amino acid in our diet, lysine.[543]

Sally Fallon of the Weston A. Price Foundation maintains that the Big Food breakfast cereal industry stifles any publications regarding the results of research regarding extruded cereals.[544] She reveals that one industry insider has broken his silence with a written publication on this issue, obviously long after he left his position in the Big Food industry, which in his case, was with the Quaker Oats Company. In his book, *Beating the Food Giants,* Paul A. Stitt shares this anecdote regarding laboratory experiments at Quaker:

> While I was doing research on my project in Quaker's library, I came across a little flyer that the company had published in 1942. It contained a report on a study in which four sets of rats were given special diets. One group received plain whole-wheat kernels, water, vitamins and minerals. Another group received Puffed Wheat, water, and the same nutrient solution. A third set was given water and white sugar, and a fourth given nothing but water and the chemical nutrients. The rats which received the whole wheat lived more than a year on the diet. The rats who got nothing but water and vitamins lived for about eight weeks, and the animals on a white sugar and water diet lived for a month. But Quaker's own laboratory study showed that rats given vitamins, water and all the Puffed Wheat they wanted died in two weeks. It wasn't a matter of the rats dying of malnutrition; results like these suggested that there was something actually toxic about the Puffed Wheat itself. Proteins are very similar to certain toxins in molecular structure, and the puffing process of putting the grain under 1500 pounds-per-square-inch of pressure, and then releasing it, may produce chemical changes which turn a nutritious grain into a poisonous substance. And Quaker has known about this toxicity since 1942.
>
> I was shocked, so I showed the report to Dr. Clark, who shared my concern. His predecessor, Dr. Graham, had published the report, and begged the company not to continue producing Puffed Wheat because of its poisonous effect on animals.
>
> Dr. Clark was so upset about finding a report like this in the company's own literature that he went right to the president of the company, Robert D. Stuart III. 'I know people should throw it on brides and grooms at weddings,' Stuart cracked, 'but if they insist on sticking it in their mouth, can I help it? Besides, we made $9 million on the stuff last year.' That's a direct quote.
>
> I have repeated similar tests with white rats, and have found that rats on a diet (sic) Puffed Wheat do worse than animals eating nothing at all. Yet despite the fact that Quaker has done its best to discredit me and intimidate members of the media interested in my message, it has yet to demonstrate that its puffed cereals can support life of any kind.[545]

Yet, we're told by the companies that make these extruded breakfast cereals that they're "healthy," "heart healthy," and "lower cholesterol." Not one of these extruded breakfast cereals is healthy. Not one. They're all just nutrient-deficient, processed foods, which are undeniably dangerous to your health. Want a healthy breakfast? Have a veggie omelet made with farm fresh eggs from pastured chickens, diced onion, mushrooms, and spinach, cooked in butter made from pastured cows that graze on organic grass, along with a banana or some other fruit. Worried about your cholesterol? Geez. We're getting to that too – in the chapter on cholesterol.

DENISE MINGER'S RE-ANALYSIS OF THE CHINA STUDY - WHEAT FLOUR & HEART DISEASE

One of my all-time favorite nutrition researchers is Denise Minger. The 20-something year-old Miss Minger is not a physician, nor does she hold a PhD in any field of science, and she is not a University researcher. Yet, when it comes to nutrition science, she is a force to be revered. Denise holds a bachelors degree in English, having graduated summa cum laude from Northern Arizona University, and she possesses an amazing mix of scientist, journalist, and artist. A self-professed "data-junkie," Denise elected to take on the monumental task of re-analyzing mountains of data from the eminent T. Colin Campbell's book, *The China Study*. Campbell is a university professor and biochemist at Cornell University. Denise undertook this task out of sheer determination to evaluate Campbell's unchallenged claims that animal foods cause not only heart disease, but cancer, diabetes and... well, what he also calls "Western-type diseases," as well as his assertion that only plant food consumption leads to good health.

Utilizing her analytical prowess and statistical wizardry, Denise, who is also the author of the brilliant and enlightening book, *Death by Food Pyramid,* debunked claim after claim made by Campbell - and when she published her results on her blog, RawFoodSOS.com,[546] she rapidly gained the respect of nutrition scientists far and wide. With that said, let's take a look at Denise's analysis of the China Study as it relates to the consumption of wheat flour. {To make sense of this, you must understand that Denise presents correlation coefficients (symbol r). An r value of 0 indicates that the two variables share no relationship at all. An r value of -1.00 indicates that the two variables move precisely in opposite directions - as one goes up, the other goes down. When the r value is +1.00, the two variable move precisely in the same direction - they're perfectly correlated.} Alright, from my all-time favorite author, let's hear how Denise tells the story:

> "When I first started analyzing the original China Study data, I had no intention of writing up an actual critique of Campbell's much-lauded book. I'm a data junkie. I mainly wanted to see for myself how closely Campbell's claims aligned with the data he drew from - if only to satisfy my own curiosity.
>
> I was a vegetarian/vegan for over a decade and I have nothing but respect for those who choose a plant-based diet, even though I am no longer vegan. My goal, with the China Study analysis and elsewhere, is to figure out the truth about nutrition and health without the interference of biases and dogma. I have no agenda to promote.
>
> I propose that Campbell's hypothesis is not altogether wrong but, more accurately, incomplete. While he has skillfully identified the importance of whole, unprocessed foods in achieving and maintaining health, his focus on wedding animal products with disease has come at the expense of exploring—or even acknowledging—the presence of other diet-disease patterns that may be stronger, more relevant, and ultimately more imperative for public health and nutritional research.
>
> Perhaps more troubling than the distorted facts in the China Study are the details Campbell leaves out. Why does Campbell indict animal foods in cardiovascular disease (correlation of 0.01 for animal protein and -0.11 for fish protein), yet fail to mention that wheat flour has a correlation of 0.67 with heart attacks and coronary heart disease, and plant protein correlates at 0.25 with these conditions?

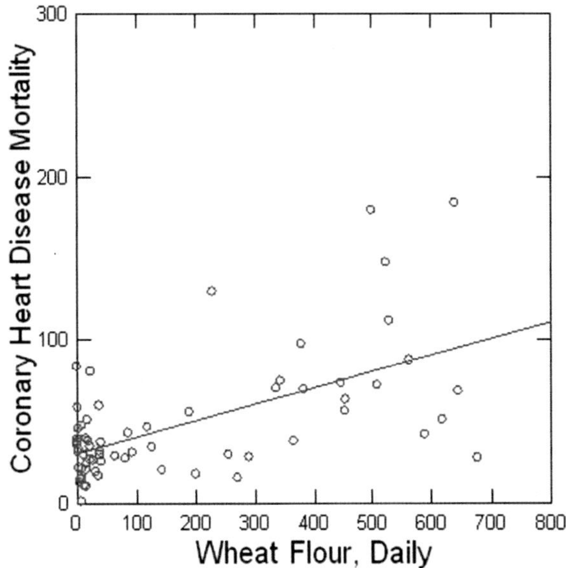

FIGURE 11.1 Coronary heart disease mortality in deaths per 100,000 population plotted against daily consumption of wheat flour in grams per day. Source: Denise Minger, RawFoodSOS.com.

> Why doesn't Campbell also note the astronomical correlations wheat flour has with various diseases: 0.46 with cervical cancer, 0.54 with hypertensive heart disease, 0.47 with stroke, 0.41 with diseases of the blood and blood-forming organs, and the aforementioned 0.67 with myocardial infarction and coronary heart disease? Could the "Grand Prix of epidemiology" have accidentally uncovered a link between the Western world's leading cause of death and its favorite glutenous grain? Is the "staff of life" really the staff of death?
>
> When we pluck out the wheat variable from the 1989 China Study II questionnaire (which has more recorded data) and consider potential nonlinearity, the outcome is even creepier.
>
> Wheat is the strongest predictor of body weight in kilograms; $r = 0.65$, $p<0.001$) out of any diet variable. And it's not just because wheat eaters are taller, either, because wheat consumption also strongly correlates with body mass index ($r = 0.58$, $p<0.001$)." [547]

Notice that Miss Minger's analysis here regards "wheat flour" - which, as we've learned, is not generally whole-grain flour. It's the typical white flour that is a highly refined food devoid of any significant bran or germ.

I stand in awe of Denise's brilliant analysis here - and this is just a little piece of it. It's factual, data-driven, and is not really subject to much interpretation. The facts stand for themselves: Today's wheat flour has a very strong association with heart disease and heart attack. Now to be completely fair, this is still epidemiological data, so we cannot conclude cause and effect. That would take a formal study wherein the variables (wheat flour consumption, e.g.) are controlled and the outcomes assessed at a later point. The problem with all such studies is simply that conditions like heart disease (and AMD) obviously take decades to develop – not a few years. Hoping for randomized, controlled, clinical trials with meaningful outcomes? Not likely to happen in any of our lifetimes. But, if we see that wheat flour consumption has a correlation of 0.67 with heart disease, that's pretty strong evidence that the two might be connected. And if they are, might we not also implicate wheat flour consumption in the vascular occlusive disease associated with macular degeneration?

On another twist to the outcome of this data, we might also consider that the consumption of wheat flour tends to "run with" the consumption of other foods that are themselves atherogenic, such as vegetable oils, trans fats, and sugar. If so, what do we call such foods? We call them processed foods!

WHOLE GRAINS IN PREVENTION OF CORONARY HEART DISEASE

David Jacobs, PhD, and Lyn Steffen, PhD, in a paper presented in the American Journal of Clinical Nutrition, discuss the benefits of whole grains as well as the reduced risk of disease with their consumption. "Benefit accrues," they state, "when all edible parts of the grain are included (bran, germ, and endosperm)." [548] They attribute much of this reduced risk to the presence of phytochemicals located in the fiber matrix. Their research suggests that risk of disease is reduced even further when the diet is "otherwise high in plant foods." [549]

As most of you already know, cardiovascular disease is the number one cause of death in both men and women in the U.S. There is very significant evidence, from both epidemiologic and clinical studies, that links increasing consumption of whole grains to reduced risk of coronary heart disease (CHD).[550] British Professor J.N. Morris and his colleagues followed 337 subjects for periods ranging between 10 and 20 years. Twenty years from the onset of the study, 45 of the men had developed CHD. The men with the least risk of heart disease were the ones that consumed the most calories (the most food) and had the highest cereal fiber intake.[551]

Though the finding that those who consumed the most food also had the least heart disease may be perplexing to many, it is a finding that recurs repeatedly. This might very well suggest that those who are the most physically active, carry the most muscle mass, and therefore, have the highest metabolic rate, also consume the most food and, therefore, greater amounts of micro-nutrients in the form of vitamins, minerals, etc., which are protective.

In the Iowa Women's Health Study, 34,492 women, all initially free of CHD and between 55 and 69 years of age, were prospectively followed for eight years, with the study concluding in 1994. Whole-grain intake was assessed based on seven items in a food-frequency questionnaire. A total of 387 developed CHD, and the data showed that those in the top two highest quintiles of whole-grain intake had a combined risk of 0.67 as compared to those in the lowest quintile with a hazards ratio of 1.0. After controlling for 15 other possible confounding variables, including fiber intake, the authors concluded that the reduced risk was not due to fiber. The authors reported, **"A clear inverse association between whole-grain intake and risk of ischemic (poor blood flow) heart disease death existed. A causal association is plausible because whole-grain foods contain many phytochemicals, including fiber and antioxidants, that may reduce chronic disease risk."** [552]

In a Finnish study, 21,930 male smokers, all between 50 and 69 years of age, were prospectively followed for just over six years. They found that those consuming the most rye products had the lowest risk of CHD death.[553] In a U.S. study of 43,757 health professionals between 40 and 75 years of age, researchers found that there was an inverse relationship between cereal fiber intake and risk of myocardial infarction (heart attack).[554]

In the Nurses' Health Study, some 68,782 women, aged 37 to 64 years, were followed prospectively for ten years, in part to examine the relationship between grain intake and cardiovascular disease. The authors here, once again, found a significantly reduced risk of CHD with higher fiber intake, particularly from cereal grains.[555]

Whole-grains have also been shown to be beneficial in body weight regulation,[556] to be strongly protective against cancer in numerous studies,[557] to help control blood glucose and reduce the risk of type 2 diabetes,[558 559 560] and to reduce all-cause mortality.[561]

The clinical evidence clearly indicates that whole-grains reduce cardiac risk, while white flour from wheat increases risk. Whole grains also reduce the risk of diabetes, cancers, overweight and obesity, and all-cause mortality. These outcomes from consuming whole grains are the polar opposites of those for wheat consumption in the form of white flour. As previously reviewed, AMD and cardiovascular disease are strongly connected, epidemiologically, clinically, and from the standpoint of biologically plausible mechanisms.

WHOLE GRAINS AND PREVENTION OF AMD...

Researchers from Rotterdam, the Netherlands, studied the risk of AMD in relation to nutrient intake. They found, "A significant inverse association was observed for intake of vitamin E, iron, and zinc." [562] Interestingly, it is the vitamin E that is sheered away via roller milling in the creation of a 75% extraction white flour and once again, in one study, this reduced the available zinc from 29 to 8 ppm, and iron from 35 to 13 ppm.

Previously, we reviewed that the isomers of vitamin E, called tocotrienols, are fairly abundant in whole grain wheat and they are found in the oil (germ). Multiple studies show that the tocotrienols suppress angiogenesis (new vessel growth) through inhibition of our old friend vascular endothelial growth factor (VEGF). This occurs through what is called *inhibition of VEGF expression*[563 564] as well as *VEGF receptor signaling*.[565 566 567] What this means is that the whole grains contain significant doses of nutrients that may help suppress the development of wet AMD, whereas white flour does not.

The last study cited also found that delta-Tocotrienol suppresses VEGF whereas alpha-tocopherol, the type of vitamin E found in virtually all supplements, does not.

I have found no available studies that look specifically at white flour or whole grain consumption and risk of AMD, however, I would submit that given the increased risk of CHD and obesity with white flour as well as the reduced risk of both conditions with whole grains, we should expect that AMD risk should be reduced with increasing whole grain consumption as well.

If nutrient deficiency is one of the primary causes for disease, white flour may be a significant contributor to such because it currently accounts for 20% of our caloric consumption, globally. For many people who consume white flour for breakfast in the form of pastries, waffles, pancakes, etc, white flour for lunch in the form of white bread or hamburger buns, and white flour for dinner in the form of more bread, rolls, croissants, or pasta, wheat may contribute up to 40 or 50 percent of their diet on a caloric basis. This much white flour in the diet would certainly greatly contribute to an overall significant nutrient deficiency. Multiple nutrient deficiencies have been associated with AMD.

SUGAR, DISEASE, AND MACULAR DEGENERATION

"Wrap your brain around this: in 1822, we ate the amount of added sugar in one 12 ounce can of soda every five days, while today we eat that much sugar every seven hours."

~ Stephan Guyenet, PhD ~

(WholeHealthSource.org)

The August, 2013 edition of *National Geographic* magazine presented a feature article by Rich Cohen, entitled "Sugar Love – A not so sweet story." The article began, "They had to go. The Coke machine, the snack machine, the deep fryer. Hoisted and dragged through the halls and out to the curb, they sat with other trash beneath gray, forlorn skies…" [568] The reference regarded the school, Kirkpatrick Elementary, in Clarksdale, Mississippi – a place where school administrators took action in 2006 towards protecting their children from the hazards of sugar and other processed foods. Cohen continues in the article, "High rates of obesity, diabetes, high blood pressure, heart disease: the legacy, some experts say, of sugar, a crop that brought the ancestors of most Clarksdale residents to this hemisphere in chains."[569] Cohen goes on to describe how sugar is addictive, an assertion that is supported behaviorally and metabolically.

Like white flour and vegetable oils, added sugar is a major displacing food of modern commerce. It displaces nutrient dense foods and has been gaining ground in that capacity for nearly 200 years. Obesity researcher, neurobi-

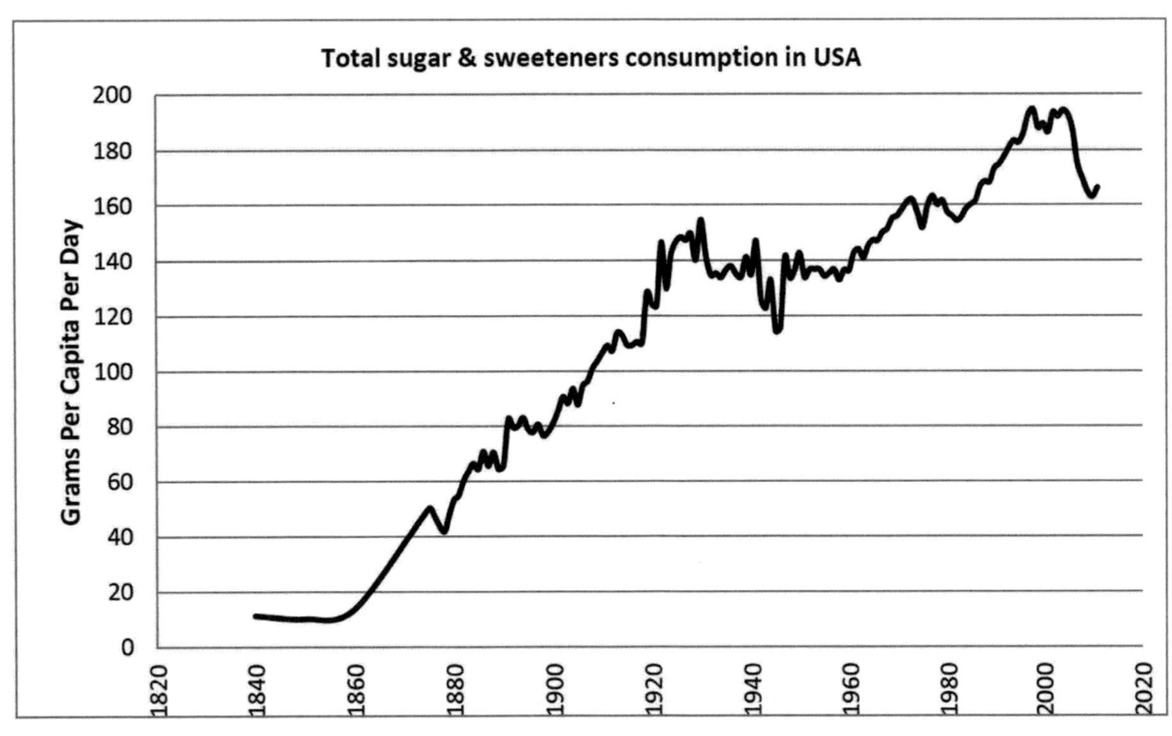

ologist, and author, the brilliant Dr. Stephan Guyenet, at the University of Washington, along with Jeremy Landen, compiled data on sugar consumption going back to 1822. They utilized statistics from "old US Department of Commerce reports and the USDA" that "represent added sweeteners such as cane sugar, high-fructose corn syrup and maple syrup, but not naturally occurring sugars in fruit and vegetables."[570] Then, Dr. Guyenet, in his usual attention to every detail, "adjusted the whole data set for post-production losses using the USDA's current loss estimate of 28.8%."[571]

Dr. Guyenet found that we consumed 6.3 pounds of sugar per person per year in 1822, rising to a high of 107.7 pounds per person per year, by 1999. This is an increase of over 17-fold during this period.[572] In 1999, this is as an average consumption of 32 teaspoons per person per day.[573]

My colleague, Marija Stojanoska, and I researched this data ourselves and Marija graphed the data on sugar consumption, above. From this analysis, one can see that sugar consumption in the U.S. was only about 12 grams a day in 1860, rising to over 190 grams per person per day by year 2000. These numbers are not fully corrected for losses, that is, non-consumption due to waste.

Most people probably think of sugar in terms of being "empty calories." In that capacity, they're right. Sugar, for the sake of this discussion, is limited essentially to table sugar, known as sucrose, and high-fructose corn syrup (HFCS), which is derived from corn. These are generally referred to as "added sugars." All natural forms of sugar, such as those found in fruits and to a much smaller extent, in vegetables, behave very differently metabolically as compared to added sugar and should not be considered along with "added sugars."

There's no question that the sugars that are added to foods truly are "empty calories," in that they are not associated with any vitamins, minerals, antioxidants, fiber, carotenoids, phytonutrients, polyphenols or any other nutrients. As such, when sugars take up a considerable portion of the diet, they can add greatly to our burden of the 'displacing foods of modern commerce'. Once again, sugars, just like white flour and vegetable oils, may contribute a significant part of the diet without any nutritional reward, thus leading to further nutritional inadequacy.

ROBERT LUSTIG, MD, ON SUGAR: IS SUGAR A POISON?

On May 26, 2009, Robert Lustig, MD, pediatric endocrinologist and leading childhood obesity expert at the University of California San Francisco, gave a lecture entitled "Sugar: The Bitter Truth." This lecture was posted to YouTube by the University of California Television (UCTV) and, as of December, 2015, has been viewed more than six million times. In this 90 minute lecture, Lustig argued that added sugars may not only be the cornerstone of our obesity epidemic, but are also a major cause of hypertension, diabetes, non-alcoholic fatty liver disease (NAFLD) and cardiovascular disease – in short – metabolic syndrome.[574] His argument is not only compelling, but is backed by enough research to fill several textbooks.

As a reminder, I'd like to point out again that macular degeneration has a long history of association with hypertension, diabetes, cardiovascular disease, and metabolic syndrome.

Now, of course, none of this issue about sugar consumption would be the case if we consumed it like a condiment, Dr. Lustig points out, but instead, we consume sugar like a complete food-group. **The 2001 to 2004 National Health and Nutrition Examination Survey (NHANES) database determined that the average intake of added sugars for Americans at that time was 22.2 teaspoons per day, which translates to about 345 calories (about 4 grams per teaspoon).**[575] On a 2,000 calorie per day diet, this much sugar would account for about 17% of the diet. In contrast, on an all-natural diet, where the only sugar would come from a small number of fruits and plenty of vegetables, the expected sugar consumption is a total of about 10 to 30 grams per day, which is only about 2 to 6 percent of the diet. This amount of sugar in the diet is consistent with the consumption of most of our 19th century ancestors, who again, had virtually no heart disease, hypertension, diabetes, or Alzheimer's disease, and in whom cancer was very rare. AMD, of course, was virtually unheard of.

The NHANES data, however, may not be as accurate as the USDA Economic Research Service (ERS), which relies on manufacturing and utilization data. By the year 1997, the USDA ERS calculated that the average American consumed 154 pounds of sugars that year in the form of sucrose (from cane and beets) and corn sweeteners (mostly HFCS), amounting to two-fifths of a pound – or 52 teaspoonfuls – per day. **The ERS estimated that approximately 20 teaspoonfuls per person per day were wasted or not consumed, *resulting in an average intake of approximately 32 teaspoons of added sugars per day*. This is a staggering amount, and would equal about 512 calories of sugar per day, or nearly 26% of the total caloric content of the diet.**[576] Contrast that with the 6 pounds of sugars consumed per person in 1822, which translates to just 7.46 grams per person per day, or less than two teaspoons of sugar per day.

According to the National Institute of Diabetes and Digestive and Kidney Diseases, **"consumption of simple sugars (sucrose, glucose, and fructose) currently is estimated at 20 percent of the U.S. diet on average."**[577]

According to Dr. Lustig, there are ten Big Food manufacturers that are responsible for 90 percent of the processed foods in the U.S.: Kraft, Coca-Cola, Nestle, PepsiCo, Proctor & Gamble, General Mills, Kellogg's, Mars, Johnson & Johnson, and Unilever.[578] In his book, *Fat Chance*, Lustig wrote, **"Barry Popkin of the University of North Carolina states that of the six hundred thousand food items for sale in the United States, 80 percent are laced with added sugar."[579] As such, sugar is actually a proxy – a marker if you will – for processed foods.**

The 2005 – 2006 NHANES data showed that the food groups contributing 5% or more of added sugars in the

American diet were sodas/energy/sports drinks (36%), grain-based desserts (13%), fruit drinks (10%), dairy desserts (7%), and candy (6%) (all numbers rounded).[580]

Sugars found naturally in foods behave very differently than added sugars and should be considered separately. In fact, the generally accepted definition of added sugars is: "Sugars and syrups that are added to foods during processing or preparation. Added sugars do not include naturally occurring sugars such as those that occur in milk and fruits." [581]

The sugar in fruits, which can be moderate, and vegetables, which is negligible, however, is "packaged" with fiber, which means that the gut has to break down the fibers and the cell walls of the plant materials before the sugars can be absorbed. This dramatically delays and prolongs the absorption of the fructose component of the sugar, thereby creating an entirely different metabolic effect since the fructose part of the sugar can only be metabolized in the liver.

Let's define fructose as well. Sucrose is a disaccharide, made up of one molecule of glucose and one molecule of fructose. It is a 50/50 mixture of glucose and fructose. HFCS is either 55 HFCS, which is about 55% fructose and 42% glucose, or HFCS 42, which is 42% fructose and 53% glucose. HFCS 55 is primarily used for sugar sweetened beverages, because it's sweeter, while HFCS 42, is used in most other processed foods, which aren't quite as sweet.

According to Dr. Lustig, in his 2009 UCSF lecture, "High fructose corn syrup and sucrose are exactly the same. They're both equally bad. Okay? They're both dangerous – they're both poison." He continues, "My charge before the end of tonight is to demonstrate that fructose is a poison. And I will do it." Further along in his presentation, Dr. Lustig states, "So they're talking about soda [a major source of fructose sugar in our diets] like it's empty calories. I'm here to tell you that it goes way beyond empty calories. Okay? The reason why this is a problem is because fructose is a poison. Okay. It's not about the calories. It has nothing to do with the calories. It's a poison by itself." [582]

In the same lecture, Dr Lustig reviews data specifically with respect to fructose consumption. His findings with regard to fructose consumption alone were presented as follows: Natural sugar consumption (from fruits and vegetables) - 15 grams per day; Prior to WW II – 16 - 24 grams per day; 1977 – 78 (USDA Data) – 37 grams per day (8% of total caloric intake); 1994 (NHANES III) – 54.7 grams per day (10.2% of total caloric intake); and today's adolescents – 72.8 grams per day (12.1% of total caloric intake). Finally, he notes that 25% of adolescents consume at least 15% of their calories from fructose alone, which means they are consuming 30% of their diet as sugar. In response to this, Dr. Lustig comments, "Twenty-five percent of the adolescents today consume at least 15% of their calories from fructose alone. This is a disaster – an absolute unmitigated disaster. The fat's going down, the sugar's going up, and we're all getting sick." [583]

Lustig's assertions are by no means the first of their kind. According to *National Geographic* author, Rich Cohen, "As far back as 1675, when western Europe was experiencing its first sugar boom, Thomas Willis, a physician and founding member of Britain's Royal Society, noted that the urine of people afflicted with diabetes tasted 'wonderfully sweet, as if it were imbued with honey or sugar.' Two hundred and fifty years later Haven Emerson at Columbia University pointed out that a remarkable increase in deaths from diabetes between 1900 and 1920 corresponded with an increase in sugar consumption." [584]

Next, British physician, scientist, researcher, and author, John Yudkin, MD, PhD, who wrote the book, "Pure, White and Deadly" in 1972, with a remake in 1986, promulgated strong warnings to the world specifically regarding the dangers of sugar. In his first book, he wrote, "First, there is no physiological requirement for sugar; all human nutritional needs can be met in full without having to take a single spoon of white or brown or raw sugar, on its own or in any food or drink. Secondly, if only a small fraction of what is already known about the effects of sugar were to be revealed in relation to any other material used as a food additive, that material would promptly be banned." [585] As early as 1957, Yudkin had begun to show that the consumption of sugar was closely associated with heart disease and diabetes. His studies indicated that sugars raise triglycerides, cholesterol, and insulin levels. In fact, in his 1972 book, he wrote, "Fructose seems to be the part of the sucrose that produces most of the ill-effects of sucrose." [586] He not only drew connections between sugar consumption and dental caries, but also diabetes, coronary heart disease, autoimmune disease, gout, and cancer. He made strong delineations linking sugar consumption with significant morbidity and early demise.

Robert Atkins, MD, author of *Dr. Atkins' Diet Revolution,* was most certainly a Yudkin acolyte. He too was convinced of the dangers of sugar, in his case, particularly with respect to its ability to cause weight gain and obesity. Of course, weight gain and obesity are linked tightly to metabolic syndrome and heart disease. In Atkins book, released in 1972, he wrote: "But, if I had to pick the single causative factor most responsible for the obesity epidemic that has spread through all Westernized countries, it would be the overconsumption of refined sugar. I think something should be done to correct this situation now." [587]

Of course, authorities didn't heed the advice of Yudkin or Atkins. Instead, they made the assertion that fat in the diet was the problem and collectively advised us to reduce our fat consumption. Quite frankly, the medical orthodoxy ridiculed Atkins and his diet. Meanwhile, sugar consumption continued to climb, rising an additional 23%, just between the years 1985 and 1999. And while the prevalence of obesity was at around 13% in 1972, when Dr. Atkins published his book, the prevalence has soared nearly three-fold to affect some 36% of the nation's adults today.

In great contrast, many thousands of Atkins' patients lost weight and reversed chronic diseases, as did millions of those who bought his book and followed his advice. Of course, though the Atkins' diet reduces carbohydrates drastically, this move virtually eliminates added sugars and white flour, and his admonition to consume all the steak, butter, and eggs desired keeps the focus of the diet on animal fats, instead of vegetable oils and their associated trans fats. The latter was, in my opinion, even far more important than the reduction of sugar and carbs.

FRUCTOSE OVERCONSUMPTION CAUSES METABOLIC SYNDROME, TYPE 2 DIABETES, HYPERTENSION & HEART DISEASE

In the same lecture by Dr. Lustig, "Sugar: The Bitter Truth," he explained how fructose uniquely causes metabolic syndrome. Glucose, unlike fructose, can be utilized by every cell in the body. Fructose, on the other hand, can only by metabolized in the liver. When we consume sugar, the enzyme sucrase in the bowel cleaves it into the two molecules, glucose and fructose. Glucose can be utilized everywhere. Fructose is transported directly and only to the liver to be metabolized. As it is metabolized, the waste product, uric acid, is produced. Uric acid blocks the production of nitric oxide, which is normally present to dilate blood vessels and thereby prevent high blood pressure. With nitric oxide being blocked, hypertension often ensues.[588] Here's a major reason for high blood pressure. Secondly, when uric acid accumulates, gout may develop, which is a type of arthritis that is often accompanied by a severely painful big toe.

Fructose is ultimately metabolized in the liver with significant proportions being converted to fats in a process known as de novo lipogenesis (DNL). This is where a high sugar diet ultimately is like a high fat diet, but *not* one of healthy fats. Ultimately, another by-product of this pathway is the production of very low density lipoproteins (VLDL), which are strongly associated with heart disease.[589] All of this occurs when we consume sugar in substantial quantities in readily digested forms, like soft drinks and candy. This isn't the situation with consumption of sugars in fruits and vegetables, regardless of the load.

In a study evaluating glucose versus fructose metabolism, Hellerstein and colleagues showed that only about 2% of an oral glucose load was converted into fat, whereas more than 30% of a fructose load was converted to fats.[590] Swiss researchers showed that, in just six days of a high fructose diet, healthy men developed high triglycerides, increased blood sugar, a six-fold increase in DNL, and they developed insulin resistance both in the liver and in fat tissue.[591] Insulin resistance is the primary marker and truly the hallmark sign of metabolic syndrome, as it is associated with the ultimate development of visceral fat, inflammation, diabetes, high blood pressure, and cardiovascular disease. And fructose has been repeatedly shown to induce insulin resistance in animal models.[592] [593] [594] When there is insulin resistance, the pancreas has to make more and more insulin to accomplish the job of glucose disposal – which is the job of getting glucose into cells.

Finally, the high insulin levels have been shown to block the action of the hormone leptin, which is normally our body's signal back to the brain that the "fat stores are full."[595] When this happens, leptin can't do its job of turning off the hunger signal because there is enough stored energy, which means that the affected individual remains hungry in spite of having consumed enough food. This mechanism explains the development of obesity in many of those who consume too much sugar.

Now some of the fat produced by de novo lipogenesis cannot make it out of the liver and this results in the accumulation of liver fat, known as non-alcoholic fatty liver disease (NAFLD). If this continues for a long enough period of time, significant liver disease ensues.[596]

Lustig and Sanjay Basu analyzed global sugar consumption in relation to disease, and found that, **"Diabetes prevalence rates rose 27% on average from 2000 to 2010, with just over one-fourth of the increase explained by a rise in sugar availability..."** They also concluded that, "In countries like the Philippines, Romania, Sri Lanka, Georgia and Bangladesh, where high and rising diabetes rates were observed in the context of low obesity rates, sugar availability rose by over 20% during the study period." [597]

The majority of sugar consumption today is a result of sugar-sweetened beverage consumption – mostly soft drinks – which have also progressively gotten larger over the past 60 years. The European EPIC Interact, a large-scale international study, determined that every can of soda consumed per day increases the risk of diabetes by 29 percent.[598] And as far as caloric consumption, for every 150 additional calories consumed per day, diabetes prevalence rises 0.1 percent, but if those 150 calories come from a can of soda, the prevalence rises 11-fold (1.1%).[599]

If we want to translate all of this concern of metabolic syndrome into cardiovascular risk, researchers representing the Centers for Disease Control (CDC) did just that, in a study that evaluated sugar consumption as a percentage of the total diet versus cardiovascular disease mortality. **They found that there was a smooth parabolic curve transitioning upward in terms of risk, with those consuming 10% or less of calories from sugar at a relative risk score of 1.0, rising to a 3-fold increased risk for those consuming 32% of calories as sugar!** [600] This, unfortunately, represents 25% of teen boys today, which means that, if they keep this up, we can expect astronomical proportions of them to be obese, have diabetes, high blood pressure, and heart attacks, by the time they're in their 30s and 40s.

SUGAR CONSUMPTION AND MACULAR DEGENERATION – A LINK?

As reviewed, high consumption of sugars that have been added to the diet, ultimately results in insulin resistance. This means that insulin doesn't function as well in doing its job of driving glucose into cells, whether they be muscle, liver, or fat. The end-result of this is higher blood sugars. When blood sugars elevate, or when particular sugars are present in greater amounts, we develop advanced glycation end products, or AGEs.[601] AGEs are proteins that have interacted with sugars, which ultimately stiffen and become modified in various ways. In the end, at the tissue level, this if often thought to be consistent with aging. AGEs can impair cell function in multiple ways and even result in premature cell death.[602]

There is significant evidence that AGEs play an important role in the outer retina, which is where macular degeneration occurs.[603] Specifically, multiple studies have shown that AGEs accumulate in both drusen and in Bruch's membrane, and are present in significantly greater quantities in patients with AMD.[604 605 606 607] Drusen, the metabolic deposits so characteristic of AMD, have also been shown to contain various lipids and proteins (apolipoprotein E, amyloid, and vitronectin)[608 609] that have undergone the Maillard reaction, the latter of which is a browning reaction that creates AGEs and can be demonstrated in various molecules.[610 611 612] The Maillard reaction is what we get when we grill meat coated with barbecue sauce – it browns or, if overdone, actually blackens. This can happen quickly, over fire, or very slowly in our bodies, at 98 degrees. More sugar means more browning!

You may recall that Bruch's membrane thickens with age, is characteristically thickened in AMD, and is less permeable.[613 614] Interestingly, basement membranes are known to thicken in relation to advanced glycation. There are two basement membranes in Bruch's membrane: the basement membrane of the retinal pigment epithelium (RPE) and the basement membrane of the choriocapillaris. It is very plausible that Bruch's membrane thickens in response to AGEs deposition, thereby decreasing its permeability. Recall that the photoreceptors have to transport metabolic waste across Bruch's membrane to the choriocapillaris, and the choriocapillaris must exchange gases and nutrients across Bruch's membrane to the photoreceptors. Accumulation of deposits, including AGEs, may be an important element of this thickening, damage, and accumulation of deposits (drusen) in Bruch's membrane, and sugars may greatly contribute to this.

Now for the clincher: fructose is tremendously more highly glycated than is glucose.[615] In fact, glucose is tremendously less likely to undergo glycation, but various other sugars, particularly fructose, are. With that said, could the damage, thickening, and therefore, the loss of diffusion potential across Bruch's membrane, as a result of sugar consumption, be a major component of the development of AMD? I would suggest that this is not only biologically plausible, but seems likely.

Whether or not this is a major factor based on population studies, will be shown in our own data, which is presented in Chapter 13 – AMD Follows Processed Foods Worldwide.

Fructose and the development of AGEs appears to play a very significant role in damage to the RPE as well. According to Professor Alan Stitt, who is the McCauley Chair of Experimental Ophthalmology at Queen's University Belfast, Ireland, "RPE cells are radically influenced by exposure to AGEs in vitro where they express abnormal levels of vascular endothelial growth factor (VEGF) and platelet derived growth factor B (PDGF-B). This may have a bearing on RPE cell function, maintenance of the choriocapillaris, and integrity of the RPE/photoreceptor complex." [616]

Researchers at Harvard showed that human RPE cells increased their VEGF gene expression (measured by determining VEGF mRNA, an indirect measure of cells' ultimate production of VEGF) after being exposed to AGEs. They determined that VEGF increased more than 4-fold when human RPE cells were exposed to AGEs at approximately the same level present in many diabetic patients' serum. However, if they combined the AGEs exposure with a low-oxygen environment, which might occur with progressive vascular disease and damage to Bruch's membrane in an AMD eye, that combination increased VEGF mRNA levels by 10.8-fold. Within 24 hours, this increased the actual VEGF protein by 1.7-fold. They found similar results when rabbit eyes were injected with AGEs and VEGF mRNA levels increased 4.8-fold.[617]

From here, the science may get pretty deep for most people, except perhaps for the vision scientists and ophthalmologists. Suffice it to say that this scenario, whereby AGEs induce increased VEGF, is then associated with the accumulation of metabolic by-products from the breakdown of photoreceptor outer segments, known as lipofuscin, and RPE cells may then have a reduced capacity to degrade these outer segments. **Here we have a mechanism by which sugars, especially fructose, induce AGEs – which ultimately damage RPE cells. The RPE cells may then become incompetent to manage the task of properly supporting the photoreceptors.**[618] Recall that AMD is characterized primarily by damage to and loss of RPE and the photoreceptors.

Finally, if all of this weren't enough, as we have reviewed in detail, sugar is a major cause of heart disease and cardiovascular mortality. We know that AMD is associated with the vascular compromise of the choriocapillaris, right? And now we know that sugar consumption is associated with a 3-fold increased risk of cardiovascular death, right? So, wouldn't it make sense that the vascular disease would also affect the choriocapillaris, which nourishes the macula, and that this might be a major cause of AMD? We've seen, over and over, that the same conditions that cause heart disease also correlate with AMD.

Perhaps the best case in point is the following: Researchers from Singapore studied metabolic syndrome and its relationship to AMD. Their conclusion? "Metabolic syndrome, obesity, high glucose, and high triglycerides were predictors of progression to late AMD." [619] The take home point is that – every last pathological detail cited in their conclusion comes from high sugar consumption. Every last one.

HIGH FRUCTOSE DIET FAVORS METABOLIC SYNDROME AND WET AMD IN EXPERIMENTAL RATS...

Researchers know that one of the fastest ways to produce metabolic syndrome in rats (or other animals) is to just give them a high sugar diet. In fact, a high fructose diet works exceedingly well. Brown rats only live about two years – so they're great for studying various diseases – but disease conditions must be induced quickly. In one study, French scientists induced metabolic syndrome in rats by feeding them a diet of 60% fructose, while control rats ate a standard diet. The rats in the experimental group gained 17% body fat within months, developed non-alcoholic fatty liver disease (liver steatosis) within 3 months, had up to two-fold increased leptin levels at one and three months, and up to two-fold increases in their insulin levels within 3 to 6 months. These are all the key features of metabolic syndrome. But, they didn't become diabetic in this time frame. The researchers then completed 5 to 7 laser spots in the retinas of these rats to cause minor breaks in Bruch's membrane. This is a method to simulate the breaks in Bruch's membrane that precede, but don't guarantee, the development of wet AMD in people. After 3 months of the fructose feeding, the rats in the experimental group developed dramatically higher rates of choroidal neovascularization (wet AMD equivalent) within two weeks after the laser treatments than did the rats in the control group (P = 0.0065).[620]

HIGH GLYCEMIC INDEX DIETS FAVOR AMD...

In the last twenty years or so, there's been much ado about the glycemic index of foods and disease. The glycemic index relates to the ability of a carbohydrate containing food to raise blood sugar. If we were to ever go down a rabbit hole, I assure you, this subject would be it. We could get lost in the chaos and confusion of this topic for the next 90 pages. Neither of us wants that.

However, I am mentioning this because quite a lot of ophthalmic research has focused on this subject. In fact, Chung-Jung Chiu, DDS, PhD, at Tufts University Laboratory for Nutrition and Vision Research, has completed an immense amount of research and a number of publications on this topic. In the first study on this subject, published in 2006, women in the Nurses' Health Study who normally consumed the highest glycemic index (GI) diets were found to have the highest risk of AMD. Those who were in the upper 30% on the GI diet scale had about a 2.7-fold increased risk for early AMD.[621] In a much larger cohort study, the Age-Related Eye Disease Study (AREDS), those who consumed diets in the upper 20% of GI compared to those in the lowest 20% of GI had greater than a 40% increased risk for large drusen (a marker for moderate AMD). This data suggests that one in five cases of advanced AMD would be eliminated with dietary GI's below the median.[622] Multiple additional studies that are in support of this general concept are reviewed by Dr. Chiu, in great detail.[623]

There's a mountain of research relating to glycemic index, but let's just cut to the chase, shall we? Do you know what a high glycemic index diet is? At the risk of making the most unscientific answer and statement thus far in this book – it is the Standard American Diet (SAD). It is loaded with two things (that are both high on the GI index): white flour and sugar. That's how we get high glycemic index diets, which are inherently unhealthy. Trust me, you won't need to worry about glycemic index for any foods, so long as they're natural and unprocessed. If that is the case, you can eat all of the (unprocessed) high glycemic index fruit, potatoes, cassava, yams, sweet potatoes, and rice that you want, without risk.

Let's look at a few examples of societies that consume lots of carbohydrates, some of which are high in glycemic index, yet are healthy and, anecdotally, until recently, have been lean, healthy, and without disease. In some of these populations, there is also evidence that they did not have AMD until converting to a Westernized, processed food-laden diet (to be reviewed in Chapter 13). For starters, let me quote Stephan Guyenet, PhD, obesity researcher at the University of Washington, whose website is *WholeHealthSource.org*, as he addresses the carbohydrate hypothesis of obesity (hypothesis that carbohydrate is intrinsically fattening, which he denies):

> "Let's start with a culture that eats more carbohydrate than any other I know: the New Guinea highland tribe at Tukisenta that was studied extensively in the 1960s and 70s. They ate 94 percent of their calories as carbohydrate, mostly from sweet potatoes, for a total calorie intake of 2,300 kcal/day in men and 1,770 kcal/day in women. Investigators found them to be fit, lean and muscular, with no sign of protein deficiency (Trowell and Burkitt. *Western Diseases.* 1981).
>
> West Nile district, Uganda, 1940s. The diet consisted of millet, cassava, corn, lentils, peanuts, bananas and vegetables (Trowell and Burkitt. *Western Diseases.* 1981). Despite food abundance, 'in the 1940s it was quite unusual to see a stout man or woman.' 'In recent years, however, a fair number of upper-class middle-aged West Nile women have begun to look rather stout, and some men have become very obese, especially those who hold lucrative posts and can purchase whatever food they like.' This corresponded with an increase in 'sugar, cooking oils, milk, fish and meat' and a corresponding decrease in 'home-grown starchy staple foods.' This same scenario has happened to hundreds, if not thousands of African communities whose traditional diets are very high in carbohydrate."[624]

Dr. Guyenet also reviews the people of the Massas (Massa) tribe of northern Cameroon, Africa, whose typical diet consists primarily of sorghum (corn-like grain) and milk. They were found to consume about 81% of their diet as carbohydrate (516 grams per day) and only 32 grams of fat per day, yet they were lean and healthy.[625]

Most Asian countries also have diets that are very high in carbohydrates, many of which would be high glycemic index. The people of China, Japan, Taiwan, and India all have had traditional diets very high in white rice (glycemic index 64 to 93)[626], yet they have traditionally been lean, healthy, with very low rates of disease.[627]

Staffan Lindeberg, MD, PhD, Associate Professor from the University of Lund, Sweden, studied and lived with the people on the island of Kitava, which is one of the Trobriand Islands in Papua New Guinea's archipelago. He completed his research during several years around 1990. The Kitavans are one of the few populations on earth that still consume a traditional diet, which is completely devoid of processed foods. Dr. Lindeberg found that they have absolutely no incidence of heart disease, stroke, hypertension, diabetes, overweight or obesity.[628] They also have no incidence of dementia or memory loss.[629] And according to Lindeberg, "Tubers, fruit, fish, and coconut are dietary staples whereas dairy products, refined fat (vegetable oils) and sugar, cereals, and alcohol are absent and salt intake is low." [630]

"In our survey in Kitava," wrote Lindeberg, "the residents were not familiar with cachexia, i.e., the long-term emaciation that lasts months or years and ends in death {consistent with cancer}. However, slow-growing visible tumors could be described as an extremely rare occurrence." [631] Lindeberg described that they have a low incidence of malignant lymphoma, superficial lymph node metastases, breast cancer, cancers of the abdomen, pelvis, stomach, GI tract, liver, uterus, and urinary tract or prostate.[632]

Lindeberg showed that protein accounts for 10% of their calories, fat for 21%, and carbohydrates for 69%. Their diet has a very high relative consumption of saturated fat at 17% of total energy intake, while the monounsaturated fats and polyunsaturated fatty acids (PUFAs) account for 2% of total energy intake each. Of the 2% of PUFAs that they do get, omega-3 fatty acids predominate over the omega-6, because they're coming mostly from fish.[633] Doesn't this resonate with the situation of our 19th century American ancestors? Lots of saturated fat (theirs from coconut, ours from animal), very low in PUFAs (they have no "vegetable oils"), and very low in monounsaturated fats too (like olive oil), right? Of course, the Kitavans consume virtually no added sugars, whereas our 19th century ancestors consumed very low (~6 lbs/yr in 1822) to relatively moderate amounts (~ 48 lbs/yr) by the end of that century (see graph in this chapter).

"The Kitava Study" gave additional details regarding their diet: "The residents of Kitava lived exclusively on root vegetables (yam, sweet potato, taro, tapioca), fruit (banana, papaya, pineapple, mango, guava, water melon, pumpkin), vegetables, fish and coconuts. Less than 0.2% of the caloric intake came from Western food, such as edible fats, dairy products, sugar, cereals, and alcohol, compared with roughly 75% in Sweden. The intake of vitamins, minerals and soluble fibre was therefore very high…" [634]

Lindeberg's research also showed that, "Three out of four Kitavans of both sexes were daily smokers and the rest were nonsmokers." This should give us great pause as we consider their cardiovascular status. The study continues, "Estimated life expectancy was 45 years at birth and an additional 25 years or more thereafter. Major causes of death were infections, trauma and complications of pregnancy…"[635] A much higher infant death rate as well as early deaths from infectious diseases brings their usual long life-spans down considerably, much like our 19th century American ancestors and most pastoralists and hunter-gatherer populations.

At Dr. Lindeberg's website, he displays a photograph of an elderly gentleman from Kitava Island, with the caption beneath, "100-year old man from Kitava, Papua New Guinea. He has never heard of spontaneous sudden death or symptoms suggestive of stroke." [636]

BRIEF SUMMARY ON SUGAR AND AMD

Remember that fructose is half of all added sugars, and this sweet molecule behaves very differently than glucose in almost every regard. Fructose is fine when consumed in fruits and vegetables where it is tied up inside of cell walls and associated with fiber, but fructose is not fine in *added sugars*. When sugars are added to foods in significant quantities, the stage is quickly set for the consumer to develop metabolic syndrome, which is associated with heart disease, type 2 diabetes, hypertension, obesity, and most importantly for our consideration, potentially macular degeneration as well.

Multiple mechanisms have been described by which high-dose sugar consumption, typical of most Americans, British, Australians and much of the remainder of the world in recent decades, may play a major role in the development of AMD. Sugar has been shown to induce advanced glycation end products (AGEs), which have been shown to accumulate in both drusen and Bruch's membrane. This process may thicken and reduce the permeability of Bruch's membrane, which could be devastating to the health of the RPE and photoreceptors. This is likely a key pathological component of AMD.

When sugar induces AGEs production and RPE cells are exposed, they may produce much greater quantities of VEGF and other growth factors, with the consequence that RPE cells may dysfunction, resulting in the accumulation of photoreceptor outer segments in the form of lipofuscin. RPE dysfunction may result in photoreceptor loss and eventually, RPE cell death, as this condition progresses.

Finally, sugar may ultimately cause choroidal sclerosis – the occlusion of the vessels in the choroid that nourish the macula. The propensity for sugar to invoke this disease process is analogous to the mechanisms behind high sugar consumption and cardiovascular disease, which has been well established.

"REFINED CARBOHYDRATES" ARE SYNONYMOUS WITH WHITE FLOUR & ADDED SUGAR

When you think of "refined carbohydrates," just translate this to white flour and added sugars, because that's what they are. We've reviewed so many reasons to avoid the two, including displacement of other nutrient-rich foods, induction of metabolic syndrome,undesirable weight gain, type 2 diabetes, heart disease, and more – but let's lump the two together and discuss one last issue.

Many times, people get a lab report back that indicates they have high triglycerides. Triglycerides are not only the bulk of fat that we eat but the dominant form of stored fat in our bodies. When triglycerides in the blood elevate, we are more prone to develop heart disease.[637] But these triglycerides don't come primarily from fat, they come from excess sugars that have not been used for energy when there is insulin resistance. And how does that begin? Overconsumption of white flour and sugar! The success of low carbohydrate diets works almost exclusively because they eliminate, or greatly reduce, these two components.

PROCESSED FOOD

"If you think you will be able to find a way to lose fat and remain in long-term health while eating mostly commercially processed food (including restaurant food), you are fooling yourself. Processed food is the main problem, and if there is a solution, it is to avoid it."

~ Stephan Guyenet, PhD ~

(WholeHealthSource.org)

As of 2006, the Pima Indians of Arizona have the highest rate of obesity and type 2 diabetes of virtually any population in the world. Their rate of obesity is approximately 70% and diabetes is 38% and still climbing, as of 2006. In contrast, the vast majority of genetically similar Pima Indians of Mexico maintain much lower weights, with just 7% obesity in men and 20% in women, and have one-fifth as much diabetes, at a rate of 6.9%, which is lower than present day Americans (at 9.3%).[638] The standard explanation would be that they eat too much and exercise too little, correct? Let's take a look at these people, because we can learn a lot from their plight.

The health of the Pima Indians of Arizona wasn't always so bleak. The U.S. Pima have lived in the desert of Arizona for at least two millennia, on the Gila River located southwest of Phoenix, where they were once a vibrant and thriving people. Up until 1849, these native Indians were both hunter-gatherers as well as agriculturalists. They hunted wild game that were abundant in the region, caught fish and clams from the river, and utilized that same Gila River to irrigate crops that they raised. They even raised some cattle and poultry. Agriculturally, they raised corn, beans, squash, and melons, and they also ate from the fruit of the saguaro cactus. According to Gary Taubes, in 1846, battalion surgeon John Griffin described the Pima as "sprightly" and in "fine health." [639] Like the many tribes and populations described by Weston A. Price, the Pima Indians of Arizona were in fine health while consuming their traditional diet.

However, in 1849, a wagon route was opened that passed right through the Pima's territory. By the 1860s, this would bring American and Mexican settlers, some of whom chose to settle on the Gila River to the Pima's north. Needing their own irrigation for crops, they diverted the river's water until it eventually dried up, leaving the Pima without irrigating water by about 1869. A famine would ensue for the next 20 to 25 years, or more. In the mid 1890s, the U.S. Government stepped in, and brought relief to the Pima in the form of "government rations" that prevented starvation, but at a huge price.

According to Stephan Guyenet, PhD, "The government provided the Pima with subsidized 'food' : white flour, sugar, partially hydrogenated lard, and canned goods. They promptly became diabetic and overweight, and have remained that way ever since." [640]

According to Gary Taubes, "...if the Pima diet on government rations was anything like that of tribes reduced to similar situations at the time on which data exist – including the Sioux on the Standing Rock Reservation in the Dakotas – then almost 50 percent of their calories came from sugar and flour." This trend persisted, in fact, Taubes continued, "By the late 1950's, according to the Indian Health Service in Tucson, 'large quantities of refined flour, sugar, and canned fruits high in sugar' were being distributed widely on the reservation, courtesy of a surplus commodity food program run by the U.S. Department of Agriculture." [641]

The Pima Indians of Arizona did have an increase in the fat in their diet when the government program stepped in, and the added fat primarily came from vegetable oils, of course.[642] As expected, some researchers who believe it's about macronutrients (fat, carb, and protein ratios), like to cite the fact that the Pima's fat consumption went up. Never mind the fact that they're getting nothing but low-nutrient density, processed food for most all of their calories. Recall that Weston A. Price evaluated hundreds of tribes and populations, and never found that macronutrient ratios (carbs:fat:protein) mattered. As long as cultures consumed their traditional diets, they remained lean and in supreme health. This was true for cultures that consumed nearly 70% of their calories as fat, like the Inuit, as well as for cultures that consumed as little as 21% of their calories as fat, such as some of the Pacific Islanders.[643 644] For reference, the average American today consumes about 33% of his or her calories as fat, about 15 to 16 percent as protein, and about 51% as carbs (NHANES 1971-2000).[645]

To this day, the Pima of Arizona receive food distributions that include canned meats, dry cereal, fruit juice, canned or dried milk, and egg mix, as well as some fruits and vegetables – really a whole bevy of processed foods. Unfortunately, the situation for the Pima Indians of Arizona has never changed.

According to Dr. Guyenet, with regard to the fact that researchers sometimes point their finger at the Pima Indians' slightly increased fat in their diet (still much lower than Americans), as though that is the reason for their plight, states "...the focus on macronutrients sometimes obscures the fact that the modern Pima diet is *pure crap*. It's mostly processed food with a low nutrient density. It also contains the two biggest destroyers of indigenous health: white flour and sugar. There are numerous examples of cultures going from a high-fat to a lower-fat "reservation food" diet and suffering the same fate: the Inuit of Alaska, the Maasai and Samburu of Kenya, tribes in the Pacific Northwestern U.S. and Canada, certain Aboriginal groups, and more. What do they all have in common? White flour, sugar and other processed food."

He continues, "The history of the Pima is a heart-wrenching story that has been repeated hundreds, perhaps thousands of times all over the world. Europeans bring in white flour, sugar and other processed food, it destroys a native populations' health, and then researchers either act like they don't understand why it happened, or give unsatisfying explanations for it." [646]

WHAT IS PROCESSED FOOD AND HOW DOES IT AFFECT US?

Processed food is any food that has undergone significant manipulation and is almost always found packaged into boxes, cans, plastic, or cardboard containers. Some 80 percent of processed foods contain substantial amounts of sugar; and numerous processed foods also contain vegetable oils and, therefore, trans fats, plus white flour from wheat, additives, artificial flavorings, and a whole slew of chemical ingredients. If you read ingredient labels, a good rule-of-thumb is that any food containing more than three ingredients is processed. Beware. These are typically dangerous foods.

Processed foods are dangerous, in fact, because they do contain vegetable oils, trans fats, refined sugars (sucrose and HFCS), and refined white flour, all of which are the antithesis of nutrient-dense. For all of the reasons given in this and the previous chapter, consuming these in any significant quantities is a recipe for disaster.

In a presentation at the Stockholm Food Forum – 2015, Robert Lustig, MD gave a presentation entitled "Processed Food: An Experiment That Failed." In that presentation, Dr. Lustig discussed the addictiveness of sugar, which is a great reason that food manufacturers put more and more of it in processed foods. He said, **"It [sugar} is also the thing that covers up the negative aspects of taste of processed food. And the food industry knows that when they add it – you buy more.** ***It is the marker for processed food because of the six hundred thousand items in the American food supply, 74 percent of them have added sugar,*** **which Dr. Popkin told you."**[647,648]

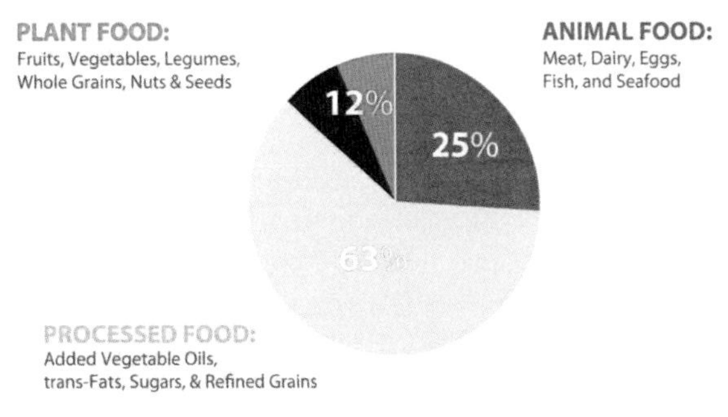

PROCESSED FOOD VERSUS NATURAL, UNPROCESSED FOODS

Below, I've compiled a table of the reasons I believe processed foods are dangerous. This, of course, reflects my own personal biases.

Too Little: Fiber, Omega-3 Fatty Acids, Micronutrients in the form of Vitamins, Minerals, Phytonutrients, etc.
Too Much: Vegetable Oils high in Omega-6 Fatty Acids, Trans-Fats, White Flour, Sugar, Emulsifiers, Preservatives, and Chemical Additives

HEALTHY FOODS DO COST MORE, BUT SAVE OUR HEALTH IN THE LONG RUN…

At the Stockholm Food Forum 2015, Dr. Lustig also presented detail regarding cost analysis for healthy versus processed food: "Healthy food costs double that of unhealthy food and it's going up at a rate of 17 pence per pound compared to processed food, which is 7 pence per pound. So you say, 'Well wait, that means that processed food is a better deal. Less healthy food is a better deal.' Well indeed, the three countries that have the lowest GDP spent on food: the U.S., U.K., and Australia, of course, are the three most obese and the three sickest countries." [649]

The study that Dr. Lustig referenced came out of the U.K and does indeed show that, as of 2012, unhealthy, processed food in the U.K. cost just £2.50 per 1000 kcal ("calories" in the U.S.) whereas healthy food cost £7.49 per 1000 kcal.[650] The healthy foods were actually three times the cost of the unhealthy ones, measured by cost per 1000 kcal (calories). I have no doubt the situation is exactly the same in the U.S.

However, if we look at the detail of this study, what it found was that, bread, rice potatoes, and pasta were the least expensive per 1000 calories, food and drinks high in fat and/or sugar were next, then meat, fish, eggs, beans, and other sources of protein, with milk and dairy foods second from the top, and fruit and vegetables at the highest cost per calorie. This is obviously a brilliant study – and it would certainly be tremendously more difficult than it might appear to be to assess a large number of foods for their healthfulness as it relates to cost. But I believe there are some serious limitations and further considerations. So, if you're on a tight budget, don't think that you can't still eat healthy. Let's look further into why and how.

Personally, most of the groceries that we purchase are organic and we try to get all meats that are pasture-raised and organic as well as wild-caught fish and seafood. I would guess our grocery bill is about double that or more as compared to cheap, processed food. However, I would submit to you that this is absolutely the best money we could ever "invest" – because it is buying (or buying back) our health. And secondly, I can virtually guarantee you that this will likely save us many times more money in the long run, with far less acute and chronic illness, metabolic disease, doctors' and hospitals' visits, medicine, surgery, and yes, of course, even macular degeneration.

And I ask you, what is your vision worth?

Secondly, I also believe you can eat quite healthy on a tighter budget. Interestingly, one of the most critical messages to take home is that, with densely nutritious food, we actually eat less food as well. As you may recall from Chapter One, Americans eat several hundred more calories per day now than we did in 1980. It is my hypothesis that this is the case, in part, because our bodies' are hungry for nutrients – vitamins, minerals, phytonutrients, etc. – and nutrient deficient foods don't satisfy that need. In short, we don't easily get "full" eating these foods because they're not satisfying our needs.

I recall that, before I began an ancestral, nutrient-dense diet, I could occasionally sit down and eat three-fourths of a container of Pringles original potato chips. These chips are 160 calories per serving with six servings in a container. It turns out that my indulgence in three-fourths of one of those containers equals 720 calories, with about 50 grams of fat, which come from the worst possible sources (corn oil, cottonseed oil, and/or sunflower oil), all while being nearly completely devoid of any micronutrients (except some vitamin E and C apparently). Now, did you ever hear of somebody sitting down to a baked sweet potato (about 115 calories for a medium size), eating the whole thing – and then eating three or four more? You can draw this analogy with virtually any processed versus whole natural food.

And some very densely nutritious foods are not that expensive. The USDA Economic Research Service (ERS) has compiled excellent data regarding the average price of fruits and vegetables and the numbers may surprise you. In the U.S., fruit prices ranged from a low of 32 cents per pound for watermelon to a high of $3.94 per pound for blackberries. A few others on the low end and their respective prices per pound were bananas, 45 cents, cantaloupe, 61 cents, oranges, 74 cents, mangoes, 77 cents, and kiwi, 90 cents. According to the ERS, "The weighted average price for all fresh fruit was $0.71 per pound." But more importantly, they state, "After adjusting for waste and serving size (because a pound provides anywhere from 2 to 14 servings), the price per serving for fresh fruits drops to a range of 11 cents a serving for apples and watermelon to 66 cents a serving for blackberries. **Almost two-thirds of the fresh fruits, 16 out of 25, cost 25 cents or less per serving, and only 2 of the 25 cost more than 50 cents per serving.** The weighted average price per serving for all fresh fruits was 18 cents per serving."[651]

In the same analysis, but with regard to vegetables, the USDA ERS states, "Among the 35 fresh vegetable items included in the analysis, retail prices ranged from 31 cents per pound for potatoes to $2.97 per pound for fresh, sliced mushrooms. The weighted-average price for all fresh vegetables was 64 cents per pound." The report continues, **"Per serving, prices ranged from 4 cents for cabbage to 91 cents for shelled green peas, with a weighted-average price of 12 cents per serving. More than two-thirds of the 35 fresh vegetables cost 25 cents or less per serving."** [652] A few of the lowest priced vegetables, on a per pound basis, includes potatoes, 31 cents, cabbage, 38 cents, whole carrots, 54 cents, onions, 55 cents, sweet potatoes, 60 cents, iceberg lettuce, 78 cents, celery, 80 cents, and broccoli, 88 cents.

As can be seen, fresh fruits and vegetables are not that expensive on a per serving basis. I've always been amazed how little bananas cost, but the reality is, they're not alone in this regard. There are quite a lot of very healthy fruits and vegetables at a low price – and whether you're exceedingly wealthy, or dirt-poor – these probably ought to be staples (for most of us). I'll have much more to say about dietary choices in chapters 19 through 21.

PROCESSED FOOD AND MACULAR DEGENERATION

Some studies have shown that AMD either has the highest prevalence in lowest income categories, or the greatest loss of vision in these categories.[653] [654] For example, in the recently published EPIC-Norfolk Eye Study, in the U.K., of 5182 participants involved, researchers found AMD in 653 of them, indicating a prevalence of 12.6%. However, those living in the most affluent 5% of areas had nearly half the odds of AMD as compared to those living in less affluent areas.[655] This was independent of education and social class.

The Baltimore Eye Survey Research Group found by regression model estimation "that for every additional $1000 of median income, the prevalence of vision worse than 20/40 declined by 0.32% (P<.005), and for every 10% rise in the proportion of families below poverty level, the prevalence of low vision rose 0.44% (P<.03)." They also found, "Subjects who reported poor general health or poor health relative to others their age had significantly higher rates of blindness and visual impairment than those who reported better health." [656]

Blindness itself is certainly more common in lower income categories and AMD is a very significant cause of blindness, globally. Some studies, however, have found no such relationship between AMD and income.[657] It is significant that people with less education and lower income have also been shown to have greater morbidity and mortality from many chronic disease conditions.[658] This is an unfortunate, but accurate, assessment. If there is an association between lower income and greater AMD, this is certainly another indicator that processed food is the major cause of macular degeneration, since processed foods are virtually always the least expensive and, therefore, purchased more often by those on vey tight budgets. But, this obviously isn't always the case – and obviously – the enormous majority of people in developed nations are consuming significant amounts of processed food.

ORIENTAL VERSUS WESTERNIZED (MORE PROCESSED FOOD LADEN) DIET

In a one-of-a-kind study, researchers at Tufts University in Boston, Massachusetts, evaluated the risk of AMD based on whether individuals primarily consumed an "Oriental pattern" or a "Western pattern" diet, wherein ethnicity itself wasn't the main focus.[659] The researchers classified some 4088 participants based on whether they primarily consumed the Oriental pattern, "characterized by higher intake of vegetables, legumes, fruit, whole grains, tomatoes, and seafood," versus the Western pattern, "characterized by higher intake of red meat, processed meat, high-fat dairy products, French fries, refined grains, and eggs." Notice that the Western diet contains more processed foods.

The results? The researchers found that a higher Oriental pattern score "was strongly associated with lower odds for both early (odds ratio 0.90) and advanced AMD (odds ratio 0.73)." [660] **For those consuming the more Oriental type diet, they enjoyed a 30% reduction of early AMD and a 60% reduction in advanced AMD.** In contrast, for those consuming the Western diet, there was a much stronger association with AMD, increasing the odds of early AMD (Odds ratio 1.15) and advanced AMD (odds ratio 1.55), quite dramatically. **For those consuming the most Western foods, there was a nearly 60% increase in early AMD and nearly a 3-fold increase in the prevalence of advanced AMD!** This study is unique and robust because it utilized a cross-section of the population and assessed risk for AMD based on the frequency of consuming 37 different diet variables, while not concerning itself so much with ethnicity.

Keep in mind, in all likelihood, although those in the Western diet category developed AMD more frequently and to a more advanced stage, I would assert that it is not red meat, high-fat dairy, or eggs that are the problem. Quite to the contrary. It is primarily that the people consuming those foods, which have been vilified for decades, tend to be the same ones who are the least concerned with their diets and, therefore, also consume the most processed foods laden with vegetable oils, sugars, trans fats, and refined white flour. This concept is known as the "healthy user bias." [661] People who tend to do one unhealthy thing, such as smoking cigarettes, also tend to be the ones that are least concerned about their diet in general. Whereas those that frequent a gymnasium, tend to also be more health conscious, choosing healthier foods in general. The ramifications of this effect are far and wide – and cannot be measured.

Wow, we've reached Base Camp Two of our Mount Everest. We're getting there!

CHAPTERS 10 AND 11 SUMMARY

Recalling from previously reviewed data in the U.S., the average person is consuming about 24% of their calories from vegetable oil, another 20% from wheat,[662] most of which is refined, nutrient-deficient, white flour, and finally, another 26% of the diet comes from added sugars in the form of sucrose and high-fructose corn syrup (HFCS). **This is about 70% of the diet – from three groups of foods (vegetable oils, white flour, and added sugars) that have virtually no nutrient content whatsoever. This is undeniably an unmitigated, metabolic and nutritional disaster – of epic proportions. This combination of foods undoubtedly created the perfect storm – one that would devastate man and his existence in countless ways.** This, and this alone, is perhaps the single most important concept in this entire book. This degree of processed food consumption results in metabolic havoc, with consequences for every single organ system there is, including the eyes.

With this type of a processed food-laden diet, only 30% of one's total caloric consumption is left to provide for all of the nutritional requirements of the entire body: all thirteen essential vitamins, all necessary minerals, the phytonutrients, essential amino acids, proteins, healthy fats, and so on – all in their necessary quantities and proportions. Bottom line: if that 30% of the diet is not of extraordinary quality, there will even more trouble – and it will likely be disastrous.

Those disastrous consequences include all of the diseases of Western civilization, in epidemic proportions. Those conditions include, but are not limited to, heart disease, stroke, type 2 diabetes, cancer, hypertension, blood lipid disorders, Alzheimer's disease, dementia, arthritis, gout, autoimmune disorders, irritable bowel syndrome, depression, ADHD, autism spectrum disorders, and many more.

Additionally, the research conclusively shows that increased vegetable oil consumption is linked to greater risk of AMD. Vegetable oils also contain trans fats – and trans fats are linked with cardiovascular disease and AMD. High sugar consumption has unequivocally been shown to have causality for cardiovascular disease, diabetes, and metabolic syndrome,all three of which are unequivocally linked to AMD. Retinal research shows that high-fructose fed rats develop wet AMD at much greater rates than rats fed standard chow, after laser treatments to induce breaks in Bruch's membrane.

It is my assertion that macular degeneration is, unquestionably, another of the diseases of Western civilization. We've seen AMD's onset historically in relation to the change in our diet, we've reviewed the pathologic mechanisms whereby processed foods could cause AMD, and coming up shortly, we'll see that wherever processed foods are consumed, AMD shows up. It just takes time – usually about 30 to 40 years or more.

12 AMD RUNS PARALLEL WITH HEART DISEASE, OBESITY, DIABETES, CANCER AND "DISEASES OF WESTERN INFLUENCE"

"The good physician treats the disease; the great physician treats the patient who has the disease."
~ Sir William Osler ~

CORONARY HEART DISEASE...

The celebrated clinician, Sir William Osler, one of the four founding physician professors of Johns Hopkins Hospital in Baltimore, Maryland, wrote quite extensively on angina pectoris, typically referred to just as "angina." Angina is the chest pain typical of myocardial infarction, or heart attack. According to author, F. Javier Nieto, "In his 1897 collection of lectures on angina pectoris given at the Johns Hopkins Hospital, Osler provided a very detailed and accurate description of the clinical features of angina as well as striking facts regarding its frequency:

> *"{A}ngina pectoris is a rare affection in hospital practice...During the ten years in which I lived in Montreal, I did not see a case of the disease either in private practice or at the Montreal General Hospital. At Blockley (Philadelphia Hospital), too, it was an exceedingly rare affection. I do not remember to have had a case under my personal care... During the seven years in which the Johns Hopkins Hospital has been opened...there have been only four instances of angina pectoris."* [663]

In this account given in 1897, Osler describes a total of 21 years of general medical practice, and perhaps around five or eight cases of angina. This is not even heart attack – just angina.

Thirteen years later, according to Nieto, "Osler delivered his famous lectures on angina pectoris at the Royal College of Physicians of London. By 1910, Osler reported having seen 208 additional cases and wondered:

> *"Has angina pectoris increased in the community? Has the high-pressure life of modern days made the disease more common? There is an impression among consultants in the United States that there has been an increase [during the] late years."* [664]

But unlike the astute William Osler, today we have the benefit of internet, historians, statisticians, and mountains of data. So we can put on our retrospectroscope, peer into the past, and ask the question: what changed between 1897, when Osler had seen less than 10 cases of angina in 21 years, to 1910, at which point he had accumulated an additional 208 cases? As previously referenced, as of 1880, wheat was being ground using roller mill technology to produce pure white flour. Second, sugar consumption had increased from about 30 pounds per person per year, in 1880, to nearly 60 pounds per year in 1910 (see graph, Chapter 11). Third, vegetable oils had been introduced in 1880. Recall that trans fats, in the form of Crisco, were not introduced until 1911. However, with regard to vegetable oil consumption, research from the LA American Veterans Trial, reported in 1969, strongly suggests that eight years on a high vegetable oil diet is not long enough to produce significant cardiovascular disease.[665]

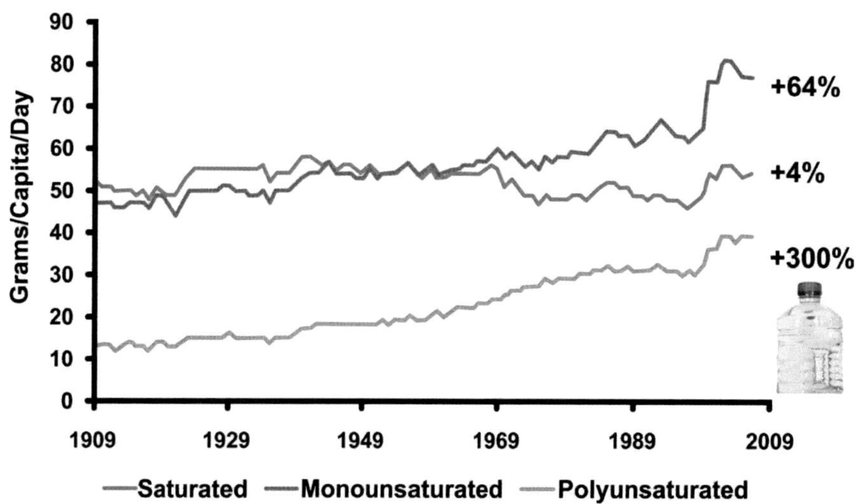

Graph courtesy of Stephan Guyenet, PhD, WholeHealthSource.org.

With that said, with regard to Osler's observation of increasing angina (but not heart attacks just yet) in 1910, it appears that we can quite reliably assert that either white flour, increasing sugar, and/or vegetable oil consumption, or possibly all three are the culprits. Recall that vegetable oils are also a very significant source of trans fats. Of course, this is still consistent with all the data we have today and, therefore, we can potentially indict any or all of these changes in the dietary for their role in heart disease.

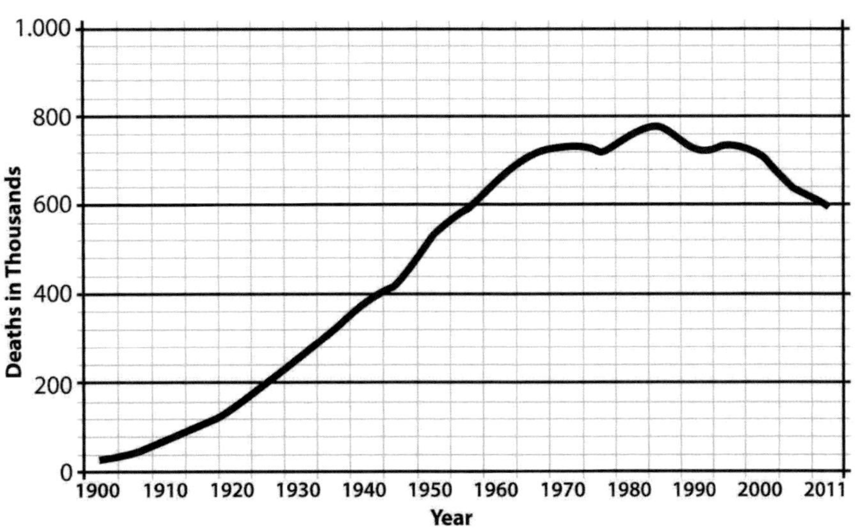

Source: National Center for Health Statistics.

Indeed, heart disease was virtually unheard of in the United States, United Kingdom, and virtually all of Europe at the turn of the 20th century, with the earliest historical reports of heart attacks generally beginning around the very early turn of the 20th century and increasing exponentially to epidemic proportions by the 1960s.[666] The escalation of cardiac disease didn't stop there, though, and despite the fact that the miracles of modern medicine are saving more and more lives from the ravages of coronary heart disease, proportionally, there's no fewer people affected. Doesn't this timeline seem eerily similar to that of AMD?

As you can see from the graph, there's no fewer heart attacks today, with the low fat diet and all the "heart healthy" items in our grocery stores and restaurants. In fact, we can see that bypass surgery is four-fold higher in 1999 than it was in 1979 and, of course, angioplasty, introduced in 1982, is through the roof. The entire reason and purpose for the advice of our government, the American Heart Association, and the American Medical Association to recommend the low-fat diet was to prevent heart disease. Did it work? Unfortunately, it did not work and, in fact, had the unintended effect of more than doubling our rate of obesity (about 14% in 1977 and nearly 37% today), nearly tripled our prevalence of type 2 diabetes (3.3% in 1980 and 9.3% in 2014 – see section and references below), and now nearly one of every three Americans age 75 and older has macular degeneration.

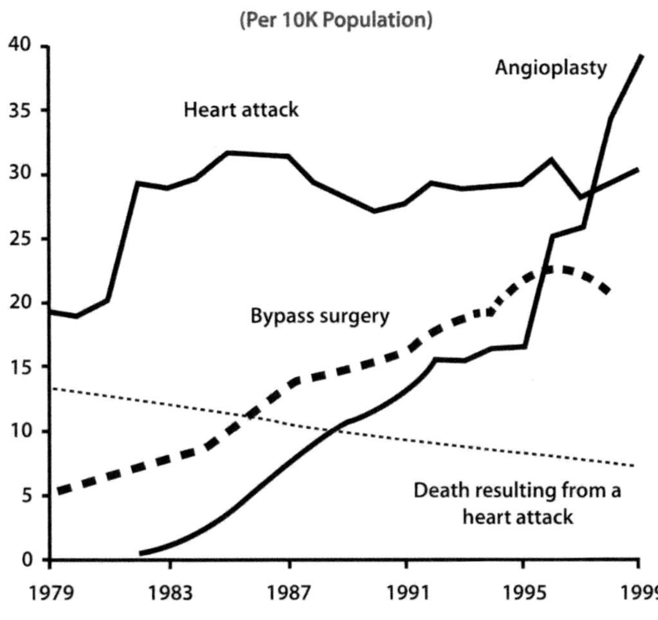

Source: NHDS sutvey-NCHS, WHO, Census Bureau..

Today, all of the cardiologists that I know are literally overrun with patients. One said to me, "I could keep my office open 24/7 and the patients would never stop." Another friend who is a cardiovascular surgeon might as well take up residence at the hospital. His wife, who teaches elementary school, says "I see him mostly for dinner – but you never know when that'll be."

AMD PREDICTS HEART DISEASE...

Interestingly, the Blue Mountains Eye Study (BMES) found that among people aged 49 to 75 years at baseline, the presence of early AMD at the beginning of the study predicted a doubling of cardiovascular mortality over the next decade, even after controlling for traditional cardiovascular risk factors.[667]

OBESITY AND OVERWEIGHT...

In 1892, not long after the introduction of cotton seed oil and "pure" white flour in 1880, the U.S. Government collected height and weight data from a representative sample of men, aged 40 to 69 years. Stephan Guyenet, PhD, University of Washington, dug up the old data and calculated the body mass index of these men. The results showed that, straight across the board, obesity remained under 4 percent from age 49 to 69.

Our rate of obesity (BMI or body mass index of 30 or greater) in the U.S. gradually elevated in the 20th century, reaching about 13% by 1960, but then it leveled off and remained at that level until about 1980. Obesity then rapidly climbed to 23% by 1988, which was within six years after the AMA, AHA, and the USDA all collectively advised Americans to consume a low fat diet. This trend continued, however, rising to 30.5% by 1999, 34.3% by 2005, and a dramatic 35.7% by 2011. An additional 34% were considered overweight (BMI of 25 – 30) by 2008.[668] The prevalence of obesity doubled in the U.S. in a span of just 24 years, between 1980 and 2004. And the number of people considered extremely obese (BMI > 40), rose more than five-fold in a span of just 44 years, from 0.9% in 1960 to 5.1% in 2004.[669] The rate of obesity in children ages 6 to 19, was under 5% in 1963, rising to about 10% by 1988, and was at 17% by 2008.[670]

Currently, in the United States alone, the rates of obesity translate into 73 million adults, with another 70 million or more people falling into the overweight category. This means that more than two-thirds of the adult population in this country is either overweight or obese. On average, the typical adult American weighs 24 pounds more today than they did in 1960.

While investigating these trends in the 1960s, Anthony Sclafani, PhD, distinguished professor and obesity researcher at the Department of Psychology at Brooklyn College of CUNY, studied the effects of various diets on rats. One day, one of his lab rats came across a Froot Loop – the delicious, sugary breakfast cereal that kids love – and Dr. Sclafani watched while the rat gobbled it down, seeming to enjoy it very much. This really intrigued Dr. Sclafani, as up until that time, his rats were mostly fed standard rat chow, which is made up primarily of whole grains with some supplemental vitamins and minerals. On standard chow, the rats would generally eat until satisfied, but rarely, if ever, would overeat.

When given additional opportunities for Froot Loops, Sclafani noted that the rats would leave the edges of the cages, where they feel secure, and venture to the center of the cage, repeatedly, in order to get more of this tasty, but highly processed, food. Sclafani decided to take this to the next level, and he went to his local supermarket and obtained some new foods for his rats. These foods consisted of sweetened condensed milk, chocolate-chip cookies, salami, bananas, marshmallows, cheese, milk chocolate, and peanut butter. Sclafani referred to this diet as "the supermarket diet," and it was obviously, a mix of foods available at any grocery store.

After just ten days of being fed the supermarket diet, Sclafani's rats weighed significantly more than they did previously.[671] This trend continued until the rats eating the supermarket foods were, on average, twice as large as rats consuming ordinary rat chow. According to Sclafani, "Feeding rats a variety of highly palatable, supermarket foods was found to be a particularly effective way of producing dietary obesity."[672] This research was published in 1976 and 1977.

The supermarket diet designed by Sclafani was later renamed "the cafeteria diet," and to this day remains the most rapid and effective way of producing dietary obesity and metabolic syndrome in rodents that are freely consuming food.[673]

If you will take notice of the foods that Sclafani chose for his supermarket diet, every single food is processed, except for the bananas and cheese, although the cheese likely didn't come from raw, unpasteurized milk. That's the point. In fact, this is exactly why some people also end up two or three times larger than they should be – because they're consuming a "cafeteria diet." And the cafeteria diet is a mixture of processed foods, right?

If this were a chapter about weight loss, I would review a boatload of research that shows that any version of cafeteria diet does exactly the same thing to people – and it can do so pretty quickly.[674,675,676,677] And, of course, as Weston A. Price found, any version of whole food, unprocessed, non-Westernized diet, prevents obesity. For our purposes, let's just leave it that processed food consumption is exactly how people gain undesirable, excess weight – in the form of both subcutaneous (under the skin) and visceral (around the organs) fat, with all of its attendant metabolic accompaniments, such as hypertension, diabetes, and metabolic syndrome.[678] And the converse is also true: People lose weight by eliminating processed foods containing any significant amounts of white flour, sugars, vegetable oils, and trans fats. In the U.S., low fat diets tend to reduce healthy animal fats even further, including eggs, beef, butter, and cream, which are nutrient-dense foods. Interestingly, low carb diets generally reduce white flour and sugar, of course, which helps to reduce or eliminate processed foods to a degree.

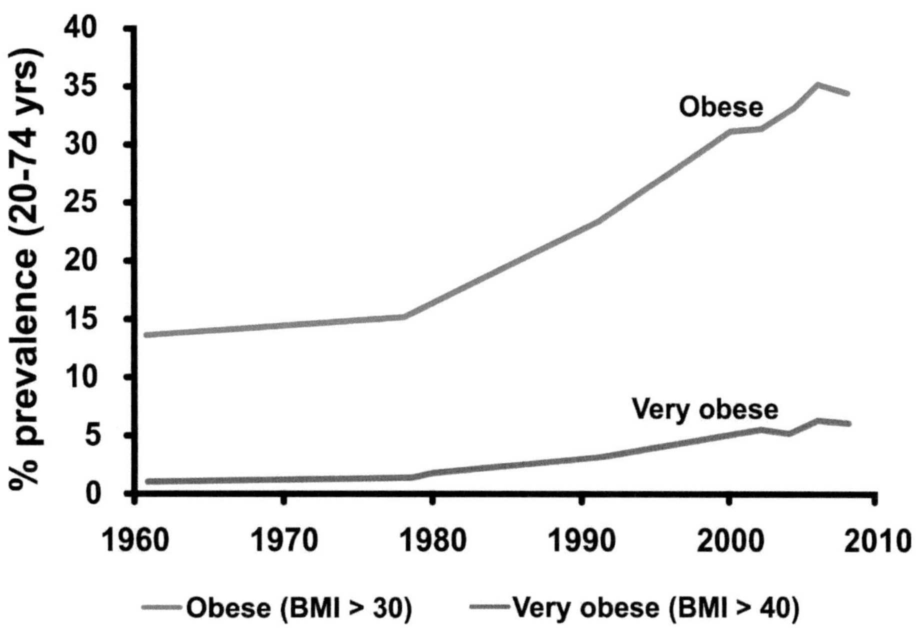

Graph courtesy of Stephan Guyenet, PhD, WholeHealthSource.org.

Numerous studies have found that obesity and being overweight are risk factors for AMD. The Beaver Dam Eye Study found that increased body mass index (BMI, which is weight in kg/height in meters squared) was associated with an increased risk of AMD and that female nonsmokers had increased risk of late AMD with increasing BMI.[679] A study from the Centre for Eye Research Australia (CERA), University of Melbourne, showed that, in men, for every 0.1 increase in waist/hip ratio, there was an associated 13% increase in the odds of early AMD.[680] Numerous other studies have associated obesity or overweight with AMD of both early and late forms.[681 682 683 684 685]

Interestingly, another Australian study followed some 15,792 men and women, aged 45 to 64 years, for six years while observing for changes in waist to hip ratios and the presence of AMD. Their conclusions? "Middle-aged persons who had a 3% or greater reduction in waist to hip ratio over time were less likely to have AMD, particularly among those who were initially obese. A decrease in waist to hip ratio of 3% or more was associated with 29% lower odds of any AMD," whereas with obese participants at baseline "a decrease in waist to hip ratio was associated with 59% lower odds of AMD." [686]

My assertion, of course, is that the exact same diets that cause an individual to become overweight or obese, also cause AMD. However, please recall that you need not even be overweight to be metabolically ill. As we've reviewed before, some 40% of the population (in the U.S.) that are "normal weight" also have metabolic syndrome. So, even if you're normal weight, if you're consuming any version of a typical Westernized diet, with its associated sugars, vegetable oils, white flour, and trans-fat laden ingredients, you're at extreme risk.

EXERCISE, OVERWEIGHT, AND AMD – EXERCISE REDUCES RISK OF AMD?

While we're on the subject of overweight and obesity, we should address the subject of exercise and AMD. Research suggests that frequent exercise may help reduce the risk of AMD. The study that showed the greatest effect of exercise on the risk of AMD, to my knowledge, was a study from Sydney, Australia, which showed that adults aged 75 and above, in the highest tertile (33%) of physical activity, compared to those in the lowest tertile of physical activity, were 79% less likely to have AMD over a 15-year period of follow-up. However, when the researchers adjusted for gender, body mass index, smoking, fish consumption, and white cell count, the association dropped into the non-significant range.[687] The Melbourne Collaborative Cohort Study showed that "frequent vigorous exercise was associated with a 22% decrease in the odds of intermediate AMD in women." [688]

Personally, I am very interested in physical fitness and I have been all my life, so I found these studies quite interesting. However, if we look at our history, we again realize that AMD was extraordinarily rare in the 19th century, when no one – I mean virtually no one – was exercising for the sake of physical fitness. In fact, the first gym in the U.S. was purportedly opened by Jack LaLanne, in 1936.[689] And, of course, we now know that AMD was extraordinarily rare in the 19th century. So how do we account for the findings of reduced AMD in those who exercise?

The answer, I believe, lies primarily within the confines of the "healthy user bias," which we have referred to previously. Almost undoubtedly, the people that are exercising are also the ones most interested in health and, therefore, diet. They're tremendously less likely to be eating as much processed food and junk foods laden with white flour, sugars, vegetable oils, and trans fats. This is the same reason that people that work-out at gymnasiums are much less likely to smoke. It's just contradictory and counter-intuitive to physical fitness.

Nevertheless, I would still recommend regular exercise for everyone that is able, particularly if you're needing to lose excess weight. Exercise can certainly help one to lose excess fat, especially the dangerous visceral fat, which is the fat around your organs.[690] The benefits of exercise are tremendous, so try to make a habit of some type of planned exercise at least 3 to 5 times a week, even for just 10 or 20 minutes. Personally, I recommend resistance exercise over "cardio," which means that I believe body-weight exercises or weight-lifting are far superior to spending your time on a treadmill, stationary cycle, elliptical machine, walking, or anything else that is "slow-go cardio."

Just four minutes of "Tabata training" (named after the Japanese scientist, Dr. Izumi Tabata), which is eight bouts of 20 seconds of intense physical activity, each followed by 10 seconds of rest, is a very brief but intense form of high-intensity interval training (HIIT) that is great for anyone. "Tabata training" is proven to increase aerobic capacity, while increasing anaerobic capacity (strength, essentially) by 28%, as well as to increase metabolism after the exercise, thereby burning calories after the workout.[691] Usually, several different exercises are completed in these 20 second intervals, such as push-ups, body-weight squats, sit-ups, running in place, burpees, split-squats, lunges, mountain climbers, etc. On days that I can't make it to the gym, I sometimes just do three sets of "Tabata's," with about 90 seconds rest in between sets, and the entire workout is complete in 15 minutes. Really short on time? Just do one four-minute Tabata workout and make it as hard as you possibly can. It will serve you well!

Having said all that, suffice it to say that no amount of exercise – even four hours a day – can overcome a bad diet. I see highly motivated people working out regularly, even for years, and remaining obese. Unfortunately, they don't know why they're that way. Discussions with numerous of these people always proves one thing – they're consuming some of the 'displacing foods,' particularly the vegetable oils. Fitness and health begins and ends in the kitchen. In fact, a mantra that I have seen recently is "abs are made in the kitchen." And it's true. We can invoke the 80/20 rule here – fitness is 80% diet and 20% exercise.

DIABETES...

Type 1 diabetes mellitus ("child onset", or "insulin dependent") was described in Egyptian manuscripts as well as by Indian physicians as early as 1500 BC. The distinction between type 1 and type 2 diabetes was made as early as 400 to 500 AD by the Indian physicians Sushrata and Charaka, who characterized type 1 as associated with youth and type 2 with obesity. Both conditions were rare throughout history, until type 2 diabetes began to become increasingly prevalent throughout the 20th century and beyond. In the U.S., the prevalence of diabetes was only 0.37 percent in 1935, rising to 0.91% in 1960, 3.3% in 1980, 8.7% by 2011, and 9.3% by 2014.[692] That translates to a ratio of 1 in every 270 people that had type 2 diabetes in 1935, whereas it is one in every 11 people today.

As reviewed previously, type 2 diabetes has frequently been shown to have associations with AMD. In one study by Korean researchers, out of 3008 participants aged 50 to 87, some 315 had diabetes and 88 had AMD. Even after adjusting for age, sex, smoking, obesity, and hypertension, subjects with diabetes were 1.8 times more likely to have AMD than those without diabetes.[693]

We should recall, at this point, that Robert Lustig and colleagues have shown causality between sugar consumption and type 2 diabetes. That is, as sugar consumption increases, so does diabetes.

CANCER...

The documentary film, *Cancer – The Forbidden Cures,* by Buenaonda Films, begins with the following excerpt: "20,000 people die of cancer every day. This translates to 8,000,000 deaths every year, half a million of whom are Americans.

At the beginning of the last {20th} century, one person out of 20 would get cancer. In the 1940s, it was one out of every 16 people. In the 1970s, one person out of 10. *Today, one person out of three gets cancer in the course of their life.* Over one million Americans are diagnosed with a new cancer every year." [694] The Centers for Disease Control (CDC) confirms these numbers are actually conservative. In fact, in the year 2013, the CDC estimated that some 1,660,290 people in the U.S. were afflicted with cancers, and this excluded the common skin cancers.[695]

Researchers at the University of Maryland found that, "Fructose intake is associated with increased risk of pancreatic and small intestinal cancers, and possibly others." [696] Other research has shown a very strong correlation between breast cancer mortality and sugar consumption in older women (correlation coefficient 0.9).[697] As metabolic syndrome develops, high insulin levels have been associated with the development of various forms of cancer.[698] Tumors are obviously big consumers of sugar – and sugar consumption has been linked to cancer development in both humans and in test animals.[699] Mary Enig, PhD, and colleagues at the University of Maryland, found that vegetable oil consumption was correlated with high rates of cancer, whereas animal fats were not.[700]

The cancers that tend to increase with Western civilization include cancers of the colon/rectum, pancreas, lung, breast, uterus, ovary, prostate, and bladder.[701]

This is worth repeating: In the United States, in the year 1900, just one person out of 20 developed cancer in their lifetime, yet today it is one in three. Billions of dollars are being spent to try to "find a cure" as though we can't figure out the connection. Could it be our diet?

DISEASES OF WESTERN CIVILIZATION...

The list of diseases and conditions that are believed to be mostly diseases of Western civilization, sometimes called 'diseases of civilization,' are numerous and far beyond our scope. Nevertheless, I believe that Weston A Price was likely the first to recognize that Westernized diets resulted not only in tooth decay, but in declining health and degenerative diseases. Other popular books that have reviewed this subject include Arnold DeVries' *Primitive Man and His Food (1952),* Walter Voegtlin's *The Stone Age Diet (1975),* and S. Boyd Eaton's *The Paleolithic Prescription (1988).*

Quite frankly, I was introduced to the "Paleo Diet" by the work of Loren Cordain, PhD, through both his first book, *The Paleo Diet* (2002), and his latest book, *The Paleo Answer* (2012). In *The Paleo Answer,* Dr. Cordain reviews all of the disease conditions that we've reviewed thus far, such as heart disease, diabetes, hypertension, metabolic syndrome,etc., but he also reviews numerous inflammatory and autoimmune disorders that might be considered diseases of civilization, such as multiple sclerosis, rheumatoid arthritis, ulcerative colitis, Crohn's disease, ankylosing spondylitis, Celiac disease, type 1 diabetes, Grave's disease, lupus erythematosus, psoriasis, scleroderma, uveitis (inflammation in the eye), vitiligo, autism, depression, bipolar disorder, asthma, migraine headaches, and more.[702] All of these conditions may find their roots in modern, Westernized, processed food-laden diets and, of course, are either known or believed to have been much less common in those consuming traditional diets.

Finally, I might mention that AMD has been conclusively linked to cognitive disorders, including Alzheimer's disease.[703] [704] In fact, Alzheimer's disease and dementia account for an enormous share of our healthcare dollars, are a tremendous burden on families and society, and are yet additional conditions that are rare or non-existent in societies consuming their traditional diets.

CHAPTER SUMMARY

It is a travesty, but without question, the enormous bulk of chronic disease today is entirely the result of "Westernization" of the diet, which is rapidly becoming a global problem. Diseases that were once rarities have become expected conditions of aging. In fact, it was this very broad scope of disease affecting our nation and, of course, now many more nations, that led me to suspect that macular degeneration might be on this long list of "diseases of Western civilization." That, along with what I witnessed in my clinics day-in and day-out, week after week, and year after year, that the same people consuming the most displacing foods were the ones most frequently affected with chronic diseases – and with AMD.

Hopefully, now it makes sense why AMD "runs with" with being overweight, having heart disease, diabetes, metabolic syndrome, Alzheimer's disease, and many other chronic disorders.

13 AMD FOLLOWS PROCESSED FOODS WORLDWIDE

"It's [AMD] becoming a worldwide problem. And something has changed to induce that."
~ Professor Alan C. Bird, MD ~
2014 (Moorfield's Eye Hospital, London)

Surgeon-Captain T.L. Cleave, M.R.C.P (Lond.) wrote the book *The Saccharine Disease,* published in 1974. Similar to Weston A. Price, Cleave recognized and further damned the consumption of white flour, sugar, and vegetable oils in their role in the "saccharine" (the 'rine' rhymes with wine, to distinguish it from the artificial sweetener) diseases, namely, coronary artery disease, diabetes, and obesity, but others as well. Cleave's emphasis was significantly greater on sugar and white flour as contributors to these disease conditions, however.

T.L. Cleave, among his other remarkable achievements, wrote eloquently regarding the incubation period for chronic diseases. The 'incubation period' indicates the length of time between exposure to an element, stimulus, toxin, etc., and the onset of the outcome, be it an illness, disease, or death. If we're exposed sufficiently to a cold-virus (rhinovirus), perhaps in 24 to 72 hours, we might come down with a cold (the risks of "catching" a cold drops precipitously with an ancestral diet, by the way). But with chronic diseases, the incubation period is much, much longer, and therefore, it is dramatically more difficult to draw cause-and-effect connections. With respect to the incubation period for diabetes, for example, Cleave wrote,

> In 1959, G.D. Campbell showed that there seemed to be a remarkably uniform period in a population exposed to a diabetogenic factor in their midst, before the disease itself appears amongst them. This period was formulated as 'The Rule of Twenty Years'. The rule was first worked out in the case of the urban Zulu [ethnic group of Southern Africa], with incrimination of sugar as the factor most likely to be involved, the data being published later in the *South African Medical Journal,* in 1960. The rule of 20 years has since been supported by other writers in other countries, as will be seen in the case of V. Albertsson in Iceland and A.M. Cohen in Israel.
>
> It is important to add that an incubation period of 20 years in the case of diabetes makes it impossible to argue, as E.P. Joslin does, against the consumption of sugar being a cause of diabetes because in the United States the consumption of sugar has been stationary in recent years, whereas diabetes has increased; and in certain other countries, where the consumption of sugar is high, the incidence of diabetes is relatively low'. Countries with a present high sugar consumption, of fairly recent origin, as in the case of developing countries, may face an outbreak of diabetes in 20 years' time. This, indeed, is exactly what is happening in Canadian Eskimos today. [705]

In like fashion, Cleave asserts that for other "saccharine diseases," the incubation period may be even longer: coronary disease, 30 years, and diverticular disease of the colon (diverticulitis), 40 years.[706]

This is exactly why we rarely see myocardial infarctions (MI, or heart attacks) in people younger than about 40 years of age, but more likely, in their 50's and 60's. Even if the diet is nutrient-deficient and replete with the "displacing foods of modern commerce" from birth forward, it still generally takes about 40 to 50 years to become severe enough to result in heart attacks, stroke, congestive heart failure, peripheral arterial disease, and so on.

The situation is identical in macular degeneration. This is the one and only reason that the condition was at least once reserved for people over age 50. However, as any experienced ophthalmologist will now tell you, we're beginning to see patients with AMD in their 30s and early 40s.[707] Type 2 diabetes was once considered 'adult onset diabetes,' but our diets have become so replete with sugar, white flour, and processed foods, that, by 2002, pediatricians, family physicians, and endocrinologists were already diagnosing type 2 diabetes - in teenagers.[708] [709]

SUGAR AND VEGETABLE OILS – THE MARKERS OF PROCESSED FOOD

The point of this previous introduction regarding incubation periods is three-fold:

1. In order to further support or refute the hypothesis that the "displacing foods of modern commerce" are the primary and proximate cause of AMD, we must analyze the processed food consumption data as far back as it is available;
2. We must understand that AMD generally takes 30 to 60 years or more to develop and, therefore, we must analyze food consumption data that long or longer, wherever available, and
3. We must understand that both sugar and vegetable oil consumption serve as the proxy markers of processed food, because these are key and primary ingredients in the vast majority of processed foods.

If we could analyze white flour consumption data as well, this would be excellent, however, I have elected not to do so because it is virtually impossible to separate out whole-grain flour from typical 75% extraction white flour in any broad fashion. We know that the great majority of wheat flour is white flour rather than whole-grain flour, but this certainly might be a point of contention. Secondly, as we reviewed previously, Barry Popkin and Robert Lustig have pointed out that sugar is the proxy marker of processed food. Thirdly, as we've seen from previous studies, vegetable oil consumption is directly and strongly linked to increasing risk of AMD and sugar consumption is indirectly linked to AMD development, as studies have shown high-glycemic index diets (think sugar and white flour) are associated with increased risk of AMD.[710 711] Finally, one should realize that white flour tends to run with sugar and vegetable oils, as these three elements are the sine-qua-non of processed food.

PREVALENCE OF AMD – COMPARING THE STUDIES

There is a striking limitation in comparing the prevalence data of macular degeneration between studies. The problem? For most of our history since AMD was first diagnosed, there have been no internationally agreed upon diagnostic criteria. To the non-ophthalmologist/optometrist, this might seem strange, but to us, this would be normal. AMD isn't an all or nothing disease. It's a little like grading aging. We don't generally call it AMD if, for example, a few small, hard-drusen exist in the macula. However, if there are soft drusen and pigmentary changes (increased pigment or decreased pigment), that's called "macular degeneration" or "age-related maculopathy" (ARM) in formal studies, and would generally be called "macular degeneration" or "AMD" by most practicing ophthalmologists. Without getting deeply technical, which would please only a few, I'll just mention that there are multiple different classification systems that are in use. These include the following:

- Wisconsin Age-Related Maculopathy Grading System (1991)[712]
- International Classification and Grading System for Age-Related Maculopathy and Age-Related Macular Degeneration (1995)[713]
- Clinical Age Related Maculopathy Staging System (CARMS) (2006)[714]
- "Three Continent AMD Consortium Global Definition" (2014)[715]

These various classification systems can make for pretty wide variations in the prevalence of the diagnosis of "Early AMD" particularly, whereas the agreements for late AMD between classification systems is much greater. For example, when a number of the world's leading authorities in the epidemiology and study of AMD, including Professor Ron Klein, MD (U.S.A.), Professor Paulus T.V.M. de Jong, MD, PhD (The Netherlands), Professor Johannes (Hans) R. Vingerling, MD, PhD (The Netherlands), and Professor Paul Mitchell, MBBS, MD, PhD (Australia), and colleagues, all came together to "harmonize the classification of AMD" on the three continents, the "adjusted prevalence of early AMD" changed as follows:

- 18.7% to 20.3% in the Beaver Dam Eye Study (U.S.)
- 4.7% to 14.4% in the Blue Mountains Eye Study (Australia)
- 14.1% to 15.8% in the Los Angeles Latino Eye Study (U.S.)
- 7.5% to 17.1% in the Rotterdam Study (The Netherlands)

As you can see, this can make a pretty big difference in prevalence data for the diagnosis of AMD. This brings us to a very critical point. In general, no attempt will be made to try to harmonize any of the data in retrospect, as this would virtually guarantee speculation and controversy. Instead, I will report all prevalence data exactly as it was presented in each study referenced, with one exception: the PAMDI studies out of Italy (see explanation under "Italy" in this chapter).

At some point, we must also realize that there are no studies of AMD prevalence for countries and regions where the condition was or is exceedingly rare. This makes perfect sense if you will consider, for example, if a study were proposed to determine the prevalence of malaria in the U.S. Any long-time citizen on the street could tell you that there is no sense in running the study, because the condition doesn't exist here. But, anyone in sub-Saharan Africa or India would understand why a study of the prevalence of malaria might be considered there, because the condition is endemic in those areas.

Well, this is exactly the situation for virtually every country or region that will be presented. At some point, the prevalence of AMD was zero or close to zero. In some regions or nations, like Japan and India, we'll observe that the prevalence of AMD has dramatically increased during our own lifetimes. In other nations, like the U.S. and the U.K., we see that the prevalence of AMD was suddently on the radar in the 1930s, with exponential increases in the late 20th century. Some countries or regions still have no formal studies, because AMD remains exceedingly rare.

In 2014, the eminent and world-renowned ophthalmologist, Professor Alan Bird, of Moorfield's Eye Hospital in London, England, in his "Distinctive Voices" lecture given at the Beckman Center, in Irvine, California said, "In world terms, WHO – until quite recently, said 'Well, we have no good data on AMD,' which is strange, but they did on river blindness and trachoma. But now it's – after cataract – glaucoma and AMD are the biggest causes of blindness in the world. So it's not just a North American and Western European problem. It's becoming a worldwide problem. And something has changed to induce that."[716]

PREVALENCE OF ARM & AMD BY NATION AND YEAR						
COUNTRY	**ARM & AMD PREVALENCE**	**YEAR**	**REF.**	**ARM & AMD PREVALENCE**	**YEAR**	**REF.**
Australia	9.1%	1991-93	717,718	15.1%	1999	719
Barbados	24.3%	1995	720			
China	5.4%	2006	721,722			
Denmark	12.2%	1989	723			
Fiji	0.2% (est.)	2010-15				
Germany	12.1%	2014	724			
Greece	14.93%	2006	725			
Greenland	13%	1977	726	52.3%	2008	727
Iceland	6.7%	1980-84	728	21.4%	2003	729
India	4.7%	1984	730	3.4%	2007	731
Israel	N/A					
Italy	14.5%**	2011	732			
Japan	0.2%*	1974-79	733	11.4%	2007	734
Kenya	12.3%	2013	735			
Kiribati	0.2% (est.)	2015				
South Korea	5.6%	2008-9	736	7.4%	2010	737
Lesotho	0.0% †	1977-79	738			
Netherlands	9.3%	1990-93	739			
New Zealand	1.3%*	1969	740	10.3% (est.)	2014	741
Nigeria	3.2%	2004	742	0.1%*	2007	743
Samoa	0.2% (est.)	2015				
Solomon Islands	0.2% (est.)	2005-15				
Thailand	2.7%	2006-07	744	12.2%	2010	745
United Kingdom	9.7%	1997	746	7.2%	2015	747
USA	8.8%	'73-75	748	20.9%	1988-90	749
Zimbabwe	1.13%	1977	750			

* Calculated from existing data; see text under appropriate heading.
† Zero prevalence disciform (wet) AMD in 12,000 patients, see text under "Lesotho."
** Calculated from the study's data; see explanation under "Italy" below.

With an observant eye, you will see that there are drastic differences between AMD prevalence in various countries and in various years, generally with increasing prevalence over time, which correlates with each country or region's consumption of sugar and vegetable oils over the previous 30 to 40 years or more. *One should absolutely, positively, not attempt to precisely compare data from one country to another or even one study to another in attempt to reconcile the data, mostly because the studies often use different grading and classification schemes. It is far more important to observe that the AMD prevalence elevates from little or none, at some point, to some very significant degree. It is the general trend that is critical to observe.* **In short, witness that the prevalence of AMD, invariably, increases within approximately 30 to 40 years or more after an increasing consumption of the "displacing foods**

of modern commerce?" Again, in this case, we'll be using the two proxy markers for processed foods: sugar and vegetable oils.

This data is drawn almost exclusively from the Food and Agriculture Organization of the United Nations (FAO), which is generally considered the single most trusted source for nutrition data among nutrition researchers.

The next characteristic with regard to this observational, epidemiologic data to keep in mind is to remember that *countries don't consume the processed foods (sugars and vegetable oils) – people do.* The point here is that, the graphs are only a loose association. Not everyone is consuming sugar and vegetable oils equally. For example, in the U.S., some people drink four sugar-sweetened beverages a day; some drink none. The same goes with vegetable oils. Some people consume them at every meal and most snacks; others prepare most all of their own meals without vegetable oils, shop and dine out very carefully and, therefore, consume much smaller amounts or even none.

With that said, let's examine the correlations between sugar and vegetable oil consumption – the markers of processed foods – and the prevalence (development) of AMD, in various countries. Please note that I've not attempted to present an exhaustive review of all prevalence studies of AMD for each nation or region as this would be overwhelming for most readers, rather, I've attempted to provide a few of the most prominent and representative studies for each nation or region.

In each graph, based on all available evidence and consultation with Chris Masterjohn, PhD, we've elected to categorize the vegetable oils into two broad categories, which we'll call "Harmful Vegetable Oils," and "Harmless Vegetable Oils." **These categories are based primarily on high content of polyunsaturated oils (harmful) versus high content of saturated and monounsaturated oils (both non-harmful).** Peanut (groundnut) oil, sesame oil, and high-oleic sunflower and high-oleic safflower oils perhaps belong in a medium risk category, because of "moderate" amounts of polyunsaturated oils. However, these last four oils are generally minor constituents in most diets and, as such, we've added them into the "Harmful Oils" category. This is the breakdown as it relates to each graph of AMD vs. Vegetable Oils & Sugar:

MOST LIKELY TO CONTRIBUTE TO DISEASE/AMD – "HARMFUL OILS":

- **Soybean Oil**
- **Corn Oil (Maize Germ Oil)**
- **Cottonseed Oil**
- **Canola Oil**
- **Rapeseed and Mustard Oil**
- **Sunflower Oil**
- **Safllower Oil**
- **Rice Bran Oil**
- **Oilcrops Oil, Other** (A category of the FAO)

INTERMEDIATE RISK OILS (BUT LISTED AMONG HARMFUL CATEGORY):

- **Peanut (Groundnut) Oil**
- **Sesame Oil**
- **High Oleic Sunflower and High-Oleic Safflower Oils**

LEAST LIKELY TO CONTRIBUTE TO DISEASE/AMD – "NON-HARMFUL OILS":

- **Palm Oil**
- **Palm Kernel Oil**
- **Coconut Oil**
- **Olive Oil**
- **Flaxseed Oil**

NATIONS WITH HIGH PREVALENCE OF AMD

UNITED STATES

The first large-scale study of AMD prevalence to be completed in the U.S. was from the Framingham Study, in Framingham, Massachusetts, between 1973 – '75.[751] In this study, as part of the definition of AMD, visual acuity had to be 20/30 or worse, which is generally not typical of most studies. **In any case, the prevalence of age-related maculopathy (ARM), which is the early dry stage of AMD, was 8.8% for people between 52 and 85 years of age, varying from 1.6% in people 52 to 64 to 27.9% in those 75 to 85 years of age.**[752]

An interesting study of the prevalence of AMD in the United States, which attempted to assess for racial differences in risk, took place in the San Luis Valley of Southern Colorado. The study was completed by re-evaluating data from some 1541 individuals that had macular photography to assess for diabetic retinopathy, beginning in 1983. The population was 47% Hispanic. The prevalence of any ARM for those between 43 and 74 years of age was 14.1% among Hispanics and 10.1% among non-Hispanic whites. There was only one advanced AMD case among the Hispanics indicating that late stage AMD in this particular population, at this particular time, was quite rare.[753] However, even in individuals younger than 43 years, 6% of the non-Hispanic whites and 6.7% of the Hispanics, were diagnosed with ARM. This is yet another example where race is no protector from disease, AMD included. Secondly, AMD – once reserved specifically for those above age 50 – by the 1980s was already affecting very significant numbers of people under 43 years of age. These people were undoubtedly consuming processed foods their entire lives.

The Beaver Dam Eye Study, completed in Beaver Dam, Wisconsin, between 1988 and 1990, found people aged 43 to 86 years of age had an overall prevalence of ARM of 20.9% and late AMD of 1.9%.[754]

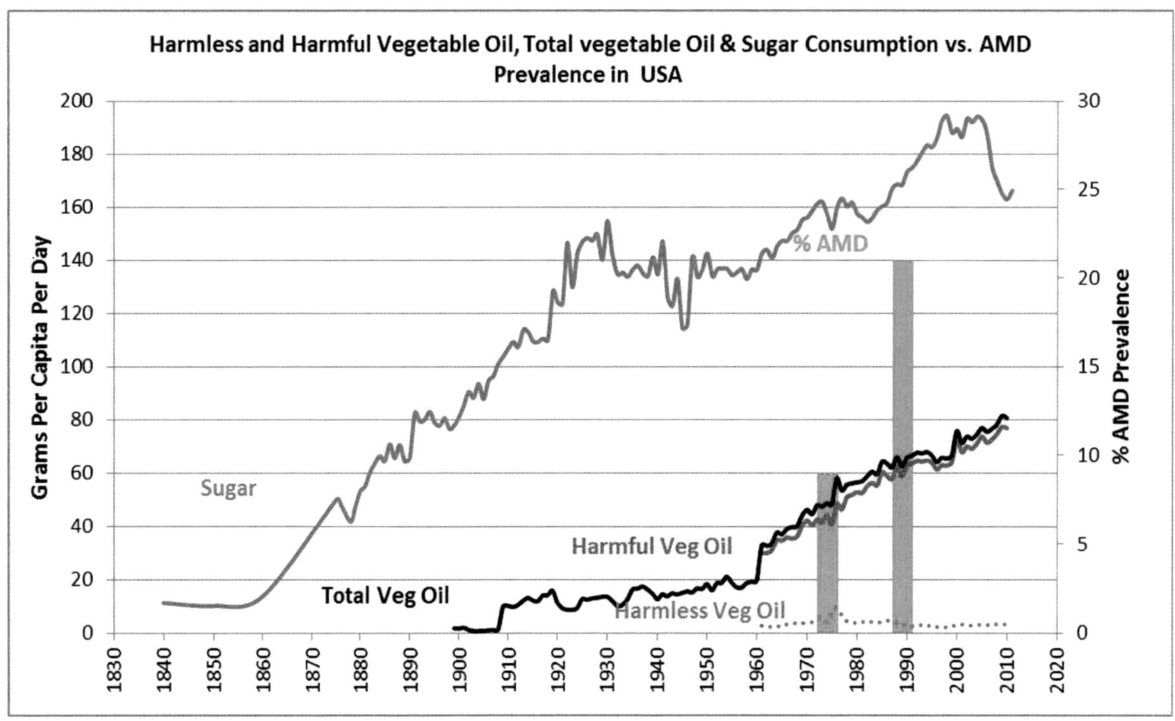

As you can see from the graph, vegetable oil consumption in the U.S., having begun in 1880, was becoming a significant source of calories nationwide by about 1909. As we know from our review in Chapter 3, AMD was definitely diagnosed more commonly in the 1930s, as evidenced by the research of Benjamin Rones (1938). Clearly, AMD was of epidemic proportions by the 1970s and still apparently climbing by 1990, with the consumption of "harmful vegetable oils" and sugar both still climbing through the 1990s. As one may observe from the graph, total vegetable oil consumption and, when the vegetable oils could be separated distinctly by type, in 1961, "Harmful Vegetable Oil" consumption, are virtually identical in character. This is because the U.S. consumes almost no saturated ("Harmless") oils, i.e., coconut, palm, or palm kernel oils. The correlation between increasing sugar and vegetable oil consumption is marked and very strong.

UNITED KINGDOM

In 1997, an AMD prevalence study was completed in Bristol, U.K., in men aged 65 to 83 years. In 934 men, early ARM was found in 9.2%, late AMD in 0.5%, for an overall prevalence of 9.7%.[755]

In 2015, a study completed in the Republic of Ireland found the prevalence of early AMD to be 6.6%, late AMD 0.6%, with an overall prevalence of 7.2% AMD in the population aged 50 and older.[756] In the European Eye Study (EUREYE), subjects in Belfast, Northern Ireland ages 65 and greater, were found to have a total prevalence of 16.68% ARM and AMD, with 3.77% being of the late AMD type.[757]

Using different grading criteria, some studies have shown very high prevalences of AMD in the U.K., particularly in the very elderly. For example, in the Melton Mowbray Study, 1980 – '82, all forms of AMD had a prevalence of 41% in patients 76 years and older,[758] while a follow up study in 1990 estimated that 50% of patients age 86 and older had any form of AMD.[759 760] Another study in western Scotland found an AMD prevalence of 38.7% in those aged 65 to 74 and 47.7% in those aged 75 to 84 years.[761]

Recall that Jennifer Evans, PhD, and Richard Wormald, MD found that, in the U.K., AMD accounted for 6% of blindness in 1933 to '43, 24% by 1970, and 49% by 1990. A separate study, in the U.K., showed that AMD was either the sole cause or contributed to blindness in 56% of those registered as blind, in 2014.[762] This is a staggering statistic, but the situation is nearly identical in the U.S. with one study confirming 54% of blindness was due to AMD, as of 2004.[763]

As we can see, the situation in the U.K. is very similar to the U.S., except that in the U.K., there is substantially less sugar and vegetable oil consumption, and perhaps a bit lower AMD prevalence than in the U.S. It appears from the graph that the prevalence of AMD is decreasing recently, however, the two studies posted on this graph utilized different AMD classification criteria, and this is not necessarily consistent with decreasing AMD prevalence. The important point to take home is that, in the U.K. in 1920, there was virtually no AMD. Yet by the 1990s and beyond, millions of people are affected. And what was the primary factor? Processed food consumption dramatically increased – as evidenced by sugar and harmful vegetable oil consumption.

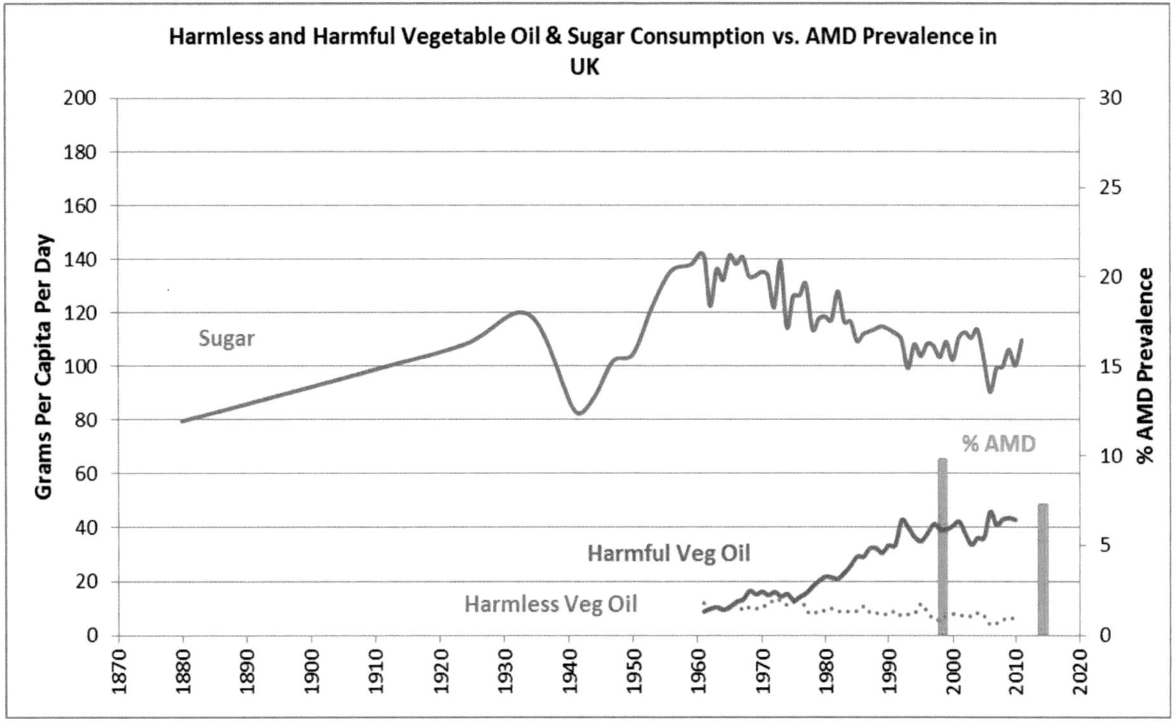

AUSTRALIA

In the Blue Mountains Eye Study (BMES) in 1995, in Australia, out of some 3647 people studied, 24 were legally blind in both eyes. Of those, 16 (66%) were blind in both eyes from AMD and in a total of 21 of the 24 (88%), AMD contributed to the blindness.[764] In the BMES, the overall prevalence of any macular degeneration (ARM and AMD) was 9.1% for people 49 years of age and older.[765,766]

In 1999, the Visual Impairment Project (VIP) of Melbourne determined that the overall prevalence of early ARM was 15.1% for people aged 40 and older. Early ARM was found in 10.1% of subjects 50 to 59 years old and 40% of those 80 to 89 years of age.[767]

As we see in the graph, sugar consumption is very high and the "Harmful vegetable oils" are moderate, with rising prevalences of AMD in the late 20th century.

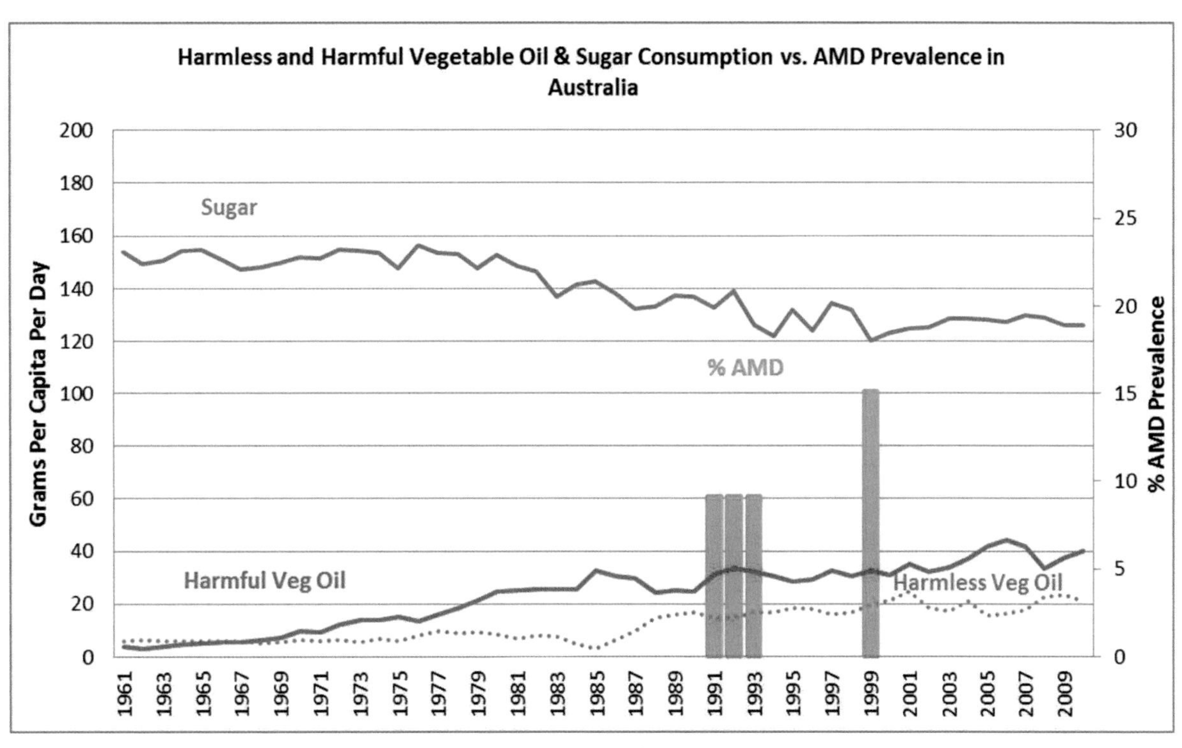

DENMARK

In 1989, researchers at the University Eye Clinic, Rigshospitalet, Copenhagen, led by Troels Vinding, MD, DMSc, completed a study on the prevalence of AMD in 1000 individuals aged 60 to 80 years. Findings consistent with AMD as well as visual impairment in at least one eye occurred with a prevalence of 12.2% overall. By age breakdown, AMD occurred in 2.3% of those 60 to 64, 5.9% of those 65 to 69, 12.1% of those 70 to 74, and 27.3% of those 75 to 80.[768]

Denmark, with a population of 5.36 million in 2001, already had more than 80,000 people with substantially impaired vision in at least one eye and more than 4,000 blind owing to advanced AMD.[769] As of 2013, there were 47,000 people in Denmark over the age of 65 with late AMD.[770]

As we can see from the graph, Denmark has had very high sugar consumption and moderately high harmful vegetable oil consumption since the 1960s, indicating substantial consumption of the 'displacing foods of modern commerce.' This has resulted in very significant AMD levels, as indicated on the graph.

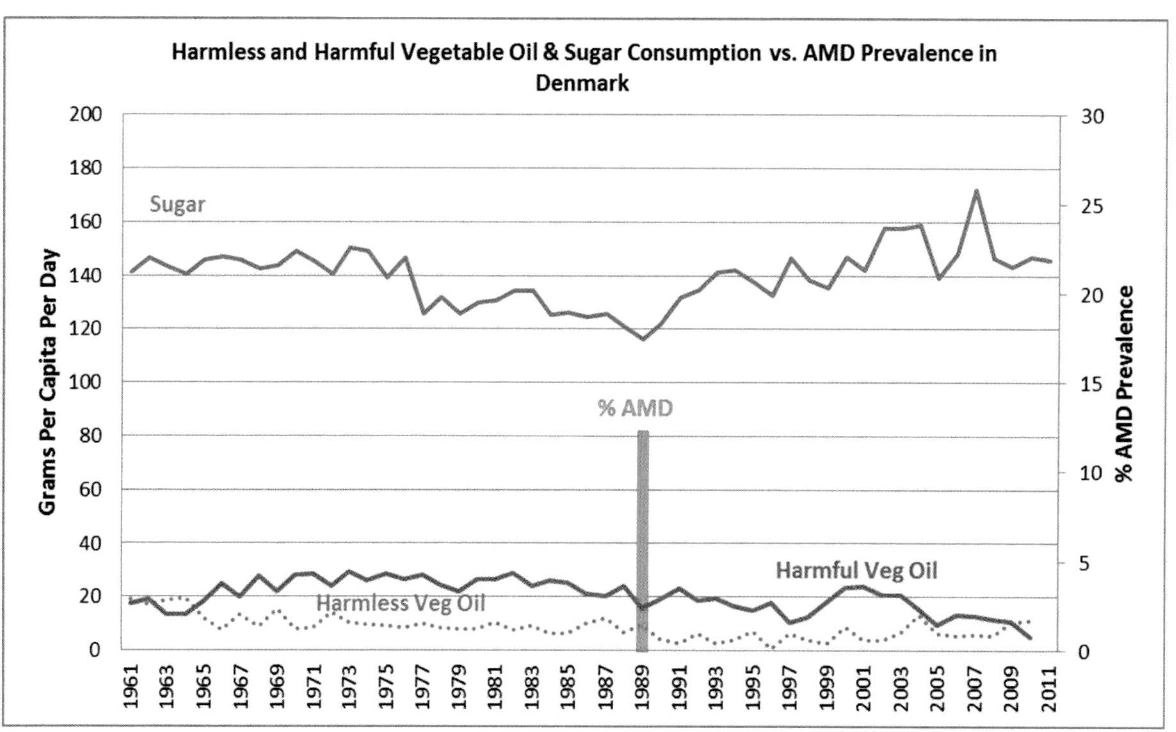

THE NETHERLANDS

The Rotterdam Study, based in Rotterdam, The Netherlands, found that of people 55 and older, evaluated between 1990 and 1993, the overall prevalence of any ARM was 9.3% with late ARM (AMD) being 1.7%.[771]

The Netherlands, very similar to much of Europe, has had very high sugar consumption for many decades, but with substantially increasing harmful vegetable oils consumption since the early 1960s. As is typical of such scenarios, within about 30 years of such, AMD develops to markedly high levels.

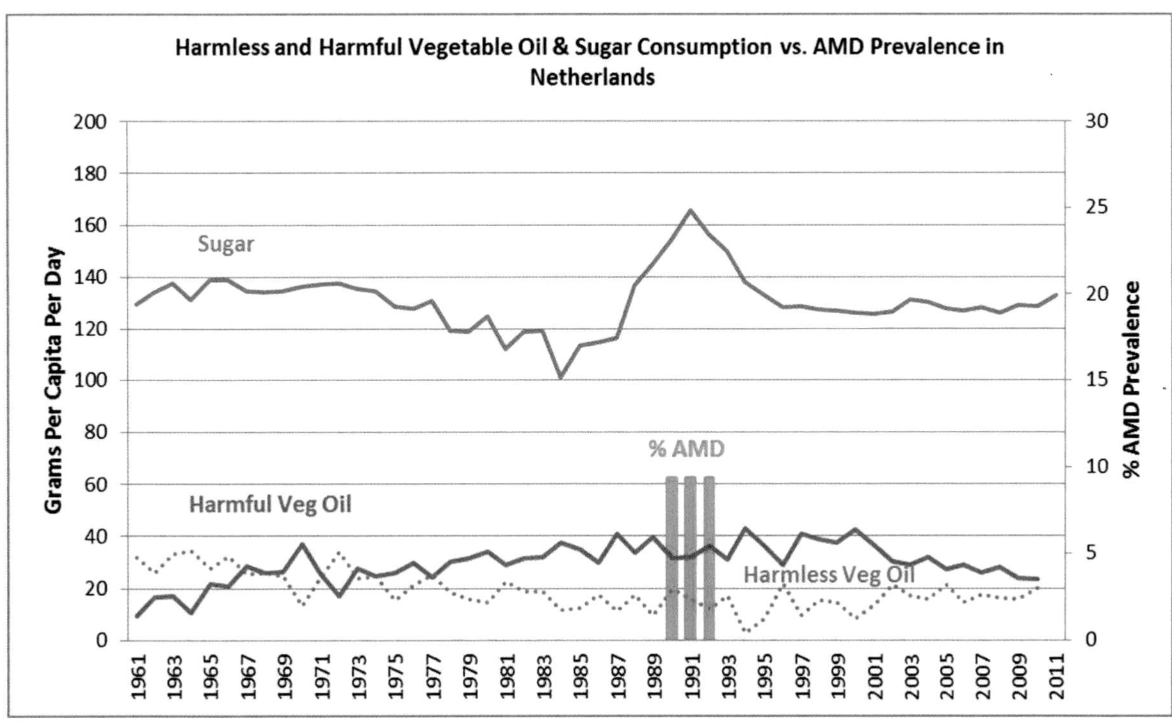

GERMANY

Perhaps the first study to assess AMD prevalence in Germany was a study that only assessed late AMD. In that study, 1.35% of people over 43 years of age had advanced AMD.[772] This is par for advanced AMD in developed nations where AMD is very common.

In 2014, a large study involving 4,340 participants, known as the Gutenberg Health Study (GHS), assessed the prevalence of AMD in participants aged 35 to 74 years. In all age groups, AMD was detected in 12.1% total, with early AMD in 11.9% and late AMD in 0.2%.[773] The range was from 3.8% in the youngest age cohort of 35 to 44 years, up to 24.2% in the oldest age cohort, of 65 to 74 years.

In Germany, we see that they've had very high sugar consumption since prior to 1961, combined with a doubling of harmful vegetable oil consumption between 1961 and 1995, with marked AMD prevalence by 2014.

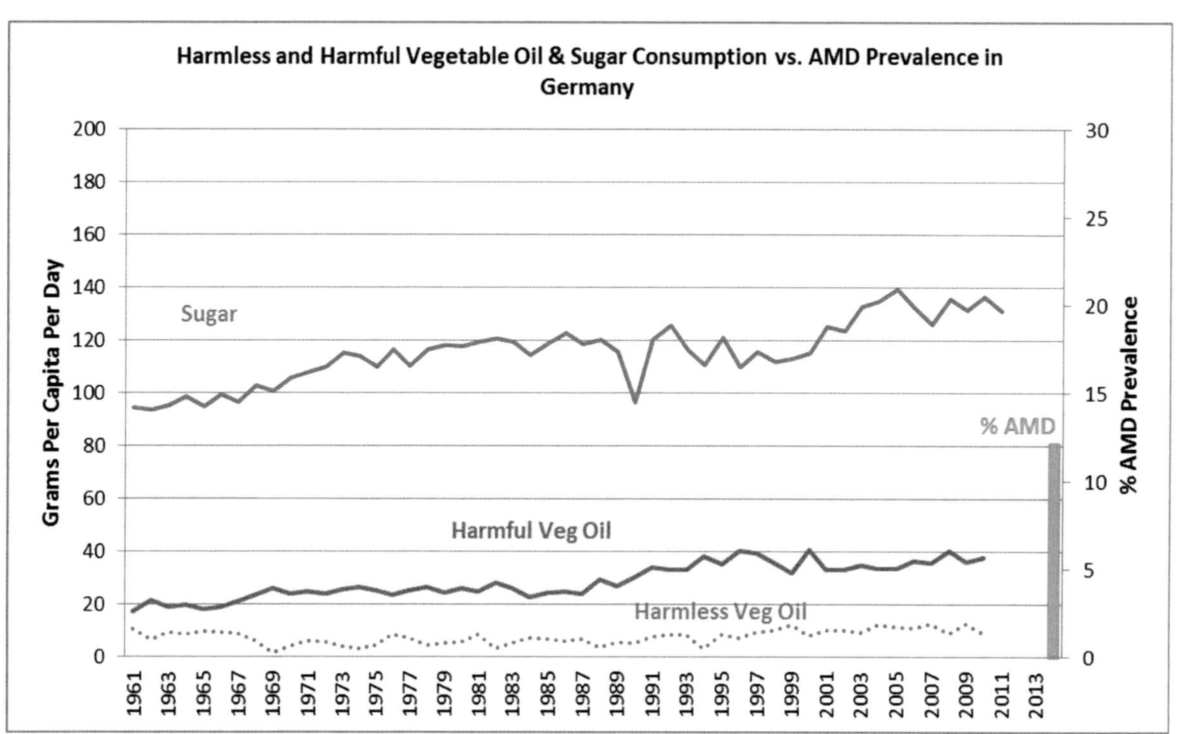

GREECE

Only one study has assessed the overall prevalence of AMD and that was the European Eye Study (EUREYE). In this study, completed in 2006, 10.22% had early ARM (Grades 1 & 2 International Classification System for ARM) and 4.71% had advanced AMD, for a total of 14.93% AMD.[774]

The Thessaloniki Eye Study was designed to assess only the prevalence of advanced AMD in Thessaloniki, which is a major urban city situtated in Northern Greece and the second largest city in Greece, second only to Athens. In this study, which evaluated subjects that were 60 years of age or older, 2.5% had advanced AMD, which was 1.3% geographic atrophy (GA) and 1.4% neovascular (wet AMD).[775]

Once again, we see high sugar consumption with dramatically elevating harmful vegetable oils since 1981, followed by high AMD levels within about 30 years.

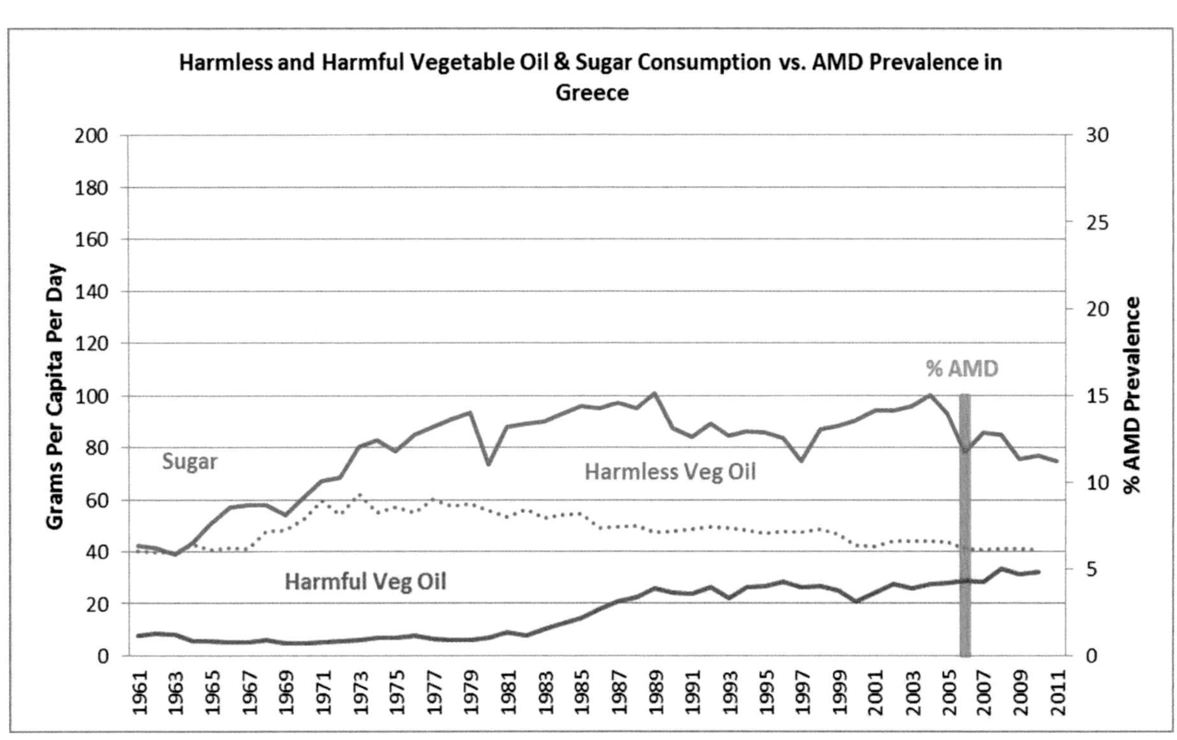

ITALY

The prevalence of age-related macular degeneration in Italy (PAMDI) study, first presented in 2011 (report 1), evaluated 1162 randomly selected subjects age 61 and above, and found "ARMD was estimated to affect 62.7% of the whole population."[776] This is a shocking statistic, as compared to all other studies and, as mentioned previously, this is the one number whereby I've reported an alternate figure in the AMD Prevalence table (above). The reason for this is that the investigators of the PAMDI studies used a definition for AMD that would result in the lowest possible threshold for calling any macular changes "ARM." And this is the whole grading mess that I never wanted to broach, but in this case, I felt it was a must.

In the PAMDI study, the researchers, who presented a brilliant study, used the definition that "ARM1 was defined by the presence of at least one medium-size druse (greatest linear dimension 63-124 μm) within 3mm of the foveal center," and "ARM2" which was defined as "the presence of at least one large druse (≥ 125 μm), with or without RPE abnormalities,"[777] which I am sure is more than most anyone wanted to know, with the possible exception of EyeMDs and ODs. The bottom line is that this results in almost anyone having drusen at all being called ARM1, which is the lowest possible threshold for calling it macular degeneration in any study that I'm aware of. If we eliminate all of those people with "ARM1" in this study, which might correlate a whole lot better to all of the other studies, I think it's much more consistent with what most researchers call ARM or AMD. I'm telling you, any attempt to harmonize all of these different grading systems would be anyone's worst nightmare – though I know a few college professors who would delight in having their students memorize these classification criteria!

Back to the PAMDI results: If we eliminate the "ARM1" category, which is 48.3% of the studied population, that leaves us with 10.4% in the ARM2 category and 4.1% in the late AMD category, for a total AMD prevalence of 14.5%. This is the number that I reported above and which I believe is the most consistent with other grading systems. As such, the prevalence of AMD in Italy is reasonably consistent with most other developed nations, such as the U.S, the U.K., Australia, and The Netherlands.

Italy, in general, has a pretty high prevalence of AMD. However, there is one study from the small community of Salandra, Italy, where AMD was quite unusual, in fact, bordering on rare. As such, I'll deal with Salandra below, under "Nations and Regions Where AMD Confirmed Rare."

Italy has had high sugar consumption and moderately high harmful vegetable oils consumption since the 1960s, with a commensurately high rate of AMD by 2011.

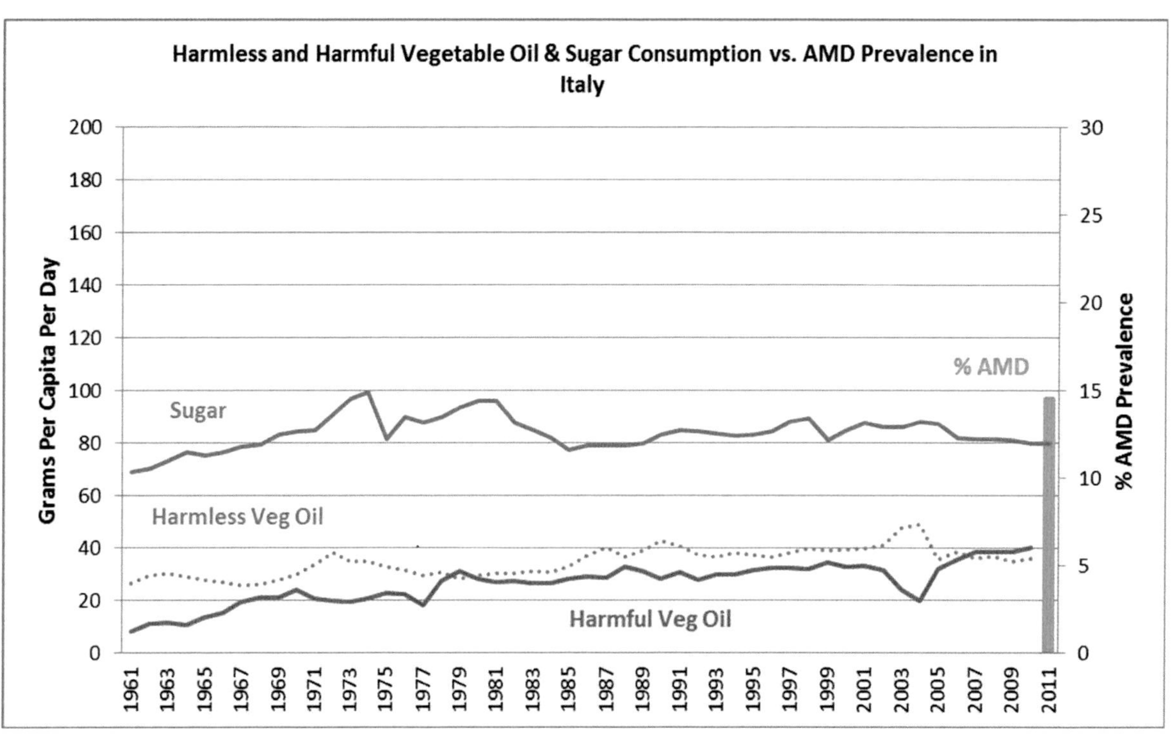

GREENLAND

As alluded to previously, for the small population of Greenland, which was 56,483 as of 2013, there is a tremendous degree and severity of macular degeneration. Understanding this data holds the potential for great insight into the cause of AMD. The population of Greenland is about 80% Inuit and only 20% of their population was born outside of Greenland.[778] As such, we'll reference the Inuit, both in Greenland and in Canada, particularly in the northeastern Canadian province of Labrador and the Northwest Territories of Canada, where some 78% of the Inuit of Canada reside.[779]

Data for Greenland is sparse, both with regard to the history of AMD prevalence as well as for diet, making firm and statistically substantiated claims much more difficult. For early data, we may rely partly on statistics relating to blindness.

According to Skydsgaard, in 1962, senile macular degeneration only accounted for 4 of 69 cases of blindness in Greenland, with 39 of those individuals being over 60 years of age.[780] At that time, glaucoma accounted for 64% of the blind. And in the Canadian province of Labrador, the study of which represented 330 Inuit, 236 people of mixed racial ancestry, and 80 caucasians, not a single one had vision below 6/12 (20/40). In short, AMD played no part in blindness in this population.[781] But by 1970 –'71, the Arctic Ophthalmological Survey examined some 4450 individuals, the majority of which were Inuit, 51 of which were diagnosed with AMD. Thomas Rosenberg, National Eye Clinic for the Visually Impaired, in Denmark, regarding the Arctic Survey, wrote, "Furthermore, it was noted that 15% of the 96 persons affected by retinal disease were legally blind... It may, therefore, appear as if an outbreak of a new disease had occurred." [782]

In 1981 AMD was identified as the leading cause of blindness in Greenland for the first time. This was confirmed once again in 1985.[783] **By the end of 1985, Rosenberg's research from the Register for the Blind in Greenland showed that blindness due to AMD varied from 5.7 per thousand males aged 65 to 69 up to a staggering 180 per thousand (18%) of men aged 80 to 84 years.**[784] In 1986, Greenland was shown to have a higher proportion of blindness due to AMD than any other reported population.[785]

By 1999, 49% of blindness in Greenland was secondary to AMD. In contrast, glaucoma accounted for 64% of blindness in 1962 but by 1999 it was responsible for only 9% of all blindness, having been usurped by AMD.[786]

There are no large, formal studies of the prevalence of AMD in the Inuit in the last millennium, however, in 1973, Wyatt presented data from 10% of the population of the Northwest Territories. Of those older than 50, including 194 Inuit, 124 Indians, 28 Caucasians, and 7 people classified as other, there were a total of 51 cases of ARM for a prevalence of 14.1%.[787] Racial categorization was not presented.

In 1977, Johnson presented data from a study in Labrador, Canada, which represented 330 Inuit, 236 biracial people (Inuit-Caucasian) and 80 Caucasians. Among those 50 and older, 12% had ARM overall, with the breakdown as 8% of Caucasians, 10% of the biracials, and 13% of the Inuit.[788] Interestingly, a study presented in 1994, of Labrador Inuit youth, aged 5 to 22 years, showed that only 3 percent were free of dental caries (cavities), while 88% had both dental caries and untreated dental decay.[789]

In 2008, Mads Varis Nis Andersen, MD, Thomas Rosenberg, MD, Professor Alan Bird, MD, and colleagues, presented "The Greenland Inuit Eye Study." This was a study that attempted to include all people over the age of 60 residing in the communities of Nuuk and Sisimiut, Greenland. There was a response rate of 74.8% with a total of 695 participants. **The prevalence of any ARM was 52.3% and advanced AMD (geographic atrophy or wet AMD) affected 9.5%.**[790] This is one of the very highest rates of ARM and, to my knowledge, the highest prevalence of advanced AMD in any population.

It might also be worth considering that, in 1988, "Erik" van Rens, MD, presented his research regarding the prevalence of AMD in Alaskan Eskimos, whose lifestyle and dietary patterns have many parallels with the Inuit; 54% of those who were older than 70 years had AMD.[791]

• So What Are the Greenlanders Eating?

Like the Eskimos, the North American Indians, and numerous other populations, the Inuit of Greenland are no longer consuming their native diet. At least up until about 50 to 100 years ago, the Inuit of Greenland would have consumed a diet very similar to the Eskimos, based largely on seal, seal oil, walrus, marine mammals, whale meat and blubber, moose, caribou, reindeer, fish, crab, very few vegetables, and very little or no fruit.[792]

Though no data is available through the Food and Agricultural Organization (FAO) directly for Greenland (and thus no graph of AMD versus vegetable oils and sugar), apparently because the data is conflated with that of Denmark, I believe our answer for their very high prevalence of AMD, resides in what will follow. In an article entitled, "The Inuit Paradox," authors Patricia Gadsby and Leon Steele detail much about the changing dietary habits of these Arctic populations. In this article, written in 2004, the authors wrote,

> No one, not even residents of the northernmost villages on Earth, eats an entirely traditional northern diet anymore. Even the groups we came to know as Eskimo—which include the Inupiat and the Yupiks of Alaska, the Canadian Inuit and Inuvialuit, Inuit Greenlanders, and the Siberian Yupiks—have probably seen more changes in their diet in a lifetime than their ancestors did over thousands of years. The closer people live to towns and the more access they have to stores and cash-paying jobs, the more likely they are to have westernized their eating. And with westernization, at least on the North American continent, comes processed foods and

cheap carbohydrates—Crisco, Tang, soda, cookies, chips, pizza, fries. "The young and urbanized," says Harriet Kuhnlein, director of the Centre for Indigenous Peoples' Nutrition and Environment at McGill University in Montreal, "are increasingly into fast food." So much so that type 2 diabetes, obesity, and other diseases of Western civilization are becoming causes for concern there too."[793]

In 2009, researchers Peter Bjerregaard, MD and Charlotte Jeppesen, MSc, University of Southern Denmark, presented a paper which confirmed that, in 1901, 83% of the energy in the Inuit diet came from the traditional foods of seal and fish, which had dropped to 37% by 1930, 35% by about 1955, 21% by 1995, and just 18% by 2006.[794] They confirmed that, by 2006, a "whole range of farmed meat, fruit, vegetables, dairy products and nutrient poor, high-calorie junk food is available." They confirmed that most of the people failed to meet the recommendations of the National Board of Nutrition and that most failed due to high intake of fat and/or refined sugar. It should be noted that, though this is not the authors of this paper's view, fat itself is never the problem, unless it is from the PUFA vegetable oils.

In 1970, two Danish physicians, Bang and Dyerberg, completed a detailed dietary study of the people of northwest Greeenland, in order to investigate the very low rate of cardiovascular disease among the Inuits existing on what was then considered traditional fare in the region.[795,796,797,798] They found that the Inuit diet consisted primarily of marine food, very rich in protein and fat, with a very high proportion of monounsaturated and omega-3 polyunsaturated fatty acids. They believed that the high proportion of fats originating from marine animals and fish protected the consumers against coronary heart disease. In 1976, Bang and Dyerberg completed another detailed dietary study, this time in western Greenland, in Illorsuit, where fishing, whaling, and seal hunting continued to be the main dietary resources. They collected 5 to 7 duplicate daily food portions, which were analyzed at the time, however, the meal samples were preserved in freeze-dried aliquots.[799,800] In 2004, Danish researchers, led by Bente Deutch and colleagues, at Aarhus University, analyzed the freeze-dried 1976 food samples against typical food samples obtained in 2004. In their own words they wrote, "Between the traditional meals collected 30 years ago and the meals from 2004, dramatic and significant changes have occurred in the dietary composition. The percentage of local food has decreased, and with it the intake of n-3 [omega-3] fatty acids."[801] They went on to state, "In the traditional meals from 1976, almost 60% of the solid weight and 40% of the energy came from local Greenlandic food items, whereas in the meals of 2004 only 23% of the weight and (20-23%) of the energy came from local products. The mean intake of seal meat in particular was lower, namely, about 60 g compared with 400 g/day in 1976, a difference of 80%... The consumption of local fish and birds was also significantly lower in 2004. In 2004, the meals from about one third of the participants comprised less than 10% Greenlandic food. In 1976 the food had a very high relative content of n-3 [omega-3] fatty acids, resulting in a mean daily consumption of 8.5 g of n-3... In 2004... the mean daily intake of n-3 fatty acids was now 3.3g... 26% of the 1976 value."[802]

In 2007, Deutch and colleagues once again completed an analysis of some 90 local meals in Greenland and compared them to the duplicate meals of 1976 as well as to other dietary studies in Greenland between 1953 and 1987. They determined that, in 2004 to 2006, the percentage of local food had dropped to only about 20%, which was associated with a large drop in omega-3 fatty acids and vitamins A, B1, B2, B12, C, iron, iodine, phosphorus, selenium, folate, and calcium, which contrasted markedly with the extremely high intakes of vitamin A, vitamin D, and iron that were present in the dietary of Greenlanders 30 to 50 years previously.[803]

In 2005, Bente Deutch and colleagues published a paper that began, "In several Arctic countries, weight gain is very evident among the local populations and the percentages of overweight and obese persons are increasing rapidly. Since the development of overweight among the Arctic populations seems to coincide with the westernization of their diet and other life-style factors..."[804] In those Greenlanders 18 to 49 years of age, they found 19% fell into the obese category, with consequent adverse effects on serum triglycerides, HDL, and cardiovascular risk indices.

Consistent with this trend of Westernization of the diet, researchers Stig Andersen, MD, PhD, Gert Mulvad, MD, and colleagues, found that, between 1963 and 1998, the fraction of overweight Inuit men, ages 50 to 69, in Greenland, increased more than 6-fold in that time frame, rising from 4.0% to 25.6% ($P < 0.001$). The fraction of overweight Inuit women more than doubled in the same time period, rising from 14.0% to 30.7% ($P<0.001$).[805]

The important point not to be missed in these studies, is that there has been a dramatic replacement of traditional foods with imported, processed foods, which are certainly foods with long shelf-lives that virtually always contain large amounts of refined white flour, sugar, PUFA vegetable oils, and trans fats. The people of Greenland reside in a region where native fruit is not available, native vegetables are scarce and, as such, these people have resorted to the consumption of 80% imported food, which, when the bulk of that food is processed, sets the stage for metabolic disaster, including macular degeneration.

ICELAND

Iceland, the southeastern neighbor to Greenland, is located in the frigid waters of the North Atlantic ocean. The population of Iceland, 329,740 in 2015, is almost exclusively white, with the descendants primarily being those of settlers from Scandinavia and the British Isles. Iceland's people are plagued by a degree of macular degeneration that approaches that of the people of Greenland. Undeniably, they share many of the same characteristics when it comes to climate and dietary issues.

In 1987, Professor Fridbert Jonasson, MD, and K. Thordarson published the results of their study of AMD prevalence in rural areas of Eastern Iceland between 1980 and 1984. Some 751 people (81.2% of the regional population) were examined, with ages ranging from 43 to greater than 83. The overall prevalence of AMD, utilizing the same criteria as the Framingham Study of 1973, was 6.7%.[806] The prevalence of those with AMD who were 73 years of age or older was 29.4%, whereas 30% of those 75 or older in the Framingham Study were affected by AMD.[807]

In 2003, Fridbert Jonasson, MD, and colleagues published results from the Reykjavik Eye Study, which is an all white population, for those 50 years of age and older, 17.9% had ARM and 3.5% had late AMD, for a total of 21.4% AMD.[808] The authors of this study point out that, according to the United Nations Food and Agriculture Organization, there is not a single European nation that consumes more fish per capita than the Icelanders.[809] The authors also assert that, "their consumption of green vegetables and fruits is relatively low by European standards, which possibly results in relatively low levels of vitamin A. Daily intake of multivitamins and cod liver oil is, however, known to be very common among elderly Icelanders... Smoking, which has been implicated as a risk factor for AMD, was relatively uncommon among those 70 years and older in our study, and fish was usually consumed several times a week."[810] It would have been very interesting to have any data on the association between those consuming cod liver oil and presence of AMD, but no such data was collected.

Iceland has one of the highest levels of sugar consumption of all nations studied, ranking only behind the U.S.A. and very similarly to Barbados, both of which have markedly high levels of AMD. Sugar, of course, is generally an excellent marker of processed food consumption, of which Iceland ranks extremely high. Relatively, their harmful vegetable oil consumption is not that high, but the combination of very high sugar and even low to moderate PUFA vegetable oils are very strong factors of AMD risk. The fact that their AMD prevalence is much higher in 2003 as compared to 1980 through1983, is consistent with a prolonged consumption of much processed foods, as indicated by high sugar and low to moderate vegetable oil consumption. Our research confirmed that the FAO data on vegetable oil consumption was artificially low in Kenya due to non-reporting of vegetable oil sales by various manufactuers, and the situation may be similar in Iceland. The FAO data should never be artificially high, but failure of reporting by manufacturers may certainly make the numbers artificially low.

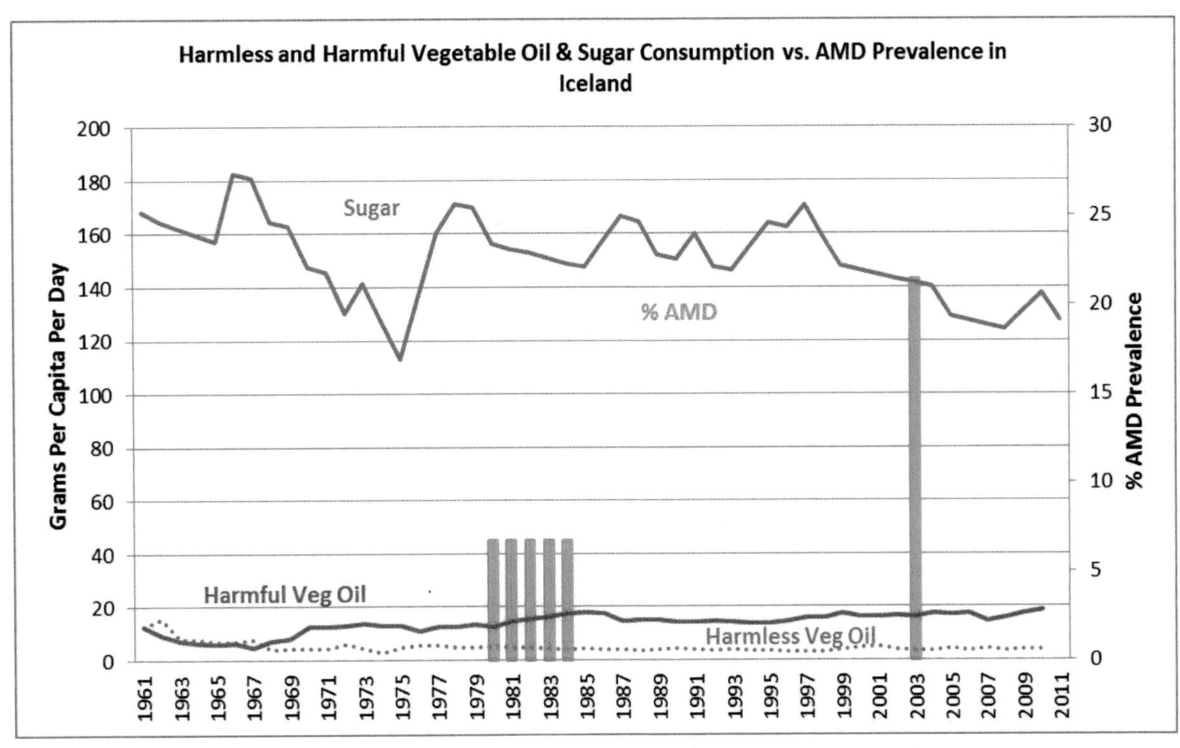

BARBADOS

Barbados, West Indies, is a sovereign island nation located in the Lesser Antilles. Though I've always thought that Barbados was in the Caribbean, technically, it is in the North Atlantic located 62 miles (100 km) east of the Caribbean Sea. It is a beautiful island with stunning beaches. However, there is much to be learned from the plight of the people of Barbados as it relates to both general health and macular degeneration.

About 92% of Barbadians, also known colloquially as "Bajans," are of African descent – the majority from West Africa. As such, this population is a good one to compare against the black populations of Africa or elsewhere. The Barbados Eye Studies were specifically designed to assess (among other conditions) macular degeneration prevalence "in a population of African descent," and that is exactly what they did.[811]

The first AMD prevalence study in Barbados was completed in 1995, and in a population of 4709 subjects aged 40 to 84 years, of which 93% were black, 4% "mixed" (black and white), and 3% white or other, early AMD was present in 23.5%, late AMD in 0.57%, and any degree of AMD present in 24.3%.[812] As you can see, these are staggering statistics for overall prevalence of AMD. In fact, for those aged 70 to 79 years, 41.7% had AMD, and for those beyond 80 years of age, 50.0% had AMD.

Nine years later, the Barbados Eye Study group re-evaluated this group of subjects. Now, unlike prevalence studies, which assess the current rate of a disease or condition, this one was an *incidence* study. Incidence is defined as the onset of a new disease or condition – one that didn't exist before. So this study evaluated, for those people that didn't have it before, the onset of AMD that didn't exist when evaluated previously, or in the case of advanced AMD, the onset of such (usually from existing early AMD) during the term of the study. **They found an overall incidence of early AMD of 12.6% and late AMD of 0.7%.**[813] **This indicates that, despite the already high prevalence of 24.3% AMD in this population, another approximately 13.3% would either develop new AMD or advance to late AMD within nine years.**

Compare the Barbadians with an overall AMD prevalence of 24.3% and 50% of their very elderly with AMD, to that of the Africans of Zimbabwe with a prevalence of 1.13% AMD for those over age 65, or a rate of AMD of just 0.01% in South Africa for all ages, or to the people of Lesotho, Africa, where some 12,000 patients presented without a single case of advanced AMD (see detail and references for all three populations below). What do you suppose is the difference?

You guessed it. The diet in Barbados is absolutely atrocious. It contains perhaps about as much processed food as anywhere on the planet – ranking right up there with Greenland and Iceland.

Barbados Today, the local news establishment of Barbados, published an article on August 7, 2013, regarding a National Seminar on Food and Nutrition Security in Barbados, where the Minister of Agriculture, Dr. David Estwick, made a presentation. According to the author of the article, Estwick asserted, "...Our awarenenss has been made even greater by our rapid dietary and epidemiological transitions," which had, according to the author,

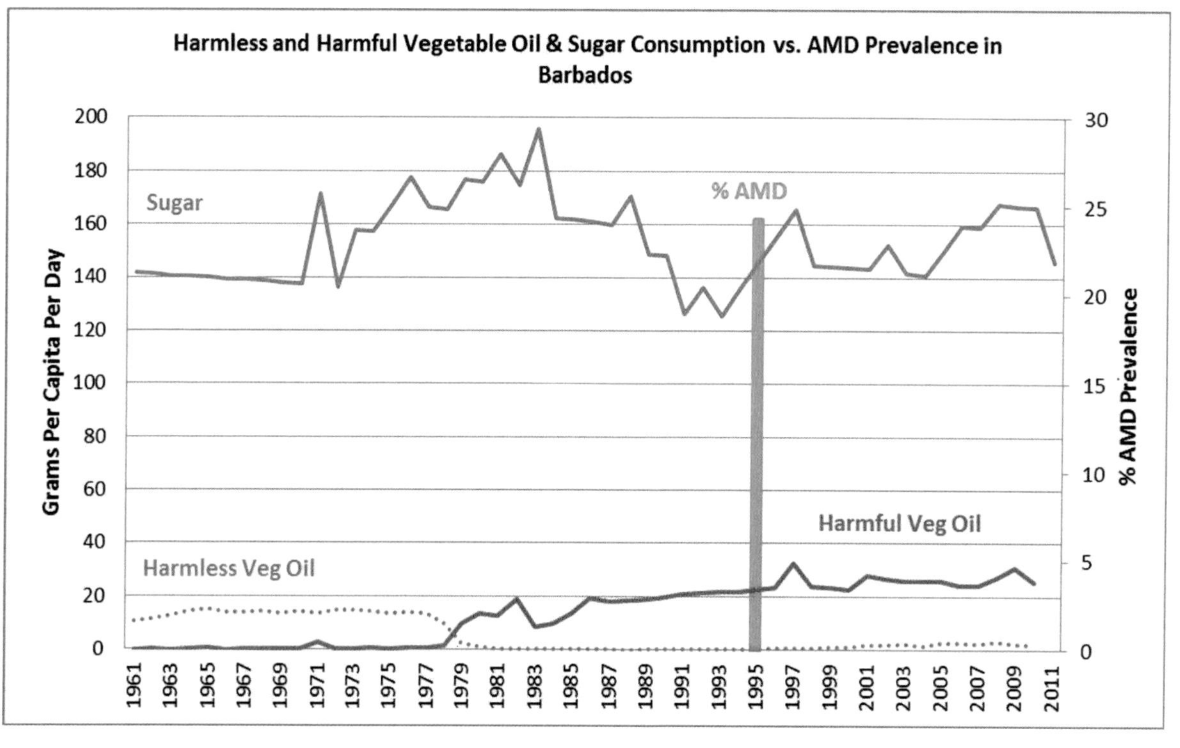

"caused nutritionists to observe a shift from foods based on indigenous staples to a more varied energy-dense diet of processed foods as well as beverages high in salt, sugar, oils, fats and alcohol."[814] Estwick added, "We've also noticed a proliferation of nutrition-related chronic non-communicable diseases such as diabetes, high blood pressure, heart diseases and cancer. And without a doubt, these have replaced malnutrition and infectious diseases as our major public health concerns."[815]

Scientific research confirms Estwick's statements. In 2008, Sharma et al confirmed that the diet in Barbados was consistent with some of the most processed food-laden diets worldwide.[816] Epidemiologist and nutrition researcher,Sangita Sharma, PhD, and colleagues published a study entitled, "Assessing dietary patterns in Barbados highlights the need for nutritional intervention to reduce risk of chronic disease."[817] The title is followed immediately in the abstract of the study by the statement, "The dietary habits of the Caribbean have been changing to include more fast foods and a less nutrient dense diet." Sugar intake exceeded the Caribbean recommendation almost four-fold, while intakes of calcium, iron (women only), zinc, and dietary fiber were substantially below recommendations. Sugar sweetened beverages and juices provided more than 40% of total sugar intake. Consistent with such a processed food-laden diet, Gaskin et al found that Barbados had developed a "world profile of chronic metabolic disease with especially high levels of diabetes and hypertension."[818] In 1993, Foster et al found that, in a random sample of the people of Barbados aged 40 to 79, some 17% were found to have type 2 diabetes and 45% were found to be hypertensive. Fifty-three percent of men and 42% of women were overweight and 10% of men and 30% of women were obese.[819] In 2005, Gaskin et al found that 27% of adolescent children in Barbados were overweight.[820]

Without question, the heavily processed food diet in Barbadoes has caused a multitude of systemic disease, diabetes, hypertension, metabolic syndrome, obesity, and one of the highest rates of macular degeneration worldwide.

NATIONS & REGIONS WHERE AMD PREVALENCE IS MODERATE

CHINA

Various studies in different locales have shown tremendous variation in the prevalence of AMD in China. For example, in 1987, Wu and colleagues found an ARM prevalence of 10.6% in people age 50 and older, whereas in late 1980s and early '90s, the Han prevalence was 6.4%, rising to 11.3% in the Uighur, 15.6% in the Tibetans, and 16.8% in the Hunan area of China for those 65 and older.[821] However, these are very small studies and study designs are not available to review, making any comparison very difficult.

In the Beijing Eye Study, published in 2006, 4439 subjects aged 40 and older were studied in the Greater Beijing region. Early ARM was present in 5.1%% of both rural and urban populations and late ARM (AMD) was present in 0.3% of subjects, for a total of 5.4% AMD.[822,823]

In October, 2009, Professor Barry Popkin, PhD, of the University of North Carolina, Chapel Hill, gave a lecture at the International Congress of Nutrition held in Bangkok, Thailand, entitled, "The World Is Fat: New Dynamic Shifts in Patterns of The Nutrition Transition." In that presentation, Dr. Popkin presented data demonstrating the rising consumption of edible "vegetable oils" in China. The

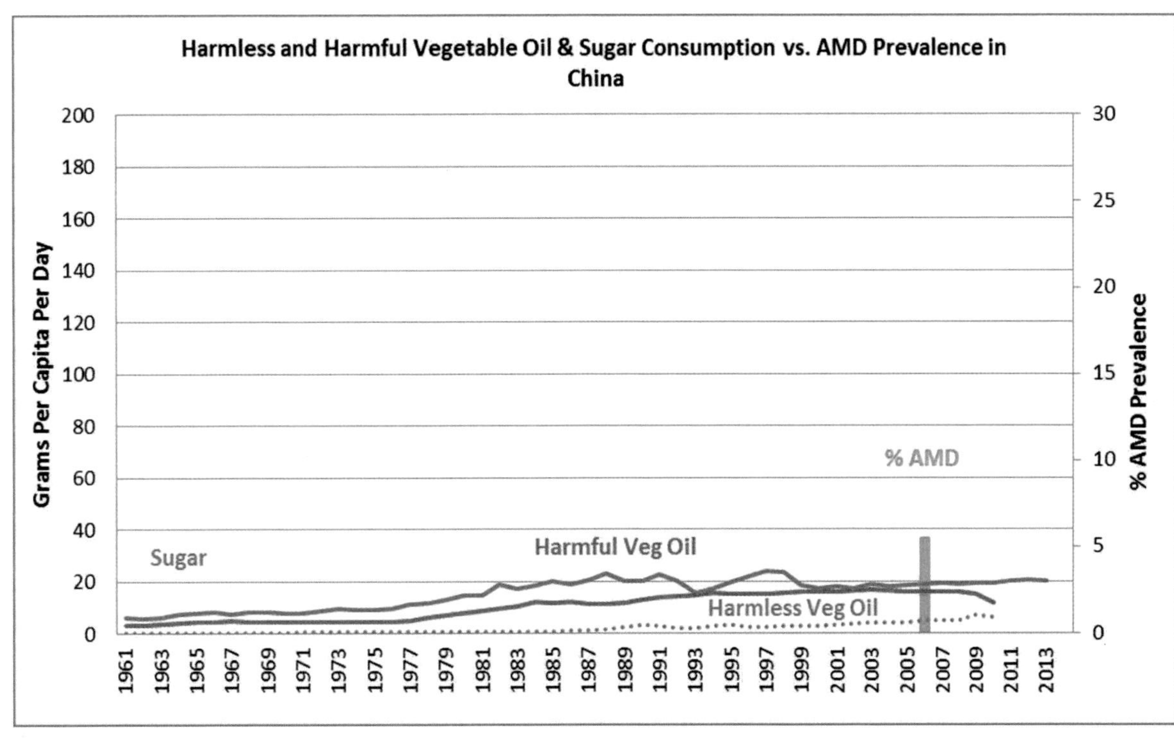

average consumption, in grams/capita/day, was 14.8 in 1989, 28.9 in 1997, and 30.9 in 2006, which is 4.9%, 11.2% and 12.4% of total caloric consumption, respectively.[824] Compare that to the average consumption in the U.S. in 2005, where vegetable oil consumption was 59.6 grams per person per day,[825] which is almost exactly twice what it was in China at the time, while the U.S., overall, has higher rates of AMD. China's increasing consumption of vegetable oils is correlated to increasing prevalence of AMD.

In China, the FAO data (FAOSTAT) from which we drew showed somewhat lower consumption of vegetable oils than did the data reviewed above by Professor Barry Popkin. The numbers are not drastically different, but it is worth noting. There is only one large study of AMD in China, as mentioned above (the Beijing study), and it is certainly possible that this is not reflective of the AMD prevalence of the nation at large. Nevertheless, the AMD prevalence there is considerably lower than most nations, consistent with their overall much lower sugar and harmful vegetable oil consumption.

ISRAEL

There have been no formal studies of the prevalence of AMD in Israel, however, one study showed that AMD accounted for 20.1% of all blindness in the country in 1998 and that in 2003, blindness secondary to AMD had elevated to 28%.[826] The authors concluded that the incidence of AMD in Israel is increasing based on this data. Blindness in Israel secondary to AMD is, however, considerably lower than in the U.K., where AMD accounts for or plays a role in 56% of all blindness.

In the graph bellow, we see that Israel has quite high vegetable oil consumption and very high sugar consumption, both of which would be anticipated given their relatively high incidence of blindness secondary to AMD.

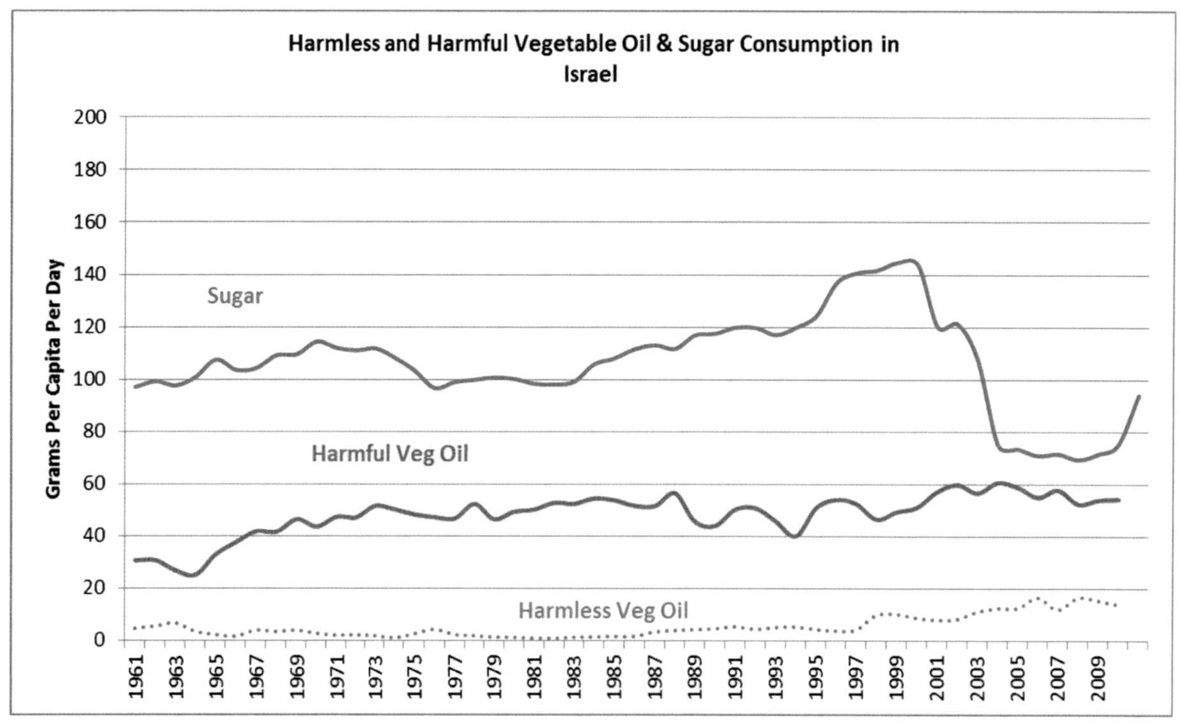

KENYA

Ophthalmologist researcher, Wanjiku "Ciku" Mathenge, MD completed the first AMD prevalence study in Kenya, in 2013. She wrote to me via email, "Until my study the teaching was... 'There is no AMD in Africa,' so no one looked for it." [827] Obviously, from the studies of Zimbabwe, South Africa, and Lesotho, there was good reason for ophthalmologists to believe that, at least at one time, there was virtually no AMD in Africa.

Dr. Mathenge, who is a native of Kenya, in a study of 4,414 subjects, found that, by 2013, 11.2% of Kenyans aged 50 and over had early AMD and 1.2% had late AMD, for a total of 12.3% overall.[828] The Kikuyu, which is the largest tribe in Kenya,[829] specifically had 12.3% early AMD and 1.1% advanced AMD.[830]

The Kikuyu tribe's people are traditionally agriculturalists, and according to the Kenya Information Guide, "In most rural Kikuyu homes, typical traditional Kikuyu food includes githeri (maize and beans), mukimo (mashed green peas and potatoes), irio (mashed dry beans, corn and potatoes), roast goat, beef, chicken and cooked green vegetables such as collards, spinach and carrots." [831]

Unfortunately, urbanized Kenya has substantially Westernized their diet in recent decades. Nakuru, the city where Dr. Mathenge's study was centered, is Kenya's 4th largest urban center with a population of 307,990 as of 2013, and Nakuru County has a population of 1.6 million. According to the Intermediate Technology Development Group, "Increasingly, overcrowding and poverty mean that most people live in congested and inappropriate homes." [832] With urbanization, of course, also came supermarkets, grocery stores, restaurants, and an abundance of cheap, processed food. Researcher, J.K. Mungati, of the Ministry of Industrialization Enterprise, presented data at the Industrialization Week conference held at KICC Nairobi in 2013. His research showed, "In 2011, a total of Ksh 1,315,671 million [Kenyan Shillings] was spent on imports out of which Ksh 106,539 million was for imports of foods and beverages (of this amount Ksh 59,133 million or 55.5% was utilized to import animal/vegetable fats and oils)."[833]

As we know from every other market, the enormous bulk of this is not animal fats – it is vegetable oils. In fact, according to the Export Processing Zones Authority, located in Nairobi, Kenya, "Kenya imports vegetable oils and fats in order to supplement its local production, which is presently inadequate to meet local demand." Further in the publication, they state, "**Kenya imports mainly vegetable oil and fats, which contribute over 95% of the total animal and vegetable oils and fats imports.** Animal oil and fats make up the balance of 5%. **At present, Kenya's domestic production of edible oils is estimated at 380,000 tonnes, only about one-third of its annual demand. The remainder is imported, at a cost of $140 million, making edible oil the country's second most important item after petroleum.**" [834]

Our research indicates that the FAO data for Kenya is incomplete and not consistent with the Export Processing Zones Authority, nor the findings and reports of manufacturers of vegetable oils in Kenya, which include Kapa Oil Refineries, BIDCO, Unilever Kenya, Pwani, and Golden Africa, all of whom market and distribute their vegetable oils in Kenya. Utilizing the statistics from the Export Processing Zones Authority, If 380,000 tonnes (metric tons) is one-third of Kenya's edible oil consumption, as they stated, extrapolating this number yields a vegetable oil consumption of approximately 24.78 Kg/person/year, which is 67 grams per person per day. This is a very high vegetable oil consumption and, of course, would be consistent with a high prevalence of AMD.

Ramona Rischke, PhD and colleagues, at Georg-August-University Göttingen, Germany, completed a study relating to supermarkets and food consumption patterns in Kenya, in 2015. Among the numerous details of this study, she and her colleagues found that "Supermarkets have been spreading rapidly throughout Kenya" and they collectively state, "We find that supermarket purchases increase the consumption of processed foods at the expense of unprocessed foods. Supermarket purchases increase per capita calorie availability, which is linked to lower prices paid per calorie, particularly for processed foods... **The consumption of processed and highly processed foods and beverages is often singled out as an important factor contributing to unhealthy diets, as this category includes high calorie foods with *poor micronutrient content*, such as sugary beverages, sweets, and all kinds of salted snacks.** Spreading supermarkets, in turn, are suspected to improve the availability of these products and to increase their desirability even among poor households in remote areas." [835]

SOUTH KOREA

The first study of the prevalence of AMD in South Korea was completed from 2008-'09 as part of the Korea National Health and Nutrition Examination Survey. From a cross-sectional, nation-wide survey and examination, for individuals over 40 years of age, the researchers found 5.1% with early AMD and 0.5% with late AMD, for a total of 5.6%.[836] The next Korea National Health and Nutrition Examination Survey, completed in 2010 – 2011 utilizing the same criteria, found early and late AMD at 6.7% and 0.7%, for a total of 7.4%,[837] which is quite suggestive of increasing prevalence even over a couple of years' time.

In South Korea, once again we see substantially rising sugar and harmful vegetable oil consumption rising since the late 1970s and with moderate degrees of macular degeneration by 2008, approximately 30 years later.

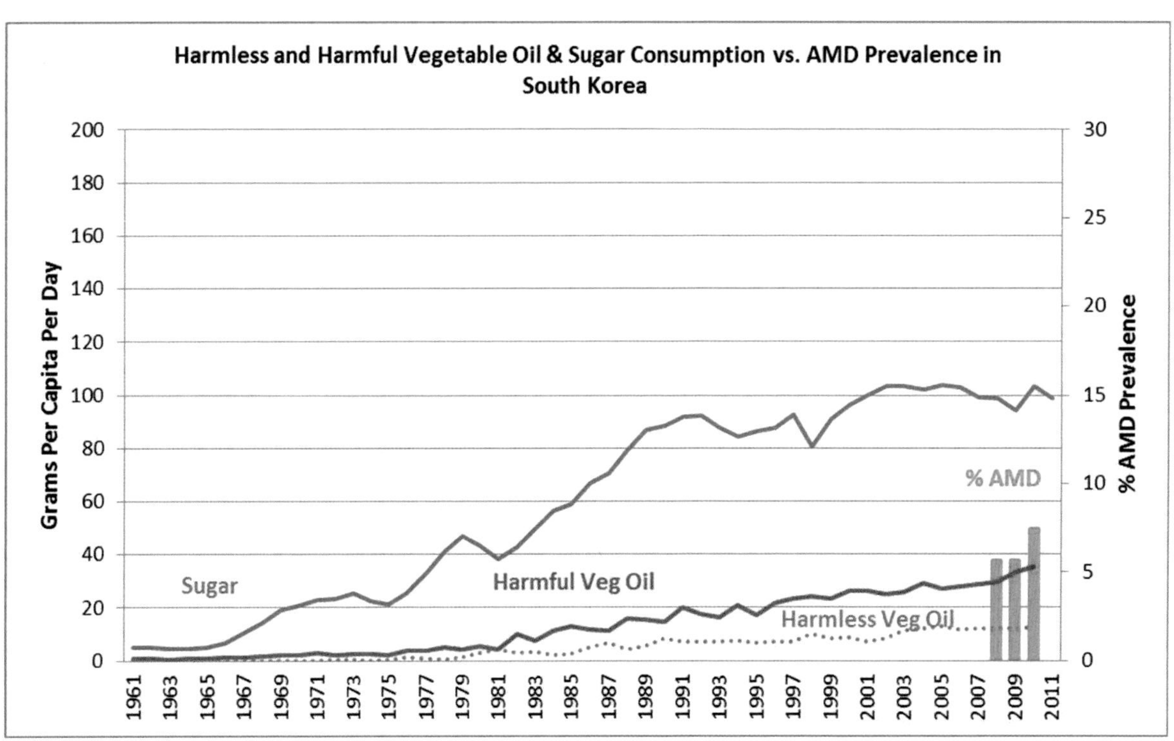

THAILAND

Thailand is a nation that appears to have had a very low prevalence of AMD until very recently, which makes it difficult to categorize for the purposes of this book. Nevertheless, typical of nations that don't have much of a problem with a disease condition, we didn't see a single AMD prevalence study from Thailand until 2011. At that time, researchers evaluated 10,788 participants from the Thailand National Survey of Visual Impairment in 2006-2007, aged 50 to 98 years (mean of 62.1), and found that only 2.7% (294 people) had early AMD and 0.3% (27 people) had late AMD.[838]

In 2015, researchers presented data collected in 2010 from 7,043 subjects aged 50 years and older. They found 12.2% to have AMD, with 94.3% of the patients affected with early AMD and very few affected by severe AMD.[839]

As we can see from the graph above, AMD has become a significant problem in Thailand as well. We see substantially rising consumption of sugar since 1964, but still very low overall consumption of harmful vegetable oils. Keep in mind that, with 12.2% of the population developing AMD in this scenario, in the face of a relatively low overall consumption of vegetable oils, may very well indicate that a small percentage of the population is consuming the bulk of the vegetable oils and, of course, this scenario is much more likely than any even distribution of consumption. This is perhaps the most critical point to consider in any evaluation of food consumption in any given population. As I've said before, remember that countries don't consume these foods – people do. And behaviors differ markedly!

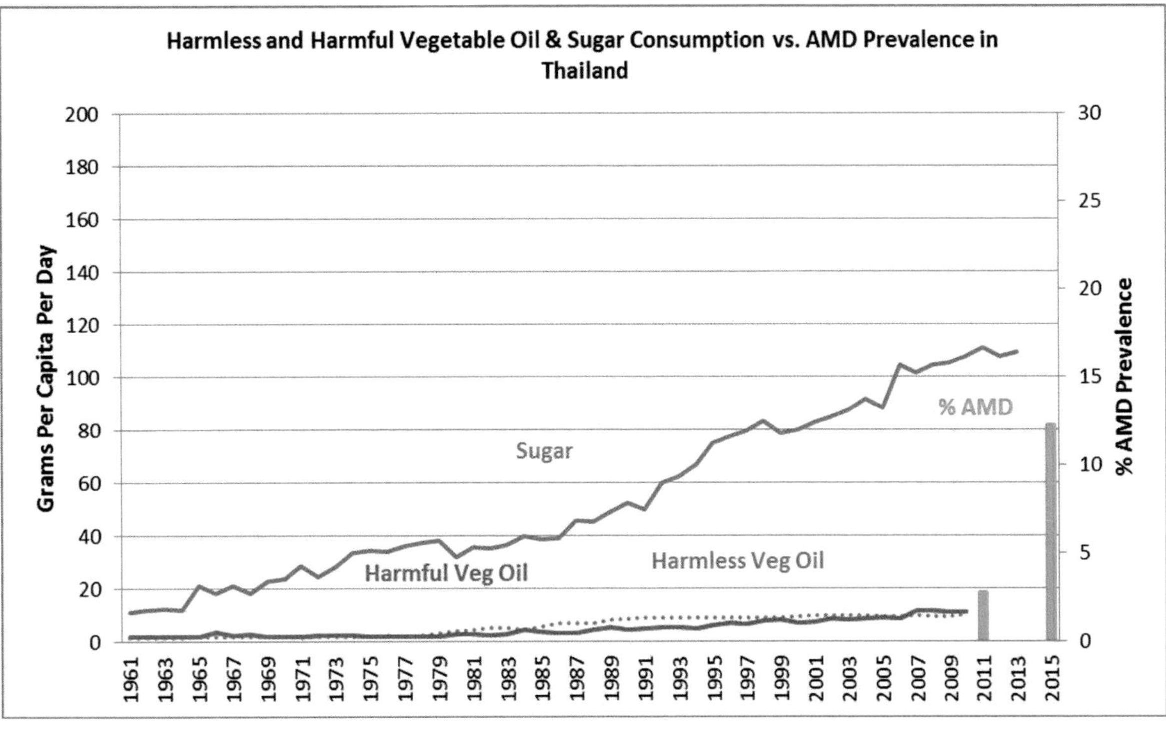

NATIONS & REGIONS WHERE AMD CONFIRMED RARE – AT LEAST AT ONE TIME!

In this section, you will see that there are nations where AMD was once confirmed rare, such as Japan and India, and whereas it is now becoming much more common. You will see that their consumption of vegetable oils and sugars was once dramatically less, but is rising in recent decades with a commensurate rise in the prevalence of AMD. In others, such as the Pacific Island countries, you will observe that AMD remains very rare and in their case, that they have very low to almost non-existent consumption of the PUFA vegetable oils, while consumption of sugar is low to very substantial, but elevating in recent decades.

JAPAN

In a paper published in 1999, Professor Alan Bird, of Moorfield's Eye Hospital in London, England, wrote, "In the past AMD was rarely recognized in Japan." [840] Some 15 years later, in 2014, in his "Distinctive Voices" lecture given at the Beckman Center, Irvine, California, he stated, "In Japan, the disorder {AMD} was very rare 40 years ago. We talked to the Japanese ophthalmologists – the elderly ones. They said, 'We never saw it forty years ago. It didn't exist.' Now it's a major problem – the same in India, they say exactly the same thing." [841]

Japan is perhaps one of the single most classic examples whereby we can observe the prevalence of AMD rise from the status of extreme medical rarity in the 1970s and '80s, perhaps as it had been in the U.S. and the U.K. in the 1920s or early 1930s, to levels nearly as high as the U.S. and U.K., all within a span of about 20 to 25 years. Preceding this drastic increase in the Japanese prevalence of AMD, you will see that their consumption of processed foods, as indicated by their increasing sugar and vegetable oil consumption, is marked.

In 1999, AMD was so rare in Japan that when Professor Ron Klein, MD, and colleagues, at the University of Wisconsin, published their paper entitled, "The Prevalence of Age-Related Maculopathy by Geographic Region and Ethnicity," Japan still had not a single major study regarding macular degeneration prevalence.[842] At the Nagoya University Hospital, only 24 eyes with dry macular degeneration and 36 eyes with wet-type degeneration were reported among 31,334 outpatients who were examined during 1974 to '79." [843] [844] Given that young patients are far less likely to present for or require eye care, this is very strong evidence that AMD was exceedingly rare at that time. If we assume 10% of the patients are under 40, that leaves 60 patients out of some 28,201 over 40, for an approximate AMD prevalence of 0.2%. This assumes that only one patient represents each eye affected, which is highly unlikely and would, therefore, make the prevalence potentially even lower.

The city of Tokyo has its own blind and visual handicap registration. Tokyo represents about 10% of the population of Japan, thus being a significant indicator of the nation's visual status. The registration detail showed that, in1968, AMD was not in the top 9 causes of registration; it was not in the top 10 causes of registration in 1978, but ranked as the 8th cause of blindness and visual handicap in 1988, indicating increasing AMD prevalence and severity.[845] By 2010, AMD was the 4th leading cause of visual impairment in Japan, accounting for 10.9% of visual handicaps.[846]

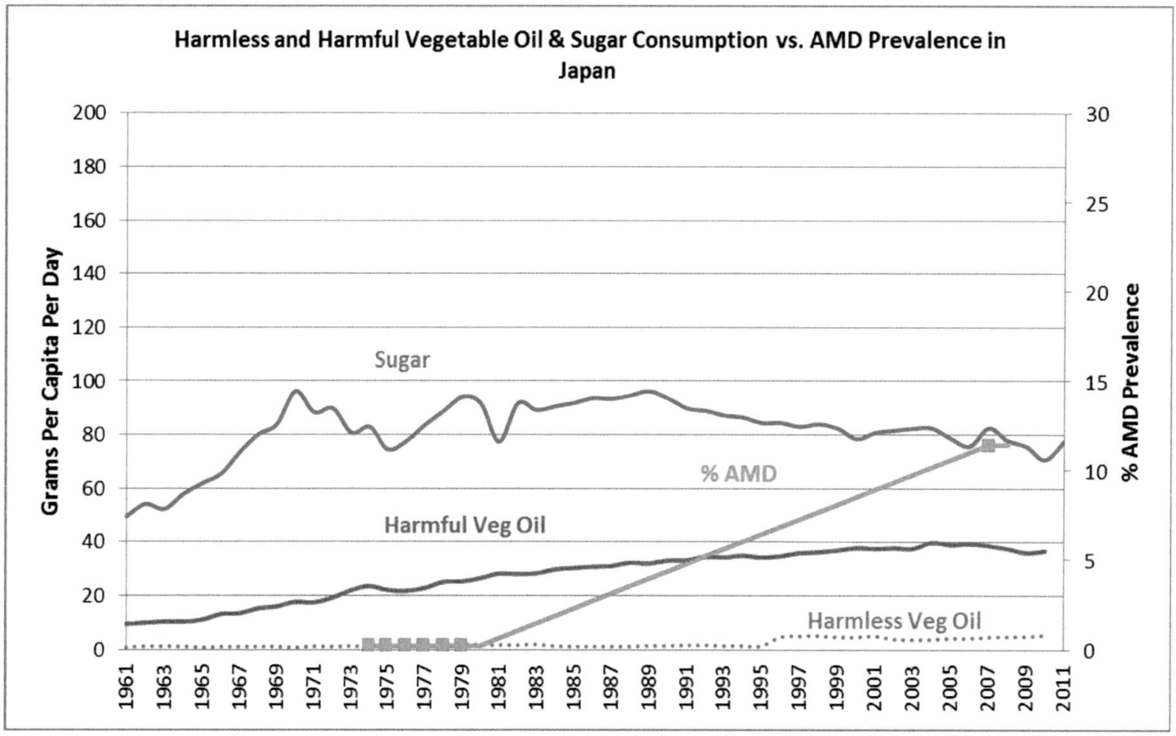

In 1993, researchers Yuzawa and colleagues ascertained the number of wet AMD cases in Japan, based on a survey of ophthalmology departments throughout the nation. Their research suggested that wet AMD would affect 35 people per 100,000 in 1993, which translated to a prevalence of only 0.035%, or just 14,400 people affected in a nation of 124.5 million people. Perhaps more importantly, the authors found that, "This number was estimated to have almost doubled over the six year period since the initial survey in 1987," adding that the "1.7-fold increase in exudative AMD represents a significant increase in the rate of this disorder." [847] Finally, the authors themselves recognized that this increasing prevalence was likely tied to their own diet, as they wrote, **"The rapid rise in this disease might reflect rapid changes in environmental factors including westernization of the Japanese life style."** [848]

By 2001, researchers in the Hisayama study had found that wet AMD, which was exceedingly rare just 14 years previously (in 1987), had risen to 1.2% in men and 0.34% in women.[849] The rate in men was suddenly competing with that of people in the U.S (see below).

Contrast the Japanese rate of wet AMD in 1993 (0.035%) to that of the U.S. Beaver Dam Eye Study of 1993, which found wet AMD in 1.2% of the population and advanced AMD in 1.6% of the population.[850] Even if we only compare the wet AMD cases and not the advanced AMD total, the prevalence in the U.S. was about 34 times greater than in Japan.

But since 2000, as the rate of AMD in Japan continued to climb, there have been at least 11 studies investigating the prevalence of AMD. In the Hisayama study, in Hisayama, Japan, researchers conducted a study of the prevalence of AMD in 1998, though they didn't report on the results until 2003. And although AMD was rare just a decade before, in this study of people older than 50 years of age, they reported, "ARM was detected in 19.5% of men and 14.9% of women." [851] In this same study, in 2003, the researchers converted to the Wisconsin Age Related Maculopathy Grading System to report subsequently, which would make results comparable to most recent U.S. studies, and they found that of residents age 50 and over, 8.5% had early ARM and 0.8% had late ARM.[852] The number rose again in 2007, to 10.0% early AMD and 1.4% late AMD.[853]

In 2013, the Nagahama study found that early AMD prevalence was 16.1% in the 50 to 59 year-old group and increased to 31.2% in the 70 to 74 year-old category. Advanced AMD was 0.27% and 0.98% in the 50 to 59 year-old and 70 to 74 year-old groups, respectively.[854]

• Japanese Immigrants to Brazil Develop Obesity and AMD Like Brazilians

Brazil has Westernized its diet.[855,856] And when otherwise healthy Japanese people move there, unfortunately, they begin to consume foods similar to the locals – with all of the attendant metabolic consequences. In fact, one recent study published in 2002 reports, "Brazil has the largest Japanese population outside Japan. Originally, Japanese showed a low prevalence of diabetes mellitus and cardiovascular disease, but nowadays such picture has been changed and they may be considered at high risk for metabolic syndrome. We previously reported the importance of type 2 diabetes mellitus, dyslipidemia and hypertension in Japanese-Brazilians. Our data are in agreement with other studies conducted in Japanese immigrants living in Washington State, Hawaii and California in the United States."[857] In fact, in this same study, the overall prevalence of obesity in these Japanese immigrants to Brazil was 40.2%, with an overall prevalence of central adiposity (high visceral fat, i.e., belly fat and fat around the organs) of 50.3% and of those with central adiposity, 19.7% had diabetes and 41.0% had hypertension.

As compared to their approximate 0.2% prevalence of AMD in Japan back in the 1970s, we should expect a dramatically higher incidence and prevalence of macular degeneration in these Japanese immigrants to Brazil, right? And indeed, that's what we see. In a study of Japanese immigrants and their descendents living in Londrina, Brazil, researchers found that, of 483 studied subjects with an average age of 71, the overall prevalence of AMD was 15.1%. The breakdown was as follows: 13.8% had early AMD, 0.4% had geographic atrophy, and 0.8% had wet AMD.[858] In São Paulo, Brazil, a study of elderly Brazilians showed that 13.9% had AMD, which is quite similar to the Japanese immigrants.[859]

• *Japanese and Other Races in America Develop AMD Comparable to Americans*

Had we been comparing AMD in Japan in the 1970s or even 1980s, which was obviously extremely rare, versus that of AMD in the U.S., which was 8.8% in the Framingham study, we would have likely concluded that "the Japanese are genetically protected against AMD." Obviously, the Japanese are not protected from obesity, metabolic disease, or AMD, as these conditions simply follow a processed food containing diet. As we will continue to see next, no race is immune to the effects of a processed food diet.

Joshua D. Stein, MD and colleagues at the University of Michigan, Department of Ophthalmology, completed an analysis of a large database of patients in the U.S under a managed care network, finding that the prevalence of dry AMD in white Americans was 5.40% while that of Japanese Americans was 4.36%. There weren't a lot of differences for other races, as the prevalence for Chinese Americans was 6.50%, Korean Americans 5.19%, Pakistani Americans 4.90%, Filipino Americans 4.77%, Vietnamese Americans 4.21%, and Indian Americans 3.54%.[860] Though certain races may have once been considered to be "genetically protected," these studies confirm that that is a fallacy.

INDIA

Recall once again that, in 2014, Professor Alan Bird, ophthalmologist from Moorfield's Eye Hospital in London, in his "Distinctive Voices" lecture, stated that the "elderly" ophthalmologists from India reflected that macular degeneration didn't exist 40 years ago and that, "Now, it's a major problem."

One senior ophthalmologist from India who was practicing in the 1960s and continues to practice today (2016), advised me that he had never heard of AMD until he attended an American Academy of Ophthalmology meeting in 1979. Only then did he learn of AMD, which in retrospect, he says was rare in those days - but much more common today. As he has asked to remain anonymous, I must respect his wishes.

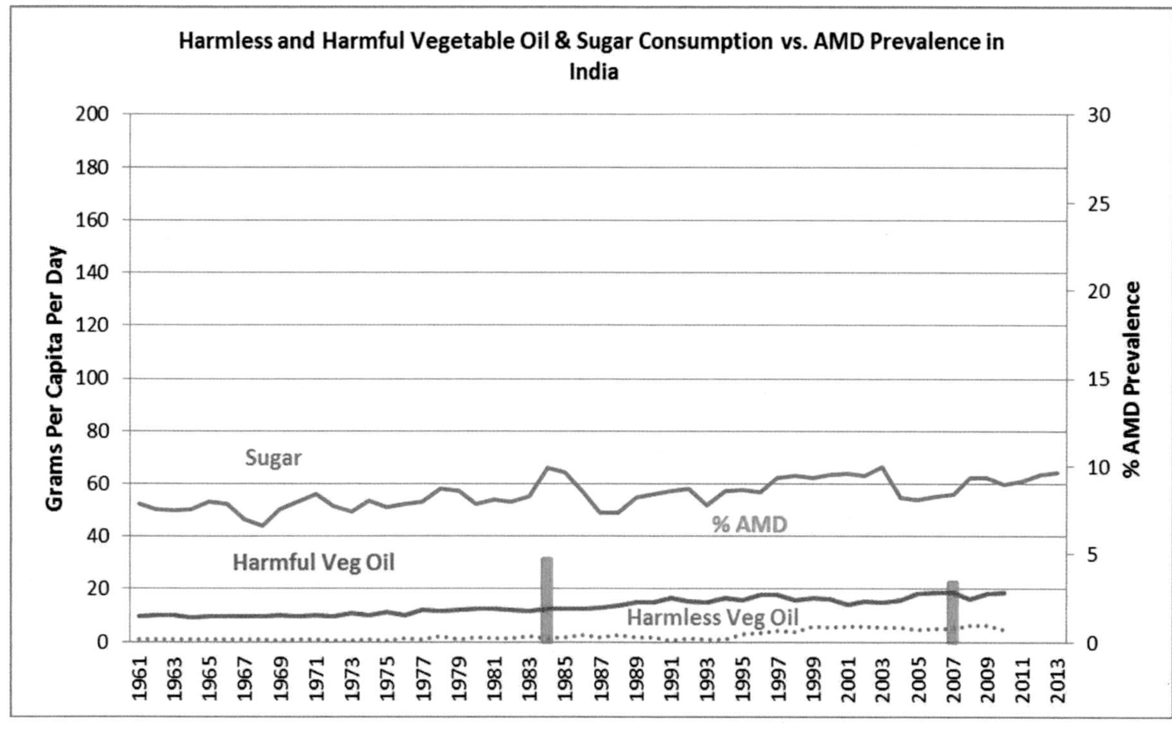

Like Japan, India has been very slow to adopt Westernized cuisine, but in recent decades and in certain regions, they too have begun to do so. Our research as well as other research indicates that, particularly since 1993, the people of India are consuming more and more soybean, rapeseed (canola), and sunflower oils – all PUFA containing vegetable oils.[861] This has obviously contributed to the development of AMD as a significant problem, while noting that the condition remains far less common than in Western nations. This, of course, resonates with their overall low consumption of harmful vegetable oils and sugar.

The earliest formal study of AMD prevalence in India was completed by I.S. Jain and colleagues, in 1984.[862] Out of 2122 patients, aged 50 and above, who were screened for AMD, 4.7% (100 patients) were found to have either dry AMD or advanced AMD. Of those 100 patients, 85 had dry AMD and 15 had a history of wet AMD (disciform disease); thus 0.7% of the population had advanced AMD. The details of patient selection criteria and geographic region selected for inclusion are not well described, and this may have greatly affected the relatively high prevalence of AMD found in this study.

In 2001, blindness was assessed in the southeastern state of Andhra Pradesh. Though blindess was very significant, at 1.84% of the population of all ages evaluated, AMD wasn't even mentioned as a cause anywhere in this study.[863] Blindness was caused mostly by cataract, refractive error, preventable corneal disease, glaucoma, complications of cataract surgery, and amblyopia. This figure stands in stark contrast to blindness in the U.K., where AMD accounted for 49% of blindness in 1990.[864]

Perhaps as an indication of the low rate of AMD, twelve years went by before the next study of AMD prevalence was even begun in India. Between 1996 and 2000, the Andhra Pradesh Eye Disease Study was completed, in the southeastern state of Andhra Pradesh. This study examined 3723 subjects 40 years and older, finding AMD in just 1.91%.[865]

Next, in 2004, came the Aravind Comprehensive Eye Study, which was completed by Dr. Nirmalan and colleagues in the southeastern Indian state of Tamil Nadu, In this study of 5150 individuals aged 40 and above, early AMD was found in 2.7% and late AMD affected 0.6.[866] In 2007, the India Eye Study (INDEYE study), by Dr. Gupta and colleagues, found AMD in 3.4% of those aged 50 and older, in a rural area of the northern state of Haryana.[867]

By 2011, AMD had risen dramatically, at least in a population in rural central India, where the prevalence of early AMD was 3.6% at age 41 to 50, 7.9% at age 51 to 60, 10.0% at age 61 to 70, but interestingly, was lower in the older age groups, at 8.3% in the 71 to 80 year olds, and 8.0% in those older than 81 years.[868] The fact that AMD is increasing in prevalence is strongly suggestive that diet is causal. I would also submit that the lower prevalence of AMD in the eldest groups is strongly suggestive that those were the groups less likely to be altering their diets as significantly.

• *When Asians from the Indian Subcontinent Relocate to the U.K.*

In 2013, ophthalmologists, Dr. Abdul Rauf, Richard Wormald, MD, and colleagues at Queens Hospital, London, completed a study on the prevalences of eye diseases in Asians from India. In this study there were 922 subjects, of which 416 were either Indian or Pakistani, and the authors note there were only a few Pakistani. This group was found to have an AMD prevalence of 8.7%.[869] This number is significantly higher than that of the Aravind Comprehensive Eye Study (3.3%), the INDEYE study (3.4%), or the Andhra Pradesh study (1.91%), suggesting that when Indians relocate to the U.K. and, hypothetically, consume a diet more like the British, their risk of AMD increases. In fact, the authors themselves wrote, "Inspection of figures from our study suggests that the overall prevalence of ARMD in British Asians is similar to other UK populations." [870]

NEW ZEALAND

In 1969, ophthalmologists Ida Mann, FRCS and Dorothy Potter, DO (Lond.) completed an investigation of 333 inhabitants of New Zealand, which are about 75% Maori by genetic heritage. Of these, 93 were between 60 and 80+ years old, and 147 were from 50 to 80+ years old. Only two patients had AMD and they were 72 and 82 years old.[871] **If we calculate the prevalence of AMD for those 50 or more years old, this would give 1.3%, and for 60 plus years old, would be 2.1%.** The authors of this study note that the New Zealanders had "rapidly attempted transition to European culture" and also stated that, "The diet, however is still somewhat lacking in protein, and obesity is a problem… Ischemic [poor blood flow] heart disease and diabetes are widespread and the expectation of life is shorter than for the white man." [872]

In 1982, AMD appears to have risen considerably, as a study by ophthalmologist, G.S. Martinez, FRCS (Edin.) and colleagues found the prevalence in some 481 subjects age 65 and above to be 6.4%.[873] By 2014, ophthalmologists Dr. David Worsley and Dr. Andrew Worsley completed a study to estimate AMD prevalence in New Zealand, finding that the prevalence had increased to approximately 10.3% for those 45 to 85 years old.[874]

As we see from the graph, sugar consumption in New Zealand has been very high since prior to 1961. However, it is only with their increasing consumption of harmful vegetable oils that their AMD has risen to very significant levels in more recent years.

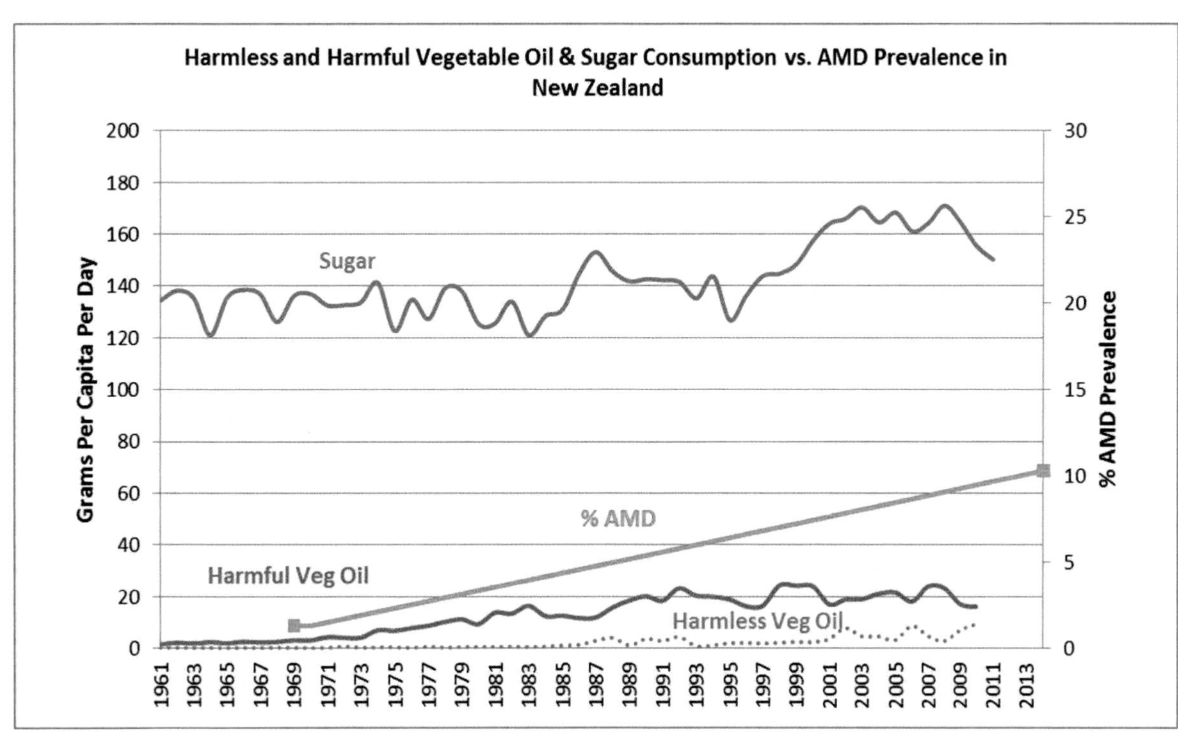

ZIMBABWE, AFRICA

In 1977, L.C. Chumbley, MD completed a study of Rhodesian Blacks located in Mashonaland, northern Zimbabwe, Africa. **During a six-month period, Chumbley found AMD in only 4 patients out of 3,350 new patients, some 353 of which were 65 or older.[875] This translated to just 1.13 percent of patients over the age of 65 and a mere 0.12% of all new patients.** Dr. Chumbley described all to be very mild cases "with mild to moderate bilateral macular pigment disturbance, moderately reduced central visiual acuity, and no other abnormality." [876] He confirmed no cases of advanced AMD.

Chumbley notes that the Bureau for the Prevention of Blindness in South Africa found that only 0.01% of all South African Blacks, of all ages, had any degree of macular degeneration.[877] Next, I'll quote Dr. Chumbley as he wrote,

> These are stunning observations when one considers that this condition is found in about 25%

of New Yorkers between 65 and 80 years of age, and in about 30 – 40% of persons aged 80 years or older. Senile macular degeneration is the commonest cause of blindness in Britain, according to one study accounting for 28.9% of all new cases of blindness during 1 year.

What factor may be operative in protecting the Shona from this condition? Host factors may be involved. On the other hand, certain environmental factors may be implicated as well.

The Shona are known to be virtually free from ischaemic coronary artery disease, unlike American Negroes, in whom an almost equal incidence to that of Whites is found. There is a markedly reduced degree of atherosclerosis among Blacks. The cultural and dietary make-up of the Rhodesian Black in Mashonaland differs widely from that of Whites, in whom generalized atherosclerosis and coronary artery disease occur with about the same frequency as among Whites in North America or Europe.

Ophthalmic pathological studies of senile macular degeneration show arteriosclerotic changes in the choroidal vessels and intercapillary connective tissue of the choriocapillaris. Some feel it is an accentuation of a normal unavoidable process of senescence. *However, like some aspects of larger vessel atherogenesis, senile macular degeneration may well be a largely preventable condition.* The answer to this problem may lie in research in preventive medicine and ophthalmic epidemiology on populations such as ours.

Arterial diseases appear to be emerging with rising prevalence in Africa...

This year we have observed the first 2 cases of central retinal artery occlusion since the Harari Eye Unit was opened 12 years ago. While this is an affection involving the retinal circulation and not the choroidal circulation, it may none the less suggest a trend of increasing vascular disease. Both these patients were expensively dressed, well-to-do urban Blacks who ate a wholly European diet and had adopted a European life style.[878] (Italics added)

In this entire passage, written some 38 years ago in 1977, Dr. Chumbley was extraordinarily close to making the connection that I am making in this entire book. He recognized the drastic differences in the prevalence data between populations, presented the vascular component of AMD, and more than once connected that the differences appeared to be in the diet. He just didn't recognize what it was exactly that made the African diet healthy, thereby preventing cardiovascular disease and AMD, while the diet of the Americans and British led to such diseases.

Note from the graph that when sugar and vegetable oil consumption were both very low in the preceding decades, AMD only affected 1.13% of patients over age 65 and 0.12% of all new patients. Compare this to Barbados, which has an AMD prevalence of 24.3% and, of course, a strikingly high sugar consumption and moderate harmful vegetable oil consumption.

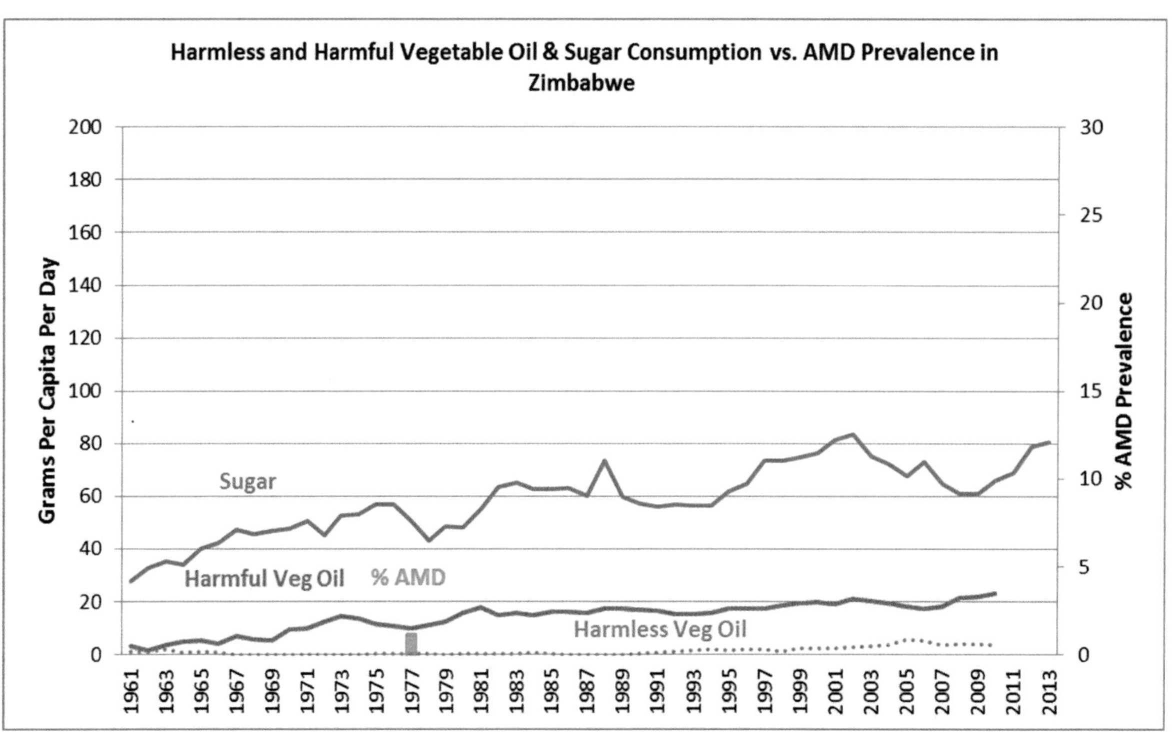

LESOTHO, AFRICA

In 1977 – '78, ophthalmologist Yitzchak J. Gordon, MD, and 'Muse Mokete, of the Hebrew University-Hadassah Medical School, of Jerusalem, Israel completed a survey of ophthalmic conditions in Maseru, the capital city of Lesotho, Africa. After completing a formal study of some 1266 ophthalmic clinic patients at 15 representative sites throughout Lesotho, they noted not a single case of disciform (presumed wet) macular degeneration cases.[879] **However, they also noted, "In Lesotho, disciform macular degeneration was not seen in this survey or in the 12,000 outpatients examined in Maseru over a two-year period."** [880]

Though the authors only reference "disciform macular degeneration," which is the advanced stage of AMD, they make no reference at all to dry AMD. Unfortunately, I have not been able to make contact with the authors of this study, which was initiated some 39 years ago as of the time of this writing. Nevertheless, I would have to assume that, if there were not a single case of wet AMD in some 12,000 patients, the prevalence of dry AMD must have fallen substantially under the one percent category. Perhaps the other consideration is that, given that Dr. Yitzchak was an ophthalmologist, it would seem odd that he would make reference to a complete lack of discoid macular degeneration and yet fail to even consider dry AMD.

According to the FAO, "Lesotho is classified as Low Income Food Deficit Country. Currently, 57 percent of the population lives below the poverty line and 14 percent is undernourished... Stunting (small for age) was found in 39 percent of children under the age of five in 2010. Maize [corn] makes up 54.8 percent of average daily calorie intake, followed by wheat with 13.7 percent and sugar with 6.6 percent. Together, these three staple crops account for 75.1 percent of the average daily calorie intake, while animal products contribute 5.9 percent of the latter." [881]

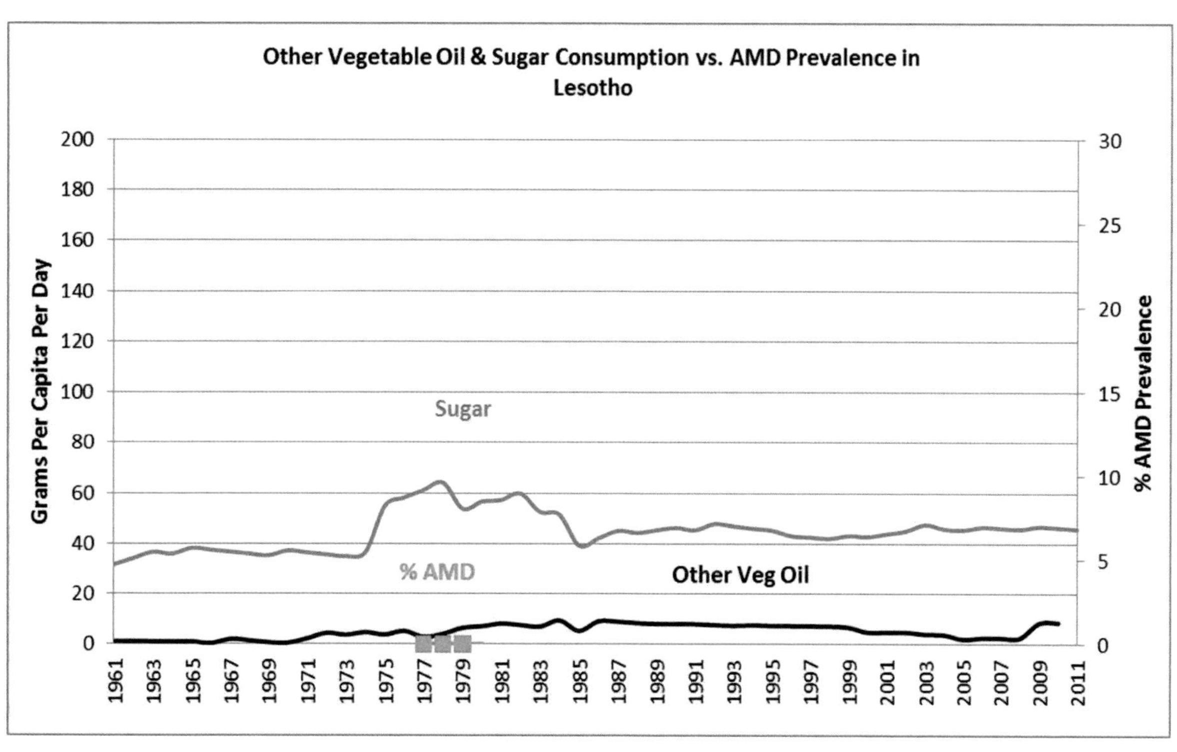

Note: In this graph, AMD is 0.0% Advanced AMD; See text above for details.

NUTRITION COUNTRY PROFILE – KINGDOM OF LESOTHO – 2010 (FAOSTAT)[882]

TREND IN PER CAPITA SUPPLY OF MAJOR FOOD GROUPS (in g/day)									
MAJOR FOOD GROUPS	**1963 - 65**	**1968 - 70**	**1973 - 75**	**1978 - 80**	**1983 - 85**	**1988 - 90**	**1993 - 95**	**1998 - 00**	**2003 - 05**
Cereals (excl. beer)	536	537	520	554	551	557	613	611	626
Starchy roots	8	9	11	34	51	77	108	123	122
Fruit and vegetables	85	84	95	109	122	134	127	104	70
Meat and offals	55	50	56	55	65	60	56	47	50
Milk and milk products	61	42	67	97	155	56	50	51	49
Sweeteners	37	36	42	58	48	46	46	42	41
Pulses, nuts, oilcrops	20	15	21	28	17	24	10	21	12
Vegetable oils	1	1	4	6	7	9	8	8	5
Eggs	3	2	3	3	2	2	2	2	2
Animal fats	2	1	2	2	2	1	1	1	1
Fish and shellfish	0	0	0	3	7	0	0	0	0
Other	110	91	95	144	116	76	71	66	59

Source: FAOSTAT

As you can see from the table above, taken directly from FAOSTAT, the average human consumption of vegetable oils for Lesotho, was 1 gram/person/day from 1963 to 1970, 4 grams/day from 1973 to 1975, and 6 grams per day from 1978-80. They also had very low sugar consumption and white wheat flour consumption is negligible. At least in the 1960s and '70s, Lesotho had virtually no processed foods, practically no vegetable oils, sugars, or white flour and, of course, they had virtually no macular degeneration.

NIGERIA

Ibadan, Nigeria is the third largest city in Nigeria with a population of over 3 million people. At the Eye and Retinal Clinic of the University College Hospital, Ibadan, researchers reviewed all cases presenting with AMD over a three-year period, from October, 2007 until September, 2010. Though the researchers didn't give any statistical analysis in this particular study, they reported that only 101 patients were seen during that period that were diagnosed with AMD.[883] This amounts to approximately 34 patients with AMD per year, or less than 3 per month, to a hospital serving a population of potentially more than 3 million people.

In a study of rural dwelling people of south-western Nigeria, which was completed in 2007, some 2201 patients, ages 8 to 92 years, were examined to determine the prevalence of various ophthalmic diseases. Of those that had ocular morbidity, 69% of them were age 41 or greater. There were only 2 patients with AMD, out of the 2201.[884] **If 69% of those examined were also 41 years or more, which would be typical for any eye clinic, then the prevalence of AMD in this population would be just two patients out of the approximate 1519 patients, for a prevalence of 0.1%, which is comparable to the findings of other populations that consume little or no processed food.**

Onitsha, Nigeria is a large city with more than 1 million people in the metropolitan area; it has a river port on the eastern bank of the Niger river and is also considered a major trading centre of Nigeria.[885] As compared to the rural dwelling people of Africa, such as those of south-western Nigeria reviewed above, we should anticipate a higher rate of AMD here in Onitsha. Just as Weston A. Price found in the 1930s, wherever one finds roads and civilization, retail stores typically pop-up, and there is bound to be man-made, processed foods and, of course, increasing consumption of processed foods. In 2004, a study of patients from the city of Onitsha, Nigeria, was completed, assessing some 7966 people for the prevalence of AMD. **This research found that 3.2% of subjects age 50 and older had AMD.** Of those with macular degeneration, early AMD was found in 71.1% with the remainder having late AMD (10.9% geographic atrophy and 18% being wet AMD).[886]

Note from the graph on the next page that the overall consumption of sugar and harmful vegetable oils in Nigeria is very low. As reviewed above, in the rural areas where there was little or no access to grocery stores and processed foods,[887] AMD was only 0.1%, but in the metropolitan area of Onitsha, where there is much greater access to grocery stores and processed foods, AMD was 3.2%.

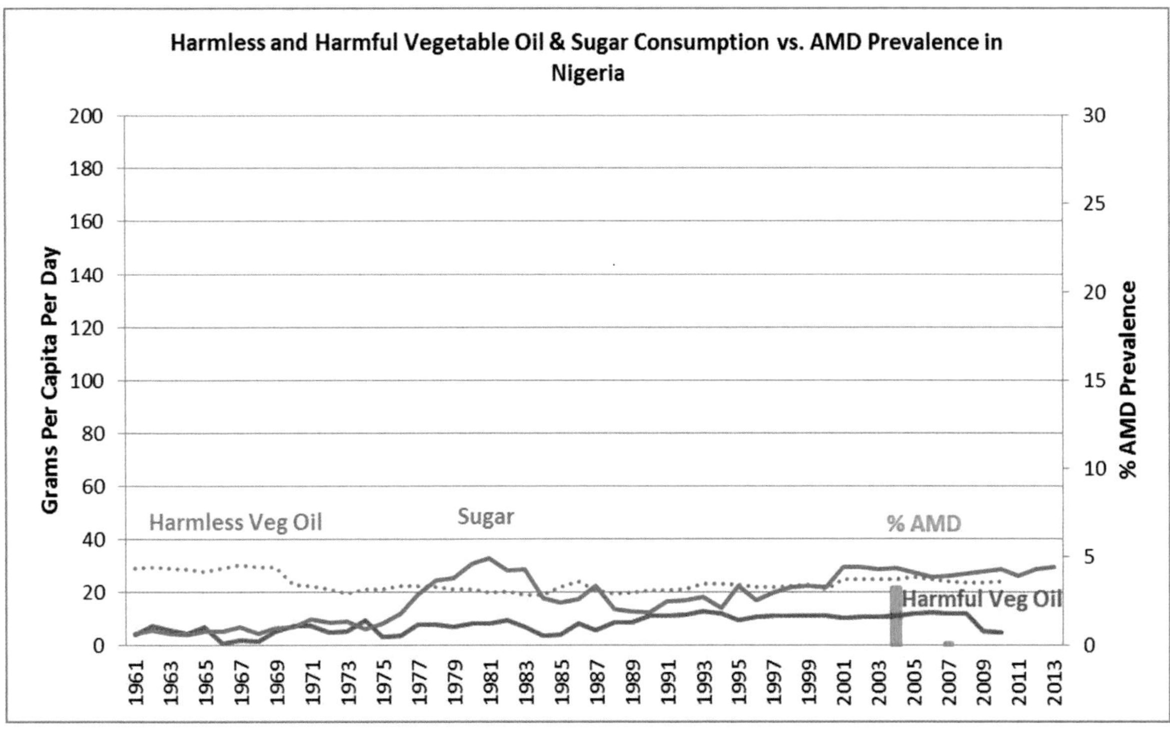

SALANDRA, ITALY - WHERE AMD BORDERS ON RARITY

Salandra, Italy is a small town with a population of 3363, located in Southern Italy in the Basilicata region. The town sits atop a hill at the end of a road and is surrounded by farmland, which is the driving force for this small community. In 1991, researchers Sergio Pagliarini, MD (Queen's Medical Center, Nottingham, England), Antonietta Moramarco, MD (Instituto di Oftalmologia, University "La Sapienza," Roma, Italy), Richard P.L. Wormald, MSc, MD, Professor Alan Bird, MD (both of The Institute of Ophthalmology, University College of London, London, England), and other colleagues collectively set out to "test the hypothesis that an environmental factor, scarce in such a remote community but ubiquitous in modern industrial societies, might modify the risk of developing ARM." [888]

In Salandra, of the subjects that were studied, 87.1% were born and raised in Salandra and both parents of 77.3% of the participants were also born in Salandra.

The ophthalmologist researchers were able to evaluate 366 of the 576 eligible participants who were older than 60 years of age (range 60 to 89), and found the following: **"The overall prevalence of ARMD [Age-related macular degeneration] was 1.1%."** [889] This 1.1% turns out to be 2 patients with signs of having had wet AMD (disciform scars) and 2 patients with geographic atrophy (GA). Without getting deep into the complexities of comparing various classification schemes to this group, it is important to consider that the

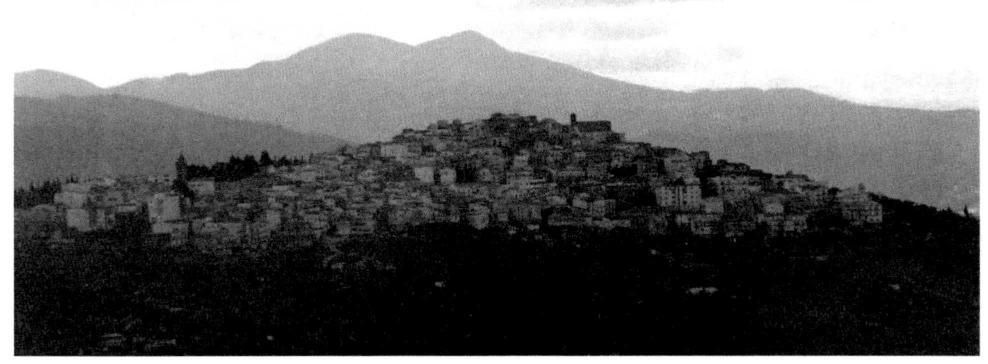

Salandra, Italy.
Image Courtesy of Antonio DiPersia.

overall prevalence would be higher in some grading systems. For example, only two of the 366 (0.6%) had soft drusen, and if these two were included in the overall classification of patients with AMD, which would be most consistent with the Wisconsin Age Related Maculopathy Grading System, this would bump up the overall prevalence to 1.7% or possibly higher depending on other factors. If one were using a much more aggressive grading system, such as the Clinical Age-Related Maculopathy Staging System (C.A.R.M.S.), then up to 4.5% of the subjects might be in the category of ARM/AMD, but this is very unlikely, since the Salandra study was counting drusen of a smaller size (50 microns) as compared to most all other studies where the threshold begins larger (63 microns). Thus, no matter how you slice it, the prevalence of ARM and AMD in Salandra was very, very low, at least compared to most developed nations as well as most of the rest of Italy.

Dr. Pagliarini and Dr. Moramarco quite carefully assessed food consumption in Salandra at that time, which is something that very few studies have done. What they found was very interesting. In their own words, "Participants tended to use local food, resorting only occasionally to industrial shelf-available products. Most stated that bottled olive oil, dairy products, meat, and vegetables were from their own resource or from local small farmers… The food consumed is produced and prepared locally, and most is eaten fresh." [890] When it came to purchased "shelf items," 99% of participants said they never consumed bottled olive oil, 85% never consumed packaged cheese, 74% never consumed cakes, 75% never consumed sausages, 89% never consumed frozen meat, 95% never consumed frozen vegetables, and 99% never consumed precooked packed food.[891]

I contacted Sergio Pagliarini, MD, lead author of the Salandra study, and I contacted Antonietta Moramarco, MD, both of whom were most gracious and helpful to me. Dr. Pagliarinit discussed (via email) the apparent AMD in Salandra based on various classification systems and the numbers those would produce, and in summary, he wrote to me, "…No matter how grouped together to categorize them into AMD subgroup definitions, [AMD prevalence] was considerably lower in Salandra." [892]

Antonietta Moramarco, MD, has been Professor of Ophthalmology at the University of Rome "Sapienza," Italy, since 1989. Dr. Moramarco was born and raised in Salandra, having moved from there when she was 13 years old. As such, she knows the people, their ways, and of course, this was a major reason she was second author on the study. She continues to travel to Salandra from Rome "every fortnight" to see patients. I asked her many questions, via email, regarding the ways and diets of the people there and she very kindly answered them all, in English – good thing, since I only speak and write one language. Let me summarize her answers.

Dr. Moramarco relayed that the people there do not buy bottled olive oil, but rather, they make their own. **I asked her, "Do the people there, to your knowledge, ever consume vegetable oils (such as soybean oil, corn oil, cottonseed oil, canola oil, sunflower oil, safflower oil, or peanut oil), all of which would have to be purchased from grocery stores?" She answered, "No, never."** [893]

She relayed that they raise their own animals and butcher according to need, consuming beef, pork, sheep, chicken, etc. The beef are raised on grass, their eggs are from locally raised chickens and at the time they ate eggs regularly. I asked, "Is sugar added to any food in any significant amounts?" to which she replied, "Everyday into the coffee, with milk, and if they make cakes." She conveyed that they make their own bread daily and make their own pasta weekly, with flour from a local "industrial floor," which is almost certainly whole-meal flour, rather than refined white flour.

I asked Dr. Moramarco if macular degeneration is still rare there in 2015 and she answered, "Yes." I asked "Is obesity rare in Salandra?" Her answer: "Really rare." I asked, "Is the obesity rate less than in metropolitan areas, like Rome?" Her answer: "Yes, much less." I asked, "Do the people use butter in their cooking, liberally?" to which she replied, "Not much." And finally, I asked, "Pork lard?" to which she answered, "Yes."

I think the conclusion here is obvious – almost none of the people of Salandra were consuming processed foods that would contain added sugars, PUFA vegetable oils, and trans fats. They were consuming much of their fat from animal fats, in the form of meats, eggs, some butter, and pork lard. Sugar was used minimally, primarily in coffee or cakes. This all sounds to me much like the diet of our 19th century ancestors, does it not? Naturally, the prevalence of AMD was very, very low in Salandra. If we might ask why is there any AMD at all, well I am sure that some people are getting a bit more processed foods, but they're obviously approximately one or two percent of the Salandra population, because any way you slice it, about 98% of the people of Salandra were protected from AMD – and this stood in stark contrast to most of the developed world.

THE PACIFIC ISLAND NATIONS: FIJI, SOLOMON ISLANDS, SAMOA, AND KIRIBATI – WHERE AMD IS EXTREMELY RARE!

In my search for the truth and anything that would support (or refute) my hypothesis, I tried to follow in the footsteps of the great Weston A. Price – and seek out populations that had little or no AMD – in order to find out what it was about their diets that could explain their protection from AMD. "Standards of excellence" is what Dr. Price called it. Of course, Price had no internet, no computer, and for most areas, no phones. It took him ten years to accomplish his worldwide studies and to this day, I still don't know how he accomplished all of that in ten years. Most all of my research is now done from the comfort of my home, and with the power of a computer, internet, and the world wide web, I have access to university libraries in every corner of the globe.

And in my search, I've contacted numerous ophthalmologists, researchers, and various support personnel to assist me. One of the people I contacted was Professor Jill Keeffe, PhD, former director of the Centre for Eye Research Australia (CERA), who had retired from her position with CERA in 2013 after 25 years at the helm. When I asked her (via email) if she was aware of any research or anecdotal evidence regarding AMD prevalence in the South Pacific islands, her first response told me I might be on to something big. **"There is very little AMD in the South Pacific Islands," Professor Keeffe wrote," – diabetes is a major problem with a number of island countries in the top 10 prevalence in the world."** She continued, "The best people to help are 2 ophthalmologists from Fiji who have a very good knowledge of eye care in the Pacific Island countries – as I said no specific data but a guestimate. They would probably be the best to make an estimate [of AMD prevalence]. They are Dr Biu Sikivou and Dr Ana Cama." [894] (It is customary not to place a period after "Dr" in the Pacific Islands)

As you will see, this contact turned out to be one of the most important pieces of the AMD puzzle of all. As Professor Keeffe said, there are no formal studies of AMD prevalence in the Pacific Island nations. **But the anecdotal evidence from these ophthalmologists, who all collectively concur, is staggering. AMD in the Pacific Island nations is rare – exceedingly rare.**

FIJI

The beautiful island nation of Fiji has a population of 881,065 as of 2013. There are four ophthalmologists who provide the great bulk of the eye care there.

I reached out to ophthalmologists Dr Sikivou and Dr Cama via email and Dr Cama replied first. Dr Cama is the Prevention of Blindness Coordinator, Pacific Sub Regional Secretariat, International Agency for the Prevention of Blindness Western Pacific (IAPB), and recent president of the Pacific Eye Care Society (PacEYES). She actively practiced in Fiji between 1999 and 2011. She wrote, "I would say that during the years of my clinical work, AMD was rare in Central Fiji." She continued, "I do recall seeing some dry AMD cases – not many. This was in the eye clinic at CWM/PEI Eye Centre in Suva [capital of Fiji]." [895] Dr Cama, an extremely gracious woman, helped me to contact all of the remaining ophthalmologists in the Pacific Islands.

Dr Biu Sikivou replied next. Dr Sikivou is the long-time Director of the Pacific Eye Institute (PEI) and lead ophthalmologist at the Fred Hollows Foundation diabetes eye clinic in Suva, Fiji. In her response to my queries, she wrote, "I recall in the early days, we hardly saw case, the few cases seen were mainly IndoFijians [from India]. In the central division, we have seen about 15 – 20 [total through the years], including some indigenous Fijians." [896]

Dr Tarai Rakabu-Hicks is the Chief Medical Officer, Department of Ophthalmology, Lautoka Hospital, Western Division of Fiji. She wrote to me, "I have been practicing Ophthalmology now for 9 years, mind you most of it was in training. However, I have noticed that AMD is indeed not something we see every day here. I have come across a few, all of them of Indian descent." She relates that the native Fijians either don't need or don't present as much for eyecare, as she also wrote, "...of the few native Fijians that have come, I have not seen AMD. Just this morning, I conducted Diabetic Retinopathy Clinic, I saw 30 patients, only 1 was native Fijian, all the other were Indians. Only one had AMD, Indian lady aged 79. This is generally what

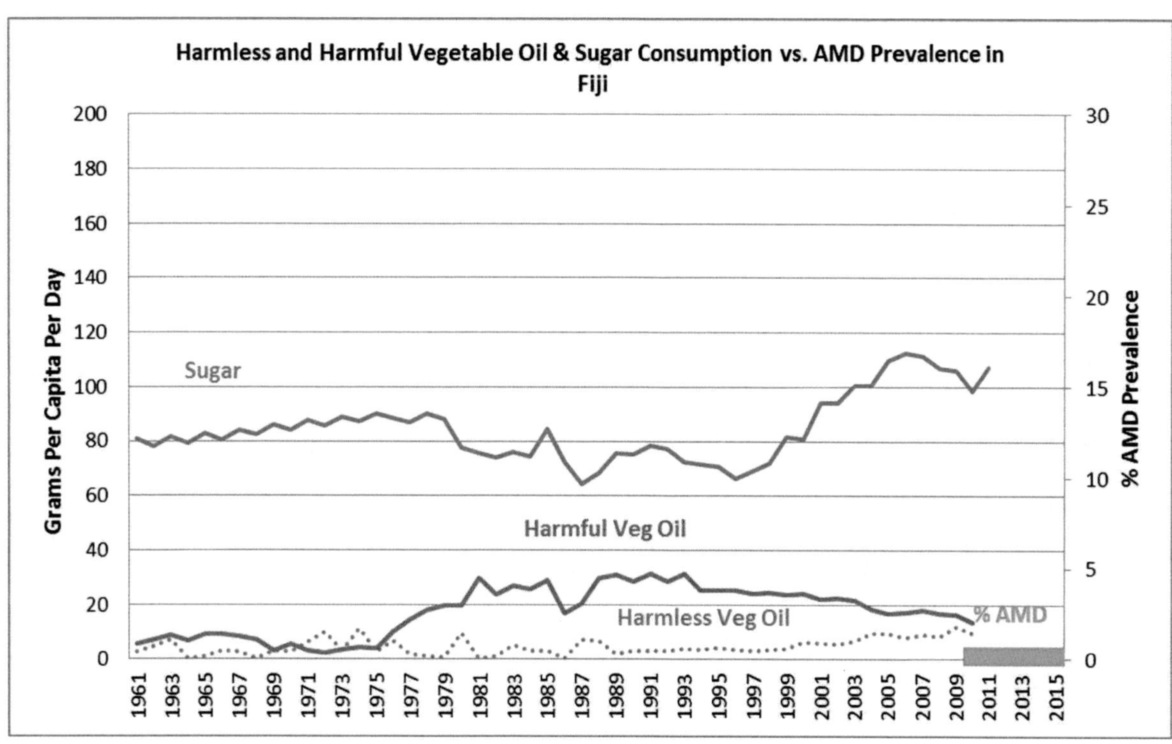

the numbers look like every week. Sometimes I don't even see any [AMD patients] at all."[897]

I asked Dr Rakabu-Hicks via email, very specifically, "Would you estimate the prevalence of AMD in Fijians, who are 60 years old or more, to be less than 1 in 200? Less than 1 in 500?" She wrote back to me, "I would say less than 1 in 500."[898]

Dr Vara Naviri practices at the HOD Ophthalmology Department, Labasa Hospital, in Labasa, Fiji, which is located in Northeastern Fiji. Labasa is a city with a population of 27,949 at the most recent census, in 2007, with a much larger drawing population. I asked Dr Naviri, "Could you estimate the percentage of Fijians in your patient population that have AMD? For people 60 years of age and older, would you estimate it is less than 1 in 100? Less than one in 200? One in 500?" Her answer: **"AMD is very rare here. I would say less than 1 in 500."** Her chart reviews confirmed the same.

One in 500 would be a prevalence of 0.2%. Compare that to the approximate 8.8% (1973-'75) or 20.9% (1988-90) found in the U.S.A. **The prevalence rate of AMD is 44 to 104 times greater in the U.S.A. than it is in Fiji.**

As you can see, all four ophthalmologists in Fiji agree that AMD is exceedingly rare there, with two of the four asserting that less than 1 in 500 people over the age of 60 is affected.

The graph and statistics above for Fiji were perhaps the most troubling initially, in terms of the hypothesis that AMD is a condition that follows processed food consumption. As we can see, sugar consumption is moderate, as is harmful vegetable oil consumption, while AMD prevalence sits at a staggeringly low 0.2%, approximately.

However, I believe this is explained by the fact that Fiji has nearly as many tourists to the nation each year as they have indigenous inhabitants. Tourism Fiji, precisely tracks tourist data, and they report 692,630 tourists in 2014.[899] The indigenous population of Fiji is only 903,000. Tourists by number and nation were as follows: Australia, 349,217; New Zealand, 123,968; Continental Europe, 30,585; USA, 61,924, China, 28,333; and South Korea, 5,676.[900] Each of these nations and regions, except China, normally consumes large amounts of sugar and vegetable oils. It is my assertion that, the tourism industry likely meets this typical consumption by serving foods higher in sugar and vegetable oils, while the natives generally continue to consume more traditional diets, at least in recent years without significant vegetable oils.

SOLOMON ISLANDS

The Solomon Islands are located about 1350 miles Northwest of Fiji, about midway between Fiji and Papua New Guinea. Dr. Claude Posala, MBBS, DO, MMED is the Head of the Ophthalmology Department, National Referral Hospital, Solomon Islands, and he represented their ophthalmology services. He wrote to me as follows: "AMD from anecdotal evidence is presumed rare [in the Solomon Islands]. For a population of 680,000 people, we get to see 20 cases each year that we presume clinically as AMD. We have been seeing this annual average for the past ten years... The 3 local ophthalmologists (including myself) working for the whole of Solomon Islands are all general ophthalmologists, hence, the AMD diagnoses made may have included other diagnoses with similar clinical findings to AMD. I have been practicing for 10 years in the eye department. One of our senior local colleagues has

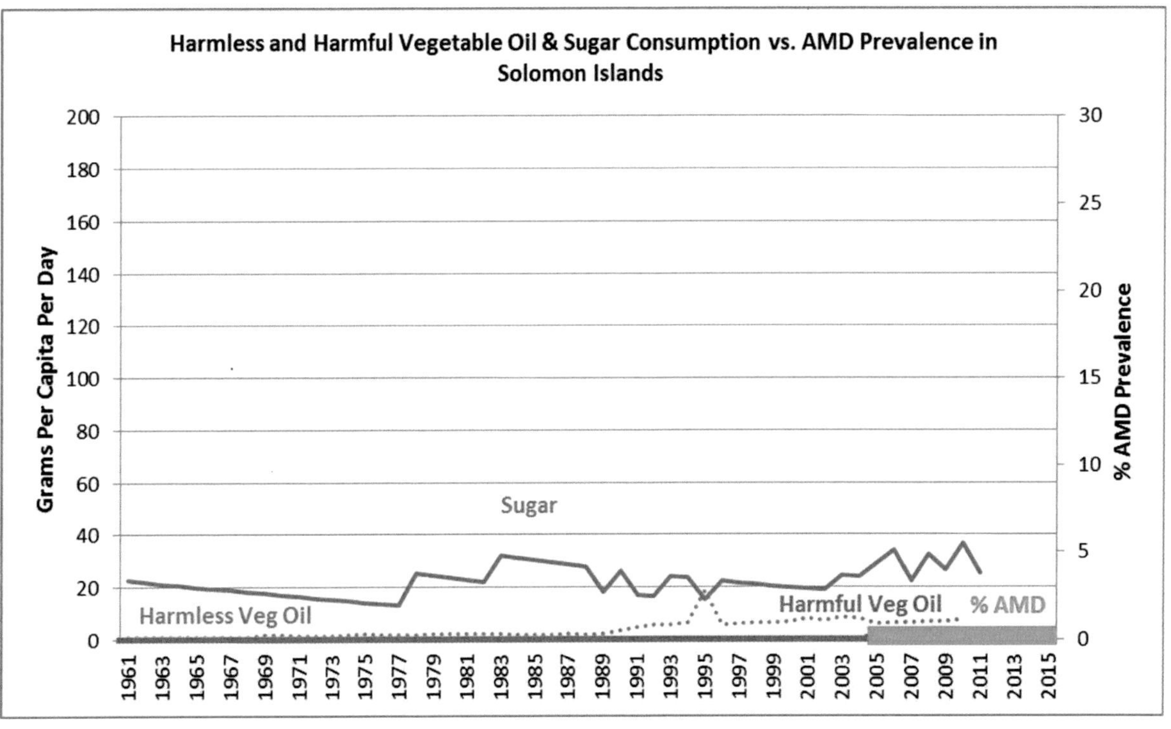

worked as an ophthalmologist for more than 20 years in Solomon Islands, and he shares the same situation which I have shared with you. The summary answer I have provided is a collective view from all of us." [901] Their collective chart analysis confirmed the same.

Twenty cases per year, for three ophthalmologists, providing for a population of 680,000, by American standards, is mind-boggling. That's about one AMD patient every two months for each doctor. In the U.S., there is about one ophthalmologist for every 20,000 people, and each one of us typically provides care for hundreds or even thousands of AMD patients each year.

In the Solomon Islands, we see that sugar consumption is extremely low and harmful vegetable oil consumption was zero grams per day from 1961 to 2001, while never greater than 1.73 grams per day since then. Compare this to the U.S. where harmful vegetable oil consumption has reached an average of nearly 80 grams per day recently and where AMD is 44 to 104 times more common.

SAMOA

Dr. Lucilla Ah Ching, MBBS, is the representative ophthalmologist for Samoa, which is a population of 190,372, as of 2013, located in the South Pacific about 700 miles Northeast of Fiji. Following my queries, Dr. Ah Ching wrote to me, "It is rare to see AMD in our clinic. There was an audit performed in 2007 which indicates 6.3% of low vision and 5.3% of blindness seen in the clinic was due to retina/AMD." [902] She references the appropriate study for her statistics and that study's data confirms her numbers.[903]

Before we had our own data and analysis of vegetable oil and sugar consumption data, I came across a study entitled "Long-Term Trends in Food Availability, Food Prices, and Obesity in Samoa,"[904] by Andrew Seiden and colleagues. As I began to read this study, I thought the results might be running counter to my hypothesis that vegetable oils, more specifically the PUFA vegetable oils, are a major contributor to AMD. In Seiden's study, the authors wrote, "Caloric availability of vegetable oil increased by 66% between 1961 and 2007, from 128 kcal per capita per day in 1961 to 214 kcal per capita per day in 2007," which is still roughly half the consumption of Americans. However, the authors then assert that, "The FAO data for Samoa do not currently distinguish between different types of vegetable oils, but a small study in Samoa in 2010 documented palm oil produced in Indonesia as being the most commonly available type of vegetable oil, both in supermarkets and small family-owned stores (McGarvey, unpublished data)." Palm, palm kernel, and coconut oil are all low risk (harmless) oils when it comes to AMD and other disease, because they are saturated oils that come from fruit. Again, in general, it is the saturated fats that are *not* associated with risk.

In Samoa, as we see the sugar consumption is low to moderate, but the harmful vegetable oils are essentially zero and, as we've just reviewed, their only significant edible oil consumption is palm oil, which is a saturated fruit oil that is safe to consume.

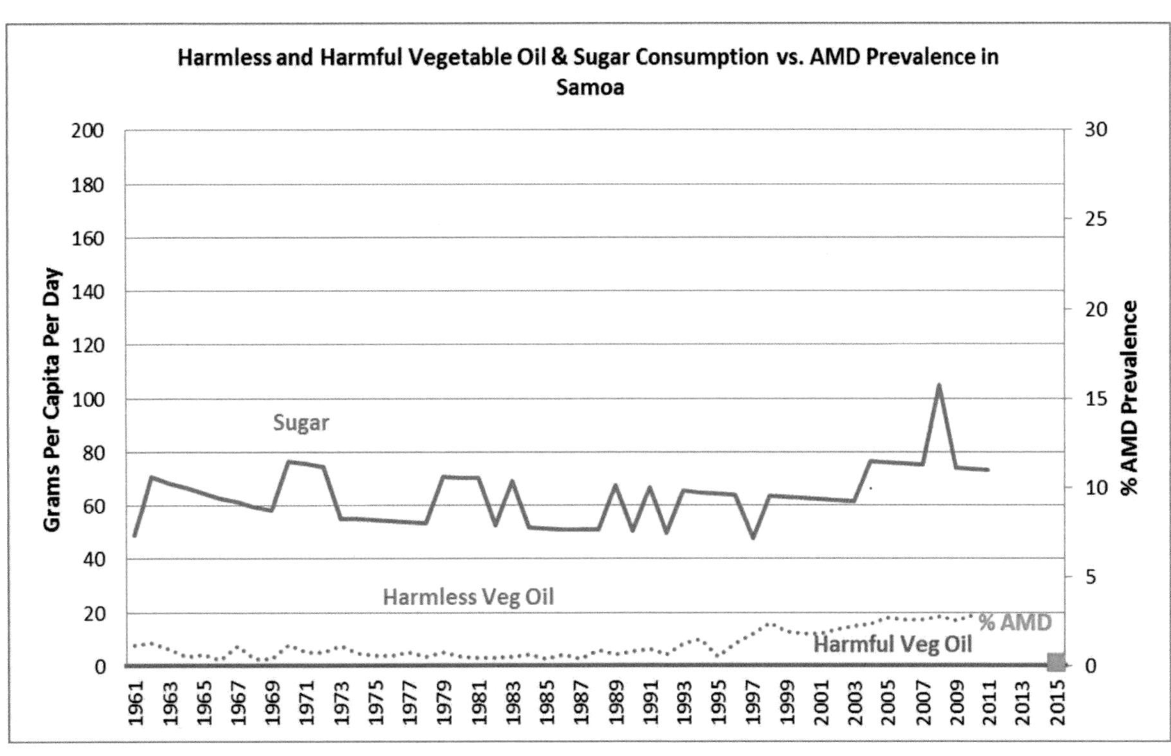

KIRIBATI

Kiribati is an island nation in Micronesia, the central Pacific, straddling the equator. It is about 1250 miles almost directly south of Hawaii and is about midway between Southern California and Sydney, Australia. According to WikiTravel, "South Tarawa [the capital of Kiribati] is one of the most densely populated, severely poverty-stricken places in the world." [905] The population of Kiribati is about 112,000, as of 2015. Though Kiribati gets few tourists, the ones that do visit typically travel to the island of Kirimati, also known as Christmas Island.

Dr. Rabebe Tekeraoi, Tangaru Central Hospital, in Tarawa, is the first and only full-time ophthalmologist for Kiribati. He completed his training in Fiji in 2014 at the Pacific Eye Institute, then returned to his home state of Kiribati to practice. Dr. Tekeraoi's native tongue is Kiribati, but he speaks and writes English as well. He wrote to me, "I am the only full-time ophthalmologist. Clinic days fluctutate from 4 patients to 30 patients. Last year, I rarely came across AMD. To what I remember I think I diagnosed 2 people with AMD." I asked Dr. Tekeraoi about his observations regarding food patterns consumption and fast food restaurants in Kiribati and he replied, "We do not have any of these fast food restaurants except a Chinese restaurant. Most people eat fresh or frozen fish most days with rice and less vegetables due to poor soil. We had few vegetables as well as root crops." **Finally, when I asked specifically what he believed was the prevalence of AMD in patients older than 60 years of age in Kiribati, he wrote, "I think it is less than one in five hundred."** [906] His chart review confirmed the same.

I find the situation in Kiribati to be more fascinating than virtually anywhere else. **The moderately high sugar consumption in Kiribati since 1961, yet the complete absence of harmful PUFA vegetable oils and nearly complete absence of AMD (0.2% of those over age 60) is perhaps the greatest evidence against the polyunsaturated vegetable oils and strong evidence of their distinct ability to cause AMD.** This, of course, is supported by similar evidence in Samoa and the Solomon Islands.

I asked my colleague friends, Bill Plauche, MD and Andrew Bossen, MD, both general ophthalmologists, who practice in Sherman, Texas, USA, at RGB Eye Associates, how many AMD patients they see on a daily, weekly, or monthly basis. They completed an analysis of their electronic medical record systems in order to provide a valid determination. Dr. Plauche provides care for an average of 15 AMD patients per day and Dr. Bossen an average of 20 AMD patients per day, practicing five days a week.[907] In terms of actual visits, that's about 3,525 patient visits per year for Dr. Plauche and 4,700 for Dr. Bossen, practicing 47 weeks of the year. They're practicing in a city with a population of 38,521, as of 2015, where two more full-time ophthalmologists practice within five miles.

My friend and collegue, Rajiv Anand, MD, vitreo-retinal specialist at Texas Retina Associates, in Dallas, Texas, has 16 partners with whom he practices in the Dallas region. When I asked what volume of patients that their practice treats that is AMD related, Dr. Anand wrote to me, "On an average day, 25 to 30% of our patients are ARMD [AMD]. Obviously, those docs that do only medical retina, see proportionately a lot more. So on an average day, 15-20

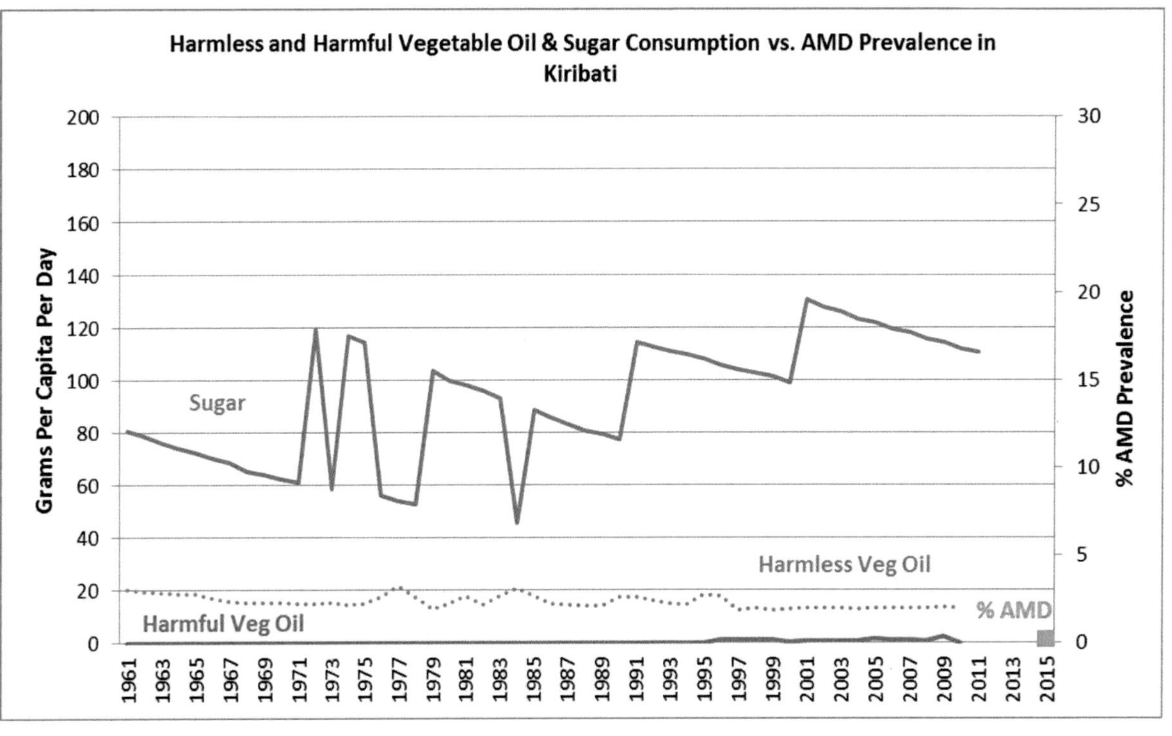

patients. With the burden of re-injecting these patients with wet ARMD, the volume exponentially increases since patients return every 6-8 weeks." [908]

Compare those numbers to Dr. Tekeraoi, who saw two AMD patients last year while providing care for the entire nation of Kiribati. The differences are staggering.

SEVERE VISION LOSS AND BLINDNESS IN THE PACIFIC ISLAND COUNTRIES

Professor Jill Keeffe, PhD, Director of CERA, was the lead author and director of a large study of blindness and vision loss in Southeast Asia and Oceania, between 1990 and 2010. In this study, published in 2014, all of the Pacific Island countries reviewed above, i.e., Fiji, Solomon Islands, Samoa, and Kiribati, are situated in Oceania and were included in the study. In 1990, macular degeneration only accounted for 3.3% of blindness in Oceania, though that number elevated to 4.6% by 2010.[909] Compare that, however, to the fact that 56% of blindness in the U.K. is caused by AMD. Also, in Oceania, macular degeneration accounted for 1.4% of Moderately Severe Visual Impairment (MSVI) in 1990, with that number nearly doubling to 2.7%, by 2010.[910] In other words, even though AMD is very rare in these countries, the number of people that are losing vision and going blind secondary to AMD is rising significantly.

CHAPTER SUMMARY

For nations significantly affected by AMD, in virtually every case what we see is that PUFA vegetable oil and sugar consumption conspicuously elevate – which is then predictably followed by the development of and/or a dramatic rise in the prevalence of macular degeneration. Now, I would be the first to tell you that correlation does not equal causation. From all of the scientific studies reviewed, as well as our data in 25 nations, this comes as close as we can get – in the field of medicine – to scientific proof that AMD is caused by the consumption of the 'displacing foods,' consisting of sugar, certain edible vegetable oils, white flour, and trans fats, primarily.

As you've also witnessed, all of the Pacific Island nations' ophthalmologists assert that AMD is exceedingly rare there, on the order of less than 1 in 500 people over the age of 60. At least in the island nations of Samoa, the Solomon Islands, and Kiribati, there are virtually no polyunsaturated vegetable oils consumed there. In the U.S. and many other developed nations, which are consuming much larger amounts of processed foods containing white flour, sugar, PUFA vegetable oils, and trans fats, the prevalence of AMD is about 74 times greater than in all of the Pacific Island nations reviewed and presented here.

Interestingly, the Pacific Island nations rank among the top 10 in the world in the prevalence of diabetes.[911] [912] This is a recent development and, as we've seen, when sugar consumption is very high, as it is in much of the Pacific Islands, diabetes develops within years. Only time will tell if this will also lead to AMD, but my educated guess is that it very well might in exceedingly small numbers – it will just take a longer exposure time to produce those results.

As reviewed in detail in previous chapters, we have biologically plausible mechanisms whereby these displacing foods, through both direct and indirect mechanisms, appear to be entirely responsible for the development of AMD.

Furthermore, what we now see is that, in the history of each country examined, what we find is that increasing vegetable oil and sugar consumption precedes the development of AMD. It is never the other way around. This meets the definition of *proximate cause.*

This is as close as we can possibly come to mathematical certainty that the 'displacing foods of modern commerce' are the primary and proximate cause of AMD. From all of the history presented, the data of 25 nations, the ten previously reviewed scientific studies correlating vegetable oils and trans fats to AMD, the constantly recurrent theme that AMD only develops when processed foods become significant, along with the biological plausibility, I believe that, without the slightest reservation at all, we can conclude that the 'displacing foods' are the causative factor for AMD. Secondarily, I believe that there is no other conclusion to derive, except that the "harmful vegetable oils," which are those containing significant polyunsaturates, are the leading cause of AMD. I believe these vegetable oils are biological toxins – in a word – poisons. Without them, AMD is extraordinarily rare. With any significant amounts, AMD drastically elevates. People are developing AMD by the tens of millions and even going blind, and the PUFA vegetable oils are the major contributor.

Part IV

Foods that Must be Exonerated

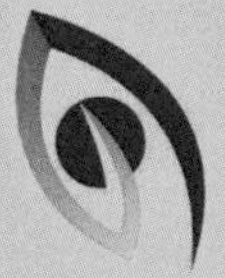

14 SATURATED FATS – COULD THEY SAVE YOUR LIFE & HELP PREVENT AMD?

For me, my eye-opener on the subject of saturated fats and heart disease came in 2007. Until then, I knew just enough about nutrition to be dangerous. But an article in Men's Health, written by Nina Teicholz, changed me forever. Her article was entitled, "What if Bad Fat is Actually Good for You?" with the sub-title, "For decades, Americans have been told that saturated fat clogs arteries and causes heart disease. But there's just one problem: No one's ever proved it." [913] Teicholz opening paragraphs were as follows:

> Suppose you were forced to live on a diet of red meat and whole milk. A diet that, all told, was at least 60 percent fat – about half of it saturated. If your first thoughts are of statins and stents, you may want to consider the curious case of the Masai, a nomadic tribe in Kenya and Tanzania.
>
> In the 1960s, a Vanderbilt University scientist named George Mann, M.D., found that Masai men consumed this very diet (supplemented with blood from the cattle they herded). Yet these nomads, who were also very lean, had some of the lowest levels of cholesterol ever measured and were virtually free of heart disease.
>
> Scientists, confused by the finding, argued that the tribe must have certain genetic protections against developing high cholesterol. But when British researchers monitored a group of Masai men who moved to Nairobi and began consuming a more modern diet, they discovered that the men's cholesterol subsequently skyrocketed.[914]

It turns out that the Masai are not the only tribe whose dietary habits and health would shock orthodox medicine's long-held belief systems regarding saturated fats. The Samburu and the Rendille, both of Kenya, the Fulani of Nigeria and Western and Northern Africa, the Inuit of Northern Canada, Alaska, and Greenland, the Eskimos of Alaska and Greenland, and the inhabitants of the island of Tokelau in the South Pacific are all just a few additional examples of cultures that, when following their traditional diets, consume enormous amounts of saturated fats. Yet, they all remain in brilliant health – and, of course, without heart disease.

THE MASAI, RENDILLE, SAMBURU, FULANI, AND OTHER TRIBES – ALL PARADOXES?

For anyone who had ever read Weston A. Price's work, none of this would even come as a surprise. In fact, Price studied the Masai as well as many other tribes in Africa, the Inuit, the Eskimos, and many South Pacific islanders, all of whom consumed tremendous amounts of saturated fats, while remaining in essentially perfect health. Price wrote extensively about these people in his two books. In fact, the people of all of these cultures remained in exuberant health as long as they continued to consume their traditional diets. And as you now know from the previous review of Dr. Price's discoveries, any of these people from cultures that began to consume the 'displacing foods of modern commerce' also began to develop degenerative diseases.[915]

We've previously reviewed the Masai, whose diet consists primarily of milk, blood, and meat, with very small amounts of vegetables. The Samburu and the Rendille tribes are very similar, while the Fulani, also pastoralists, consume significant grains in the form of millet, sorghum or corn, along with soups or stews that might contain tomatoes, peppers, bone, meat, onion, and other vegetables. All of these tribes are pastoralists – and their food comes almost exclusively from the cattle that they raise, which includes camels, goats, and cows. The fats in the diets of the Masai and the Samburu comes almost exclusively from animal fat – and animal fat accounts for 66% of their total calories, yet they do not suffer from heart disease.[916] [917] A typical Masai member will consume about 3,000 calories per day and generally between one to one-and-a-half gallons of raw milk per day. The animal fat in that quantity of whole raw milk is about two-and-a-half sticks worth of butter per day! The adult Masai warriors would consume even more – up to the equivalent of three sticks worth of butter per day. Yet, despite this extraordinarily high consumption of animal fat, the research concludes, "The aortas and coronary arteries of the Masai show little atherosclerosis." [918] Are all of these tribes just "paradoxes" to the saturated-fat-causes-heart-disease hypothesis?

THE "FRENCH PARADOX"

Physicians, scientists, and authors – for decades – have discussed the "French paradox," referring to the fact that the French consume large amounts of saturated fats and yet have a very low prevalence of heart disease. Of course, if an additional review of both the anthropologic and epidemiologic evidence is completed, one rapidly begins to notice that there isn't just a French paradox, there would also be a "Masai paradox," a "Rendille paradox," a "Samburu paradox," an "Inuit paradox," and a "Tokelau paradox," just to name a few. If the data doesn't fit their hypothesis, many authorities refer to this as a "paradox," but of course, if the data is deemed to be accurate, then any paradox should make one question their hypothesis.

The French consume saturated fats in the form of butter and cream, but also from eggs, meats, cheese, and of course, they're the people that made *pâté* famous. *Pâté* is a mixture of ground meat and fat minced into a paste that can be spread. In France, the most common *pâté* is *pâté de foie gras*, which is made from the livers of fattened geese. The French have a relatively low rate of heart disease. According to the research of Sally Fallon, "In the United States, 315 of every 100,000 middle-aged men die of heart attacks each year; in France the rate is 145 per 100,000. In the Gascony region, where goose and duck liver form a staple of the diet, this rate is a remarkably low 80 per 100,000." [919]

Researchers in recent years have attempted to attribute this "French paradox" to their consumption of wine,[920] resveratrol (a polyphenol present in red wine),[921] folate in fruits and vegetables,[922] cheese,[923] smaller portion sizes,[924] and even the French people's "attitudes to food and the role of food in life." [925] Had any of these researchers known of the research of Weston A. Price, they would have quickly realized that the reason for the "French paradox" is simple: They were one of the last industrialized nations to succumb to the temptation to supplant their traditional foods with significant Westernizing foods – white flour, sugar, and vegetable oils. Indeed, even the French have begun to do this to a much greater degree in recent decades, which is gradually whittling away at their resistance to Western diseases.

THE INUIT AND ESKIMOS – ALSO PARADOXICAL?

The Inuit and the Eskimos, on their traditional diets, consumed large amounts of animal fats too. In the previously referenced Discover magazine article, "The Inuit Paradox," by Gatsby and Steele, the authors interviewed Patricia Cochran, an Inupiat (Eskimo) of Northwestern Alaska. In discussing the cuisine of her childhood, Cochran stated,

> Our meat was seal and walrus, marine mammals that live in cold water and have lots of fat. We used seal oil for our cooking and as a dipping sauce for food. We had moose, caribou, and reindeer. We hunted ducks, geese, and little land birds like quail, called ptarmigan. We caught crab and lots of fish—salmon, whitefish, tomcod, pike, and char. Our fish were cooked, dried, smoked, or frozen. We ate frozen raw whitefish, sliced thin. The elders liked stinkfish, fish buried in seal bags or cans in the tundra and left to ferment. And fermented seal flipper, they liked that too.[926]

For traditional Inuit and Eskimos, surviving in Arctic and sub-Arctic zones, fruits and vegetables were a rarity. For the enormous majority of the year, no edible plant life was available. They consumed a very large portion of their diet as fat, particularly from seal oil but also from moose and caribou. The fat of the animals was always saved and eaten. Yet, as Weston A. Price found, these people also were brilliantly healthy and without chronic disease, including heart disease.

THE INHABITANTS OF TOKELAU – THE GREATEST PARADOX OF ALL?

According to obesity researcher, Stephan Guyenet, PhD, at the University of Washington, the population of the three South Pacific atolls, collectively known as Tokelau, has traditionally dined on seafood, wild fowl, coconut, fruit, and after about 1863, breadfruit (much like plantains), pulaka (a starchy tuber), and pigs and chickens. **The unique dietary situation with the people of Tokelau is that they consume an extraordinary 54 to 62 percent of their calories from coconut, the fat of which is 87% saturated. According to Dr. Guyenet, "This gives them perhaps the highest documented saturated fat intake in the world."** [927] **This indicates that the Tokelauans consume 40 to 50% of their calories as saturated fat.** Obviously, this would be a great population to further test the hypothesis that those much-maligned saturated fats cause heart disease, right?

With regard to their pre-Westernization of their diet, the Oxford Science text, *Migration and Health in a Small Society – The Case of Tokelau,* written by Albert F. Wessen states,

> Their populations [of Tokelau] are notable for their low levels of blood pressure, high rates of infectious disease {mostly, parasitic}, and low rates of coronary heart disease, obesity, and diabetes. At the other end of the spectrum are those Polynesian societies, such as the Hawaiians and the Maori of New Zealand, who were submerged by 'Western' settlers and the dominating cultures they brought with them. These populations have inevitably acquired the diseases of the 'West', sometimes to an exaggerated degree.[928]

Again, according to Dr. Guyenet, beginning in the 1960s Tokelau began to be visited by cargo ships that brought sugar, white flour, and other imported sweetened foods. In 1968, only 2% of their calories came from sugar, but by 1978, that number had risen to 14%. In 1961, the ships delivered 12 pounds of flour per person per year to Tokelau, which increased to 60 pounds per year by 1980. Dr. Guyenet stated that this "correlated with an increase in several non-communicable disorders, including overweight, diabetes and severe tooth decay. Further modernization as Tokelauans migrated to New Zealand corresponded with an increase in nearly every disorder measured, including heart disease, weight gain, diabetes, asthma and gout. These are all 'diseases of civilization', which are not observed in hunter – gatherers and certain non-industrial populations throughout the world." [929]

THE U.K. AND THE U.S.A. CONSUMPTION OF SATURATED FAT & HEART DISEASE – PARADOXES FROM THE PAST

As noted by data from prior to 1966, in southeastern England, substantially more butter, milk, meat, and total fats were consumed per person than in Scotland,[930] but the Scots had a far higher death rate from coronary heart disease (CHD) than did the inhabitants of SouthEast England.[931] Similarly, going back to the 19th century, the Victorian middle and upper classes were prodigious consumers of animal fats, just like Americans of the same era, yet CHD among them was extremely rare.[932]

As shown by Stephan Guyenet, PhD, the consumption of polyunsaturated fats in the form of vegetable oils in the United States rose 300% between 1909 and 2009;[933] in the first 50 years of this period alone, we experienced a dramatic increase in the death rate from coronary heart disease.[934] In fact, between 1940 and 1954 alone, the age-adjusted death rate from coronary artery disease rose approximately 40 percent.[935] There's been no decrease in the prevalence or incidence of heart disease since then, by any measures.

HOW WAS SATURATED FAT EVER INDICTED AS THE CAUSE OF HEART DISEASE?

For those who are not "graph savvy," the above graph shows that heart disease deaths in the USA were a medical rarity in 1900, substantially climbing decade after decade until the 1970s, when bypass procedures, coronary stents, and coronary angioplasty began saving lives. As we see, the consumption of saturated fat was nearly a flat line during this period, at 50 grams per day in 1910 and about 55 grams in 1995. The difference is almost negligible. However, vegetable oil consumption was at about 2 grams per day in 1900, rising to 80 grams per day by 2010.

I know what you must be thinking. How in the world did we ever indict saturated fat as the cause of heart disease, especially in light of all of the above evidence, which is obviously diametrically opposed to any such indictment? This boggles my mind as well. Did our government not once take a few weeks or months to develop such a correlation as the above graph? Wouldn't this eliminate saturated fat as a cause – or *the cause* – of heart disease, in fifteen seconds of examination?

In fact, the single body of research from the Masai tribe – the data that concluded that the Masai likely consumed more saturated fat than any other known culture, and yet were completely free of heart disease – from way back in 1971 – should have been enough to summarily dismiss the diet-heart hypothesis, right? If you're not familiar, the "diet-heart hypothesis" is the hypothesis that cholesterol causes heart disease (the "lipid hypothesis"), saturated fat raises cholesterol, and therefore, saturated fat causes heart disease. The whole hypothesis was founded on one premise: a correlation was drawn between higher cholesterol and heart disease, and research showed that saturated fat could raise cholesterol, and voila – suddenly, saturated fat was the culprit in heart disease.

Indeed, there was a *slight correlation* between higher cholesterol and greater heart disease. But the most important thing in science is this: *Correlation does not equal causation.*

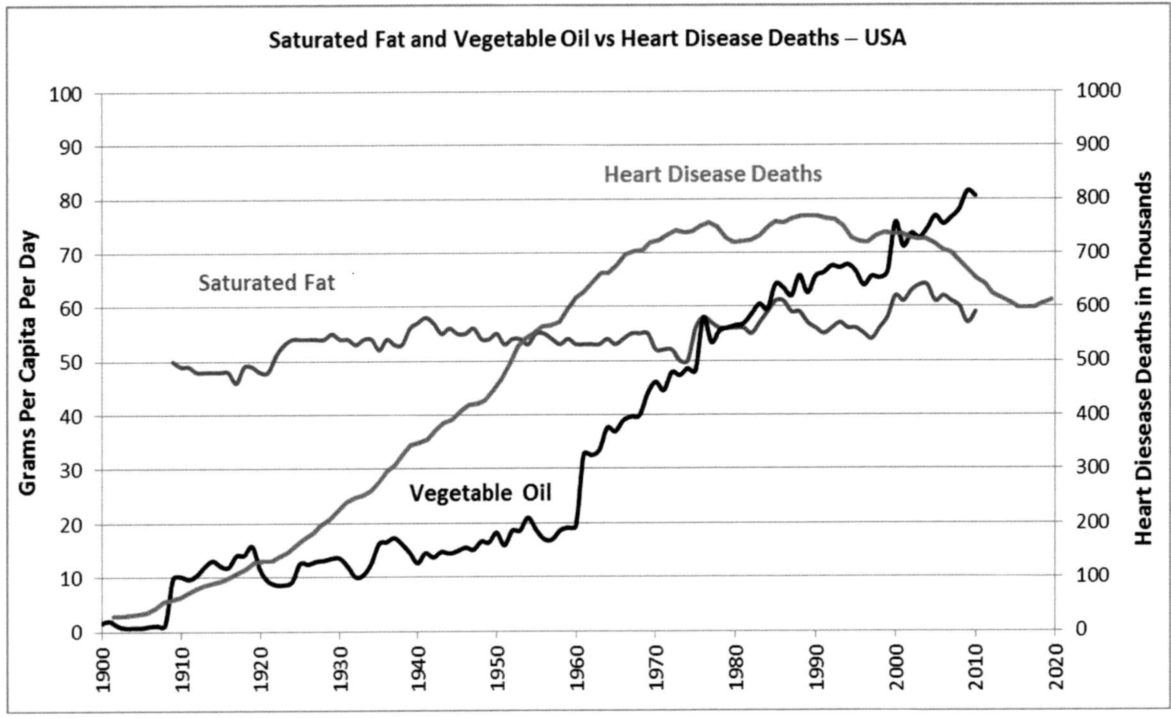

Saturated Fat & Vegetable Oil Consumption vs. Heart Disease Deaths – USA.

If we complete a study that finds that 16 to 17 year old boys who drive red cars are more likely to crash than those driving white cars, should we conclude that red cars are more likely to cause accidents? Instead, we might consider the hypothesis that boys driving red cars are more likely to be driving sports cars at high speeds, correct? The point is, correlations can only suggest hypotheses, which can be further tested.

In tribe after tribe, population after population, what we witness is that for those people who replace saturated fats from animals with vegetable oils that contain high percentages of polyunsaturated fatty acids (PUFAs), plus sugar and possibly white flour, the results are predictably the same – heart disease, cancer, and other degenerative diseases.

But again, how was the diet-heart hypothesis, ever considered plausible? The answer? One man. And his name was Ancel Keys.

ANCEL KEYS AND HIS "DIET-HEART HYPOTHESIS"

My all-time favorite author, the brilliant Denise Minger, in her book, *Death by Food Pyramid,* begins this story as follows: "ONCE IN A GREAT WHILE a figure emerges boldly from the abyss and spends eternity saddled with equal parts love and hate, prestige and controversy, reverence and angst. AT&T commercials had their Carrot Top. Seinfeld had its Newman. And the world of nutrition had a man named Ancel Keys." [936]

In 1951, Ancel Keys, a physiologist from the University of Minnesota, had begun to develop a hypothesis that was born partly out of a trip he and his wife had made to Naples, Italy. This was post WWII and Italy was not only recovering but remained in the depths of a war-torn Europe. Food was scarce. The Neapolitans were living in a severely depressed economic climate. They had little meat, eggs, butter, or milk, not by their choosing, but because those foods were luxuries they couldn't afford. A survey taken in 1951 ranked Italy and Greece as having less food available per capita than any other countries in Europe: a mere 2400 calories per person, as compared to some 3800 calories per person available in the U.S. at that time (available food is not equivalent to consumed food).[937]

Indeed there was little heart disease in Italy at the time but, of course, there was also little food. Nonetheless, Keys hypothesized that the lack of dietary fat was the link. In 1953, Keys published a highly influential paper under the title "Atherosclerosis, a Problem in Newer Public Health." His assertion? The death rate in the U.S. was climbing – and heart disease was the cause. In what has colloquially been known as his "Six Countries Study," Keys presented a graph of heart disease plotted against dietary fat consumption for the United States, Canada, Australia, England, Italy, and Japan. Americans consumed the most fat and had the most heart disease. The Japanese consumed the least fat and had the least heart disease. The other four countries fell neatly between the two. Keys called the correlation a "remarkable relationship." [938]

The curious thing was that Keys didn't have data for just six countries –he had data for 22. In 1957, some four years later, two researchers by the names of Yerushalmy and Hilleboe, took Keys' data, plotted a new graph with all 22 countries represented and, suddenly, Keys' dramatic correlation rather began to fall apart at the seams. Sure, there was a relationship, but not nearly so dramatic and with glaring inconsistencies. Yerushalmy and Hilleboe summed up their analysis in one sentence: "The suggested association between national death rates from heart disease and percentage of fat in the diet available for consumption cannot at the present time be accepted as valid." Worse still for Keys' hypothesis, these researchers showed that there was data that would run contrary to the hypothesis. For example, in Finland the death rate from heart disease was 24 times as high as that in Mexico, but the two had nearly equivalent levels of fat consumption.[939]

But their analysis might have been several years too late. Keys had already made a dramatic impact upon a nation that was hungry for answers about heart disease – and now they had something they could point their fingers at. After all, people could just look at pork or beef fat and surmise that it might just very well end up clogging their arteries – a simplistic and inaccurate observation that, quite frankly, would be laughable to any vascular disease researcher since the 1920s.

> Cholesterol and other lipids don't deposit on the inside lumen of the artery wall, which is the pop- science version of vascular disease. When and if they deposit there, they do so beneath the endothelium, which is the inner lining of the vascular wall. The deposits end up in the intima layer of the vessel wall.

But Keys' assertions were accepted without scientific evidence by many, including some authorities, and he soon became a public figure. Next, he found his way onto a seat at the American Heart Association (AHA). Keys influence there was equally powerful. And despite the fact that the AHA had scorned the diet-heart hypothesis in 1957, four years later in 1961 with Keys on their board – and without a single study in support – they too followed the low fat mantra of Keys, recommending that Americans lower their consumption of fats in order to reduce their risk of heart disease.

In 1971, Keys published his "Seven Countries Study." [940] This one had conclusions that were remarkably similar to the "Six Countries Study," however, Keys recommended reduction of saturated fat, specifically. This time, Keys admitted to selecting countries on this study, but nevertheless, on deeper inspection, his conclusions didn't hold up even within countries. For example, the intake of saturated fat was about equal in the populations studied from Turku and North Karelia, in Finland. Yet, mortality from heart disease was three times higher in North Karelia than in Turku. Eastern Finland had five times as many heart-attack fatalities and twice the heart disease prevalence as western Finland, but the difference in animal fat consumption and cholesterol levels between the two regions were negligible. The saturated fat consumption was also equal on the Greek islands of Crete and Corfu, but mortality from heart disease was nearly 17 times higher on Corfu than on Crete.

In an ironic twist of fate, Keys' assertions resulted in even more consumers substituting margarine and Crisco, for butter and lard. As has been the case ever since the introduction of newfangled foods, each introduction came at the expense of our health.

One might think that most scientists were on board with this diet-heart hypothesis proferred by Keys, but nothing could be further from the truth. There were storms of protests all along the way. Didn't matter. The finale came when George McGovern's Senate Select Committee on Nutrition and Human Needs, along with a few of McGovern's staff members, that Keys dietary fat hypothesis would become dogma. In 1977, the "Dietary Goals for Americans," a government recommendation for diet, would be released nationwide. The goals, astonishingly, were written by none other than Nick Mottern, a labor lawyer who had no scientific background at all. The goals advised Americans to eat less fat, less cholesterol, less refined and processed sugars, more complex carbohydrates and fiber, and drink alcohol in moderation.[941]

Of course, there was no recommendation to avoid vegetable oils, trans fats, or white flour. And the emphasis was and always has been – on fat – particularly saturated animal fat. The irony here is that heart disease – the very disease that the dietary goals aimed to reduce – would be dramatically worse as a result. Obesity, metabolic syndrome, diabetes, heart disease, cancer, and Alzheimer's disease, just to name a few, all dramatically elevated as a result of these admonitions.

For those who want an in-depth review of this history, Gary Taubes brilliantly chronicles all the details in his book, *Good Calories, Bad Calories.* Just as historically and scientifically accurate, while equally entertaining, is Denise Minger's review in her book, *Death By Food Pyramid.*

META-ANALYSES – ONCE AGAIN PROVIDE THE FINAL WORD...

In 2010, researchers from both the Oakland Research Institute in Oakland, California and from the Harvard School of Public Health, completed a meta-analysis in which they reviewed twenty-one different studies to assess whether a reduction in saturated fat would improve cardiovascular health. Some 347,747 subjects were followed for anywhere between 5 and 23 years and 11,006 of them developed either coronary heart disease or stroke. Their conclusion? **"A meta-analysis of prospective epidemiologic studies showed that there is no significant evidence for concluding that dietary saturated fat is associated with an increased risk of coronary heart disease or cardiovascular disease."** [942]

Another major meta-analysis study (in case one wasn't enough) that bears review was that of Doctors Micha and Mozaffarian at the Harvard School of Public Health, in

Boston, published in 2010. This review evaluated the effect, among other things, of substituting carbs in the diet for saturated fat, which was our government's recommendation some 33 years earlier. After exhaustive review, the authors concluded with, "Replacing saturated fat with carbohydrate has no benefit" and further stating, "Evidence for the effects of SFA [saturated fatty acids] consumption on vascular function, insulin resistance, diabetes, and stroke is mixed, with many studies showing no clear effects." Next, one of the most profound statements ever made on this subject, after examining all of the available evidence: **"These meta-analyses suggest no overall effect of saturated fatty acid consumption on coronary heart disease events."** [943]

This Harvard School of Public Health Study, which examined the results of decades of studies on saturated fat consumption and its relationship to heart disease – and the conclusion is that there is none.

PROFESSOR CHRIS MASTERJOHN, PHD, BROOKLYN COLLEGE, WEIGHS IN ON PUFA'S AND THEIR RELATIONSHIP TO CORONARY HEART DISEASE

Chris Masterjohn, PhD, Assistant Professor of Health and Nutrition Sciences at Brooklyn College in New York, is lauded as one of the most knowledgeable and prolific authors on the subject of heart disease today. He has written numerous and brilliant articles for his own website, *Cholesterol-and-health.com*, as well as for the Weston A. Price Foundation at *WestonAPrice.org*, and authored or co-authored numerous scientific studies. From his article titled "Understanding the Essential Fatty Acids," which is posted at the Weston A. Price Foundation's website, in which Professor Masterjohn discusses the untoward effects of vegetable oils, he writes, "The obvious implication of these studies {vegetable oils and heart disease} is that the oxidative destruction of PUFAs in the LDL membrane, but not the concentration of cholesterol carried in the blood by these LDL particles, determines the development of atherosclerosis. It is no wonder, then, that trials attempting to prevent heart disease with diets rich in polyunsaturated vegetable oils failed so miserably." [944] And after reviewing the results of six studies evaluating the effects of substituting vegetable oils for animal fats on heart disease, he concludes, **"These six studies clearly show that vegetable oils are not capable of reducing total mortality and strongly suggest that they may raise the risk of heart disease and cancer."** [945]

SO WHAT ABOUT SATURATED FAT & AMD DEVELOPMENT?

Somewhere along the line, somebody is going to raise the issue that a study or two found an association between increased saturated fat consumption and AMD.[946 947] Indeed, they have. I believe we can invoke the healthy user bias here, as the second of these studies found an increased risk for AMD not only with saturated fats, but with polyunsaturated, monounsaturated, and transunsaturated fats. Well, that's all the fats. So should we just indict fat in general? This is a great example whereby we can be sure that they're not all the problem, but regression analyses cannot separate out these risks when most everyone is consuming either the problem food or some variety of the problem foods. It just doesn't work. Once again, this is exactly why the historical and anthropological studies are invaluable.

WHEN PUFA (VEGETABLE) OILS & SUGAR REPLACE SATURATED FAT – WE SEE MORE AMD, AND WOMEN ARE AT GREATER RISK. WHY?

We've previously reviewed in detail that greater consumption of vegetable oils, which invariably displace animal fats, is unequivocally associated with more AMD. In many studies, AMD has been found to be more prevalent in women – and without a satisfying explanation. In the words of the authors of the PAMDI study, which was an AMD prevalence study in Italy, "With the exception of ARM1 {the earliest possible definition of AMD}, any form of ARMD {age-related macular degeneration} is more prevalent in women than men, as reported in the Beaver Dam Eye Study, Blue Mountains Eye Study, and Rotterdam Study, despite none of the studies providing any convincing explanation." [948]

However, I believe the hypothesis in this book, once again, supports the definitive answer. The gender disparity issue on AMD takes us as far back as the 1950s, or at least back to 1977, when the U.S. promulgated its "Dietary Goals for the United States," because the boiled down take home message to most Americans seemed to be, "Eat less fat – especially saturated fat." A by-product of this dogma also seemed to be, "Eating fat makes you fat." This was a message that gradually found its way around most of the world.

Women particularly, to this day, seem to adhere to this unfounded and misdirected admonition. Adam Drewnowski, PhD, in an article published in *Nutrition Reviews*, put it this way: "The conventional dietary advice is to replace fats with low-calorie fruits, vegetables, and grains. However, a diet devoid of fats seldom tastes good and consumers have become adept at replacing one source of fat with another. For example, nutritional survey studies conducted by the United States Department of Agriculture (USDA) show that the consumption of meat by women dropped by 34% between 1977 and 1985. Similarly, the consumption of meat (mostly sandwiches and stews) decreased by 35% between 1977 and 1985, while the consumption of skim and low-fat milk increased by as much as 60%. The consumption of cheese and frozen desserts also increased substantially. It appears that consumers have learned to avoid overt sources of fat (meat, butter, and milk), replacing them with food products in which the presence of fat is either less obvious or more difficult to detect by sensory means." [949]

I witness this constantly. Women, more than men, seem to try to avoid the obvious sources of fat. A slab of butter, a marbled steak, whole fat yogurt, whole milk – all out. Yet, they often choose pastries, desserts, creamy pasta dishes, etc., instead, many of which are just loaded with those hidden destroyers of health – vegetable oils, sugars, and white flour. These, of course, not only displace the natural saturated fats that are sources of the extraordinarily important fat soluble vitamins, but the vegetable oils are a huge source of undesirable omega-6 fats and even trans fats, while sugar consumption leads us down the path of metabolic syndrome and all of its attendant risks, which include AMD. This, I believe, almost assuredly answers the question as to why women tend to be at greater risk for AMD. It all boils down to fear of fat – particularly animal fat – the same fat that once kept us so healthy.

CHAPTER SUMMARY

Personally, it took me two years to be able to look at the fat on my steak – or lard – and to finally realize that those are the heart-healthy fats. Fifty years of repetition, no matter how absurdly incorrect, isn't easy to undo. But, hopefully, you realize that the typical study in most developed nations lasts up to a few years, controls only a variable or two, and is completed using groups of people that are already all in the "experimental group" (they're all consuming versions of the Standard American Diet, for example). These studies are fraught with problems, uncertainties, and unreliable outcomes. Personally, I would rather trust in the "world's laboratory," where people have consumed similar diets for decades, or even for centuries, and whereby we can assess the outcomes based on the health of their people. Isn't this more logical, particularly for diseases that take decades to develop, like heart disease and macular degeneration?

So while scientists continue to argue over the cause of heart disease, obesity, diabetes, and metabolic syndrome, one thing is clear. These diseases either don't exist – or are extremely rare – in societies that don't consume the 'displacing foods.'

The reality is this: Saturated fat consumption is not associated with heart disease by all available studies and, of course, by all available historical evidence. However, polyunsaturated fat consumption is. This is absolutely critical to understand, because after all, if you don't accept the fact that animal fats are the health-promoting fats, you're destined to consume the only other fats that are available in any significant quantities in most countries (like the U.S.) – and that's the PUFA containing vegetable oils (nut oils aside). In some countries, saturated fats from palm, palm kernel, and coconut oils are much more prevalent and, of course, we see dramatically better health in those countries.

We've seen, repeatedly, in study after study, that PUFA vegetable oil consumption is associated with increasing risks of AMD. The history of food consumption from the U.S., the U.K., Japan, India, the South Pacific island countries, and essentially every country presented in Chapter 13 supports this conclusion as well. The development of AMD in the "world's natural laboratory" is incontrovertibly associated with vegetable oil consumption, and by all accounts, *appears to be protected against by saturated fat consumption* of the natural type, i.e. from animals and plants. Almost every piece of evidence that I can find is supportive of this conclusion and not one piece of solid evidence contradicts it.

CHOLESTEROL – IS MORE BETTER?

The fact that cholesterol, to this day, is blamed for causing heart disease – and vascular disease in general – is perhaps the single most absurd and erroneous concept that is currently held in medicine. This is barely a step up from blood-letting due to "bad humors," practiced as recently as the 19th century. Cholesterol, a molecule so vitally important to life, that it is a component of every single living cell, can be manufactured by every cell in our bodies, is the precursor to the steroid hormones, sex hormones, and vitamin D, and is a major component of bile acids so important to fat absorption in the gut. In fact, some 25% of our total cholesterol is found in our brains, which only account for 2% of our body weight, and yet, this normal cholesterol molecule is blamed for heart disease – simply because it is there physically and a slight association has been drawn for young men with higher levels?

Quite frankly, any component of cell membranes, or perhaps any number of molecules or even minerals, could have been blamed for heart disease using the logic that went into this theory. In fact, today we could be blaming anything that happens to be present in atherosclerotic plaques, such as phospholipids, triglycerides, various lipids, elastin, aspartic acid, threonine, serine, glutamic acid, lysine, histidine, arginine,[950] macrophages, lymphocytes, smooth muscle cells,[951] or even phosphorus or calcium – for heart disease.[952] The "calcium score," which is a measure of the coronary artery calcium present in a patient's coronary arteries, is a better predictor of coronary heart disease (CHD) events, such as heart attacks, abnormal heart rhythms, and congestive heart failure (CHF), than is the measurement of cholesterol.[953]

With that knowledge, maybe calcium should have been indicted for its role in heart disease? In fact, if Ancel Keys had indicted calcium as the culprit in heart disease instead of cholesterol, today, we might all be trying to figure out how to get our blood calcium levels down – and avoiding calcium like the plague! Instead of statin drugs to lower our cholesterol, we might have anti-calcium drugs – drugs that would bind calcium in our blood or in our bowel and escort them from our bodies. We probably would have been far better off with that blundering mistake instead. Over the past 25 years, I have witnessed well over a hundred patients injured, many apparently permanently, by the anti-cholesterol campaign and it's associated arsenal – known as the cholesterol-lowering drugs (typically, the statins). And none of them were ever helped.

THINK FOR YOURSELF...

When I was in my last year of college, we had a visiting professor come to lecture at Colorado State University, where I attended. Though I don't remember his name, he was a physicist, and physics happened to be my favorite subject. Toward the end of his lecture, he said this:

> "Did you ever notice which way the water circles as it's going down the toilet – or your bathroom sink? Did you ever think – that it might have something to do with which direction the earth is revolving? Now, do you suppose that it would make a difference depending on which hemisphere of the earth you're on?" He paused for several moments, then continued. "I'm just trying to get you to think."

That stuck in my head, forever. It's a mental exercise that's fun to do – and you can figure this out by watching the water circle down your toilet – and then, if you think carefully, you will be able to determine which way the earth is rotating, even if you don't already know. I'm not going to reveal the answer, as the professor did not. He left it to us to ponder. The point is this: This chapter, like so many, needs a book. But, I can only provide a brief overview and highlight a few facts. So, I am going to ask you to think for yourself.

The best way to analyze any situation is to ask questions – poignant questions. Ask yourself the questions that you should, for your own sake: For example, if we didn't have heart disease in the 19th century and prior, should we suddenly indict a molecule (cholesterol), common to every cell in our bodies, for its cause? Or saturated fat for that matter, of which we consumed just as much in the 19th century? Would it make any sense at all to indict the cholesterol molecule for heart disease, when it is so vitally important, that without it, we would die? Wouldn't it make more sense to examine the history of our diet, ascertain what has changed, and consider those elements as the possible villains, instead?

CHOLESTEROL FACTS AND STATS – TO MAKE US THINK

- More than 20 studies clearly show that elderly people with high cholesterol live longer than elderly people with low cholesterol.[954]
- In the Framingham Study, which is the longest running study of cholesterol and heart disease that exists, those who had high cholesterol and were older than 47 years of age lived just as long or longer than those with low cholesterol.[955] If you're 48 years old or older, higher cholesterol is better!
- In the largest study of MI (heart attack) patients and associated cholesterol levels ever published, at UCLA Medical Center, 136,905 patients admitted to 541 hospitals with MI's had total cholesterol

levels lower than average (174.4 mg/dl) and LDL ("bad cholesterol") lower than average (104.9 mg/dl). The researchers conclude with the following: "These findings may provide further support for recent guideline revisions with even lower LDL goals…"[956] In other words, since the heart attack patients already had LDL at what the researchers were convinced was the perfect level (100mg/dl), instead of questioning the hypothesis (high LDL cholesterol causes heart disease), they decided the LDL level just wasn't low enough – and advised patients that they need even lower levels of LDL cholesterol. The Rx? Statins, of course!

- No relationship between total cholesterol and heart disease or stroke has <u>ever</u> been established in women.[957] Women with cholesterol of 350 mg/dl have no higher risk of heart attack than those with cholesterol of 150.
- If you consume much cholesterol, your liver produces less, and if you consume little, your liver produces more, which is why diets generally have minimal effect on total cholesterol. Every day, we typically produce 3 to 5 times more cholesterol than we eat. We cannot consume enough cholesterol to supply our needs.[958]
- The Japanese first noted high rates of cerebral hemorrhage (stroke) with low blood cholesterol levels.[959]
- Low total cholesterol levels and higher risk of cerebral hemorrhage was confirmed in additional studies in Japan,[960 961 962 963] Honolulu,[964 965] and the Multiple Risk Factor Intervention Trial (MRFIT).[966]
- High cholesterol has never been shown to be a risk factor for stroke.[967]
- Nine studies have shown that high cholesterol is not a risk factor for arterial disease in the legs.[968]
- Many countries have shown decreased saturated fat consumption in recent decades, with increasing rates of type 2 diabetes, including the U.S. Type 2 diabetes is a strong risk factor for heart attack and other vascular disease.[969]
- The Masai peoples in East Africa have the lowest average cholesterol ever measured in healthy people, yet more than 60% of their calories are derived from animal fats, approximately 50% of which is saturated fat.[970]
- In 30 or more studies, patients who had suffered a heart attack or stroke had not eaten more saturated fat than those without heart attack or stroke.[971]
- People with familial hypercholesterolemia, a genetic disease associated with extremely high total and LDL cholesterol levels, on average, live just as long as people with low or normal cholesterol.[972]
- People with familial hypercholesterolemia are more likely to die at an early age of heart disease, but are much less likely to die of cancer and infectious diseases.[973] Their higher MI rate might also be partially explained by the fact that they often have higher blood levels of the clotting factors, prothrombin, fibrinogen, and factor VIII. Nevertheless, people with familial hypercholesterolemia, cannot be classified as to risk of heart disease in the same categories as people without this inherited disorder.
- Perhaps the most damning evidence against the cholesterol hypothesis, as put forward by Uffe Ravnskov, MD, PhD, is that there is no exposure-response (dose-response) with cholesterol and coronary disease as demonstrated by angiography;[974] that is, if cholesterol were the causative factor, the higher the cholesterol, the worse the progression of coronary atherosclerosis, right? But there is no such relationship. In three studies, no correlation was found,[975,976,977] and in two others, a decrease in cholesterol was associated with a higher risk of atherosclerosis.[978,979]

Professor Chris Masterjohn, PhD, eminent authority on heart disease at Brooklyn College in New York, in his article entitled, "Foods High in Cholesterol Could Save Your Health!" wrote the following:

> Since we cannot possibly eat enough cholesterol to use for our bodies' daily functions, our bodies make their own. When we eat more foods rich in this compound, our bodies make less. If we deprive ourselves of foods high in cholesterol – such as eggs, butter, and liver – our body revs up its cholesterol synthesis. The end result is that, for most of us, eating foods high in cholesterol has very little impact on our blood cholesterol levels.
>
> In seventy percent of the population, foods rich in cholesterol such as eggs cause only a subtle increase in cholesterol levels or none at all. In the other thirty percent, these foods do cause a rise in blood cholesterol levels. Despite this, research has never established any clear relationship between the consumption of dietary cholesterol and the risk for heart disease.[980,981]

THE STATINS: ENEMIES WITH FEW BENEFITS

The Cochrane Collaboration independently reviewed 18 randomized controlled trials with 19 different trial arms, which included 56,934 patients, between 1994 and 2008, to evaluate the effect of statins on cardiovascular disease (CVD). The mean age was 57 years and at the conclusion of the study, the authors reported, "Of 1000 people treated with a statin for five years, 18 would avoid a major CVD event which compares well with other treatments used for preventing cardiovascular disease."[982] Put another way, there is a 1.8% chance that, after taking a statin drug for five years, that the treatment will actually help to prevent a cardiovascular event, such as a heart attack. This miniscule benefit may be little or no different than taking an aspirin. In fact, the benefit is not based on cholesterol-lowering, but presumably because of favorable effects on inflammation, the vascular endothelium, and on the coagulation (clotting) cascade.[983]

Yet the potential side-effects of statins may be devastating. Statins poison the CoQ10 production system, which may drastically cripple energy production. Up to 20% of patients taking statins experience muscle weakening,[984] which ironically, contributes to greater congestive heart failure in patients on statins. The statins may rarely cause rhabdomyolysis, which is a severe form of muscle breakdown with potential kidney failure. In fact, Baycol, the statin drug which blocks the HMG CoA reductase pathway – exactly the same as all the other statins – was pulled from the market when it was found to be responsible for 31 deaths.[985] One study showed that for every 10,000 normal, healthy people taking a statin drug, there were 23 additional patients with acute kidney failure, 74 extra patients with liver dysfunction, and another 307 additional patients with cataracts.[986] The statins negatively impact memory, thought, and concentration – with one study showing a negative effect on cognitive function in just six months worth of therapy,[987] and another showing decrements in attention and psychomotor speed, both of which were clinically significant.[988] Statins may cause peripheral neuropathy, with associated tingling, numbness, and burning pain, particularly in the lower legs. This condition may not resolve after stopping the statin.[989] The authors of one study found that "the majority of the literature suggests an increased risk of new-onset diabetes in patients treated with statins," and that "a dose-response curve has been shown between statin treatment and the development of diabetes."[990] Statin drugs inhibit testosterone production by 40% in rat Leydig cells in vitro, which is probably why these drugs have been so strongly tied to erectile dysfunction.[991] Pfizer, the makers of Lipitor, reported that more than 29 million people in the U.S. alone had been prescribed Lipitor.[992] Lucky for Pfizer, the New York Times reported that more than 35 million men had already filled prescriptions for Viagra, which Pfizer also makes.[993] According to the FDA-Adverse effect reporting system database, for every 10,000 reports of a statin-associated adverse event, approximately 40 reports were for the dreaded lung condition known as interstitial lung disease.[994] This condition is the result of fibrosis, or scarring, of the lung tissue. The end result is potentially severely reduced lung capacity, leaving the patient like that of a chronic smoker with chronic obstructive pulmonary disease (COPD, or emphysema). Given the nature of cholesterol and its critically important effects in the brain, it's also no great surprise that Parkinson's disease has been associated with reduced cholesterol levels. In fact, the association is so strong that each mmol/L increase in total cholesterol has been associated with a 23% decrease in the risk of developing Parkinson's disease. This reduction of risk has been shown to be significant in women, but not in men.[995]

One of the greatest ironies of all, the statin drugs have been shown to worsen coronary artery calcification – the very arteries these drugs are designed to protect. The Confirm (Coronary CT Angiography Evaluation for Clinical Outcomes: An International Multicenter) Registry found shocking evidence that the statin drugs have been associated with greater prevalence and degree of calcification of coronary artery plaques.[996] Furthermore, the use of statins has been associated with an increased incidence of coronary artery stenosis and a greater incidence of coronary vessels developing obstruction. Five different prospective studies have determined that statin therapy does not cause coronary artery calcium regression and that coronary calcium deposition continues unabated despite statin therapy.[997] [998]

Other reported adverse side effects of statins include mood disorders, hemorrhagic stroke,[999] depression, irritability, headaches, joint pains, abdominal pain, nausea, upset stomach, sleep problems, sexual function problems, fatigue, dizziness, and a sense of detachment.[1000]

To get all the nitty-gritty details on heart disease, cholesterol, and saturated fat, strongly consider reading the brilliant works of Chris Masterjohn, PhD, at www.cholesterol-and-health.com. I also am a huge fan of the following books on cholesterol: *Ignore the Awkward – How the Cholesterol Myths are Kept Alive,* by Uffe Ravnskov, MD, PhD, *The Great Cholesterol Myth,* by Jonny Bowden, PhD, and Stephen Sinatra, MD, and *The Great Cholesterol Con,* by Anthony Colpo. I've also written a much more thorough review in my upcoming book, *Ancestral Diet Rx.*

Finally, it should come as no surprise, but statin drugs also do not help AMD. In fact, it looks like they may make it worse. Israeli researchers, Nadia Kaiserman, MSc, and colleagues at the Hebrew University Medical School, in Jerusalem, evaluated the data from some 139,894 subjects and the need for photodynamic laser therapy (PDT) for wet AMD during the years 1999 to 2002. They found that those being treated with statins required PDT, the primary treatment for wet AMD at that time, nearly twice as often (0.27%) as those not taking statins (0.16%).[1001]

CHAPTER SUMMARY

I've just scratched the surface regarding cholesterol and how beneficial and essential this molecule is to our health. Once again, it might be worth repeating that LDL cholesterol may have associations with heart disease, but apparently only because of the oxidized form, LDL-OX, which develops secondary to consumption of vegetable oils. Otherwise, LDL is our friend, just like HDL. There's nothing inherently bad about cholesterol – only what we attach to it because of a processed-food laden diet, replete with dangerous vegetable oils. Blaming cholesterol for heart disease is like blaming red blood cells (RBCs) for carbon monoxide poisoning in the case of severe exposure, because the red cells are the ones carrying the carbon monoxide.

As you can also see, there are many risks with cholesterol levels that are low, including greater risk of stroke, cancer, and depression – and only a slightly reduced risk of heart attack, but for men and only those under age 50. Elevated cholesterol levels, on the other hand, are associated with longer life, less cancer, better memory, less depression, and only a slightly higher risk of heart attack, but again, only in men under age 50.

With regard to macular degeneration, the point of this chapter is that you must not fear cholesterol, especially not its consumption. You must also embrace the consumption of saturated fat, particularly animal fats. To reduce the risk of AMD, we must absolutely be consuming the foods that we've been told not to eat, including saturated animal fats, eggs, butter, and, of course, I would strongly recommend consumption of liver, either from beef, chicken, or fish (cod liver oil). These are the foods that supply us with tremendous levels of the fat-soluble vitamins (A, D, and K) – and you cannot get them in adequate amounts from any plant foods, or for that matter, even from the lean animal meats.

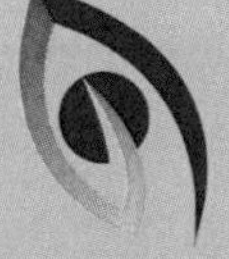

Part V

More On Molecular Mechanisms for AMD

16 VITAMIN A, D, & K, PLUS LUTEIN AND ZEAXANTHIN – DEFICIENCIES ASSOCIATED WITH AMD

"Vitamin K2 works synergistically with the two other "fat-soluble activators [Weston A.] Price studied, vitamins A and D. Vitamins A and D signal to the cells to produce certain proteins and vitamin K then activates these proteins."[1002]

~ Professor Chris Masterjohn, PhD ~
Brooklyn College, New York

In a New York Times "In Depth Report" segment, approved by the American Accreditation Healthcare Commission and fully referenced to scientific articles, the authors wrote, "A low dietary intake of vitamins A, C, E, and beta carotenes has been linked to heart disease. All of these nutrients have antioxidant effects and other properties that should benefit the heart. However, there is now clear evidence that *supplements* of these vitamins, singly or in combination, do *not* protect against heart disease or cancer. Deficiencies in the B vitamins folate (known also as folic acid) and B12 have been associated with elevated blood levels of homocysteine, an amino acid that has been associated with a higher risk for heart disease, stroke, and heart failure. However, there is now clear evidence that *supplements* of these vitamins do *not* reduce the risk of heart disease (italics mine)." [1003] These associations are mentioned first, since we know that AMD has been strongly associated with heart disease, as well as because the two may share numerous causative factors. And as is nearly always the case, vitamins provided in supplement form (pills) don't help.

AN EPIDEMIC OF VITAMIN DEFICIENCIES

There are 13 essential vitamins that are critical to humans: The fat-soluble vitamins, A, D, E, and K (K1 and K2), and the water soluble vitamins, which includes the "B complex," which is B1 (thiamine), B2 (riboflavin), B3 (niacin), B5 (pantothenic acid) B6 (pyridoxine), B7 (biotin), B9 (folic acid), and B12 (cobalamin), and vitamin C. If any of these are consumed in amounts less than ideal, there are consequences, and they may be severe.

In 2011, researchers from Tufts University in Boston published a study entitled, "Foods, Fortificants, and Supplements: Where Do Americans Get Their

Nutrients?" These researchers found that large percentages of the population had dietary intakes of multiple vitamins and minerals that were below the estimated average requirement (EAR). **In fact, they reported that 34% were below EAR for vitamin A, 25% for vitamin C, 70% for vitamin D, and 60% for vitamin E, while 38% were below EAR for calcium and 45% below EAR for magnesium. Only 3% consumed potassium greater than the EAR and only 35% consumed vitamin K greater than EAR.**[1004]

In fact, the authors also calculated what percentage of the subjects would have failed to meet the ERS if they did not have supplements as well as enriched and fortified products. In this scenario, they found that 100% would fail to meet the ERS for vitamin D, 74% for vitamin A, 46% for vitamin C, 93% for vitamin E, 51% for thiamine, 22% for vitamin B6, and 88% for folate.[1005] As one can see, our population has come to rely tremendously on fortified and enriched foods.

Mind you, with these figures, they referenced the EAR, which is just the average requirement for people. In contrast, the recommended daily allowances (RDAs) are defined as "the levels of intake of essential nutrients that, on the basis of scientific knowledge, are judged by the Food and Nutrition Board to be adequate to meet the known nutrient needs of practically all (~ 98%) healthy persons."[1006] As one can see, if the RDA were used to define the percentage of population undernourished, even these numbers would have elevated dramatically.

The NHANES 2001-2002 study corroborates these numbers, indicating that very large percentages of Americans are undernourished (table below).

PERCENTAGE OF AMERICANS WITH INADEQUATE INTAKES FROM FOOD BASED ON ESTIMATED AVERAGE REQUIREMENTS

QUESTIONS OF THIS CHAPTER:

The questions of this chapter are these:

- What is the effect of all of these vitamin deficiencies on AMD?
- Are there specific nutrient deficiencies that are consistently linked to AMD?
- If there are vitamin deficiencies linked to AMD, wouldn't this – and this alone – be very strong evidence for the hypothesis that the displacing foods of modern commerce are the primary and proximate cause of macular degeneration? After all, as we now understand, it is these 'displacing foods' that are the cause of our nutrient deficiencies, correct?

This is not to assert that the nutritional deficiencies are the only problem associated with consuming the 'displacing foods,' but these deficiencies are a major problem. Let's dig into this…

LUTEIN AND ZEAXANTHIN – REDUCED CONSUMPTION IN THOSE WITH ADVANCED AMD

The Age Related Eye Disease Research (AREDS) Group showed that dietary lutein and zeaxanthin intake was inversely associated with advanced stages of AMD or even large or extensive intermediate drusen.[1008] Two previously published studies also found associations between reduced lutein and zeaxanthin in the diet and advanced AMD.[1009][1010] There are actually three xanthophyll carotenoids that are found in the macula, which include lutein, zeaxanthin, and meso-zeaxanthin. When these carotenoids accumulate there, they are referred to as macular pigment (MP). They are known to not only filter and absorb short wavelength (blue) light,[1011] but also to have antioxidant properties.[1012] Studies indeed confirm that MP increases in response to

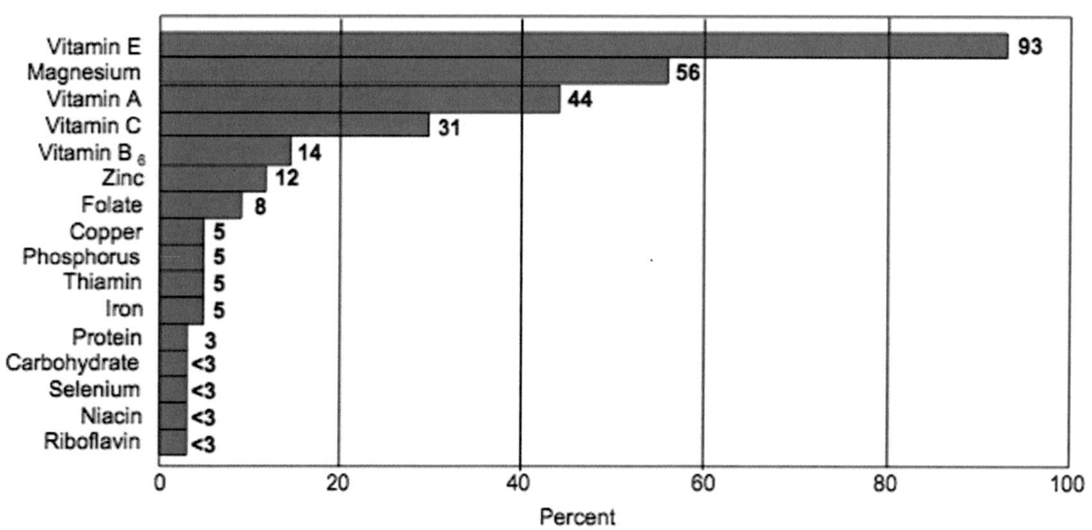

Source: What We Eat in America, NHANES 2001-2002, 1 day, individuals 1+ years, excluding breast-fed children and pregnant or lactating females (USDA)[1007]

supplementation with carotenoids, but evidence indicating that this reduces the risk of AMD is still lacking.[1013]

Nevertheless, given that lutein, zeaxanthin, and meso-zeaxanthin accumulate as macular pigment, it certainly stands to reason that they are beneficial and would contribute to protection against AMD.[1014] Researchers Professor John Nolan, Professor Stephan Beatty, and colleagues, of the Macular Pigment Research Group, Waterford Institute of Technology, in Waterford, Ireland, have shown that, of the three major established risk factors for AMD – age, genetic background, and smoking – all are associated with a relative lack of MP before the disease of AMD begins.[1015] Another recent study showed that advancing age and smoking are associated with a precipitous central dip in macular pigment.[1016]

Researchers Sarah Sabour-Pickett, John Nolan, and colleagues, noted that of the eight observational studies that have investigated dietary intake of carotenoids and AMD, five reported inverse relationships between carotenoid consumption and AMD, that is, high carotenoid intake was associated with lower risk of AMD.[1017] This is strongly suggestive that we should consume foods that would sustain and enhance our macular pigment, despite the fact that the research hasn't made this conclusion just yet.

Lutein and zeaxanthin are found abundantly in dark, leafy-green vegetables such as spinach, kale, and collard greens.[1018] As a percentage of total carotenoids, however, egg yolk and maize (corn) contain the highest percentage, at more than 85% of total carotenoids. Orange pepper is the vegetable with the highest quantity of zeaxanthin, at 37% of total. Lutein and zeaxanthin also make up some 30 to 50% of kiwi fruit, grapes, spinach, zucchini, and certain types of squash. Unquestionably, consuming a variety of fruits and vegetables, plus eggs, will increase the dietary intake of lutein and zeaxanthin, and this may contribute to protection against developing AMD.[1019]

This is yet another major reason to consume eggs and for those that do, I would strongly recommend that you buy eggs from pastured chickens if at all available. In this case, because the chickens are consuming a natural diet containing grass and insects, the eggs will contain substantially more vitamin A, E, beta-carotene, and omega-3 fatty acids. Kris Gunnars, BSc, researcher from Authority Nutrition (*AuthorityNutrition.com*), references Mother Earth News magazine and their study of pastured versus conventionally raised eggs. Their results? The pastured eggs contained about 8 times more beta-carotene (and presumably other carotenoids), and three times more omega-3 fatty acids than supermarket eggs.[1020] Plus, the vitamin K2 in just one to two pastured eggs a day will greatly reduce your risk of cardiovascular disease, by promoting calcium deposition into your teeth and bones, rather than in your arteries![1021] [1022]

If we may return to the AREDS findings, with regard to other vitamins and nutrients and their possible link to AMD, the authors reported, "No clear associations with other nutrients were seen."[1023]

However, we know from the research of Weston A. Price, presented in *Nutrition and Physical Degeneration* (1939), previously reviewed in Chapter 7, that Americans subsisting on typical diets of that era (1930s) routinely consumed approximately 10% or less of the fat-soluble vitamins (A, D, E, and K), about 4-fold less water soluble vitamins (B complex and C),[1024] and many-fold less minerals, than did 14 different major populations and hundreds of tribes from around the world consuming their traditional diets – and who remained in brilliant health and virtually free of degenerative disease. And we also know that AMD in the U.S. was extraordinarily rare in the 19th century when we were consuming far less processed foods and, therefore, substantially higher proportions of vitamins, especially fat-soluble vitamins.

With regard to the findings of the AREDS research just reviewed, i.e., no associations between vitamin consumption and AMD, I would like to invoke the principal that we cannot ascertain potential differences in the presence or consumption of nutrients and their association to a disease (AMD) when everyone is in the "experimental group." That is, in any typical and recent U.S. study, most all subjects are in the nutrient-deficient group. These types of studies are, once again, tantamount to attempting to ferret out the cause of lung cancer in a society where 100% of the inhabitants smoke, but where some smoke three packs a day while some only smoke a pack. The only appropriate comparison of nutrient intake and risk of AMD, once again, would be to evaluate the consumption of all of these vitamins and minerals in a society that is still existing on their traditional diet – perhaps Masai warriors, Kitavans, or the Tarahumara Indians of Mexico – who presumably have no AMD (no studies available yet), and compare them to a cohort group of Americans consuming the typical standard American diet. I am very confident that, in this hypothetical scenario, there would be associations between vitamin consumption and AMD – and the differences would be astonishing. Today's food consumption patterns in the U.S. are almost definitely even less nutrient-dense than they were in the 1930s, when Price did his research, and our prevalence of AMD has gone up dramatically since then.

Moving forward, besides lutein and zeaxanthin in the diet, the AREDS group (reviewed above) didn't find other nutrient deficiencies in the diet, in those with AMD, but numerous other studies have. Let's move on to those next.

LOW VITAMIN D STATUS – AN EPIDEMIC AND A HUGE RISK FACTOR FOR AMD

There's a lot of evidence that when vitamin D status is low, the risk of AMD elevates – and it may do so quite drastically. Researchers at the University of Wisconsin, led by Amy Millen, PhD, assessed some 913 women for vitamin D status and presence of AMD. With regard to the status of vitamin D in their blood, they categorized the women as "adequate" if they had 20 or more nanograms per millileter (ng/mL), "inadequate" at levels between 12 and 20 ng/mL, and "deficient" if they were under 12 ng/mL. They found that of the 913 women, 550 had adequate levels, 275 had inadequate levels, and 88 had deficient levels. Now here is the clincher: **Those women that were in the deficient class of vitamin D status had a 6.7-fold increased odds of having AMD, if they also had two copies of a certain gene (Y402 of the CFH gene).**[1025]

However, compared to the "referent group," which had serum vitamin D above 30 ng/mL and no specific genes that increase risk of AMD, **those with no specific genetic risks and deficient vitamin D status still had a 2.6-fold greater odds of AMD, those with inadequate vitamin D status had a 1.5-fold increased odds of AMD, and those with adequate vitamin D status still had a 1.6-fold increased odds of AMD.** The authors of this study convey that vitamin D is hypothesized to suppress a pro-inflammatory state in the retina via multiple mechanisms and to effect immune-modulating properties, which ultimately protects against the development of AMD.[1026] Furthermore, both the receptor for vitamin D and the enzyme to convert it to the active form have been discovered to be present in the retina.[1027]

Multiple other studies have found inverse relationships between vitamin D levels and AMD, that is, high vitamin D levels are protective while low levels carry increased risk.[1028,1029,1030,1031]

So how does vitamin D decrease risk, or lack of vitamin D increase the risk for AMD? In one study, researchers gave aging mice vitamin D3 for just six weeks, and these mice "showed significant reductions in retinal inflammation and levels of amyloid beta (Aβ) accumulation, which is a hallmark of aging." [1032] The authors wrote, "These changes were reflected in a significant improvement in visual function, revealing that vitamin D3 is a route to avoiding the pace of age-related visual decline. Excess amyloid beta deposition and inflammation are risk factors leading to age-related macular degneneration (AMD)..." [1033]

Dr. Amy Millen, who was the lead researcher at the University of Wisconsin on the vitamin D status and AMD risk study that we reviewed (above), sat for an interview with editor Maxine Lipner for the journal EyeWorld. In the interview, Dr. Millen said, **"This is just another bit of evidence suggesting that nutrition is important to eye health. But, it's hard in an observational study to tease out or control for the many lifestyle factors that are also related to vitamin D levels – so someone with high D status probably has a healthy diet and is physically acive."** [1034]

SOURCES OF VITAMIN D

Humans can get all of their vitamin D from the exposure of their skin to varying amounts of sunlight, with darker skin requiring more exposure time than lighter skin. However, for the enormous majority of people living and working indoors, this source is negligible – for most people – and for most of the year. There are essentially no significant plant sources of vitamin D in the human diet, though certain mushrooms may provide D2.[1035] **Of the animal sources of vitamin D, there are not many, with oily fish (salmon, herring, mackerel, and sardines), offal, which is organ meats such as liver, kidneys, heart, etc., meats, and eggs being the primary sources.**[1036] **Fish liver, however, is an excellent source, which is why extra virgin cod liver oil (EVCLO) is a tremendous source of vitamin D3.**[1037] Fish eggs are also an excellent source of vitamin D as well as other vitamins. Though I have not been able to locate a scientific study that shows the vitamin D levels in fish eggs such as caviar and salmon roe, Weston A. Price made the following observation: "A chemical analysis of the dried fish eggs that I brought to my laboratory from Alaska as well as of samples brought from other places has revealed them to be a very rich source of body-building minerals and vitamins." [1038]

Toxic levels of vitamin D do occur, however, I am only aware of this adverse event in those consuming synthetic vitamin D supplements. If this occurs, the result will be deposition of calcium into soft tissues – particularly the arterial walls of vessels in the kidney.[1039] However, there is no reason to suspect that this wouldn't also occur in the coronary arteries and in the choroid of the eye. For this reason, *I would strongly advise against taking vitamin D supplements in any form.* Higher doses of vitamin D depend on higher levels of vitamin A and vice versa. This is why supplementing with non-food based vitamins is risky business.

VITAMIN A STATUS – ANOTHER EPIDEMIC OF DEFICIENCY, WHICH MAY CONTRIBUTE TO AMD?

As you can see from the NHANES 2001 – 2002 study and the table above, some 44% of Americans are not consuming adequate vitamin A from their foods, based on the Estimated Average Requirement (EAR). The EAR is based upon the Dietary Reference Intakes (DRIs), which are nutrient reference values developed by the Institute of Medicine of the National Academies. The EAR for vitamin A was set at 625 ug/day (~2,083 IU) and 500 ug/day (~1667 IU), for men and women 19 years of age and older, respectively.[1040,1041] To arrive at this figure, the National Academies assumes that a certain amount of pro-vitamin A, in the form of carotenoids from plants, will be converted to vitamin A. This is correct, but nevertheless, the conversion itself is highly variable, as will be discussed briefly.

Contrary to popular opinion, vitamin A is only present in animal foods.[1042] There is none in any plant foods. Nonetheless, in many grocery stores and elsewhere, I see signs above some vegetation, such as spinach, kale, and others, which states, "Great Source of Vitamin A." These, of course, are false statements, but FDA regulations allow foods with carotenoids to be labeled as such. Vegetation may include any number of some 60 bioavailable carotenoids, which may be converted to vitamin A in the liver, but we should be aware that plants do not contain vitamin A and that the conversion of carotenoids to vitamin A is a highly inefficient process.

SOURCES OF VITAMIN A AND FEAR OF TOXICITY

The only natural sources of vitamin A come directly from the animal kingdom and primarily include liver and other organ meats, egg yolks, full-fat milk, butter from grass fed cows, and cod liver oil.[1043]

There is significant fear of vitamin A toxicity and this comes almost exclusively from - you guessed it - synthetic vitamin A. Isn't this a recurring theme? Researchers from Belgium collected data on 41 cases of liver damage caused by excessive vitamin A consumption. They reported, "The smallest continuous daily consumption leading to cirrhosis was 25,000 IU during 6 years, whereas higher daily doses (greater than or equal to 100,000 IU) taken during 2 ½ years resulted in similar histological lesions." [1044] In the scientific literature, there are a couple of reports of vitamin A poisoning in Arctic explorers who ingested significant amounts of polar bear or seal liver. The liver of these animals may contain up to millions of units of vitamin A in relatively small quantities and the liver of these animals should generally not be eaten.[1045]

THE PROBLEM WITH CAROTENOIDS AS PRECURSORS TO VITAMIN A

Beta-carotene, the most abundant carotenoid, looks like two vitamin A molecules joined at their tail ends. At one point, researchers believed that beta-carotene could be cleaved apart in our bodies, providing two molecules of vitamin A. As usual, things are not so simple in our bodies.

Alfred Sommer, MD, Dean Emeritus and renowned ophthalmologist at Johns Hopkins Bloomberg School of Public Health, spent years grappling with the science of vitamin A while he served on a panel that made recommendations to the World Health Organization (WHO) regarding nutritional blindness. Over a half a million children per year still die of vitamin A deficiency in the world. As told by Catherine Price, in her book *Vitamania,* Dr. Sommer attended a vitamin A conference in 1974 where an Indonesian scientist presented his research that showed that feeding people an abundance of dark leafy-green vegetables for three months didn't even alter their vitamin A status.[1046] Considered heretical at the time, later in the 1990s a Dutch group replicated the work, feeding huge amounts of dark leafy greens to women and children, again for three months. Though the leafy greens contained lots of beta-carotene and other carotenoids, once again, their vitamin A status was unchanged.[1047]

It turns out that, as Sommer has described, the conversion is perhaps 3 to 4 molecules of beta-carotene to one molecule vitamin A under the most desirable circumstances - when the food is eaten with an oily base. But under less ideal circumstances, the conversion ratio is much worse - as low as 6:1 or 12:1.[1048] He confirmed that, in the U.S., the Institute of Medicine has settled on a conversion rate of 12:1. According to Sommer, however, the conversion may still be far lower. In the words of Dr. Sommer, from Catherine Price's *Vitamania:*

> "What the researchers found is that if you feed someone a fruit that's rich in beta-carotene—papaya, mango—it takes about 18 molecules, not 6, to get one molecule of vitamin A," said Sommer. "And if it's a dark leafy vegetable like spinach, it takes about 27 molecules of beta-carotene to make one of vitamin A. So if you put together what a kid might get from fruits and leafy vegetables, it'll take about 24 molecules of beta-carotene to make one molecule of vitamin A." Other recent papers have come up with slightly different conversion factors, but the basic range is the same.[1049]

The Institute of Medicine of the National Academies uses the following conversions, taken directly from their Dietary Reference Intakes (DRIs) tables:

1 Retinol Activity Equivalent (RAE) = 1 μg retinol, 12 μg β-carotene, 24 μg α-carotene, or 24 μg β-cryptoxanthin.[1050]

Thus, with regard to the research and experience of Dr. Sommer, it appears that even the National Academies formulae may overestimate the conversion of pro-vitamin A carotenoids into active vitamin A, which might indicate that the numbers of people that are deficient in vitamin A is even higher than the 44% that is estimated by the NHANES 2001-2002 data.

In a three-year study that evaluated the main types of fruit, vegetables, and the top 10 dietary sources of vitamins A, C and E in five ethnic groups, in Los Angeles county and Hawaii, researchers found that, "Carrots were the primary source of vitamin A, accounting for 17.0- 34.5% of total intake across all ethnic-sex groups. Cereals [with synthetic vitamin A} and dark greens were also among the major sources of vitamin A for all groups, except for Latino-Mexican men and women for whom dark greens contributed 4.0 and 3.7%, respectively. Combined meat-vegetable dishes were among the top contributors to vitamin A for all groups, except for Latino-Mexican women." [1051]

The point of all of this is that, the animal-based foods that once supplied us with abundant vitamin A, such as liver, eggs, cod liver oil, and butter, have all been demonized as a result of the anti-saturated fat, anti-cholesterol campaign. Vitamin A is found only in and associated with animal fats and, even then, it is present in significant quantities only when the animals have had substantial sources of carotenes in the diet, such as green pasture, insects, or fish meal.[1052] The only other good source of vitamin A in the diet is shellfish, but shellfish are certainly not staples for most people. Could it get much worse in terms of our vitamin A consumption? Well, possibly...

To make matters worse, the polyunsaturated oils (PUFAs), which have largely supplanted lard and butter in cooking, cause destruction of carotene in the gut unless sufficient antioxidants are present.[1053,1054] Recall that, by 2005, animal fats, such as butter, lard and edible tallow {beef fat}, made up only 14 percent of our added fat consumption in the U.S., with the rest being vegetable oils, margarine, and trans fats - and, of course, margarine and trans fats are derived from vegetable oils.[1055]

IS AMD, IN PART, A VITAMIN A DEFICIENCY DISEASE?

At this point, I'd like to recall from Chapter 6 that researchers Gregory R. Jackson, PhD, Cynthia Owsley, PhD, and colleagues found that patients with early AMD had significantly delayed rod-mediated dark adaptation times, actually - 13 minutes longer on average – than those without AMD.[1056] In a separate study, Owsley and colleagues also found that a 30-day course of high-dose vitamin A improved dark-adaptation times in people with AMD as well as those without AMD.[1057] Finally, this research group also showed that those people with delayed dark adaptation times were approximately twice as likely to develop AMD within just a three-year window.[1058] This is strongly suggestive of a vitamin A deficiency, or at least a perturbed mechanism to get vitamin A to the photoreceptors.

Let me also recall that Weston A. Price found, in 14 major populations, that the traditional diets of people on five different continents contained at least ten times as many fat-soluble vitamins (A, D, E, and K) as did American diets of his day.

Clearly, all of this evidence is adding up to look as though, in general, vitamin A deficiency is very common – perhaps at least half of the population, if not much more. So why are we not bombarded with studies, magazine articles, and newspaper articles advising us that we're vitamin A deficient, just as we see regarding our vitamin D deficiency? After all, as you've seen, many of the foods that contain vitamin D, such as liver and other organ meats, eggs, and cod liver oil, are also the foods high in vitamin A. The answer is simple. *There is no blood test to accurately assess our vitamin A stores. The only reliable test to accurately measure vitamin A status is a liver biopsy.* However, liver biopsy is a very invasive test that would rarely be used to determine one's vitamin A status.[1059] The risks would be pretty significant, since a long needle with a large bore would have to be inserted through the right upper quadrant of the abdomen right into the liver.

Professor of Nutritional Sciences, Sherry A. Tanumihardjo, PhD, at the Vitamin A Assessment Laboratory, University of Wisconsin – Madison, wrote in a paper presented in the *Journal of Nutrition*, in 2004, "In healthy individuals, serum retinol [vitamin A] concentrations are homeostatically controlled and do not begin to decline until liver reserves of vitamin A are dangerously low." [1060] Dr. Tanumihardjo reviews the fact that the present indicators of vitamin A status are all ophthalmic. These include xerophthalmia (dry eye syndrome), abnormal conjunctival impression cytology smears (from the ocular surface), night blindness, which is associated with AMD, and delayed dark adaptation, which we've also reviewed and is associated with AMD. Interestingly, for those of you not aware, we currently have an epidemic of dry eye syndrome, with at least tens of millions of Americans affected.[1061] And multiple studies have shown that vitamin A treatment is effective for dry eye disease, including autologous serum (a person's own serum) eye drops, which contain significant vitamin A.[1062,1063,1064,1065] One study even shows that vitamin A eye drops are as effective for dry eye as topical cyclosporine (Restasis).[1066]

This review of dry eye syndrome has two possible conclusions: 1) An epidemic of dry eye syndrome might indicate generalized vitamin A deficiency, and 2) Dry eye syndrome would not be responsive to vitamin A treatments if we were not already vitamin A deficient.

Until a couple of years ago, I had been plagued by dry eye syndrome for more than 30 years, since I was about 20 years old. After reading Price's *Nutrition and Physical Degeneration,* I decided I ought to start eating liver. I hadn't eaten liver since my Dad last made it when I was about 12 years old. One winter night back in 2014, I made and ate beef liver and onions, seasoned with salt, pepper, thyme, and Rosemary, chopped up into small pieces just the way my Dad used to prepare it. In any case, that night I had to get out of bed at 2:00 a.m. to pick up my daughter some 20 miles away as she returned from a ski trip. Having not even considered that my dry eye syndrome might be affected, I awoke in the night to find that my dry eyes were dramatically improved. Nearly as amazing, my night vision had obviously improved, and since that night, I've had only mild and occasional dry eye issues. It was remarkable. Naturally, my family and I continue to eat liver and we eat organically raised chicken liver and pasture raised beef liver, both cooked with onions in butter from pastured cows. I've recommended this to numerous dry eye sufferers and every one has reported substantial improvement or even complete resolution of their dry eyes.

In my view, there is ample evidence to indicate that, in general, vitamin A deficiency is common, based on the relatively recent change in our diets, the NHANES studies, the dark-adaptation studies, the research of Weston A. Price, and perhaps even the epidemic of dry eye syndrome. The fact that delayed dark adaptation predicts AMD onset is yet another reason to strongly suspect vitamin A deficiency might be implicated in the cause of AMD.

BLOCKING VITAMIN A TO TREAT AMD?

When researchers dig into the molecular detail of what's going on in AMD, one of the situations they find is that there is accumulation of a substance called lipofuscin within the RPE cells.[1067] Lipofuscin, in turn, contains significant amounts of a molecule called N-retinylidene-N-retinylethanolamine, better known as A2E. A2E essentially consists of two molecules of vitamin A connected to a molecule of ethanolamine. A2E accumulates in the RPE cells in patients with macular degeneration and is also suspected of being toxic to the RPE cells themselves.[1068] As such, researchers have attempted to block the development of A2E by preventing vitamin A (retinol) from reaching the RPE.[1069] This is being accomplished in studies using drugs like fenretinide. Fenretinide is a vitamin A analogue which, from a molecular standpoint, looks a lot like vitamin A.[1070] Therefore, this drug can bind to the retinol-binding protein

(RBP), which normally carries vitamin A in the blood and delivers it to the RPE cells. This, in turn, prevents much of the use of vitamin A in the retina.

So does this drug work in terms of delaying AMD progression? Well, as far as delaying the progression from dry AMD to wet AMD, at least in one study, it did. The incidence of wet AMD was 2.2-fold greater in the placebo group versus the fenretinide group after two years of treatment.[1071] It is important to realize that patients treated with the fenretinide had significant side effects, for example, 2.5% withdrew because of delayed dark-adaptation, meaning they had trouble seeing in the dark. Some had visual disturbances, abnormal color vision, and reduced vision.[1072]

This study and others like it, certainly perplexed me when I initially read them, particularly because there is some success with these drugs. My question was: How could a drug that prevents delivery of vitamin A – the most necessary vitamin in the visual cycle – help delay progression of AMD? The answer, I believe, lies with the fact that these types of drugs literally attempt to shut down metabolism within the retina. It's a bit like putting an obese person on a starvation diet – just stop feeding them. It works, for a while, but at what expense? It doesn't address the etiology – the underlying problem. And with AMD patients, of course, this comes with the side effects, namely, visual disturbances, night blindness, etc. And we don't know what the long-term consequences would be by drastically reducing serum retinol (vitamin A) levels in the blood, but it will likely be devastating, contributing to much other disease.

For example, we know that diet is not only a modifiable risk factor for disease,[1073] but as reported in the *European Journal of Clinical Nutrition,*[1074] improving the nutrient density of the diet, particularly by increasing the consumption of fruits and vegetables, and other sources rich in the antioxidant vitamins A, C, and E, results in a decrease in the incidence and mortality from cardiovascular disease, cancer, and other chronic disease.[1075,1076,1077,1078,1079,1080,1081,1082,1083]

Returning to fenretinide and any other drugs intended to literally remove vitamin A from our bodies, my concern is, first of all, they don't address the main problem. That is, they don't address what is causing AMD in the first place. I'm pretty certain none of these researchers would implicate vitamin A as the bad guy here, at least in terms of initiating AMD – as that would just be counterintuitive to everything we know about vision and metabolism, in general. And I certainly hope they're not convinced that we're getting too much vitamin A.

After all, once again, we know from everything we just reviewed and an abundance of research, such as that from Weston A. Price, which proved that the natives of tribes all around the world consumed more than 10 times as much vitamin A as we do. Yet, the research strongly suggests that they did not have eye disease or vision loss. On the contrary, their vision was often found to be superb.

For example, in 1919, J. N. Roy, MD, Professor of Ophthalmology at the University of Montreal, Montreal, Canada, published a study in *The Canadian Medical* journal entitled, "The Eyesight of the Negroes of Africa."[1084] Professor Roy visited 22 different colonies in Africa, examining about 5,000 Africans from one hundred different tribes, to evaluate their eyesight. This led him to many conclusions, including that vision "is better in Africa than in Europe," "refraction [to evaluate need for glasses] shows that their eyes are almost all emmetropic [indicating little or no need for glasses]," that "simple myopia [nearsightedness] is found in the proportion of about 1.5 per 100, and then it is always of a mild degree," "myopic astigmatism is found in about the same proportion as simple myopia, i.e., 1.5 per 100," and "simple hypermetropia [farsightedness] and hyperopic astigmatism are found in about 2.5 per 100."[1085]

Roy continued, "In a general way, I have been surprised at the excellent eyesight of the negroes," stating further, "My statistics show that the average vision of the natives of Africa is 12-5," which translates to 20/8, or actually 20/8.3 to be exact. This level of vision is astonishing to me as in my 24 years of clinical experience in ophthalmology, I have only seen two or three patients who could read the 20/10 line in my offices, which is vision that is twice as good as 20/20. Roy further stated, "The highest normal vision recorded was one of 20-5 [20/5], and this was in a man affected with sleeping sickness."[1086] For comparison, eagles have been shown to have vision of approximately 20/4, which is purportedly good enough to see a toothpick in a man's mouth a quarter-mile away.[1087] "The negroes have a great power of vision in the dark," Roy wrote after he formally tested their night vision against whites. He continued, "My experiments, repeated frequently and at different places, show that the negroes see at night from two to four times better than the whites."[1088]

Roy made no recorded observations of failing vision in the elderly. "In concluding," he said, "Let me once more call to your attention the marvelous visual apparatus of the negroes," and he appropriately compared the caucasian population as he wrote, "For the whites, their mode of life has a deleterious influence on their physique. The hygiene of the sight and hearing is defective on account of the use of strong artificial light and injurious noises."[1089] Though, obviously, I would vehemently disagree with his last assertion of connecting our failure of vision and hearing to "strong artificial light and injurious noises," Roy's findings are nevertheless entirely consistent with the findings of Weston A. Price. That is, those people consuming their traditional diets developed supremely healthy bodies, even with superior sense organs, and were virtually free of degenerative disease.

VITAMIN K2 DEFICIENCY: LIKELY ANOTHER CONTRIBUTOR TO AMD!

Weston A. Price did not know it's name, but he discovered the vitamin that was the difference between straight and healthy teeth, lack of cavities, and well-proportioned faces, versus narrowed dental arches, crooked teeth, cavities, and an endless list of bone problems. **Societies on five different**

continents had discovered uniquely beneficial sources of that vitamin (and all the other fat soluble vitamins), which included liver and other organ meats, fish liver oils, fish eggs (roe), and cheese and butter from cows consuming rapidly growing green grass, simply because they astutely followed the traditions of their fathers for hundreds, if not thousands, of years. Dr. Price called this vitamin "activator X." [1090]

Seven or eight decades later, we're beginning to understand the extraordinary implications of a lack of "activator X," which is now known to be vitamin K2 – and we're finally beginning to link the synergies between the fat soluble vitamins, D, A, and K2, which Price so eloquently described in 1939.

Vitamin K comes in two primary forms: vitamins K1 and K2. Vitamin K1 comes exclusively from plants, such as green leafy vegetables. It is utilized by the liver to activate calcium-binding proteins important in blood clotting. K2 comes mostly from animal sources, as reviewed above, but is also found in the Japanese dish, natto, which is a type of fermented soy.[1091] Natto, by the way, has a pungent odor that is not well accepted by many societies. **Vitamin K2 has been shown recently to play a critical role in depositing calcium into teeth and bones, where it should be, rather than in soft tissues such as arteries, where it shouldn't be.**[1092,1093,1094]

Knowing that, we see that vitamin D and vitamin K have carefully orchestrated synergies: vitamin D is critically important in pulling calcium from the gut, while vitamin K2 makes sure that calcium goes to where it should be going. The problem? We're beginning to see that, for those consuming a Westernized diet, we're severely deficient in vitamin K2.[1095] No surprise, right? It's another fat soluble vitamin and it's best sources for most diets come from animal foods which have been demonized. But like vitamin A, there's no blood test that can easily measure it.

Cees Vermeer, PhD, Maastricht University, The Netherlands, is one of the world's leading researchers on the subject of vitamin K. He founded the Division on Vitamin K Research at Maastricht University, in 1975, and has studied the biochemistry of vitamin K since then. In a landmark study by Dr. Vermeer and associates, in 2004, the researchers followed 4807 subjects without history of heart attack, beginning between 1990 and 1993, until 2000. They evaluated dietary intake of vitamins K1 and K2, and found that the relative risk of coronary heart disease risk was 0.73 for those in the upper two thirds of dietary K2 consumption versus those in the lower third. They also found that intake of K2 was inversely related to all-cause mortality and to aortic calcification. Vitamin K1, on the other hand, was not related to any of the outcomes.[1096]

As for deficiencies of vitamin K2 as it relates to dietary patterns, researchers Elke Theuwissen, Egbert Smit, and Cees Vermeer, in a paper published in *Advances in Nutrition,* in 2012, wrote, "We conclude that the Western diet contains insufficient vitamin K to ascertain the requirements of extrahepatic tissues [those besides liver], such as bone and the vascular wall." [1097]

In April of 2011, nutrition researchers at the University of Auckland, New Zealand, published a study in the British Medical Journal that was quite shocking – calcium and vitamin D supplements increased the risk of heart disease. According to the study, women who supplemented with calcium to help prevent osteoporosis had a higher risk of atherosclerosis, heart attack, and stroke, than those who didn't supplement. The hazard ratios for those that supplemented was 1.22-fold greater risk of MI (heart attack) and 1.17-fold greater risk of stroke, than those who didn't take the supplements.[1098] Based on this research, the authors found in conclusion that, for every bone fracture that calcium supplementation would prevent, two cardiovascular events in the form of MI or stroke were precipitated. In examining relevant data, the authors wrote, "When the results for calcium and vitamin D are taken together with those from trials of calcium used as monotherapy, they provide consistent evidence from 13 randomized, placebo controlled trials involving about 29,000 participants with about 1400 incident myocardial infarctions and strokes that calcium supplements with or without vitamin D increase the risk of cardiovascular events." [1099]

Suddenly, it becomes crystal clear why Price's "activator X," which is vitamin K2, is so critical. Price strongly advocated that no amount of minerals in the diet could be properly absorbed and utilized, without the "fat soluble activators," which is the fat soluble vitamins. In this case, consuming calcium, with or without vitamin D, when there is lack of vitamin K2, drives that calcium right into the vessel walls, increasing the risk of heart attack and stroke, while osteoporosis runs rampant. And as you can now see, deficiencies of the fat soluble vitamins all tend to run together. So the same people deficient in vitamins A and D are likely to be deficient in K2. Perhaps now the epidemic of heart disease, stroke, and other vascular diseases, along with osteoporosis – weak and fragile bones – is beginning to make sense?

The question now becomes: Could vitamin K2 deficiency increase the risk of macular degeneration as well? As I alluded to in Chapter 6, I believe the answer is a resounding yes. Here's why.

Do you recall at this point that Bruch's membrane lies squarely between the choriocapillaris (the blood supply) and the RPE – and that Bruch's membrane thickens much more significantly in those with AMD than it does in those without AMD? **Well, we also know from at least seven different studies that Bruch's membrane may thicken and calcify with age and it does so much more significantly in patients with AMD.**[1100,1101,1102,1103,1104,1105,1106] **When Bruch's membrane thickens and calcifies, it creates a relative barrier between the choriocapillaris and the RPE, as we reviewed in Chapter 6.** Researchers call this increased "hydraulic conductivity" in Bruch's membrane, meaning that it is much more difficult for the exchange of fluids, nutrients, and even gases between the choriocapillaris and the RPE.[1107] From this, we may infer as to why there is the accumulation of waste products in and around the RPE.[1108,1109,1110] This looks like a significant and currently missing part of the AMD puzzle.

If this is true, then we might expect that vitamin K antagonists, like warfarin (Coumadin), might be associated with increased risk of AMD because they block the effects of both vitamins K1 and K2. There is only one study that I have found, but indeed, the link is there. The authors of this one study found that the number of people using vitamin K antagonists like coumadin were statistically significantly higher in those people with drusen and wet AMD.[1111]

What I am postulating here is that this is part of the molecular link between cardiovascular disease and AMD. This hypothesis, however, subsumes some significant similarities between Bruch's membrane and the walls of arteries. But, do Bruch's membrane and the vessel walls of the coronary (or other) arteries share any commonalities? Indeed, scientists believe that they do. Researchers, Sobha Sivaprasad, FRCS, Tracey A. Bailey, PhD, and Victor N. Chong, FRCS, from King's College Hospital, London, UK, published a paper in 2005, entitled, "Bruch's membrane and the vascular intima: is there a common basis for age-related changes and disease?" In the abstract of this article the authors wrote, "**The vascular intima and the Bruch's membrane share several age-related changes and are the seat of many common molecules. Diseases of these structures may represent parallel responses to the tissue injury induced by multiple intercalated factors...**" [1112]

Larry Donoso, MD, PhD, Gregory Hageman, PhD, and colleagues at Wills Eye Hospital, Eye Research Institute, in a study presented in *Survey of Ophthalmology* (2006), wrote, "The association between cardiovascular disease and AMD is inferred from the histological [tissue] similarity of atherosclerotic deposits within arterial vessels to those of drusen, the hallmark of AMD, in the eye. Furthermore, a local inflammatory response has been implicated in the etiology of both macular drusen and drusen-like deposits in arterial vessels." [1113]

WHAT ABOUT OCCLUSION OF VESSELS IN THE CHOROID AND CHORIOCAPILLARIS – IS THIS RELATED TO VITAMIN K2 REDUCTION AS WELL?

If you will recall from Chapter 6, we reviewed multiple studies that showed one of the main findings in AMD is occlusion of the vessels of the choroid. Recall, for example, that Juan Grunwald, MD, Professor of Ophthalmology at the University of Pennsylvania, and investigator at the Scheie Eye Institute, found that, in subjects with AMD, choroidal blood volume was 33% lower than that of control subjects ($P = 0.005$) and that average choroidal blood flow in subjects with AMD was 37% lower than those without AMD ($P = 0.0005$). [1114]

If we dig just a little deeper into the detail of how vitamin K2 prevents the calcification of arteries and other soft tissues, it turns out that, **of the numerous proteins involved in preventing soft tissue calcification, many studies have shown that matrix Gla-protein (MGP) is the dominant one.**[1115 1116 1117] But MGP must be activated in order to accomplish this job, and that requires vitamin K2.[1118] In fact, Cees Vermeer's group states, "It is generally accepted that MGP is a potent inhibitor of arterial calcification.[1119]

So how does this relate to the closure of vessels in the choroid and choriocapillaris? Well, it turns out that the vasculature of the choroid and, in fact, the entire eye, contains smooth muscle cells.[1120] **And MGP is significantly present and active in normal vascular smooth muscle cells.** [1121 1122] **This means that, in the face of deficient vitamin K2 and oxidized LDL, the choroid may begin to calcify and occlude, thereby leading to loss of blood flow to the RPE as well as the photoreceptors!**

The only other question that might arise here is this: Does calcification of vessels correlate with occlusion, i.e., atherosclerosis? I think the answer to this is best summed up by the eminent cholesterol and vascular disease researcher, Uffe Ravnskov, MD, PhD, who wrote, "Degree of coronary calcification seems a good surrogate for degree of coronary atherosclerosis, because it correlates strongly with total plaque volume and obstructive coronary disease, and is a powerful predictor of clinical outcome." [1123]

So now, hopefully, you can see that we've finally tied together the cause of coronary heart disease and macular degeneration!

SO WHAT'S THE SIGNIFICANCE OF DEFICIENCIES OF VITAMINS A, D, AND K2? IN FACT, WHY NOT JUST TAKE A VITAMIN K2 PILL?

Ahhh, and these questions take us back to the introduction in Chapter 1 and reductionist thinking – which always gets us in trouble. And secondly, now we finally get to discuss, if ever so briefly, the amazing symphony that these fat soluble vitamins play together. For this, we need the genius of Chris Masterjohn, PhD, Nutritional Sciences Professor at Brooklyn College in New York. Dr. Masterjohn brilliantly ties together the synchrony of vitamins A, D, and K2 in an article he wrote for the Weston A. Price Foundation, entitled, "On the Trail of the Elusive X-Factor: A Sixty-Two-Year-Old Mystery Finally Solved." In part, he wrote,

> {Weston A.} Price showed Activator X (vitamin K2) to exhibit dramatic synergy with vitamins A and D. Chickens voluntarily consumed more butter and died more slowly on a deficiency diet when the butter was high in both vitamin A and Activator X than when it was high in vitamin A alone. Cod liver oil, which is high in both vitamins A and D, partially corrected growth retardation and weak legs in turkeys fed a deficiency diet, but the combination of

cod liver oil and high-Activator X butter was twice as effective. Likewise, Price found that the combination of cod liver oil and a high-Activator X butter oil concentrate was more effective than cod liver oil alone in treating his patients for dental caries and other signs of physical degeneration.

Vitamin K2 is the substance that makes the vitamin A- and vitamin D-dependent proteins come to life. **While vitamins A and D act as signaling molecules, telling cells to make certain proteins, vitamin K2 activates these proteins by conferring upon them the physical ability to bind calcium.** In some cases these proteins directly coordinate the movement or organization of calcium themselves; in other cases the calcium acts as a glue to hold the protein in a certain shape. In all such cases, the proteins are only functional once they have been activated by vitamin K.

Osteocalcin, for example, is a protein responsible for organizing the deposition of calcium and phosphorus salts in bones and teeth. Cells only produce this protein in the presence of both vitamins A and D; it will only accumulate in the extracellular matrix and facilitate the deposition of calcium salts, however, once it has been activated by vitamin K2. Vitamins A and D regulate the expression of matrix Gla protein (MGP), which is responsible for mineralizing bone and protecting the arteries from calcification; like osteocalcin, however, MGP can only fulfill its function once it has been activated by vitamin K2. While vitamins A and D contribute to growth by stimulating growth factors and promoting the absorption of minerals, vitamin K2 makes its own essential contribution to growth by preventing the premature calcification of the cartilaginous growth zones of bones... The synergy with which vitamin K2 interacts with vitamins A and D is exactly the type of synergy that Price attributed to Activator X.[1124]

VITAMIN DEFICIENCY, DENTAL DECAY, AND MACULAR DEGENERATION

I might forget where my keys are, a city I visited, or even what I ate yesterday, but I couldn't forget that I would reveal the connection between dental decay and AMD, which I alluded to in Chapter 3. Recall from that chapter that the eminent Sir Stewart Duke-Elder, in his 1940 *Text-Book of Ophthalmology,* wrote "...it is significant that a very large number of such cases [of AMD] suffer from a chronic and long-standing streptococcal toxaemia, originating, for example, from the teeth, the throat and the bowel." [1125] It turns out that Duke-Elder's observations, that patients with AMD also tend to have dental disease and more infections in general, is now backed by scienctific studies. We don't think of this connection as much today, because we have dentists fixing up the teeth by the millions. Let's look at this research.

In 2008, Professor Ron Klein's group at the University of Wisconsin found that patients with increased retinal pigment had a 1.68-fold greater risk of having periodontal disease.[1126] And in 2015, the NHANES III Survey found that, for patients under age 60, the presence of periodontal disease was independently associated with nearly twice the risk (1.96 greater odds) of having AMD. This association wasn't present for those older than 60.[1127]

The association of AMD with various systemic infections has been previously reported. In fact, infections with Cytomegalovirus (CMV), Helicobacter pylori (H.pylori), and Chlamydia Pneumoniae have all been recognized as significantly associated with AMD.[1128] [1129] One of these studies even found the organism Chlamydia pneumoniae in the choroidal neovascular membranes (the wet AMD anatomy) that were excised from the eyes of patients with a history of wet AMD.[1130] And in fact, these microbes were also shown to be able to produce a variety of inflammatory mediators, including cytokines, such as interleukin-8 IL-8), monocyte chemotactic protein-1 (MCP-1), and vascular endothelial growth factor (VEGF),[1131] which we've discussed as being instrumental in the development and growth of wet AMD tissue.

Interestingly, there's also been a strong connection drawn between cardiovascular disease and periodontal disease, as well as other systemic inflammatory conditions.[1132] In fact the authors of this last cited research, make the following statement in their abstract:

> Observational studies to date support an association between periodontal disease (PD) and atherosclerotic vascular disease (ASVD) independent of known confounders. They do not, however, support a causative relationship. Although periodontal interventions result in a reduction in systemic inflammation and endothelial dysfunction in short-term studies, there is no evidence that they prevent ASVD or modify its outcomes.[1133]

I agree. Treating the dental disease, such as cavities, abscesses, etc., won't prevent heart disease. And there isn't a causative relationship between dental disease and heart disease. The logic, I hope you're seeing, takes us back to the mountain of evidence discovered by Weston A. Price. Dental decay and disease is associated with consumption of significant amounts of the 'displacing foods of modern commerce,' right? This is exactly what Dr. Price found caused dental decay. And heart disease is also caused by the consumption of significant amounts of the 'displacing foods.' They're both caused by the same thing, which is exactly why fixing a mouthful of cavities with fillings doesn't solve the heart disease – since you haven't changed the diet.

Likewise, I submit to you that dental decay and AMD go hand-in-hand because they're also caused by the same thing – namely, a diet with significant amounts of the 'displacing foods.'

CHAPTER SUMMARY

First, we see that most people on a Western diet with significant amounts of 'displacing foods,' will be deficient in lutein and zeaxanthin, which normally accumulate in and appear to protect the macula, along with meso-zeaxanthin. Perhaps much more importantly, many or even most people consuming a Westernized diet will be deficient in the fat soluble vitamins, A, D, and K2. Weston A. Price showed that it is the synergy of these three vitamins that is so crucially important to preventing degenerative diseases. Vitamins A and D signal cells to make proteins, but it is vitamin K2 that activates those proteins. Herein lies the crux of a multitude of degenerative diseases, which includes heart disease, cancer, and, in my opinion, macular degeneration.

And so lack of vitamin K2, particularly, is the huge missing link in this puzzle. Somewhat oversimplified, but lack of K2 may lead to thickening and calcification of Bruch's membrane, which creates a diffusion barrier between the choriocapillaris and the RPE. The RPE gradually accumulates waste in the form of lipofuscin and A2E, drusen form as a result of accumulation of lipids and other debris, and water even collects underneath the retina (known as pigment epithelial detachments to ophthalmologists) because the RPE is still pumping water out of the retina against the now damaged barrier (thickened and calcified Bruch's membrane), as postulated by Bird and Marshall.[1134] Now, the RPE – sickened and starved of nutrients – can't supply the demands of the photoreceptors, which might then lead to their death or malfunction.

Deficiency of vitamin K2 may also lead to failure to activate matrix Gla-protein (MGP), which normally acts to prevent arterial calcification. Because the choroid of the eye (as well as the optic nerve, retina, heart, kidney, and numerous other structures) are lined by vascular smooth muscle cells that contain MGP, a lack of vitamin K2 may lead to choroidal calcification and sclerosis, which leads to occlusion. If this occurs, there is failure of blood supply to the RPE, followed by RPE cell death, which immediately results in photoreceptor death. Each RPE cell is responsible for the lives of about 30 photoreceptors (rods and cones). When RPE cells start dying in significant numbers (atrophy), we get what is called atrophic AMD – and this is associated with a far worse prognosis for vision.

This entire proposed hypothesis ties together cardiovascular disease and AMD at the population level, vascular level, and at the molecular level as well. And guess how all of this can be prevented? The answer: Any type of ancestral diet, any one of which would include great sources of vitamins A, D, and K2, such as liver, extra virgin cod liver oil, and fish eggs. Notably, none of the ancestral diets contained supplements; nor did they contain white flour, sugar, vegetable oils, or trans fats, in any form or fashion. That's it! There it is, in a nutshell.

17 SMOKING AND AMD – ANOTHER BIG SURPRISE!

There is no question – smoking is a very significant *risk factor* for AMD. In fact, smoking is a risk factor for heart disease, other vascular diseases, lung cancer, chronic obstructive pulmonary disease (COPD), and so much more. I think this habit is one of the worst things you could do to yourself.

However, a review of the history of smoking, along with data from the Pacific Island countries and territories, strongly supports the conclusion that smoking is not a *primary cause* of macular degeneration. Let's review why.

We need to look at the history of smoking in its relation to AMD, just like we do diet. And the first thing I came across that raised my antennae was from CNN, in an article entitled, "A brief history of tobacco." The article begins,

> Tobacco was first used by the peoples of the pre-Columbian Americas. Native Americans apparently cultivated the plant and smoked it in pipes for medicinal and ceremonial purposes. Christopher Columbus brought a few tobacco leaves and seeds with him back to Europe… The first successful commercial crop was cultivated in Virginia in 1612 by Englishman John Rolfe. Within seven years, it was the colony's largest export. Over the next two centuries, the growth of tobacco as a cash crop fueled the demand in North America for slave labor.
>
> Cigarettes, which had been around in crude form since the early 1600s, didn't become widely popular in the United States until after the Civil War… sales surged again with the introduction of the "White Burley" tobacco leaf and the invention of the first practical cigarette-making machine, sponsored by tobacco baron James Buchanan "Buck" Duke, in the late 1880s.[1135]

Jordan Goodman, chapter author in the book *Ashes to Ashes: The History of Smoking and Health* wrote, "In the United States, cigarette smoking was a rare event in the years before the Civil War [1861-1865]. Even by 1869, in which year the country manufactured two million cigarettes, it was still an uncommon sight. Ten years later, however, once Bright flue-cured tobacco came to be used as the filler, the new cigarette fashion began to take hold as output soared to 300 million units."[1136]

Smoking obviously became increasingly popular after the invention of the cigarette-making machine, however, this evidence clearly indicates that there was at least a small, but significant, prevalence of smoking long before the 1930s when macular degeneration first hit the ophthalmologists' radar screens as something with prevalence. That suggested to me that smoking may not play a strong and direct role in AMD, but perhaps more of a secondary role.

In numerous studies, smoking has been shown to increase the odds of macular degeneration, generally anywhere from about two-fold up to five-fold.[1137,1138] In the majority of studies, smoking increases the risk of AMD anywhere from 2.39 to 4.22-fold.[1139,1140,1141] Not only that, but smoking is also proven to be a risk factor not only in the development of AMD but also in the progression to late AMD.[1142,1143,1144,1145,1146,1147,1148]

Cigarette smoke contains more than 7,000 chemicals, including some 400 toxins, and at least 70 known carcinogenic (cancer causing) compounds.[1149,1150] It contributes to oxidative damage, vascular alterations, inflammation, and has been shown to negatively impact the retinal pigment epithelium (RPE).[1151] Among the whole bevy of chemicals produced by lighting up, cigarette smoke also contains dioxins, which are a class of dangerous chemicals that are formed primarily during combustion processes.[1152] Though dioxins are toxic, as usual, our bodies have a way of dealing with these. In this case, there are cellular receptors known as aryl hydrocarbon receptors (AhR), to which dioxins attach,[1153] but nevertheless, there are ramifications: dioxins promote vascular endothelial growth factor (VEGF) in human RPE cells, and they've been shown to exacerbate the development of wet AMD in laser-treated mice.[1154]

Now this is where things really get interesting. The ingenious physiological design of the human body can deal reasonably well with dioxins and, as it turns out, this requires substantial vitamin A.[1155 1156]

Cigarette smoking is associated with a reduction in the serum level of retinol, which is the primary form of vitamin A that we consume, as well as a reduction in all of the following carotenoids: b-cryptoxanthin, c-carotene, b-carotene, and lycopene.[1157,1158] In further support of the fact that vitamin A and the carotenoids are utilized in the detoxification of dioxins (and perhaps other toxins in smoke), research also shows that total carotenoids are lower in current smokers than in past smokers, which is strongly suggestive that this is highly unlikely to be due to lower dietary consumption of the carotenoids in smokers.[1159]

Researchers Richard Baybutt, Agostino Molteni, and colleagues at Kansas State University have shown that just six weeks of vitamin A deficiency in rats produces emphysema and profound damage to the liver, *without smoking.*[1160] Baybutt, Ting Li, and Molteno found that, benzo(a)pyrene, another constituent of cigarette smoke, induces vitamin A depletion.[1161] The researchers found that vitamin A levels in the serum, lung, and liver of smoke-treated rats were significantly reduced and that there was an inverse relationship between vitamin A in the lung and the severity of emphysema ($P < 0.03$).[1162] In the abstract of this study, the authors summarize with, "The results of this research indicate that exposure to cigarette smoke induces vitamin A depletion in rats, which is associated with the development of emphysema."[1163]

Researchers have also shown that in actively smoking mothers, during pregnancy, versus non-smoking mothers, the fetal cord blood in the smoking mothers carried substantially more vitamins A and E than in the non-smokers.[1164] Those expectant mothers who were non-smokers but exposed to passive smoke had higher levels of vitamin A in their cord blood as well. The authors interpret this as follows:

> Active and passive maternal smoking behaviour during pregnancy increases the fetal demand for antioxidant compounds in order to counteract the oxidative burden by cigarette smoke. Against this background, the observed increase in umbilical cord serum levels of vitamins A and E may subserve antioxidative processes in response to tobacco smoke-induced oxidative stress. This would reduce the availability of vitamins A and E for fetal maturation, which is critical inasmuch as both compounds are indispensable for the developing fetus.[1165]

To simplify this a bit, the mother's body mobilizes vitamins A and E via the placenta to the baby (in the cord blood) in order to protect the baby who is also being exposed to the dangerous compounds of cigarette smoke. This is very compelling evidence that vitamin A is critical to our defense against cigarette smoke and would, therefore, be reduced in smokers.

Additional research has also shown that diets poor in vitamin A increase the risk of emphysema, or chronic obstructive pulmonary disease (COPD) in smokers.[1166 1167] Smoking also seems to actively depress serum levels of vitamin D,[1168] vitamin C,[1169] B complex vitamins, selenium, and possibly vitamin E.[1170]

Returning to the concept of vitamin A and smoking, in essence, vitamin A and some of the carotenoids that are vitamin A precursors are used to detoxify such dangerous chemicals as dioxins and benzo(a)pyrene. The question is: Could it be that smoking reduces our vitamin A (and some other vitamin or nutrient reserves) and for those who are already vitamin A deficient, the risk of AMD elevates even further? Let's examine this hypothesis further – to see if it might potentially hold water.

If this hypothesis is valid, then smokers who consume a traditional (or more traditional) diet, as opposed to the nutrient-deficient, Westernized diet, should be able to smoke more cigarettes, and yet still have a low prevalence of AMD because their vitamin A (and possibly E and carotenoid) reserves are greater. Agreed?

If this is the case, the aforementioned data regarding vitamin A and carotenoid status is strongly indicative that deficiencies of vitamin A and/or carotenoids may be risk factors for AMD in and of themselves. Correct? So let's look at the evidence regarding AMD prevalence and smoking.

SMOKING AND AMD IN THE U.S. VS. SOUTH PACIFIC ISLAND COUNTRIES

As you will recall from Chapter 13, AMD is exceedingly rare in the South Pacific island countries of Fiji, Samoa, and the Solomon Islands, as well as in the Central Pacific island nation of Kiribati. In all of these island countries, the prevalence of AMD is estimated as less than one in 500 (0.2%) and this is for people aged 60 and above. Compare that to prevalence data of the U.S where the Framingham study found 8.8% of people aged 52 to 85 with AMD and the U.S. Beaver Dam Eye Study, which found 20.9% of people aged 43 to 86 with some degree of AMD. Averaging those two U.S. studies' prevalence data shows that approximately 14.85% of people older than about 48 years have some degree of macular degeneration. *This indicates that the U.S. has approximately 74 times the prevalence of AMD as compared to the Pacific island countries of Fiji, Solomon Islands, Samoa, and Kiribati.*

So let's look at the prevalence of smoking in these countries. In the U.S. Beaver Dam Eye Study, Wisconsin, (1992), 27% of the subjects were former smokers and 12.5% were active smokers.[1171] In the Framingham Study, however, which is in Framingham, Massachusetts, the researchers found that, in 1988, 55.6% of men and 36.1% of women were smokers at both examination 1 and examination 4, which were some 26 years apart.[1172] Smoking was obviously less prevalent in much of the United States than it was in Framingham, as the overall prevalence for smoking among U.S. adults aged 18 years or more was 46% in 1965, steadily falling to 37.4% in 1970, 33.2% in 1980, and 25.5% by 1990.[1173]

Shockingly, cigarette smoking in the Pacific Island nations is dramatically more prevalent than in the U.S. In fact, the Centers for Disease Control (CDC) states that,"Pacific countries have some of the highest prevalences of current tobacco smoking [in the world]." [1174] Of the rural Melanesians (Fijians) of Fiji, between 1975 and 1981, 88% of the men and 50% of the women smoked, while 66% of the men and 33% of the women in urban areas smoked. Fewer of the Asian Indians (from India) in Fiji smoked; 62% of the men and 22% of the women in rural populations, and 42% of the men and 4% of the women in urban areas.[1175] In 2002, 49% of men and 21% of women were still smoking.[1176] Yet, in the last 15 years or more, the ophthalmologists from Fiji all conclude that macular degeneration is a medical rarity there – approximately 1 in 500 people of those older than about age 60 is affected.[1177,1178,1179]

Out of all of the Pacific island nations, the prevalence of smoking is the highest in Kiribati. Between 1975 and 1981, in urban areas 88% of the men and 74% of the women smoked, dropping only slightly in rural areas to 84% of men and 66% of women.[1180] In 1999, the situation had improved, however, 57% of men and 32% of women were still smoking.[1181] Yet Dr Rabebe Tekeraoi, Kiribati's only ophthalmologist for 113,000 people, diagnosed two cases of AMD last year (2015), and estimates their prevalence of AMD as "less than 1 in 500" people over the age of 60.[1182]

The situation is quite similar in Samoa, where in the rural areas, 75% of men and 27% of women smoked, and in the urban areas, where 57% of men and 17% of women smoked, in 1978.[1183] In 2004, 49% of men and 18% of women still smoked, indicating little change in prevalence.[1184] The population of Samoa is 193,580 as of 2016, yet Dr. Lucilla Ah Ching, ophthalmologist for Samoa, has advised that, "It is rare to see AMD in our clinic." [1185] AMD has approximately the same prevalence in Samoa, apparently, as the other South Pacific island countries, which is probably in the range of one in every 500 for those 60 years and older.

Specific smoking prevalence data wasn't available for adults in the Solomon Islands, however, research published in The New Zealand Medical Journal in 2007 states that, "Smoking prevalence in Pacific Island Countries and Territories ranges from 22% - 57% (males) and from 0.6% - 51% (females)." [1186] And research from the CDC found that, in 2011, approximately 28% of males and 18% of females, aged 13 to 15 years, were already smoking.[1187] However, once again, ophthalmologists there report AMD as extremely rare, likely less than one in 500 people over the age of 60. Three ophthalmologists caring for the whole of the Solomon Islands report seeing about 20 AMD cases per year over the last ten years, coming from a population of 680,000 people.[1188]

As you will recall, the consumption of vegetable oils in the Pacific island nations is extremely small, with the exception of Fiji. However, as reviewed, Fiji has a very large tourist population, numbering almost as many as the indigenous peoples, and this may be where the vegetable oil consumption is being served. Otherwise, PUFA type vegetable oils are virtually non-existent in Samoa, the Solomon Islands, and Kiribati.

CHAPTER SUMMARY

In most all studies, smoking is associated with a 2- to 5-fold increase in the prevalence of AMD. However, these studies were mostly completed in nations where the diets have been Westernized with significant displacing foods of modern commerce, including white flour, sugar, vegetable oils, and trans fats.

Smoking is associated with reduced micronutrient levels, particularly vitamin A and the carotenoids, but also vitamins of the B-complex, C, selenium, and possibly vitamin E. Vitamin A is known to be reduced in response to exposure to toxins in cigarette smoke, including dioxins and benzo(a)pyrene. Vitamin A consumption is an important element of traditional diets, and is severely reduced in Westernized diets.

The populations of the South Pacific Islands and territories, including Fiji, Samoa, the Solomon Islands, and Kiribati, have some of the highest prevalences of smoking in the world, and this has been confirmed for more than 40 years, yet they also have the lowest prevalences of AMD in the world, to my knowledge. What do they *not have*? Not nearly as much processed foods, particularly those containing vegetable oils and trans fats. This is a very strong indictment of the dangers of vegetable oils in the causation of AMD – as well as some of our strongest evidence of all that traditional diets prevent AMD even under adverse conditions.

With regard to smoking and AMD, all of this data suggests that it is not smoking per se that causes the much greater increase in the prevalence of AMD – it is that smoking depresses the micronutrients that are so critical in preventing AMD – perhaps particularly, vitamin A. Without question, a nutrient-dense diet protects from the development of AMD, even in the face of smoking.

My advice: Consume a nutrient-dense diet, which does not contain the 'displacing foods of modern commerce' – and never, ever, ever smoke.

Part VI

Eating to Prevent & Treat AMD

18 SYNTHETIC VITAMINS AND MULTIVITAMINS – SHOULD WE STEER CLEAR?

The discovery that tables may groan with food and that we may nevertheless face a form of starvation has driven home the fact that we have applied science and technology none too wisely in the preparation of food.

~ *New York Times EDITORIAL, 1941* ~

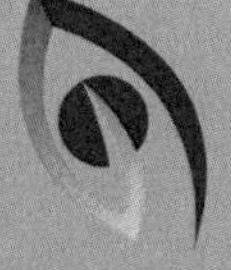

Are we starving, actually? In so many regards, I believe the answer is yes. We're starving for nutrients – micronutrients, that is. We're severely deprived of vitamins and minerals, as I hope you're beginning to see.

Today, when we hear the term "vitamin" or "multivitamins," most of us immediately envision a pill or a tablet. It's a tragedy that we've somehow bought into this erroneous fallacy that great sources of vitamins come in bottles, pills, and "fortified" foods. We've been led to believe by the Big Food manufacturers and the supplement industry that a whole slew of vitamins listed on a label somehow makes for a healthy product. Few people, I am sure, envision chicken or beef liver, fish eggs, butter from cows grazing on green grass, or extra virgin cod liver oil, when they hear the phrase "rich in vitamins." Yet, our pre 20th century ancestors and all the "tribes" and cultures that Weston A. Price found to be so vibrantly healthy somehow not only knew this, but they knew of the life-giving, health-providing properties of these foods – and without ever knowing the term "vitamin."

Interestingly enough, all wildlife instinctively know where the micronutrients are. When lions capture and kill their prey, they tear open the belly and devour the liver, heart, and kidneys first, unless they can't get there due to competition from other animals.[1189] The liver, which is the most nutrient-dense food available, is their most desired food. Alaskan fisherman tell me they've witnessed bears catch salmon, squeeze out their roe (eggs), eat the roe, and toss the fish back in the water still alive and well. Eagles often kill their prey and eat the organs of the belly, while leaving the remainder of the carcass behind. Even insects know where the nutrient-dense foods are, which is why you won't find them in most any white flour, polished white rice, or sugar. But, leave a little access to true 100% whole-grain flour or sprouted brown rice, and you'll soon have bugs.

Somehow, we've abandoned these instincts. We've developed a sort of collective amnesia for the health-providing properties of *whole food.*

In an article entitled "The Vitamin Myth: Why We Think We Need Supplements," published in *The Atlantic*, author Paul Offit wrote,

> On October 10, 2011, researchers from the University of Minnesota found that women who took supplemental multivitamins died at rates higher than those who didn't. Two days later, researchers from the Cleveland Clinic found that men who took vitamin E had an increased risk of prostate cancer. 'It's been a tough week for vitamins,' said Carrie Gann of ABC News.
>
> These findings weren't new. Seven previous studies had already shown that vitamins increased the risk of cancer and heart disease and shortened lives. Still, in 2012, more than half of all Americans took some form of vitamin supplements. What few people realize, however, is that their fascination with vitamins can be traced back to one man. A man who was so spectacularly right that he won two Nobel Prizes and so spectacularly wrong that he was arguably the world's greatest quack.[1190]

The scientist that Offit was referring to in this passage was Linus Pauling, a scientist that believed mega-doses of vitamin C would not only prevent the common cold, but cancer as well. He urged the public to take 3,000 milligrams of vitamin C daily (about 50 times the recommended daily allowance – RDA) while taking 18,000 milligrams (18 grams) daily himself. His books, Vitamin C and the Common Cold (1970) and *Vitamin C, the Common Cold and the Flu* (1976) were best sellers. Vitamin C sales more than quadrupled and drugstores couldn't keep up with the demand. But, was he right? Would anyone dare question the assertions of a Nobel Prize winner? Indeed, researchers set out to affirm or disaffirm Pauling's claims. Their findings? As Offit correctly states, "At least 15 studies have now shown that vitamin C doesn't treat the common cold." [1191] Mind you, this is synthetic vitamin C. These studies weren't about eating oranges, tangerines, and kiwi.

Linus Pauling's claim that high-dose synthetic vitamin C cured cancer was also ousted – by two controlled clinical trials.[1192] Sadly enough, Pauling's wife died of stomach cancer in late 1980. Pauling himself died with prostate cancer, in 1994.

Pauling's anecdote illustrates a common theme: Vitamins that come in synthetic form not only fail to provide impressive results, they make us significantly less healthy. Worse yet, they cause us to die a little sooner.

A BRIEF HISTORY OF VITAMINS

In 1747, James Lind, a Scottish physician who also served as naval surgeon on the HMS *Salisbury*, set out to determine a cure for Scurvy. Until then, scurvy, which is caused by a vitamin C deficiency, generally caused the death of about half of the men in any voyage between Europe and the Caribbean Islands. In what was likely the first controlled experiment, Lind divided sailors up into groups of two, and administered to each pair of sailors one of either hard cider, vitriol (sulfuric acid and alcohol), vinegar, seawater, two oranges and a lemon, or an "electuary," which was a creative mix of garlic, mustard seed, balsam of Peru, dried radish root, and gum myrrh. Though the experiment was supposed to last two weeks, the pair that received the lemon and oranges ran out of their supplement within a week. However, those two men recovered so rapidly from their early onset of scurvy that they were able to assist Dr. Lind in the care of the others who were sick.[1193] Eventually, vitamin C containing citrus fruits would come to be known as "antiscorbutics," which literally translates into anti-scurvy foods. But it would be nearly 200 years, in the year 1932, before vitamin C was actually isolated and identified.[1194] [1195]

Beriberi, a dreaded condition of neuropathy, found its roots in a monotonous diet consisting primarily of highly polished white rice. When steel roller mill technology began being utilized for polishing the bran from rice, converting brown rice to white rice, yet another refined food was created. This entire concept has similarities to that of wheat milling and the difference between whole-grain flour and white flour. Milling of rice in this fashion may have come a little sooner than that for wheat, and though the disease beriberi was described as early as the 17th century, the condition spread quickly following the mass production of polished white rice, particularly in Asia. Between 1878 and 1882, a third of the Japanese navy was ill with beriberi. This condition presents as either "wet beriberi," with congestive heart failure and massive edema (swelling) of the legs, or "dry beriberi," with a peripheral neuropathy characterized by pain and weakness in the legs, numbness, and severe lack of appetite despite extreme weight loss. The condition often led to death by suffocating convulsions.[1196]

Between 1878 and 1933, the etiology of beriberi remained highly elusive. Numerous physicians and researchers would be involved in unlocking the cause of this dreadful disease. During most of this period, the concept of vitamins had not yet been developed. As such, most physicians held the popular opinion of that time that an infectious agent was the cause. However, Dutch physician, Christiaan Eijkman (1858 – 1930), noted that chickens fed polished white rice developed the disease, but they did not when fed brown rice. He considered the possibility of a nutritional deficiency, but then rejected the hypothesis. In 1912, Casamir Funk suggested a deficiency of a "vitamine," a substance present in brown rice, but not in white rice. Eventually, there was agreement that a diet consisting largely of white rice could induce beriberi, whereas brown rice or even the "polishings" left over from the white rice could treat the condition. In 1933, Robert Runnels Williams (1886-1965), a dedicated chemist, would finally isolate the nutrient missing in the diet of those affected, which was thiamine.[1197] The vitamin was eventually mass produced and used to "fortify" foods to prevent beriberi.

Catherine Price, author of *Vitamania,* regarding the elusive nature of finding vitamins in scenarios such as that of beriberi, wrote, "...Germ theory's central tenet—that disease is caused by the *presence* of something—hid the idea that disease could also be caused by something that is *lacking*. Germ theory's light was so bright, so illuminating, that it blinded scientists to the idea that disease could be caused by something that wasn't there." [1180]

As Dr. Price repeatedly found in those consuming traditional diets, the presence of fat-soluble vitamins was ten-fold greater than that of modernized diets, while both water soluble vitamins and minerals were also dramatically greater. And, of course, those that consumed the 'displacing foods,' with their associated lack of vitamins and minerals, developed a myriad of degenerative diseases.

More than a century ago, animal feeding experiments showed that a diet based on pure carbohydrates, fats, and proteins, supplemented with minerals and water, could not sustain growth in animals, nor survival.[1198] However, just adding small quantities of whole, unpasteurized milk to the diet restored normal growth and survival. These observations eventually led to the concept of 'vitamines,' a term coined by Casimir Funk, in 1912. The term 'vitamines,' was derived from the term 'vital amines' and later shortened to vitamins.[1199] Vitamins, it was determined, were the substances present in foods in vanishingly small quantities, which allowed growth, vitality, and even sustained life.

After physicians and scientists discovered cures for scurvy, beriberi, and pellagra (to be reviewed), and vitamins could be synthesized and produced en masse, governments began to "fortify" various foods, which is the addition of synthetic vitamins, thereby attempting to eliminate such diseases. And it seems that, ever since, we've had an obsession with synthetic vitamins.

In fact, though fortification of foods is no longer mandatory in the United States, many manufacturers continue to fortify their foods, just as they did many decades ago. The majority of bread and other grain products are made with flour that has been enriched with thiamin, niacin, riboflavin, and iron. Ready to eat cereals are typically made with added iron, B vitamins, including folate and most all milk is fortified with vitamin D and has been since 1933.[1200] The same is true of breakfast cereals, rolls, pastries, protein bars, and tens of thousands of other foods. But, as Catherine Price discusses in her book, *Vitamania,* this has increased our dependency on synthetic vitamins while allowing us to consume otherwise nutrient-deficient, processed foods. She wrote,

> Indeed, the so-called standard American diet—high in refined grains and sweets, and associated with "Western" diseases like heart disease and cancer—could not have developed without the help of synthetic vitamins. This has led to an odd paradox. Given the limitations of the global food supply and consumer preferences, synthetic vitamins are truly essential for the prevention of nutritional deficiency diseases—not just in the developing world, but here, too. In America, however, where synthetic vitamins are widely used to correct nutritional deficits caused by processing, they've also contributed to the very problem they were meant to fix. While they're designed—and now often required—to keep us healthy, synthetic vitamins also enable the very products and dietary habits that are making us sick.
>
> That itself is unnerving. But vitamins haven't just shaped our food supply; they've also shaped our minds. More so than any other component of food, vitamins are responsible for our current approach to nutrition, a perfectionist attitude that's simultaneously misguided and fantastically naïve." [1201]

'Fantastically naïve' is correct and, despite my own intense investigation of nutrition for nearly two-and-a-half years, I myself remained just as naïve regarding our severe lack of vitamins and minerals, particularly the fat soluble vitamins – until I read Weston A. Price's *Nutrition and Physical Degeneration* back in 2013. And if we consider that Americans, like many developed nations today, are consuming 64% to 70% of their calories from three nutrient-deficient foods (white flour, sugar, and vegetable oils), we come to the sobering realization that, if it weren't for the synthetic fortification of foods, we would have vitamin deficiency diseases far, far worse than at anytime in the history of the world. Catherine Price hit the nail on the head: fortification of our foods with synthetic vitamins contributes to the very problems they were intended to resolve. But the question remains, are we seeing a plethora of disease and disease conditions, despite fortification? Is fortification of our nutrient-deprived, processed food, allowing us to dig ourselves deeper into nutritional deprivation?

THE FUNDAMENTAL QUESTIONS OF THIS CHAPTER ARE THESE:

- Should we be consuming synthetically produced vitamins, or multivitamins? Perhaps this question might be rephrased as follows: Which one is *most beneficial*: Synthetic vitamins – or the vitamins contained in natural food?
- Despite the oft repeated phrase, "Vitamin deficiencies are rare in the U.S," is this actually a fallacy? Are we, in fact, significantly depleted in many vitamins as well as the minerals and other cofactors that act synergistically with them, despite consuming synthetic vitamins and fortified foods?
- Could multiple vitamin deficiencies play a role, possibly even a pivotal role, in the development of macular degeneration – despite our near obsession with consuming synthetic vitamins?

DO SYNTHETIC VITAMINS PREVENT AMD?

Ophthalmologists, like most everyone else, have long held the hypothesis that AMD is caused, at least in part, by reactive oxygen species – that is, charged particles or free radicals that are produced during metabolism. As the theory continues, if this is so, what we must do is consume (synthetic) antioxidant vitamins, which "will quench these free radicals, thereby limiting the damage." The theory certainly sounds plausible, and it has been tested quite extensively, but *almost always using synthetic vitamin supplements, rather than whole food*. Let's see what the research shows.

Cochrane, formerly known as the Cochrane Collaboration, is an organization of some 37,000 scientists, researchers, professionals, and others who work as a global independent network to provide credible, unbiased health information to the collective scientific body of work. When Cochrane has reviewed anything, you can be sure that the conclusion will be about as fair, unbiased, scientifically rigorous, and without commercial influence, as any study available. It doesn't mean necessarily that even Cochrane is always correct, remember, it's "science." It's a search for the truth, which is often pretty hard to find.

That said, fortunately for you and I, the Cochrane Eyes and Vision Group, London School of Hygiene & Tropical Medicine, lead by Jennifer Evans, MSc, PhD, has reviewed all of the available research regarding synthetic vitamin supplementation and AMD, which was published in 2012.

Their first task: "To examine the evidence as to whether or not taking antioxidant vitamin or mineral supplements prevents the development of AMD." Their results: "We included four randomized controlled trials in this review; 62,520 people were included in the analyses. The trials were conducted in Australia, Finland and the USA and investigated vitamin E and beta-carotene supplements...**People who took these supplements were not at decreased (or increased) risk of developing AMD.**" Their final conclusion: **"There is accumulating evidence that taking vitamin E or beta-carotene supplements will not prevent or delay the onset of AMD. There is no evidence with respect to other antioxidant supplements, such as vitamin C, lutein, zeaxanthin, or any of the commonly marketed multivitamin combinations."** [1202]

Clearly, synthetic vitamin supplements do not prevent the development of AMD.

DO SYNTHETIC VITAMINS SLOW THE PROGRESSION OF AMD?

The next question: Do multivitamins delay the progression of AMD that is already established? The trials that most ophthalmologists rely on here are the Age Related Eye Disease Studies (AREDS). The first AREDS trial, published in 2001, involved 3640 subjects, 55 to 80 years old, who were randomized to receive either a daily antioxidant supplement (PreserVision, Bausch & Lomb), which consisted of vitamin C (500mg), vitamin E (400 IU), beta carotene (15mg), zinc oxide (80mg), and copper (2mg cupric oxide), or placebo. **The experimental group that received the antioxidants had a reduced rate of progression of intermediate AMD to advanced stages of AMD by 25% over a period of 5 years, with an associated 19% reduction in the risk of moderate visual loss.**[1203] The researchers concluded that, if all Americans with either intermediate AMD or advanced AMD in one eye were to consume these synthetic vitamin supplements, more than 300,000 people might avoid the development of advanced AMD over the next five years.[1204]

The AREDS 2 trial sought to determine whether adding the carotenoids found in dark leafy green vegetables, lutein and zeaxanthin, long-chain omega-3 fatty acids (docosahexaenoic acid {DHA} and eicosapentaenoic acid {EPA}), or both might further reduce the risk of progression of AMD. Their conclusion? **"Addition of lutein +zeaxanthin, DHA + EPA, or both to the AREDS formulation in primary analyses did not further reduce risk of progression to advanced AMD. However, because of potential increased incidence of lung cancer in former smokers, lutein + zeaxanthin could be an appropriate carotenoid substitute in the AREDS formulation."** [1205]

Just so we're clear, neither adding in lutein and zeaxanthin, nor the long-chain omega-3 fatty acids, had any positive effect. However, in this study, the researchers noted an increased risk of lung cancer in smokers and former smokers, i.e., there were 23 lung cancer cases in the beta-carotene group (2.0%) versus 11 in the no beta-carotene group (0.9%), which was statistically significant ($P = .04$).[1206]

Once again, Jennifer Evans, PhD and the Cochrane collaborative team worked their magic to evaluate whether synthetic vitamin supplementation might be of benefit to those who already have AMD. They systematically evaluated 13 randomized controlled trials that included 6150 participants, including five trials in the USA, two in the UK, two in Austria, and one each in Australia, China, Italy, and Switzerland. Their conclusion? **"The review of trials found that supplementation with antioxidants and zinc may be of modest benefit in people with AMD. This was mainly seen in one large trial [AREDS] that followed up participants for an average of six years. The other smaller trials with shorter follow-up do not provide evidence of any benefit." They add, "Although generally regarded as safe, vitamin supplements may have harmful effects."** [1207]

The evidence is clear. Of the 13 trials that looked at whether or not antioxidant synthetic vitamins would benefit patients with existing AMD, primarily just one trial – the AREDS1 trial – found any benefit at all, and that benefit was only for one out of every four patients that already had intermediate AMD or advanced AMD in one eye. If it weren't for that one trial, no ophthalmologist could recommend synthetic vitamins based on any science at all.

Another study showed that supplementation with beta-carotene conferred a relative 17% increased risk of lung cancer in smokers.[1208] And a large international trial, lasting about seven years, showed that high-dose (400 IU) vitamin E consumption, which is the same as that in the AREDS trial, was associated with an increased risk of heart failure and hospitalization for heart failure, among people with diabetes or existing heart disease.[1209]

THE PARADOX OF MULTIVITAMINS AND PROGRESSION OF AMD

It is worth reviewing the fact that, the AREDS vitamin supplements have not been shown to prevent AMD. They've only been shown to help prevent progression of AMD in 25% of people that already have intermediate AMD or advanced AMD in one eye. Yet, many eye care providers and patients alike, believe that they should take the vitamins to *prevent* AMD. This is, in my opinion, quite the paradox. On the one hand, based on one single study, we're advising patients to take multivitamin supplements (AREDS formula) to prevent progression of AMD, but yet at the same time, that formula cannot help prevent the condition? Just think about that one… and I'll provide my position in the Chapter Summary.

COULD THE AREDS SUPPLEMENTS MAKE AMD WORSE?

Carl Awh, MD, ophthalmologist and vitreo-retinal specialist at Tennessee Retina in Nashville, Tennessee, and colleagues, evaluated data from the patients in the AREDS participants based on certain genotypes. They found that a certain subset of patients, those with high CFH and low ARMS2 (both genotypes that affect AMD risk), which was 13% of the entire group of subjects, had a 135% higher chance of progressing to advanced AMD if they were in the supplement group.[1210] [1211] In an interview with Dr. Awh published in Medscape, he said "It's something to keep in mind as we recommend nutritional therapy for people with macular degeneration. We don't want to give a therapy to an identifiable subgroup of people that more than doubles their risk of disease progression." [1212]

SYNTHETIC VITAMIN MANUFACTURERS CLAIMS ARE INCONSISTENT WITH THE SCIENTIFIC EVIDENCE…

A recent study by Jennifer J. Yong and colleagues at Yale-New Haven Hospital-Waterbury Hospital, in Waterbury, Connecticut, reviewed the fact that manufacturers of multivitamin supplements for individuals with AMD are routinely making claims that are inconsistent with the results of the AREDS study. Not only are manufacturers producing vitamin supplements that contain different amounts of vitamins and nutrients than those used in the AREDS or AREDS2 study, but some also add minerals and herbal extracts that were not part of the AREDS formulas. Quite frankly, I find this only minimally concerning, but what is much more alarming is the fact that the researchers find that the manufacturers claims are not scientifically accurate. The authors of this study report that, of eleven ocular nutritional supplements reviewed, "All the individual supplements claimed to 'support,' 'protect,' 'help,' or 'promote' vision and eye health, but none specified that there is no proven benefit in using nutritional supplements for primary prevention of eye disease." [1213]

Recall that the AREDS trials provided no evidence at all that these supplements prevent AMD and, in fact, the studies show that they only potentially benefit some of those who already have intermediate AMD or advanced AMD in one eye. The bottom line here? Be cautious of the claims made by the manufacturers. Collectively, the supplement makers are selling 36 billion dollars worth of supplements per year in the U.S alone. Their motivation may not always be altruistic.

SYNTHETIC VITAMINS – DO THE META-ANALYSES INDICATE THAT MULTIVITAMINS RESULT IN AN INCREASED RISK OF DEATH?

Cochrane researchers worked diligently for a long, long time on this one. In 2012, they published their systematic review of some 78 randomized clinical trials to evaluate whether antioxidant supplements prolong life, are neutral, or demonstrate harmful effects and shorten our lives. The 2008 Cochrane review had already demonstrated that multivitamin supplements increase the risk of death from all causes.

Back to the 2012 Cochrane review. In this systematic review, 78 trials involving 296,707 participants who were randomized to either antioxidant supplements that included beta-carotene, vitamin A, vitamin C, vitamin E, and selenium, or placebo, or no intervention at all (not even placebo), were analyzed. **When the researchers analyzed only the studies with a "low risk of bias," (e.g., not funded by companies that profit from the sales of multivitamins), they found that those people taking the supplements were 1.04 times as likely to die as were the controls.** The authors wrote, "The increased risk of mortality was associated with beta-carotene and possibly vitamin E and vitamin A, but was not associated with the use of vitamin C or selenium. The current evidence does not support the use of antioxidant supplements in the general population or in patients with various diseases." [1214]

The take home message: None of us should be taking synthetic multivitamin and mineral supplements, except under very unusual circumstances, for example, if we cannot for any reason, eat whole foods. There is a far superior alternative…

THE DILEMMA WITH WHOLE FOODS VERSUS 'VITAMINS' AND FDA PROMOTION…

Author, lecturer, and filmmaker, G. Edward Griffin, who wrote the book *World Without Cancer*, made the following statement in a lecture given regarding his book: "Anything that comes from nature cannot be patented. They [the pharmaceutical industry] are not interested in that. So, we translate that into the real world of FDA approval – surely these drug companies aren't going to spend 20 million dollars or more testing any substance from nature – because it can't be patented. That and, of course, the FDA says 'It's illegal to use unless its been tested for efficacy and safety.' Now you see the catch-22 you're in there. Nothing from nature, regardless of how effective it might be, will ever be proven safe or effective according to the FDA. It'll never be! Because nobody's going to spend the money to go through the tests. So therefore, everything from nature will always be condemned by the FDA as unproven." [1215]

He's right. This is why there are no trials that spend hundreds of millions of dollars testing a whole, unprocessed food diet, complete with pastured meats from organic farms, against the typical processed food-laden Standard American Diet. Who would benefit? We the people would. But, who's going to pay for it? If the healthy diet proves – after a ten year billion dollar trial – that it helps prevent all sorts of chronic disease, there is nothing to sell at the conclusion except organically raised crops and pastured meats and eggs. There's no drug that can be sold for a few hundred million or a couple billion dollars a year. Hence, the reason there are no such trials and why we're unlikely to ever see such trials – so don't look for them. This is why we must also look at epidemiologic data, that is, the population studies and our history. There's an enormous ongoing trial in the USA and many other nations – except that almost everyone in the entire nation is in the experimental group – and no one signed informed consent.

CHAPTER SUMMARY

The data is clear. If you want to have optimum nutrition, there is only one way to get that: whole, natural, organic, unprocessed foods. Multivitamins in pill form are a pathetic substitute for the brilliant nutrition of whole foods, raised in traditional fashions, and prepared according to the traditions of our ancestors.

However, if after reading this book, you elect to continue a Westernized diet, with plenty of processed foods, then you might want to consider taking the original AREDS formula vitamins, if and only if, you already have AMD. Keep in mind these vitamins are associated with a higher risk of heart failure in diabetics and those already affected with cardiovascular disease; also, anything with beta-carotene will likely increase the risk of lung cancer in smokers or former smokers. You should also keep in mind that there is only a one in four chance they will help you and, if you're among the 13% with high CFH and low ARMS2 genes, these supplements will more than double your risk of progression. The bottom line? Even AREDS formula multivitamins might be associated with greater risks to your health and will likely cause your earlier demise. Seventy-eight studies proving a higher death rate from all causes for people consuming multivitamins cannot be wrong.

The fact that multivitamins helped 25% of the people consuming them in the AREDS trials is testimony to one thing: the 25 percent of those that benefitted had nutrient deficiencies so great, that even synthetic vitamins helped them. For that segment of the population, they worked. *The fact that the consumption of multivitamins had no effect on the prevention of macular degeneration in the first place, yet helped to prevent progression of AMD in 25% of the people that already had moderate AMD, is further evidence that those people who are at this stage of AMD have the greatest nutrient deficiencies.* I ask you, can any other reasonable and logical conclusions be drawn from this data?

If you want to be healthier and prevent, control, or reverse AMD, then multivitamins are definitely not your best choice. For that, you need, once again – at the risk of sounding like a broken record – whole, unprocessed foods, straight from nature – and as natural as you can get them (possibly a reason to consider organic options).

To suggest that nutrition scientists currently have limited understanding of the interactions of vitamins, minerals, and a whole slew of other cofactors would be the understatement of the century. In fact, I would submit that we don't understand as much as one-tenth of one percent of the inconceivable complexity of the interactions between vitamins, minerals, cofactors, phytonutrients, polyphenols, and numerous other biologically active molecules that come from none other than whole foods. Weston A. Price offered similar sentiment, which is why he continually advocated for the consumption of whole, natural foods. In his book, *Nutrition and Physical Degeneration,* he wrote, "Great harm is done, in my judgment, by the sale and use of substitutes for natural foods." [1216]

Congratulations, we've reached Base Camp 3 of our Mount Everest! We're headed for the summit!

19 WHOLE UNPROCESSED FOODS: PASTURED MEATS, PASTURED EGGS, RAW MILK, AND WILD-CAUGHT FISH – ALL PREFERRED

Unlike the real Mount Everest, the last of our climb – the trek to the summit – is the easiest. We've covered all of the history, the fundamental science, the prevalence data, the data correlating sugar and vegetable oils (as markers of processed foods) to AMD, and now finally, in Part VI, we're mostly putting together the details into an actionable plan.

In this chapter, we will deal with a few issues that may not directly have an effect on developing AMD, but nevertheless, play an important role in our general health. As such, I believe it's worth including these details.

One of the characteristics of healthy diets that might be worth reiterating is that we find from all of the available research, beginning with the research of Weston A. Price, to numerous contemporary studies of various populations and tribes all around the world, that you can be healthy choosing almost any variety of macronutrient ratio (protein: fat: carbs). We've reviewed this before. So, if you prefer lots of meat, like I do, then eat that way. If you prefer a diet that's mostly all carbs, like potatoes, rice, cassava, yucca root, plantains, etc., then of course, eat that way. If you prefer an extremely high fat diet, loaded with butter, cream, eggs, heavily marbled steaks, then eat that way! *Every one of those diets will be perfectly healthy, as long as you virtually eliminate the five "foods" that are an abomination to society and to our health: White flour, sugar, vegetable oils, trans fats, and all processed, man-made foods.*

Once those five groups of "foods" are eliminated, the next step is to try to consume food in a way that is consistent with what Nature intended. It might be best if your fruits and vegetables are raised organically (we'll review this shortly), but the most important thing is soil conditions, because that is where those foods get their nutrients. Strongly consider trying to get your fruits and vegetables locally, especially if available from a local farmer. With regard to animals, it is far better to eat meats raised in pastured conditions that have consumed foods from their natural habitat, and we'll review this in detail.

WHOLE UNPROCESSED FOODS – ORGANIC VERSUS CONVENTIONAL

I've repeated the term "whole, unprocessed organic foods" so often in this book you're probably beginning to cringe when I write it again. Well, perhaps the point is taken, but it's a huge point, and those four words underlie the very foundations of this book and the treatment of macular degeneration.

Over the past few years, without actually investigating the research, we've been purchasing organic options most of the time. Seems reasonable that avoiding pesticides, herbicides, and genetically modified organisms (GMOs) would be the best choice, right? But, is organic truly different and, if so, is it worth the extra cost? Will it make a difference in our health? Let's look at the available research before we just give organic the 'ole thumbs up and conventional the thumbs down.

In 2012, an article published in *Scientific American*, entitled "Are lower pesticide residues a good reason to buy organic? Probably not." The article may have found its roots in a study completed at Stanford University, which found no nutritional benefit to organic foods. Of course, according to *Scientific American* author, Christie Wilcox, organic food supporters say that "'Stanford missed the point... it's not about what organic foods have in them, it's what they don't.' After all, avoidance of pesticide residues is the #1 reason why people buy organic foods."[1217]

And that is exactly right. There are real and potential benefits in avoiding pesticides and herbicides, that may not have been appreciated by the Stanford produced study. In the Stanford study, Smith-Spangler and colleagues assessed some 17 studies in humans and 223 studies of nutrient and contaminant levels in foods, "finding no significant differences between populations by food type for allergic outcomes (eczema, wheeze, atopic sensitization) or symptomatic Campylobacter infection."[1218] The study authors purported that pesticide residues were 30% lower in organic versus conventionally raised produce and they also acknowledged that "the risk for isolating bacteria resistant to 3 or more antibiotics was higher in conventional than in organic chicken and pork (risk difference, 33%)."[1219] The study also found that 38 percent of conventional produce tested contained detectable pesticide residues, versus only 7 percent for the organic produce.[1220] The latter may come by cross-contamination from conventional to organic fields.

Austrian researchers, Dr. Alberta Velimirov and Dr. Thomas Lindenthal, published a highly critical appraisal of the Stanford study, citing a number of oversights and other issues with the study. For example, Smith-Spangler et al acknowledged that the risks of contamination with pesticide residues was lower in organic produce, but they purportedly used an unusual metric that reduced the level of risk to just 30% lower, whereas this figure would have been 81% if conventional statistical analyses were used.[1221] Velimirov and Lindenthal list the following additional issues with the study:

- There was a significantly lower risk of eczema in young children who consumed organic dairy.
- The reduction in pesticide residues is trivialized in the discussion on the basis that the risk of exposure that exceeds allowable limits is relatively low.
- The organic produce, overall, contained higher levels of phenols, which are believed to help prevent cancer.

- The authors of the Stanford study minimize the importance of bacterial antibiotic resistance developing as a result of consuming animal products treated with antibiotics.
- The authors correctly assert that phosphorus levels are higher in organic produce, which is beneficial, but fail to list increased beneficial fatty acids in breast milk in their summary.
- The authors fail to mention in their summary that organic products have higher levels of phenols.
- The authors fail to list in their summary that organically produced cow's milk has higher levels of omega-3 fatty acids and vaccenic acid (a healthy naturally occurring trans fat).
- The authors fail to list in their summary that organic produce has lower levels of mycotoxin deoxynivalenol in cereals. [1222]

The Stanford study was further critiqued by Professor Charles Benbrook of the Center for Sustaining Agriculture and Natural Resources at Washington State University.[1223] In addition to perhaps echoing the findings of Velmirov and Lindenthal, Professor Benbrook cited a fundamental flaw of the study as follows: "The team's answer to the basic question, 'Is organic food more nutritious or safer?,' is based on their judgment of whether published studies provide evidence of a clinically significant impact or improvement in health. Very few studies are designed or conducted in a way that could isolate the impact or contribution of a switch to organic food from the many other factors that influence a given individual's health. Studies capable of doing so would be very expensive, and to date, none have been carried out in the U.S." [1224] Benbrook went on to state,

> Over time, I believe that unbiased analysis coupled with modern-day science is likely to show with increasing clarity that growing and consuming organic food, especially in conjunction with healthy diets rich in fresh, whole foods, is one of the best health-promotion investments we can make today as individuals, famiiies, and a society.[1225]

Benbrook also reviewed that, studies spanning the duration of a woman's pregnancy through the first few years of a child's life "provide encouraging evidence that organic food can reduce the odds of some adverse health impacts, including birth defects, neuro-behavioral and learning problems, autism, and eczema."[1226 1227 1228 1229 1230 1231 1232]

In the states of Minnesota, Montana, North Dakota, and South Dakota, where most of the spring durum wheat is grown in the U.S., more than 85% of the acreage is treated with chlorphenoxy herbicides, such as 2,4-dichlorophenoxyacetic acid (2,4-D) and 4-chloro-2-methylphenoxyacetic acid (MCPA). For counties where the applications are highest, the research shows that infants conceived during the months of April – June, which is when the herbicides are applied, had significantly increased chances of being born with circulatory/respiratory malformations (not heart) compared with births at other times of the year. Infant death from congenital anomalies also increased signifantly in high-wheat counties for males, but not for females. The authors point out that the chlorphenoxy herbicides are in widespread use on wheat crops.[1233]

There's a mountain of additional research, but the point is, even for those of us who are not going to have children again, perhaps we might be concerned for our grandchildren or great grandchildren to be? And if herbicides and pesticides can cause so much harm in fetuses, infants, and young children, could they even possibly be good for us?

My suggestion is this: If you can afford the additional cost to go organic, by all means do so. If you cannot, just realize that you're still far better off consuming lots of conventionally raised fruits and vegetables than you would consuming processed foods with any significant amounts of white flour, sugar, vegetable oils, and trans fats.

EGGS – SUPERMARKET, CAGE-FREE, ORGANIC, FREE-RANGE, OR PASTURED?

First of all, there are multiple terms regarding eggs that I imagine has resulted in a lot of confusion – it certainly was confusing to me until I researched this a bit. Here's the situation: If eggs are not labeled otherwise, you can anticipate that they're from hens kept in battery-cages, which is the worst possible scenario and the least healthy eggs for us to consume. If they're labeled "Cage-Free," this means that they're likely kept indoors, in huge buildings, with no outdoor access. If labeled "Free-Range" or "Free Roaming," that means they have outdoor access, though the access may be incredibly limited, mostly unavailable, and the chickens may not even know how to get there. The "Certified Organic" label means that they're not in battery cages, the hens have outdoor access, and their feed is organic, vegetarian, and free of pesticides and antibiotics. **There's only one more category, and that is "Pasture-Raised." This is the category you want.** Ideally, this means that the hens are walking around outdoors with lots of room, they're eating grass and insects, like they should, and they're happy hens.[1234] Their eggs are by far the healthiest, which we'll look at next.

According to SELFNutritionData, one cup worth of eggs (approximately three eggs) contains the following percentage of RDA of the following vitamins and minerals: 16% of vitamin A, 41% of riboflavin, 7% of vitamin E, 15% of folate, 25% of B12, 19% of pantothenic acid, 23% of phosphorus, 10% of zinc, and 60% of selenium.[1235]

When it comes to egg quality, one study divided hens into either pastured groups consuming alfalfa, red and white clover, or mixed grasses, with all three receiving some hen mash versus caged hens consuming a commercial diet. In this study, the eggs of pastured hens had twice as much vitamin E, twice as much long-chain omega-3 fats, 2.5-fold more total omega-3 fatty acids, and less than half the ratio of the omega-6 to omega-3 fatty acids. Vitamin A concentration was also 38% higher in the pastured hens' eggs, though the total concentration didn't differ.[1236] Clearly, pastured hens produce much more nutrient-dense eggs.

MILK – PASTEURIZED MILK IS PROCESSED & RAW MILK IS FAR SUPERIOR

Paleo diet authors may subscribe to the principle that milk cannot be safely consumed because "we're not adapted to drinking milk from an evolutionary standpoint." However, Weston A. Price and many others since have found that many societies drink raw milk as a staple of their diet and they either are, or were, extremely healthy. The first example noted by Price was the Swiss villagers of the Loetschental Valley, followed by the Masai of East Africa, and we now know that the Rendille and the Samburu of East Africa are virtually identical to the Masai in this regard.

According to *RealMilk.com*, "Real milk is milk that comes from pastured cows, that contains all the fat and that has not been processed in any way—it is raw and unhomogenized. Real milk that has been produced under sanitary and healthy conditions is a safe and healthy food. It is important that the cows are healthy (tested free of TB and undulant fever) and do not have any infections (such as mastitis). The cows should be eating food appropriate to cows, which is mostly grass, hay or silage, with only a small amount of grain, if any. The milk should be full-fat milk, as many important anti-microbial and health-supporting components are in the fat." [1237]

Mainstream authorities have held that pasteurization is required to make milk safe to consume, but this belief system runs counter to centuries of history in not only the safety of raw milk consumption, but much evidence for associated health benefits. According to the research of Sally Fallon of the Weston A. Price Foundation, "All outbreaks of salmonella from contaminated milk in recent decades—and there have been many—have occurred in pasteurized milk. This includes a 1985 outbreak in Illiinois that struck over 14,000 people causing at least one death... Raw milk contains lactic-acid producing bacteria that protect against pathogens. Pasteurization destroys these helpful organisms, leaving the finished product devoid of any protective mechanism should undesirable bacteria inadvertently contaminate the supply."

Summarizing other issues presented by Sally Fallon:

- Pasteurization alters the amino acids lysine and tyrosine, reducing protein availability
- Pasteurization reduces vitamin C by 50 percent or more and B-complex vitamins up to 80%
- Milk consumption in civilized societies is linked to diabetes
- Pasteurization destroys the natural enzymes in milk, which normally help one to assimilate the minerals in the milk
- Vitamin D2 or D3 is added to pasteurized milk, while the former is toxic and has been linked to heart disease and the latter is difficult to absorb
- Powdered skim milk is often added to commercial mik, the cholesterol of which is known to be oxidized, thereby contributing to atherosclerosis.[1238]

Bottom line? If you want to consume milk, try to get raw milk from a qualified supplier (lists available at *RealMilk.com*). If you're extremely sensitive to the lactose of milk, i.e., lactose intolerant, this condition may resolve with raw milk. Notably, even people that are extremely sensitive to milk can virtually always safely consume ghee, which is a form of clarified butter without any milk proteins.

For more on this subject, I would strongly recommend Sally Fallon's brilliant book, *Nourishing Traditions (1999, 2001)*. Mrs. Fallon has more knowledge about the benefits of raw milk and the dangers of pasteurized milk than anyone I am aware of. *RealMilk.com* is also an excellent online reference, with links to available suppliers for raw milk. At the time of this writing, raw milk is available retail in 10 of the U.S. states, with on-farm sales legal in 15 states, and herdshares available in 4 states.[1239]

MEAT – CAFO RAISED VERSUS PASTURE RAISED

It is such a travesty that people have been led to believe that meat, particularly red meat, which is synonymous with beef or lamb, is inherently bad. Animal meats contain all 13 essential vitamins[1240] – and if we specifically consider organ meats, such as liver, heart, kidney, pancreas, etc. – the animal meats are huge sources of vitamins. Animal meats, particularly with their associated fats, supply all of the amino acids necessary for life and all the essential fats. It's no wonder the Masai, Rendille, Samburu, the Eskimos, and the Inuit were so healthy. They were getting tons of nutrients. But remember, the fat soluble vitamins are in the fat! That's why liver, eggs, butter, and whole-fat, raw milk are brilliantly healthy. The only vitamin missing in significant quantities in the meats mentioned above – is vitamin C.

Dr. Price found that white man, living in the Arctic north, would sometimes develop scurvy from lack of vitamin C. But the North American Indians did not. When Dr. Price inquired as to how the Indians avoided it, they advised that they ate the adrenal glands – very small glands that sit atop the kidneys. Generally, only highly educated anatomists and physicians would know exactly where to find these glands. Subsequent research found that "the adrenal glands are the richest sources of vitamin C in all animal or plant tissues." [1241] The brilliance of the so-called "primitive tribes" never ceases to amaze me.

But on to the question of CAFO raised animals versus pasture raised. Let me just ask the question: Does it make sense that cows, which normally feed on grass, should be eating corn and soy as their staples? Do you suppose a cow would naturally eat corn from corn fields and soy beans from soybean fields? But, there's a great reason for feeding cattle corn and soy – they fatten rapidly on it. It's also a lot like feeding vegetable oils, sugars, white flour, and pasteurized dairy to people – they tend to fatten quickly on it.

In CAFOs, from where the enormous majority of people are getting their beef, the cattle are often given hormones to make them grow faster along with antibiotics, the latter because cattle in these conditions have weakened immunity and because the conditions are deplorable.

When it comes to our health, the nutrients from grass-fed beef, including the fats, antioxidants, and precursors to vitamins, are drastically different than grain-fed beef.[1242] Grass-fed beef usually contains several times more healthy omega-3 fats, in fact, as much as five-fold more than grain-fed beef.[1243] [1244] [1245] And the conjugated linoleic acid (CLA), which has been associated with reduced body fat in humans, is approximately twice as concentrated in grass-fed beef.[1246] The total omega-6 fatty acids, which are the dangerous inflammatory ones, have been found to be higher in grain fed cattle and the longer they consume grain, the greater the omega-6 fat concentrations.[1247] According to Patricia Whisnant, DVM, of Americn Grass Fed Beef, the main reason grass-fed beef is more expensive is because it takes about 18 to 24 months - almost twice as long – to raise the animals to full size when they're consuming grass as when they're consuming grain.[1248]

FISH – IT'S ALL GOOD, WITH WILD-CAUGHT EVEN BETTER

With all of the controversy and disagreements regarding diets, the one thing even all contemporary researchers agree on is that fish consumption is good. Well, there are a few vegans out there who will even argue against that! Nevertheless, as reviewed in Chapter 10, numerous studies conclude that consuming fish decreases the risk of AMD.

But the question of this segment is whether or not farm-raised fish is as healthy as wild-caught. By now, you've probably guessed the answer. Natural is virtually always better. In general, farm-raised fish have more fat, while the wild-caught fish generally have higher proportions of omega-3 fats as well as higher proportions of the long-chain omega-3s, DHA and EPA,[1249] which are all tremendously beneficial in the prevention of AMD. And for those concerned about contaminants present in some fish, research shows that the benefits of fish consumption far outweigh the risks.[1250] For concerns of mercury, just avoid regularly consuming lots of very large fish, such as shark and tuna, as these are the fish that contain the most mercury.

THE MORE HUMANELY AND NATURALLY THE ANIMALS ARE TREATED, THE HEALTHIER THEY ARE FOR US TO EAT, BE IT EGGS, MILK, MEAT, OR FISH

I'm only going to scratch the surface, but over the last few years I've learned of some of the gory details of CAFOs – Concentrated Animal Feeding Operations. My sentiments? Appallng. Absolutely appalling. Chickens kept in "battery cages" too small for them to turn around, intensively confined for their entire lives in a space less than a single sheet of letter-sized paper;[1251] the situation is not much different for most pork, being confined to steel cages so small they can barely move forward or back, and cannot turn around their entire lives unless for a moment to be moved to another building;[1252] cattle that live in and walk in their own manure in crowded, cramped, horrendous conditions. This treatment of animals is nothing short of deplorable. None of these animals, by the way, are consuming their natural feed. And that means that, even if we have no concern at all for their welfare, their meat, milk, and eggs are vastly inferior to those of animals raised in more natural habitats.

If for no other reason than the inhumane and cruel treatment of animals confined to most CAFOs, I will not support these organizations. To these producers, animals are a means to revenue – and nothing more. They have no respect for the animals – or their welfare. If more people take this tact – and these mega-producers running CAFOs that resemble Nazi concentration camps – lose just 10% to 20% of their business, they're likely to change business practices. But as long as we buy milk, eggs, chicken, pork, and beef from the grocery stores and the restaurants that offer them, the more we keep these unethical operations running. If nothing else – vote with your dollars. Support the organic farmers and ranchers that care about the animals; the ones who treat animals with care and concern and not just a means to a sale based on nothing more than their weight or what they can produce. In the long run, it benefits us as well as the animals.

CHAPTER SUMMARY

In general, I believe it is much safer to consume organic produce than conventionally raised produce, because conventionally raised is generally treated with pesticides, herbicides, or both. Optimal nutrition would include pasture raised beef, chickens, and pork, eggs from pastured chickens, raw milk and/or raw milk products, such as cheeses, and wild-caught fish.

But, if organic produce and pasture raised meats and wild-caught fish are beyond your budget, just choose these exact same foods conventionally raised. That alone, will be a thousand-fold greater for your health, for your eyes, and for preventing AMD or AMD progression, than choosing foods from the categories of the 'displacing foods of modern commerce.'

20 GRAINS: WHICH ONES TO EAT & PROPER PREPARATION IF YOU DO

Loren Cordain, PhD, Professor Emeritus at Colorado State University and modern founder of the Paleo Diet, asserts that for optimal health we must eliminate the foods that we aren't evolutionarily adapted to consume, which would include the foods that are new to us in the last ten-thousand years, i.e., since the end of the Paleolithic Era. The foods that are new to us since then would include grains, dairy, legumes (beans), and tubers (potatoes).[1253]

I have very deep respect for Dr. Cordain, whom I hope to meet one day, as if it weren't for him, his research, and his books, I may have never been led down this path. After all, it was the Paleo Diet that got me started on this journey and helped me to begin to recover from arthritis and perhaps avoid the whole onslaught of "Western diseases." However, once I read Weston A. Price's research, not only was I forever changed, but I then understood that all of the foods that are discouraged in the Paleo Diet either were or are still consumed by various societies existing on traditional diets while remaining in brilliant health. For example, the Swiss villagers of the Loetchental Valley consumed huge quantities of rye bread, the Gaelics of the Outer Hebrides consumed oats as staples, and many African tribes consumed corn (maize). But, they didn't prepare these grains like we do! With that said, I believe it is vindicating to know that almost all *traditional* foods can be eaten, while it is really the newer "food products" (i.e., vegetable oils and trans fats) and refined foods (white flour and sugar) that are the true villains.

WHEAT – ONE LAST TIME!

In Chapter 11, we reviewed the grain of wheat in much detail. Given that wheat plays such a huge role in the diet of billions of people around the world, I feel it's worth giving a final summation on my consumption recommendations. By way of that, it might be worth quoting the brilliant, Dr. Stephan Guyenet, who wrote, "White flour, pretty much wherever it shows up throughout the world, metabolic havoc ensues." Dr. Guyenet also wrote, "I'm not aware of any truly healthy traditional culture that eats wheat as a staple. As a matter of fact, white flour has left a trail of destruction around the globe wherever it has gone. Polished rice does not have such a destructive effect, so it's not simply the fact that it's a refined carbohydrate. Hundreds, if not thousands of cultures throughout the world have lost their robust good health upon abandoning their traditional foods in favor of white flour and sugar. The medical and anthropological literature are peppered with these stories." [1254]

Of course, it is my assertion that the history of the U.S. and the U.K., for example, proves that we were once healthy eating wheat, albeit before 1880 when roller mill technology entered the picture, and long before the 1940s, when many farmers began to spray their wheat crops with herbicides (to be reviewed below).

Of course, as I reviewed in the last chapter, I believe much of the destructive capabilities of wheat lies with two inherent problems: 1) Wheat is usually consumed as white flour, rather than whole grain flour, thereby being a refined, processed, nutrient-deficient food, and 2) Traditionally raised wheat, as reviewed by Holm and Johnson, is typically sprayed with herbicides, particularly since the 1940s.[1255] The effects of this may be devastating, including birth defects and possibly even increased risks of infant death.[1256]

I would advise anyone who is not in perfect health or with lots of energy to consider a three or four week trial off of wheat for evaluation. Then, one might experience whether or not any symptoms might resolve, such as arthritis, headaches, abdominal issues, constipation, diarrhea, etc., all of which could indicate gluten sensitivity. Wheat consumption, because of its potential role in leaky gut, ought to be eliminated in virtually anyone with an autoimmune condition, in my opinion.

My advice is that, if you're going to eat wheat, I would try to consume whole grain type flour (most grocery store "whole wheat" breads contain little actual whole grain), and one that is organic. If you eat bread and you're adventurous enough to make your own, you might consider a guide article entitled, "Our Daily Bread," by Katherine Czapp at the Weston A. Price Foundation's website.[1257] If you purchase already prepared bread as most do, consider an organic, whole-grain type bread, preferably one that is from sprouted grains. Sprouting helps to reduce the levels of phytates in grains and legumes, which otherwise tie up minerals in grains making them unavailable for absorption, even if they're in the food.[1258] [1259] [1260] Great examples of healthy breads include Ezekial bread, FoodForLife bread, and Manna Bread, all of which are excellent and healthy for those without gluten sensitivity. For a great review, consider the article, "10 Healthy Ways to Replace Conventional Wheat Bread," on *AuthorityNutrition.com*,[1261] as well as the article "Before You Ever Buy Bread Again…Read This! And Find the Healthiest Bread On the Market," by Vani Hari (*FoodBabe.com*).[1262] Vani's website name might not sound too scientific, but this young lady is a diligent researcher and is highly respected. She's received plenty of accolades too, not to mention that some huge food producers, including Chick-fil-A, Chipotle, Subway, Kraft, and General Mills have changed recipes and eliminated harmful ingredients in foods, because of her. [1263]

WHOLE GRAIN PREPARATION

In the United States and many industrialized nations, there is a common theme of advice to "consume plenty of whole grains," which is an attempt to advise against consuming refined white flour. Nevertheless, this advice is still flawed and and may even be downright counterproductive. The reason being is that this leads one to believe that any version of whole grain is "healthy." This just isn't the case, because of the fact that whole grains need proper preparation. Whole grains, such as wheat, rye, corn, oats, rice, millet, and sorghum contain phytic acid, which combines with various minerals in the food, including iron, zinc, and calcium, rendering significant quantities of those minerals unavailable for absorption; this, in turn, may promote mineral deficiencies.[1264] This is similarly true for legumes (beans, peas, lentils).[1265] There are other antinutrients (defined as natural or synthetic components in food that interfere with the absorption of nutrients) in grains, lentils, and legumes that I won't delve into but I think that some understanding of phytic acid is really essential because minerals play central and critical roles in metabolism of every cell, right along with the other micronutrients, i.e., vitamins. This is critical to the metabolism of vision as well.

Phytic acid, also known as phytate, may be most problematic in grains, but all edible seeds, nuts, and legumes contain some quantities of phytate. Phytic acid serves as a storage form of phosphorus, which breaks down when, for example, the seeds sprout (germinate) as this releases not only the phosphorus but also makes other minerals such as calcium and magnesium available for use by the growing plant.[1266] This is the reason that sprouted grains, including sprouted wheat, rice, corn, quinoa, etc., are far more nutritious – because the phytate is neutralized to a degree making the minerals in the grain much more absorbable. Some authors mistakenly assert that phytates will negatively impact absorption of minerals from other foods in the diet, but this is not true. They'll only affect absorption of the minerals in the food that they're actually residing in. But, when those foods account for a significant proportion of the diet, which they often do, failure to properly prepare the grains can lead to mineral deficiencies.

According to Atli Arnarson, PhD, of Authority Nutrition.com, there are three commonly used methods to reduce the content of phytates in foods:

- "**Soaking:** Cereals and legumes are often soaked in water overnight to reduce their phytate content.
- **Sprouting:** The sprouting of seeds, grains, and legumes, also known as germination, causes phytate degradation.
- **Fermentation:** Organic acids, formed during fermentation, promote phytate breakdown. Lactic acid fermentation is the preferred method, a good example of which is the making of sourdough." [1267]

As always, one of the best sources for an excellent review of proper grains preparation is Sally Fallon's book, *Nourishing Traditions*. Her review is impeccable, historical, and chock-full of real-world advice too. This takes all the guess-work out of the proper preparation of grains and legumes, and includes lots of recipes.[1268]

CHAPTER SUMMARY

For those who will consume grains, particularly wheat, caution must be exercised and great consideration should be given to the potential health risks versus benefits. For those who choose to consume wheat, in my opinion, they themselves should be completely free of disease, at a healthy weight, and have absolutely no autoimmune or inflammatory disease conditions, such as Lupus, multiple sclerosis, rheumatoid arthritis, Crohn's disease, irritable bowel syndrome, etc. Those with leaky gut may be at greater risk for macular degeneration given the inflammatory component of such a condition.

Most all grains and legumes may be able to be consumed by the majority of people, however, I would recommend to purchase organic options if possible, and to prepare them properly. Some people will not tolerate some or all grains or legumes. All of the healthy tribes and populations that Weston A. Price evaluated in the 1930s that did consume grains, on five different continents, took great care to properly prepare them. This is key. The methods used in proper preparation include soaking, sprouting, and fermentation. No wonder true organic sourdough bread, which has undergone fermentation, is so amazing – it's not only delicious, it 's healthy too.

THE LIFE-GIVING "SACRED FOODS" – FOR AMD TOO!

In Chapter 7, I reviewed the "sacred foods" of various tribes and populations that Weston A. Price evaluated in his world travels and studies. This is such an enormously important concept, however, I wanted to just provide a brief review in a separate chapter. Understanding the concept of densely nutritious foods, which is the sine-qua-non of "sacred foods," is of paramount importance.

The "sacred foods" were those foods that Dr. Price discovered "primitive tribes" considered literally as "life-giving" foods. These were foods held in the highest of regard and tribe members would often be willing to risk life and limb in order to get them. To the Swiss villagers of the Loetschental Valley, it was the butter from cows that grazed on the rapidly growing grass of Spring and late Summer. To the Gaelics of the Outer Hebrides, it was the chopped cod's head and cod's liver. To the Massai, the African tribe of Kenya and Tanzania, it was the milk, meat, and blood of the cattle they herded. To the Eskimos and Inuit, it was seal meat, seal oil, organ meats (not seal liver), and fish. To the Indians of the far North of Canada, in the Rocky Mountains, it was the organ meats of moose and caribou. To the South Sea Islanders, it was shellfish and an abundance of sea life. To the Peruvian Indians of the Andes Mountains, it was fish eggs (roe) that they would travel more than one hundred miles and from elevations as high as 18,000 feet to procure.[1269]

Collectively, the "sacred foods" are the ones that provide what Dr. Price called the "fat soluble activators," which are the fat soluble vitamins, A, D, E, and K. Of these, it is A, D, and K2 that are the vitamins so critically important to health and, of course, found in such great quantities in the "sacred foods." Just as importantly, these three fat-soluble vitamins are not well distributed in the food supply. Hence, the critical need to consume very specific animal foods that contain them in abundance.

I would summarize the "sacred foods" as follows:

- **Butter** – From cattle grazing on rapidly growing green grass
- **Eggs** – From pasture-raised chickens or other fowl consuming grass and insects
- **Organ Meats** – Such as liver, heart, kidneys, pancreas, etc., preferably from organically raised, pastured animals
- **Fish Eggs (Roe)** – From wild-caught salmon, sturgeon (caviar), flying fish roe (Japanese "tobiko"), and any and all others
- **Shellfish and Seafood** – Particularly fatty fish, such as wild-caught salmon, herring, mackeral, and sardines. Whole small fish, including the head, bones, etc., e.g., sardines & anchovies, are excellent.
- **Extra Virgin Cod Liver Oil & Pastured Butter/ High-Vitamin Butter Oil** – Note that these are not supplements, but are both whole food items.

If you include these categories of foods in your diet every week, you're very likely to begin to experience health benefits – and perhaps dramatically. If one consumes butter from cows grazing on green grass (pastured butter), eggs from pastured chickens, organ meats such as liver once a week or so, and some seafood or shellfish a couple of times a week, then I don't believe extra virgin cod liver oil (EVCLO) and high-vitamin butter oil are necessary. However, if one were eating all of those foods except the organ meats (e.g. liver), I would strongly advise regular consumption of EVCLO. Note that primitive societies generally did not have any form of cod liver oil or high-vitamin butter oil. However, cod liver oil was once a very commonly consumed food in the U.S., the U.K., and other societies, particularly before World War II.

In his 1939 textbook, *Nutrition and Physical Degeneration,* Price wrote, "It is unfortunate that as the white man has come into contact with the primitives in various parts of the world he has failed to appreciate the accumulated wisdom of the primitve racial stocks."[1270] He was referring, of course, to the brilliance of the "primitives," for which Price had great reverence. If you read his book, undoubtedly, you will gain that reverence too, as I have.

In Dr. Price's research on the effectiveness of the fat-soluble vitamins in their ability to allow absorption and utilization of minerals, he wrote,

> Extensive laboratory determinations have shown that most people cannot absorb more than half of the calcium and phosphorus from the foods eaten. The amounts utilized depend directly on the presence of other substances, particularly fat-soluble vitamins. It is at this point probably that the greatest breakdown in our modern diet takes place, namely, in the ingestion and utilization of adequate amounts of the special activating substances, including the vitamins needed for rendering the minerals in the food available to the human system… Adult individuals vary in the efficiency with which they absorb minerals and other chemicals essential for mineral utilization. It is possible to starve for minerals that are abundant in the foods eaten because they cannot be utilized without an adequate quantitity of the fat-soluble activotors [vitamins A, D, and K2]."[1271]

In Chapter 16, we reviewed that vitamin K2 is the critical micronutrient required to deposit calcium into bones and teeth, while keeping it from depositing into arteries, the latter of which plays a critical role in the development of atherosclerosis. I've hypothesized that a lack of vitamin K2 may be a significant component of AMD development by way of causing Bruch's membrane to calcify, which may contribute to the diffusion barrier problem between the choriocapillaris and the RPE. We've reviewed that increased consumption of vitamin K2 protects against heart disease, reduces coronary heart disease mortality, and reduces calcification of the aorta.[1272] The next logical question is: Could consumption of vitamin K2 help to reverse that calcification, thereby reducing one's risk of heart attack and heart disease in general? Fortunately, it looks like the answer to that question is yes. Researchers from Maastricht University in The Netherlands treated rats, in which they had induced arterial calcification, with vitamin K2 and found that calcification can be reversed![1273]

If reversal of vascular calcification is possible, it is theoretically plausible that the same scenario might occur with Bruch's membrane in the eye, thereby treating AMD. Perhaps this is in part why we witness AMD reverse when people "clean up" their diet, which I'll review in the next chapter.

Recall from Chapter 16 that, even without any particular genetic risk factors, those people who were deficient in vitamin D status had a 2.6-fold greater odds of having AMD, while those with inadequate vitamin D status had a 1.5-fold increased odds of having AMD, as compared to the "referent group" that had serum vitamin D above 30 ng/mL. Amy Millen, PhD, and her group had hypothesized that vitamin D deficiency might lead to increased inflammation and even angiogenesis (wet AMD).

The point is simply that processed food-laden diets, deficient in the fat-soluble vitamins, are obviously associated with AMD, as we've witnessed time and time again in 22 countries. And now we see an entirely plausible mechanism whereby both vitamin K2 deficiency and vitamin D deficiency may both play a role. With the brilliant synchrony that vitamins A, D, and K2 play together, I would assert that collective deficiencies in these fat soluble vitamins very likely play a huge role in the development of AMD. It would only make sense that the best way to manage this scenario is to enhance one's nutrient consumption by consuming the "sacred foods."

History tends to repeat itself – and what we've seen, over and over, is that many societies have developed collective amnesia for the fundamentals of nutrition through whole foods. The consequences, unfortunately, are often disastrous. We need to firmly implant in our minds that degenerative diseases don't necessarily occur because something is there, but perhaps as much or moreso because something isn't there. And a huge part of that *something* is vitamins, particularly the fat soluble vitamins.

In our society, we've largely replaced healthy, wholesome, organic foods, with processed, nutrient-deficient foods that have been "enriched" with synthetic vitamins. We've also spent billions of dollars on vitamin supplements. And I ask, where has that gotten us?

There are just two final foods in our diets that I haven't reviewed yet. Those are cod liver oil and organ meats. In the latter case, I'll focus on liver. Let's review these just briefly.

TRADITIONAL COD LIVER OIL VS. EXTRA VIRGIN COD LIVER OIL

In the United States, until the end of World War II, consumption of cod liver oil was commonplace, having once been known for its great ability to prevent rickets (weakening and bowing of the bones, secondary to vitamin D deficiency) as well as for its ability to prevent infections (secondary to its vitamin A content).[1274] The situation was quite similar in the U.K., with cod liver oil consumption having been common since the 19th century.[1275] With the advent of antibiotics to treat infections and the regular fortification of milk and other foods with vitamin D, cod liver oil was largely abandoned as a relic from the past.

But, as you probably expected, not all cod liver oil is the same. Not even close. Sally Fallon, founder of the Weston A. Price Foundation (WAPF), has written quite extensively on the various cod liver oil products and has listed a number of products to be considered. She reported that one industry founder, in his quest to evaluate cod liver oil (CLO) production processes worldwide, made a trip to Norway where he made a shocking discovery. Most of today's standard CLO production practices – destroy the naturally occurring vitamins in the oil during the molecular distillation process. The vitamins are then replaced in the CLO with synthetic vitamins. This process, of course, is not at all consistent with a cod liver oil cold extraction process, wherein the naturally occurring vitamins are retained in the oil, while the oils themselves remain protected from oxidation.[1276]

Cod liver oil comes from extracting the oils from the livers of cod and other fish, which are very rich in the fat-soluble vitamins. However, as briefly reviewed above, there are vastly different methods of extracting the oils. In one product, i.e., most current conventional cod liver oils, the process to create them utilizes alkali refining, bleaching with clay or natural earth elements, "winterization," which is either a cold press or filter operation, deodorization, which removes most of the vitamin D and significant amounts of vitamin A and, finally, the addition of either natural or synthetic vitamins.[1277] This sounds a lot like a processed food preparation with "enrichment" to me.

Contrast that with the process to create cold-extracted, extra virgin cod liver oil (EVCLO). Summarizing the ancient and traditional process, published by F. Peckel Möller in his book, *Cod Liver Oil and Chemistry,* in 1895, the fishermen would, upon returning from the sea, separate the liver and roe (fish eggs) into barrels, which were closed and the oils allowed to separate for several months through the winter into the early Spring. This would allow the cellular walls to break down under cold conditions, releasing the oils, which would float to the surface.[1278] The oil rising to the surface would be consistent with today's "extra virgin cod liver oil," which is particularly rich in vitamins A, D, B12, and other nutrients. In 1895, Möller wrote, "Cod-liver oil is undoubtedly one of the most valuable medicinal agents known to man." [1279]

Currently, I am particularly impressed with the transparent production process and laboratory testing, presented by Rosita Real Foods, regarding their EVCLO. This product appears exceptionally produced, with excellent independent lab testing for the omega-3s DHA and EPA, vitamins A and D, as well as remarkably low levels of rancid or oxidized end products, dioxins, and PCBs (RositaRealFoods.com).

EVCLO, which is a great source of vitamins A and D, combined with high-vitamin butter oil, which is a great source of vitamin K2, make for a great duo for those who are not consuming organ meats, such as liver, plus "grass fed" (pastured) butter. These two (EVCLO and high-vitamin butter oil) are the essential combination that Dr. Price used to rescue children and adults from the depths of nutritional deficiency, in some cases literally at the brink of death.[1280]

Sally Fallon, president of the Weston A. Price Foundation, made recommendations for makers of cod liver oil, updated in November, 2015 (as of the time of this writing), under the title, "Cod Liver Oil Basics and Recommendations." [1281] In this article, she recommends as the "Best" cod liver oils, the following companies: Green Pasture (GreenPasture.org), Radiant Life (RadiantLifeCatalog.com), Natural Health Advocates (Building-Health.com), Traditional Health First, NutraPro International virgin cod liver oil (NutraProIntl.com), and Rosita Real Foods extra virgin cod liver oil (Corganic. com). Personally, I give my highest recommendation to the Rosita Real Foods EVCLO, combined with pastured butter, which provides an excellent source of the fat-soluble vitamins (A, D, and K2).

LIVER & OTHER ORGAN MEATS (OFFAL)

Sure, my palate would certainly prefer cedar plank salmon, sushi, or a prime steak cooked medium rare, but every week, I eat some organ meats. For my family, these usually include eating the liver, heart, and gizzard (the giblets) of a pasture raised chicken, or we'll eat some pastured chicken liver with onions, seasoned with salt and poultry seasoning and cooked in grass-fed butter. About half of the time that we consume organ meats, we eat pastured beef liver and onions as well, which I cook in pastured butter, seasoned with salt, pepper, thyme, and rosemary. The reason we eat liver and other organs, also known as offal (it's terrible that it sounds like awful), is because there is nothing – I repeat, nothing – that is more nutritious, than liver. As you will see, the micronutrient density is beyond compare.

The misunderstandings regarding vitamin A and the consumption of liver are legion. And not unlike the saturated-fat-causes-heart-disease myth, this dogma is repeated often enough that there are far more concerns about vitamin A overdose and toxicity than the millions-of-fold greater likelihood of vitamin A deficiency.

There are two often quoted concerns regarding liver consumption, 1) that liver is the "storage depot for toxins," and 2), that there is a putative risk of vitamin A toxicity. Both assumptions are proved to be invalid.

With regard to toxins, let's just see if this concern is valid. In one study completed in Spain, researchers assessed the levels of three common toxins, arsenic, cadmium, and lead, in liver and muscle, among other tissues. They found that arsenic was 10.8 μg/kg in calves' liver and 3.75 μg/kg in calves' muscle – both values extrtremely low. Cadmium was 7.78 μg/kg in calves' liver and 0.839 μg/kg in calves' muscle. Lead was 33.0 μg/kg in calves' liver and 6.37 μg/kg in calves' muscle.[1282] In all cases, the numbers are extraordinarily small, but generally a little higher in the liver. I think this is most consistent with the logic and common belief system that the liver is not a storage depot of toxins, but rather a place where toxins are rendered inert and prepared for excretion, usually via the kidneys. The concentrations of toxins does increase significantly in the liver of cows as compared to calves, however, so if one is concerned about consuming as low a toxin load as possible, calf liver would be better. This, I don't believe, was ever a concern of the healthy cultures that Weston A. Price visited. In fact, in general, they attempted to hunt older animals since they would carry more fat, which is the part of the animal that most traditional societies consumed *instead* of lean meat.

If one desires to avoid toxic heavy metal exposure by avoiding liver and other animal foods, they might be surprised to find that these same heavy metals also accumulate in various plants, which brings us to the realization that a large variety of food is contaminated.[1283] This isn't surprising, since these heavy metals are both naturally occurring as well as a common part of the earth's crust.[1284] Interestingly enough, just as we've seen that vitamin A is required to detoxify dioxins and benzo(a)pyrenes in cigarette smoke, perhaps this is the case for numerous toxins. Could it be that the very combination of vitamins and minerals in liver and other organ meats are the same ones that lead us to manage toxins in general?

As reviewed previously, reports of vitamin A toxicity from consuming liver are extremely rare, primarily having occurred in Arctic explorers who consumed polar bear and seal liver. It is those who consume synthetic versions of vitamin A that have extraordinarily higher risks of toxicity.[1285]

Liver is an excellent source of vitamin A as we've reviewed. According to Professor Chris Masterjohn, PhD, "Vitamin A has traditionally been understood to promote healthy vision, promote healthy fertility in males and females, and allow for proper embryonic development. More recently researchers have found vitamin A to be important to many other processes. These include preventing childhood mortality, preventing childhood asthma, promoting pubertal development, protecting against oxidative stress, protecting against environmental toxins, preventing kidney stones, regulating the amount of fat tissue in the body, regulating blood sugar, and protecting against fatty liver disease." [1286] Many traditional societies consumed (or still consume) organ meats, particularly liver. The Japanese, who are phenomenally healthier than we are (though more recently Westernizing their diets), still consider liver an important food for pregnant women.[1287] Given the enormous health benefits, including healthy pregnancies and healthy babies, it's no wonder. Once again, we should take heed to so many cultures' ancient and accumulated wisdom.

In keeping with the findings of Weston A. Price, one study of the Inuit people of Greenland, showed that, in 1953, they consumed an average of 30,000 IU of vitamin A per day.[1288] The current U.S. RDA for vitamin A is 3,000 IU daily for men, which indicates that the Inuit were consuming ten times this much, again, typical of societies consuming traditional diets. The health of these societies and particularly their natural fat-soluble vitamin consumption should lead us to question the validity of our own RDAs. These findings suggest that the U.S. RDA numbers, in some cases, are far too low. Below is a table showing the comparison of nutrients in 100 grams of apple, carrots, and red meat, versus beef liver.

As one can see, liver is a tremendous source of numerous vitamins and minerals, including phosphorus, magnesium, potassium, iron, zinc, copper, and of course, vitamin A, multiple B vitamins, and even vitamin C. Note that carrots have no vitamin A (same as all plant foods) and 100 grams (about 3 ounces) of red meat contains 40 IU vitamin A while 100 grams of liver has 53,400 IU of vitamin A. Liver is not the best source of vitamin D, which is yet another reason why sun exposure, cod liver oil, and/or consumption of fatty fish is warranted.

CHAPTER SUMMARY

All of the supremely healthy societies that Weston A. Price studied were consumers of certain foods that were particularly rich in the "fat-soluble activators," which is the fat soluble vitamins, A, D, and K2. These were, of course, not consumed to the exclusion of the water soluble vitamins, which are the B-complex and C vitamins. But, the fat soluble vitamins are not abundant and widely distributed throughout the food supply. Very specific animal foods are required in order to consume them in any significant quantities.

It behooves us to learn from these brilliantly healthy societies with their collective and accumulated wisdom, and make "sacred foods" a part of our everyday meals. This, obviously, is critical to our health. I believe that this is a significant component of preventing AMD, as well as the therapeutic treatment of existing AMD. The first component, of course, is to eliminate the processed foods.

I would recommend that we consume butter from organically raised cows grazing on grass whenever possible, eat pastured eggs regularly, consume organ meats like liver at least once every week or so (even in small quantities), and eat fish and shellfish frequently (2 – 3 times a week, minimum). For those who eat plenty of these foods on a regular basis, one will likely fulfill all the requirements for the fat soluble vitamins. For those who do not consume organ meats, I would strongly recommend to consume fermented cod liver oil and high-vitamin butter oil, regularly.

	APPLE (100 g)	CARROTS (100 g)	RED MEAT (100 g)	BEEF LIVER (100 g)
Calcium	3.0 mg	3.3 mg	11.0 mg	11.0 mg
Phosphorus	6.0 mg	31.0 mg	140.0 mg	476.0 mg
Magnesium	4.8 mg	6.2 mg	15.0 mg	18.0 mg
Potassium	139.0 mg	222.0 mg	370.0 mg	380.0 mg
Iron	.1 mg	.6 mg	3.3 mg	8.8 mg
Zinc	.05 mg	.3 mg	4.4 mg	4.0 mg
Copper	.04 mg	.08 mg	.18 mg	12.0 mg
Vitamin A	None	None	40 IU	53,400 IU
Vitamin D	None	None	Trace	19 IU
Vitamin E	.37 mg	.11 mg	1.7 mg	.63 mg
Vitamin C	7.0 mg	6.0 mg	None	27.0 mg
Thiamin	.03 mg	.05 mg	.05 mg	.26 mg
Riboflavin	.02 mg	.05 mg	.20 mg	4.19 mg
Niacin	.10 mg	.60 mg	4.0 mg	16.5 mg
Pantothenic Acid	.11 mg	.19 mg	.42 mg	8.8 mg
Vitamin B6	.03 mg	.10 mg	.07 mg	.73 mg
Folic Acid	8.0 mcg	24.0 mcg	4.0 mcg	145.0 mcg
Biotin	None	.42 mcg	2.08 mcg	96.0 mcg
Vitamin B12	None	None	1.84 mcg	111.3 mcg

22 YOUR ULTIMATE PLAN TO PREVENT, TREAT, AND POSSIBLY REVERSE EARLY AMD

"If I have seen further it is by standing on the shoulders of giants."
~ Isaac Newton ~
(written February 15, 1676)

I'd like to begin this last chapter with a historical anecdote regarding the disease pellagra that I believe is a great analogy to what we could potentially encounter with the cause of AMD.

Pellagra is a disease characterized clinically by the "Four D's": photosensitive dermatitis, diarrhea, dementia, and death. The dermatologic features include desquamation (peeling of the skin), erythema (red patches), scaling, and keratosis (thickening and drying) of sun-exposed areas. After 1902, pellagra became a disease endemic to the Southern U.S. There were many theories as to its cause. Many physicians suspected it was an infectious disease, perhaps brought to the U.S by immigrants from Europe and particularly, Italy, where the disease was quite common. Other physicians blamed the disease on the buffalo gnat. Still others observed that the disease afflicted members of the same family and, therefore, concluded that the disease was hereditary. By 1911, pellagra was the leading cause of death in asylums for the insane and by 1912, there were an estimated 25,000 cases that had been diagnosed in the previous five years with a mortality rate of 40 percent.[1289]

In 1914, Joseph Goldberger, MD, a New York physician employed by the U.S Public Health Service, was sent to the South to determine the infectious nature of pellagra. After all, Goldberger had already been successful in his works with other infectious diseases, including yellow fever, dengue, typhus, hookworm, and diphtheria. He began to study pellagra, and identified that people affected by the disease were consuming a diet very high in maize (corn) and seemed to generally be consuming a poor diet, low in vegetables, meat, and milk. He also noted that the nursing and support staff that cared for victims of pellagra rarely seemed to contract the disease. The typical diet of the Southern poor at the time consisted of the "three Ms" – which was meat, meal, and molasses. The meat was generally pork fatback and the meal was cornmeal. This was a cheap, filling, and monotonous diet. Goldberger was convinced that this nutritionally deficient and atrocious diet was the problem.

In 1914, Dr. Goldberger filed a report presenting his theory, which was not well received by physicians of the South who stated they had already considered a nutrient deficiency and ruled it out. This didn't stop Goldberger, however. He persisted by treating affected children in two orphanages and adults in one asylum in Jackson, Mississippi, by changing their meager diets with the addition of fresh vegetables, meats, milk, and eggs – foods rich in vitamins and proteins.[1290] The children affected by Pellagra who were given the healthy diet recovered and unaffected children given the same healthy diets didn't contract Pellagra. Findings with adults in asylums were similar. Some of those confined to asylums recovered from their dementia and were released. This wasn't enough to convince most, however, and Goldberger's funding for the diets soon ran out.

Goldberger convinced Governor Earl Brewer of Mississippi to pardon any convicts who agreed to be a part of a controlled dietary experiment. The governor agreed and the Rankin State Prison Farm, near Jackson, Mississippi was selected as the site to conduct the experiment. There were virtually no known cases of Pellagra in the prisons, where the food was often better than the poor, the institutionalized, and even those in some hospitals. Twelve volunteers were selected to be in the experimental group and all volunteered and were made aware that the dietary regime might place them at risk of developing pellagra.[1291 1292]

In her review, Frances Rachel Frankenburg, MD, author of *Vitamin Discoveries and Disasters: History, Science, and Controversies,* wrote:

> "In April 1915 the convict volunteers were housed in a scrupulously clean building separated from the other prisoners. They were fed a highly controlled diet. Breakfast consisted of biscuits, fried mush [porridge of cornmeal], grits, brown gravy, cane syrup, and coffee. Lunch included corn bread, collards, sweet potatoes, grits and syrup. Supper was similar to lunch. The usual Rankin prison diet was better in that it contained meat of some sort at all meals, buttermilk, peas, and beans. Prisoners on the experimental diet became ill and weak within two weeks of beginning the diet. The prisoners hated the diet, yet this diet was the standard diet of the southern poor. By the fifth month of the study, in September 1915, six of the volunteers had developed dermatitis and 'nervous and gastro-intestinal symptoms.' Other physicians confirmed that in five of these prisoners, these changes were consistent with the diagnosis of pellagra. The experiment had succeeded. Goldberger had induced pellagra by feeding otherwise healthy men a diet lacking fresh milk, meat, and vegetables. In retrospect, the prisoners were probably also suffering from other dietary deficiency syndromes, such as riboflavin deficiency, but the point had been made: the poor diet common in the South caused pellagra." [1293]

Goldberger told the inmates what to eat to cure their pellagra and, of course, they obliged and their pellagra resolved. But the Southerners weren't accepting of Goldberger's findings, as their pride kept them from believing that a Southern diet could be at fault. Some even accused him of perpetrating a hoax. When he linked the scourge of pellagra to low-paying jobs that caused people to eat poorly, many took offense to what might be considered "social criticism." Goldberger was stunned by their lack of acceptance and irrational reactions.

He returned to the lab in attempt to isolate the nutrient lacking in the diets of those afflicted, despite the fact that he had already knew how to both prevent – and to cure – pellagra. It would be some 11 years, 1926, before Goldberger would isolate the lacking nutrient. He and his colleagues determined on the basis of animal experiments, that "pellagra-preventive factor" (P-P Factor) was the waters-soluble B-vitamin that was missing in the typical poor Southerner's diet.

Unfortunately, Goldberger died of cancer in 1929, and it wasn't until 1937 that Conrad A. Elvehjem, a biochemist at the University of Wisconsin, finally determined that P-P Factor was actually niacin, or vitamin B3.[1294] By the 1940's, the Food and Nutrition Board had recommended "enrichment" of bread and flour not only with niacin, but with iron and thiamine, the latter of which would prevent beriberi. It wasn't until 1945, at the end of World War II, that pellagra would be forever eliminated and become a disease of historical interest.[1295] Goldberger's cure wouldn't be accepted and the preventive treatment promulgated to the public until some 30 years after he had discovered the remedy for the condition – a remedy that was found in nothing less than a healthy diet with varied whole foods – fresh meat, vegetables, milk, and eggs. But how soon we forget…

THERE IS NOT AND WILL NEVER BE A SINGLE SMOKING GUN FOR AMD – UNLESS THAT "SINGLE CAUSATIVE FACTOR" IS A FAULTY, PROCESSED FOOD LADEN DIET

Take this hypothetical scenario: Let's say I take 400 rats and randomly divide them up into two groups. Group 1 rats are placed into a very natural habitat – let's say a barn and a contained yard where they can run free and eat their "wild" diet – grains, fruits, vegetables, and their favorites, seeds and insects. In Group 2, the rats are contained and given breakfast cereal, pasteurized milk, potato chips, bologna, pizza, peanut butter, and ice cream, all made with "appropriate" amounts of vegetable oils, trans fats, white flour, and sugar. Oh yeah, and let's give some of the rats in the latter group some cigarettes to start smoking – perhaps some will like it. Nine months later, all of the rats in Group 1 are lean, healthy, and free of disease. Group 2 rats have tremendous illness. Most are overweight or obese, they've gotten infections, and some even have had tumors, and 15% of them are already dead. What variable in Group 2 are you going to point your finger at?

The scenario with people is exactly the same. Beginning in 1880 and shortly thereafter, we've witnessed that a number of major components of the Western diet began to change. We suddenly had "edible" cottonseed oil, trans fats in the form of Crisco, roller mill technology that created a highly processed white flour instead of whole-grain flour, increasing sugar consumption, and finally, putting all of these components together into various combinations in the form of processed foods. With this "experiment," if you will, there were a tremendous number of variables introduced. I can't even list them all, but for starters, this introduced increasingly higher omega-6 fats and possibly even omega-3 fats, highly unstable polyunsaturated fatty acids, trans fats coming from Crisco and the vegetable oils, and substantially increasing sugar consumption. But it doesn't end with what we've added. It's just as important, and perhaps more so, what we've removed.

The addition of the newfangled, invented foods, caused a replacement of natural, organic foods. Suddenly, the consumption of butter and lard were reduced and whole grains were replaced by this new refined white flour. Sugar consumption was also on the rise. With this came diminished consumption of the fat-soluble vitamins, A, D, and K, in highly variable patterns. We lose some B-vitamins and fiber with the replacement of whole wheat flour with refined white flour. Canned food consumption is on the rise, sometimes treated with preservatives such as sodium benzoate (still used today) and formaldehyde (a known carcinogen). And because we start mixing all of these newfound ingredients together, we now have some of the first completely processed foods in our diet – and they're taking up a large portion of our daily ration.

Taken together, we now have an "experiment" with 37 variables (I'm making up the number) – so when these people start getting sick, with heart disease, cancer, Alzheimer's disease, and macular degeneration, what are you going to point your finger at? In the ideal experiment, you change only one variable at a time. For example, you take two sets of mice, both virtually the same in every regard, and then you randomize the mice into two groups. They both live in the exact same environment, they both eat the exact same healthy food, etc. Then, you introduce one variable – say, maybe you give one group regular doses of the pesticide 2,4-D. At the end of the experiment, you assess for differences and if there are differences, you can be pretty sure why they exist. But you don't introduce nine different variables into your experimental group, and then try to sort out the differences using sophisticated statistics and regression analyses. Yet, this is the task that researchers are left to try to sort out with people, where it's even much more complex than in this mice analogy.

Secondly, there are acute toxins – and chronic toxins. Carbon monoxide and cyanide are acute toxins. Give a significant dose – and whoever is exposed will soon be dead. It's easier to figure out. Chronic toxins take decades – maybe even a lifetime – to cause their ultimate harm. This is exactly why cigarette smoking with its increasing popularity from the year 1900 until around 1970, wasn't definitively blamed for lung cancer in the U.S. until 1964. Specifically, that reason is because cigarette smoking takes decades to have its full impact – in the form of emphysema and cancers.

So, if you take two sets of perfectly healthy 20 year olds, and you start one group of them smoking while the other does not, will you see definitive differences in them in 5 years? Ten years? Twenty? Or thirty? The answer is more like 20 or 30 years. That's right, in fact, it generally takes about 30 years of smoking to produce "fatal emphysema," which occurs when more than 60% of the lung tissue is destroyed.[1296] However, they'll obviously gradually be reducing lung function, no doubt. With regard to lung cancer, according to United Kingdom's website "netdoctor," if a person begins smoking in their teens and smokes until they're 30 years old, then quits, their chance of lung cancer by age 75 is 1.8 percent. Quit at age 40 and the risk increases to 3 percent by age 75. Quit at age 50, the risk is 6 percent, and quit by age 60 and the risk of cancer by age 75 is 10 percent.[1297] So with those kinds of odds, a lot of smokers are just willing to role the dice. If, on the other hand, 80 percent of smokers got lung cancer or fatal emphysema within three months or maybe even three years from the onset of smoking, I think cigarettes might have been banned as poisons a century ago, or at least few people would choose to smoke them.

The point is, it is exactly the same scenario with what has happened to our Western diet since year 1880 and its associated afflictions. There were drastic changes to our diet at the beginning of the 20th century, which we've reviewed repeatedly. By the 1920's, there were beginning to be a few heart attacks, a little higher rate of cancers, and perhaps a few more cases of macular degeneration. By the 1930's, we were seeing significantly more heart disease, more cancers, and macular degeneration was suddenly on the ophthalmologist's radar as a significant disease. By the 1960s, heart disease, cancer, and macular degeneration were exceedingly common, at least in the U.S. and the U.K. By year 1980 to 1990 and beyond, all of these conditions and so many more are of epidemic proportions, particularly in the elderly, and around the world. The effects of such dietary changes are slow to onset, chronic in nature, and insidious. That's why it's been so difficult to ferret them out.

MACULAR DEGENERATION...

History tells us that AMD prevalence was close to zero between 1850 and the 1920s, becoming prevalent enough in the 1930s that, in 1940, Sir Stewart Duke-Elder wrote *"SENILE MACULAR DEGENERATION... is a common cause of failure in central vision in old people."* [1298] He did not give any statistics relating to the incidence of dry AMD, however, with respect to wet AMD, he did cite *"only some 130 cases have been reported in the literature,"* with the earliest case having been reported in 1923 (Neame, 1923).[1299] So, we are left to speculate that, perhaps AMD was responsible for a few percent of the vision loss in the elderly, presumably far behind cataracts and glaucoma, the primary causes of vision loss in that era (1930s).[1300]

Yet today, we see that AMD afflicts anywhere from 17 to nearly 40 percent of those people aged 75 and beyond, based on seven different studies of populations in the U.S., Australia, the Netherlands, and Barbados, West Indies.[1301] We see that nearly 196 million people are afflicted with AMD worldwide, with two million of those people already blind in both eyes from the condition.

I am submitting one final graph for your consideration. The graph is total vegetable oil (more than 99% PUFA) and sugar consumption in the U.S. versus population in millions affected by AMD. We see that there was virtually no AMD until 1930s, approximately some 30 years after vegetable oils became a significant component of the diet, and while

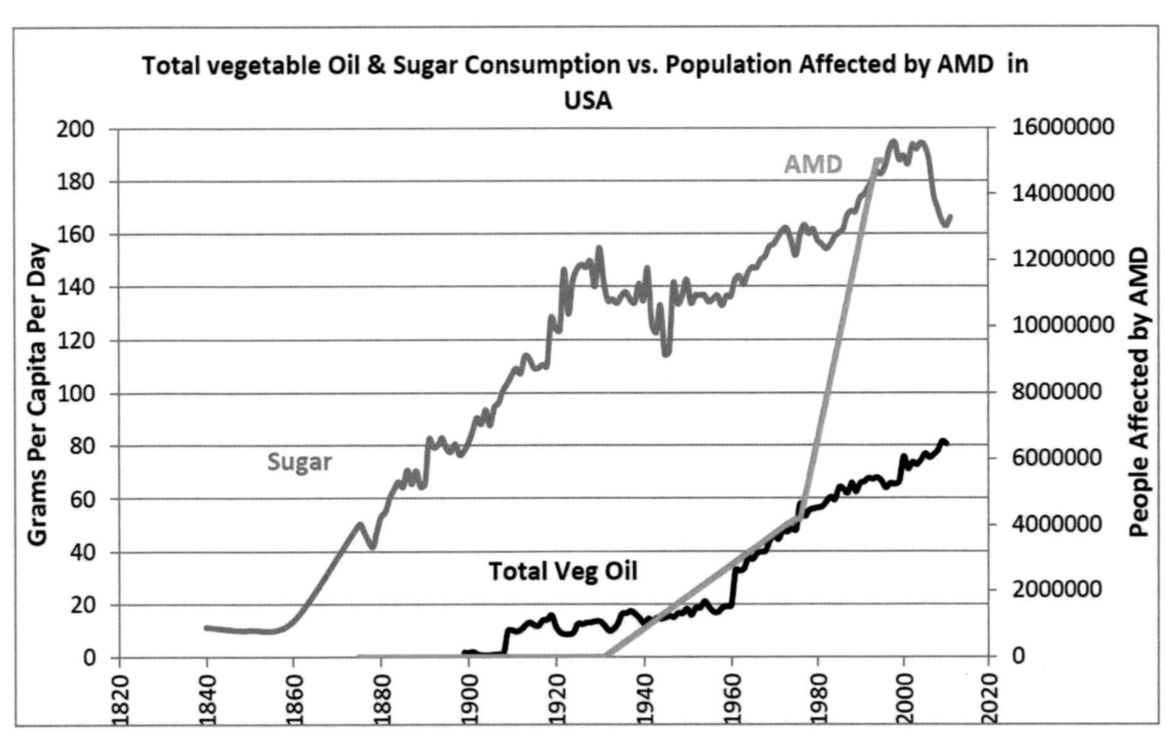

sugar consumption continued to climb. We see then that AMD reaches a staggering 15 million people affected by 1994, with dramatically increasing sugar and vegetable oil consumption.

If we cannot accept the fact that the collective and dramatic alteration in our food, including the replacement of whole, organic, densely nutritious cuisine with processed, nutrient-deficient, inflammation-mediating food, is the primary and proximate cause of not only AMD but numerous other afflictions of "civilization," then I believe we've reached the nadir of rational and logical thought.

This hypothesis is strongly supported by temporality, pathologic and pathogenic mechanisms, and abundant epidemiologic evidence beginning in the United States, the United Kingdom, and Australia, followed by numerous other population studies in Europe, and eventually, Japan, India, China, the Caribbean (Barbados, West Indies) and even Africa, which was once heralded as the place where "macular degeneration does not exist." The facts speak for themselves. Macular degeneration essentially did not exist in any of these populations or in any of these countries, including the United States and Great Britain - less than a century ago. For Japan and India, AMD was a rarity just about 40 years ago, just as Professor Alan Bird, MD, said. For the South Pacific islanders, who until recently consumed little to no processed foods, macular degeneration is a medical rarity. But if they continue to Westernize their diets, they'll soon have all of the diseases of civilization as well, including AMD. Unfortunately, for many nations who began to Westernize their diets four or five decades ago, they're developing heart disease, obesity, cancer, and macular degeneration, just as we have seen. China, Japan, and other Asian countries, some African nations, the Caribbean Islands, and anywhere else who has bought into our nutrient-deficient diet, replete with vegetable oils, trans fats, refined sugar, white flour, and thousands upon thousands of nutrient-depleted, dangerous, processed foods, are all perfect examples.

No nation, in fact, no population and no person should aspire to the Western diet as it is currently practiced. It is self-evident - our diet maims and destroys. It is truly an abomination of what anyone should consider "healthy." **I believe there is ample evidence to indict a processed food laden diet, replete with the 'displacing foods of modern commerce', as the cause of macular degeneration.** Now if anyone wants to argue that we don't have a randomized, double-blind, controlled clinical trial, then this is how to accomplish that. Just take two groups of similar, healthy ten year olds and randomly divide them into two groups - say 5000 per group. Start one group on an organic, whole food diet, with meats, organ meats, and eggs coming from pasture raised animals living on organic farms, combined with plenty of fresh whole fruit and vegetables, nuts and seeds, and possibly some organically raised whole grains prepared with fermentation or sprouting (when tolerated). Start the other group of ten year olds on a typical Westernized diet, with plenty of processed foods, fast foods, and well... the typical standard American diet. Make sure the latter group gets plenty of white flour, sugar, vegetable oils, and trans fats. Then, keep things that way and assess them 20, 30, 40, 50, 60, and 70 years later. Probably 30 to 50 years into the study, you will have your answers - and you will have it from a randomized controlled clinical trial (RCCT).

Sound ridiculous? It is, sort of... but I hope it illustrates the point. We're not going to have evidence based on a randomized controlled clinical trial anytime soon - just as we don't have that sort of proof for heart disease. In fact, it would be harder to "prove" than it has been for research to "prove" that cigarette smoking is dangerous for our health, where no randomized, controlled, prospective, clinical trial has ever been done to conclusively demonstrate that smoking causes emphysema and cancer. Imagine, who would sign up for such a study, where you're randomized to smoking versus not? But, it's no different with processed food. Most all Americans, Australians, and Europeans, unfortunately, are in the "experimental group," that is, they're the ones receiving the most processed, dangerous foods. If you're one of them, do you want to stay in that group?

Let me ask you a question: How many Jack LaLanne types am I speaking to right now? That is, how many of you have chosen to consume nothing but whole, unprocessed, organic foods of both plant and animal origin as your staples at every single meal or snack, every single day of your lives? I believe, unequivocally, that this is the best commitment that you can make to improve your health, to reverse damage, and to provide the best possible nutrition for every single organ and every cell in your body, including your eyes. This, I am convinced, is the key to both preventing and treating macular degeneration. It is self-evident.

And as for genetics, race, color, creed, ethnicity or any other factor regarding a genetic basis for macular degeneration - attempting to find a genetic basis for macular degeneration is like trying to find the genetic basis for lung cancer - in smokers. Genetic heritage is not the basis for lung cancer - smoking is. Likewise, genetic heritage is not the basis for macular degeneration - DIET IS.

YOUR OPHTHALMOLOGIST'S TREATMENT & ADVICE

When it comes to your ophthalmologist, optometrist, physician, or any other healthcare professional's advice regarding nutrition and supplements, I hope you will strongly consider every word in this book. Three years ago, my advice to my own patients would have been wrong. I didn't know what I have since learned and conveyed to you in this book. All of this began with the knowledge I had gained from reading and studying the writings of Weston A. Price as well as that of many other studies, the collective experience of observation and discussions with thousands of my own patients, and a hypothesis. All I can ask is that you act according to your own beliefs.

With regard to your ophthalmologist's recommendations for direct treatment of wet AMD, in general, I would follow every last word of that advice and treatment recommendation. The VEGF inhibitors, such as Avastin, Lucentis, Macugen, and Eylea, which are all injected into the eye when wet AMD rears its ugly head, are absolutely essential.[1302] I would just combine that with the appropriate dietary regime recommended herein.

REVERSING MACULAR DEGENERATION

During my career, I've witnessed at least nine patients reverse early AMD rather completely and over a long period of time. That's not many, but every one of them did that by "cleaning up" their diet on their own – and generally without any advice from me. These were people that had documented early AMD, notably reversed, and followed for years in most cases. I didn't know how to advise these patients – they simply did it on their own, often for a number of reasons. But, always being inquisitive about nutrition, it was my asking what they had done and it was, in part, their answers that further spurred me to consider the hypothesis proferred in this book. If they can do that, many of you can too. But, it takes a very concerted effort and a great commitment.

Reversal of macular degeneration, to various degrees, is also supported by scientific studies. In 1973, world renowned ophthalmologist and retina specialist, the late J Donald M. Gass, M.D., of Bascom Palmer Eye Institute of Florida, in a study of the natural progression of AMD wrote, "There was fading or disappearance of some of the drusen in five patients on whom follow-up studies were done for an average of five years." [1303]

R. Theodore Smith, MD, PhD, and colleagues at the Retinal Image Analysis Laboratory, NYU Schoool of Medicine, in New York, found that there is "dynamic soft drusen remodeling" in AMD, wherein drusen have been shown to not only develop anew but to undergo resorption as well.[1304]

In 1995, the eminent Neil M. Bressler, MD, Professor of Ophthalmology at the Johns Hopkins University School of Medicine, along with colleagues, carefully observed 483 men over the age of 30, over a 5-year period, evaluating for either appearance or disappearance of signs of AMD. They found that disappearance of large drusen occurred in 16 (34%) of 47 participants, increased macular pigmentation (hyperpigmentation) disappeared in 11 (58%) of 19 participants, and disappearance of AMD-3 occurred in 17 (28%) of 61 participants, as documented photographically. In this study, "AMD-3" was defined as large or confluent drusend, focal hyperpigmentation of the RPE, or non-geographic atrophy of the RPE." [1305]

"FOR THE WORDS OF TRUTH ARE SIMPLE"

Aeschylus, the first of classical Athens' great playwrights, wrote "for the words of truth are simple" for one of his plays. The phrase became repeated so often that it became proverbial in ancient Greece. We should adhere to the principle whenever possible. Why complicate it? We've gotten pretty deep into the science of macular degeneration at times in this book. But to understand why we have an epidemic of AMD today while the condition virtually did not exist just a hundred years ago – is simple. What were we eating then? And what are we eating today? And how are they different? And because the incubation period for AMD is probably 30 to 50 years or more, generally, that's how far one has to look back at diet with our retrospectroscope to find the answers. As we've seen, this really comes down to just four main things that were altered, while I will add a fifth for good measure:

FOODS TO AVOID

1. **White Flour**
2. **Sugar** (Sucrose or table sugar and high-fructose corn syrup)
3. **Polyunsaturated Vegetable Oils** (Primarily Soy, Corn, Cottonseed, Canola, Rapeseed, Grapeseed, Sunflower, Safflower, Ricebran, Mustard oil, and anything labeled "vegetable oil")
4. **Trans Fats** (hydrogenated and partially hydrogenated oils, most common in shortening, margarine, and PUFA vegetable oils)
5. **Processed Foods –** Which Are Mostly A Mix of The Previous Four, Pasteurized Dairy, Plus Hundreds or Thousands of Proprietary "Mystery Ingredients," Often Labeled "Artificial Flavor" [1306]

The five groups above succinctly represent the 'displacing foods of modern commerce.'

Just last night, my daughter, Kyla, age 17, argued that "It's just too hard for most people to figure out how to eat healthy." At many levels, I think she's right. It can get pretty confusing. So, in wrapping up, here is my best shot to keep it really simple.

TWENTY-ONE DIETARY RULES TO PREVENT & POSSIBLY REVERSE AMD

1. 'If man made it, don't eat it.' Eat everything the way Nature gave it to us, without compromise, just as Jack LaLanne advised.
2. Eat muscle meats as desired, but also eat organ meats (liver, heart, kidney, pancreas, tongue, etc.) from animals that have *not been* processed, at least once or twice a week. If you can afford it, opt for pasture-raised, always.
3. If you don't eat organ meats (such as chicken or beef liver) regularly (at least once every week or two), strongly consider an excellent source of cold-extracted extra virgin cod liver oil on a daily basis as well as fish roe (eggs) at least once or twice a month or more.
4. If available, eat fish and/or seafood at least two to three times a week. Buy wild-caught, if you can afford it.

5. Eat about 6 to 12 eggs per week or more – preferably one to two or more per day. Eggs from pasture-raised chickens are by far the best.
6. Eat fruits and vegetables of various colors, every day, particularly seasonal and local. Try to eat at least one citrus fruit (oranges, grapefruit, kiwi, etc.) each day. If you can afford it, always buy organic options.
7. If available, eat some dark, leafy-green vegetables such as spinach, kale, and collard greens, at least several times a week.
8. Dairy (milk and cheese) that comes from raw sources and from cows grazing on grass, particularly green grass, and in organic conditions, is brilliantly healthy. On the other hand, dairy that comes from cows raised in CAFOs (concentrated animal feeding operations), which are grain fed (soy or corn), plus treated with antibiotics and hormones, is a disaster. Furthermore, pasteurized, homogenized milk is processed food – just avoid it. Drink raw milk from cows raised on pastures, or drink none.
9. Eat some nuts and seeds in small portions. Be sure they have not been processed. If they contain any other vegetable oils, including peanut oil, look elsewhere.
10. Avoid GMOs: In the U.S., most all corn, soy, canola, sugar from beets (not cane), cottonseed, and some zucchini and yellow squash at the time of this writing, is GMO. Genetically modified organisms are atrocious and, although we don't have evidence yet that they cause or contribute to AMD, you must avoid these like the plague to stay healthy.[1307]
11. Make every attempt to avoid PUFA "vegetable oils" like the plague. These are *biological poisons*, elevating the risk of AMD dramatically, and include soybean, corn (maize), canola, cottonseed, rapeseed, grapeseed, sunflower, safflower, rice bran, and mustard oil.
12. Never consume anything with trans fats, i.e., hydrogenated or partially hydrogenated vegetable oils. This includes almost all PUFA containing vegetable oils, reviewed above. Any type of margarine or shortening falls into this category and should be strictly excluded.
13. Expeller pressed coconut oil, red palm oil, and palm kernel oil, which are mostly saturated fats, are fine and can be used either in cooking or in cold foods, but don't allow these to significantly displace animal fat consumption (e.g. butter, lard, or beef tallow). Peanut oil and expeller pressed sesame oil are certainly much lower risk than the PUFA oils, but should be used cautiously, in small quantities.
14. Cook foods almost exclusively in butter, lard, beef tallow, duck fat, other animal fats, or possibly unrefined, expeller pressed coconut oil, palm oil, or palm kernel oil. Butter from pasture-raised cows raised on organic green pastures not only tastes great and is stable for cooking purposes, but is brilliantly healthy because it provides the vitamin K2 we so desperately need. Butter or lard should be your first choices for cooking.
15. For salads, try to use small amounts of extra-virgin olive oil, avocado oil, expeller pressed sesame oil, or possibly very small amounts of peanut oil. Generally, it is best to make your own salad dressing, using very small quantities of olive oil that is both "virgin" and "cold-pressed." Olive oil must come from a trusted source, as most products currently on the market are not genuine, having been adulterated with the cheap polyunsaturated vegetable oils. These oils still have high ratios of omega-6 to omega-3, so strictly limit their intake to small quantities.
16. Never "take" synthetic vitamins (pills), except under extreme circumstances (e.g., vegans, individuals on a feeding tube, etc.) and be extremely cautious of any advice to take them. Get your vitamins the natural way – from whole foods (note: cold extracted extra virgin cod liver oil is a whole food and not a "supplement").
17. Never "take" fish oil capsules or liquid, flax seed oil capsules or liquid, or any other supplemental oils. These are polyunsaturated oils and our requirements for these are exceedingly small. The poluunsaturated oils consumed should be obtained from natural sources, particularly wild-caught fish and grass-fed beef.
18. Get off the drugs! If at all possible, once you've begun to consume an ancestral diet without any of the 'displacing foods of modern commerce' for a few weeks or so, work with your physician to determine if any medicines you are taking can be eliminated. This might include, but is not limited to, medicines for high blood pressure, cholesterol, type 2 diabetes, arthritis, and low thyroid. You may find these are no longer necessary.
19. Exercise regularly. Try to get some significant exercise at least four to five times a week, preferably including some resistance exercises such as weight-lifting or body-weight exercises. This will help to maintain muscle mass, enhance metabolism, and will cause you to consume more food, thereby enhancing micronutrient (vitamin and mineral) consumption.
20. Get enough sleep. Most of us should get at least 7 to 8 hours of sleep per night. This should come much more naturally once vitamin and mineral deficiencies are corrected with an ancestral diet.

Try to eliminate any type of synthetic sleep aids as much as possible.

21. Have fun and enjoy life! Once you complete the first 20 steps here, the 21st will come more naturally. Take time to just relax, have fun, and enjoy your family, friends, hobbies, church, or any other activities that make life more enjoyable and rewarding. This is key!

ANOTHER BOOK COMING SOON...

Over a period of about three years, I wrote a different (clandestine) book by the name of *Ancestral Diet Rx* - which is still to be released. This book was the culmination and summation of much of my studies about weight gain and health as it relates to our diet, exercise, and lifestyle. That book had its beginnings based on the Paleo Diet but morphed into what I would call "Ancestral Diets." The latter is simply a term that is being used to refer to the diets of our ancestors, even the more recent ones. But, before I could quite finish that book, my mind was overtaken by the hypothesis for AMD that I have presented in this book. I strongly believe that this hypothesis, research, and book had to take precedence. Too many people are losing vision to this disease on a daily basis – and this is happening needlessly. In any case, I hope to release *Ancestral Diet Rx* soon, and hopefully, this will make a great accompaniment to *Cure AMD.*

THE FINALE...

Let me, finally, restate my hypothesis and the corollary:

> **The 'displacing foods of modern commerce' are the primary and proximate cause of age-related macular degeneration.**
>
> **Corollary: Ancestral diets prevent AMD (and may reverse early AMD).**

So, finally I ask you: Do you believe that there is enough evidence to support this hypothesis? If indeed you do, follow the advice shared in this book. As I said to you in the beginning, I think you will be amazed.

It is my goal to spread this knowledge and the hypothesis proffered in this book. I am asking you, if you agree that this hypothesis has validity, to assist me in this mission by sharing your knowledge with your family, friends, and colleagues. If you are a health care practitioner, please share your knowledge with your patients as well. No matter who you are, taking as little as a few seconds to just one to two minutes of your time, enthusiastically sharing your knowledge, can forever change people's lives. Remember to "pay it forward."

Thank you for your attention, for buying this book, and for sticking with me to the end. Take heed and apply to your life the three main concepts from this book, the final one from yours truly:

"Life in all its fullness is Mother Nature obeyed."
~ Weston A. Price ~

"If man made it, don't eat it."
~ Jack LaLanne ~

It is not Age-Related Macular Degeneration (AMD), it is Diet-Related Macular Degeneration (DMD).
~ Chris A. Knobbe ~

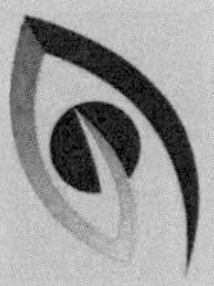

References

1 Jacobs DR and Steffen LM. Nutrients, foods, and dietary patterns as exposures in research: a framework for food synergy. Am J Clin Nutr. 2003; 78(3): 5085-5135.

2 Cordain, Loren. The Paleo Answer. Hoboken, New Jersey: John Wiley and Sons, Inc., 2012.

3 Egan KM, Seddon JM. (1994) *Albert & Jakobiec: Principles and Practice of Ophthalmology. Basic Sciences* (Philadelphia: W.B. Saunders Co.), p. 1273.

4 Mayo Clinic Staff. Mayo Clinic. Available at: *http://www.mayoclinic.org/diseases-conditions/macular-degeneration/basics/risk-factors/con*-20075882

5 Age-Related Macular Degeneration Overview. *WebMD.com*: *http://www.webmd.com/eye-health/macular-degeneration/age*-related-macular-degeneration-overview

6 Duke-Elder, WS. *Textbook of Ophthalmology. Vol. III, Diseases of the Inner Eye*. St. Louis: The C.V. Mosby Company, 1941. p. 2373.

7 Egan KM, Seddon JM. (1994) *Albert & Jakobiec Principles and Practice of Ophthalmology. Basic Sciences* (Philadelphia: W.B. Saunders Co.), p. 1266.

8 Bressler SB, Bressler NM, Gragoudas ES. (1994) *Albert & Jakobiec Principles and Practice of Ophthalmology. Vol. 2 Retina and Vitreous*. Philadelphia: W.B. Saunders Co. p. 832-3.

9 Taubes, Gary. Why We Get Fat. (New York: Alfred A. Knopf, 2011) p. 9.

10 Wright, JD., et al. Trends in intake of energy and macronutrients – United States, 1971-2000. Feb 2004. MMWR Morb Mortal Wkly Rep 53 (4): 80-2.

11 Adams, KM, Lindell KC, et al. Status of nutrition education in medical schools. Am J Clin Nutr. 2006 Apr; 83(4): 941S-944S.

12 Ibid.

13 Chen, Pauline W. "Teaching Doctors About Nutrition and Diet." *The New York Times*. Sep. 16, 2010. Available at: *http://www.nytimes.com/2010/09/16/health/16chen.html*

14 Ibid.

15 "How Much Does the U.S. Spend on Health and How Has It Changed?" The Henry J. Kaiser Family Foundation. May 1, 2012. Available at: *http://kff.org/report-section/health-care-costs-a-primer-2012-report/*

16 Murray CJL, Frank J. Ranking 37th – Measuring the Performance of the U.S. Health Care System. N England J Med. 2010; 362: 98-99.

17 Moyer, Christine S. "U.S. found to be unhealthiest among 17 affluent countries." American Medical News. Jan. 21, 2013. Available at: *http://www.amednews.com/article/20130121/health/130129983/4/*

18 Khan, A. America Tops List of 10 Most Obese Countries. *U.S. News & World Report*. May 28, 2014. Available at: *http://health.usnews.com/health-news/health-wellness/articles/2014/05/28/america-tops-list-of-10-most-obese-countries*

19 Grundy SM, Brewer HB, et al. Definition of Metabolic Syndrome. Circulation 2004; 109: 433-38.

20 Lustig, Robert H. *FAT CHANCE – Beating the Odds Against Sugar, Processed Food, Obesity, and Disease*. New York: Hudson Street Press, 2013. *p. 93*.

21 Beltran-Sanchez H, Harhay MO, et al. Prevalence and Trends of Metabolic Syndrome in the Adult U.S. Population, 1999-2010. J American College of Cardiology. Aug 20, 2013. 62 (8): 697-703.

22 Cheung N, Wong TY. Obesity and eye diseases. Surv Ophthalmol. 2007; 52(2): 180-95.

23 Peeters A, Magliano DJ, et al. Changes in abdominal obesity and age-related macular degeneration; the Atherosclerosis Risk in Communities Study.

24 Schaumberg DA, Christen WG, et al. Body mass index and the incidence of visually significant age-related maculopathy in men. Arch Ophthalmol. 2001; 119(9): 1259-65.

25 Klein R, Peto T, et al. The epidemiology of age-related macular degeneration. Am J Ophthalmol. 2004; 137(3): 486-495.

26 Katsi VK, Marketou ME, et al. Essential hypertension in the pathogenesis of age-related macular degeneration: a review of the current evidence. J Hypertens. 2015; 33(12): 2382-8.

27 Sun C, Klein R, Wong TY. Age-related macular degeneration and risk of coronary heart disease and stroke: the Cardiovascular Health Study. Ophthalmology. 2009; 116(10): 1913-1919.

28 Tan JS, Mitchell P, et al. Cardiovascular risk factors and the long-term incidence of age-related macular degeneration:

the Blue Mountains Eye Study. Ophthalmology. 2007; 114(6): 1143-1150.

29 Klein R, Deng Y, Klein BE, et al. Cardiovascular disease, its risk factors and treatment, and age-related macular degeneration: Women's health initiative sight exam ancillary study. Am J Ophthalmol. 2007; 143(3): 473-483.

30 Clemons TE, Milton RC, Klein R, Seddon JM, Ferris FL 3rd. Risk factors for the incidence of Advanced Age-Related Macular Degeneratino in the Age-Related Eye Disease Study (AREDS) AREDS report no. 19. Ophthalmology. 2005: 112: 533-539.

31 Hahn P, Acquah K, Cousins SW, et al. Ten-Year Incidence of Age-Related Macular Degeneration According to Diabetic Retinopathy Classification Among Medicare Beneficiaries. Retina. 2013; 33: 911-919.

32 Mitchell P, Wang JJ. Diabetes, fasting blood glucose and age-related maculopathy: The Blue Mountains Eye Study. Aust N Z J Ophthalmol. 1999; 27: 197-99.

33 Topouzis F, Anastasopoulos E, et al. Association of diabetes with age-related macular degeneration in the EUREYE study. Br J Ophthalmol. 2009; 93: 1037-1041.

34 Seddon JM, Gensler G, Milton RC, et al. Association between C-reactive protein and age-related macular degeneration. JAMA. 2004; 291(6): 704-710.

35 Maralani HG, Tai BC, Wong TY, et al. Metabolic syndrome and risk of age-related macular degeneration. Retina. 2015; 35(3): 459-66.

36 Van Bol L, Rasquin F. [Age-related macular degeneration]. Rev Med Brux. 2014; 35(4): 265-70.

37 Pascolini D, Mariotti SP. Global estimates of visual impairment: 2010. Br. J Ophthalmol 2012; 96: 614-618.

38 The prevention of blindness. Report of a WHO Study Group. Geneva. World Health Organization, 1980 (WHO Offset Publication No. 54).

39 Resnikoff S, Pascolini D, Etya'ale D, et al. Global data on visual impairment in the year 2002. Bulletin of the World Health Organization. 2004; 82: 844-851.

40 Congdon N, O'Colmain B, et al. Causes and prevalence of visual impairment among adults in the United States. Arch Ophthalmol. 2004; 122(4): 477-485.

41 Pascolini D, Mariotti SP. Global estimates of visual impairment: 2010. Br J Ophthalmol. 2011; 96: 614-618.

42 Bourne RRA, Jonas JB, et al. Prevalence and causes of vision loss in high-income countries and in Eastern and Central Europe: 1990-2010. Br J Ophthalmol. 2014; 0: 1-10.

43 Klein R, Klein BE, Linton KL. Prevalence of age-related maculopathy. The Beaver Dam Eye Study. Ophthalmology. 1992; 99: 933-943.

44 Wong WL, Su X, et al. Global prevalence of age-related macular degeneration and disease burden projection for 2020 and 2040: a systematic review and meta-analysis. Lance Glob Health. 2014; 2: e106-16.

45 The number of ophthalmologists in practice and in training worldwide; a growing gap despite more than 200,000 practitioners. International Council of Ophthalmology. Jun 1, 2012, Available at: *http://www.icoph.org/resources/271/The-number-of-ophthalmologists-in-practice-and-in-training-worldwide-a-growing-gap-despite-more-than-200000-practitioners.html*

46 Global need for vision care indicates need for more optometrists. Primary Care Optometry News. Aug. 2012. Available at: *http://www.healio.com/optometry/primary-care-optometry/news/print/primary-care-optometry-news/%7B-5dee8831-92d1-49bf-9108-f8457cd4cf6e%7D/global-need-for-vision-care-indicates-need-for-more-optometrists*

47 Wong TY, Chakravarthy U, Klein R, et al. The natural history and prognosis of neovascular age-related macular degeneration: a systemic review of the literature and meta-analysis. Ophthalmology. 2008; 115(1): 116-26.

48 Age-Related Eye Disease Study Research Group. A randomized, placebo-controlled, clinical trial of high-dose supplementation with vitamins C and E, beta carotene, and zinc for age-related macular degeneration and vision loss: AREDS report no. 8. Arch Ophthalmol. 2001; 119: 1417-1436.

49 Risk factors for choroidal neovascularization in the second eye of patients with juxtafoveal or subfoveal choroidal neovascularization secondary to age-related macular degeneration: Macular Photocoagulation Study Group. Arch Ophthalmol. 1997; 115: 741-747.

50 Hageman, Gegory S. Age-Related Macular Degeneration (AMD) by Gregory S. Hageman. Webvision. Available at: *http://webvision.med.utah.edu/book/part-xii-cell-biology-of-retinal-degenerations/age-related-macular-degeneration-amd/*

51 Seddon JM, Ajani UA, et al. Dietary carotenoids, vitamins A, C, and E, and advanced age-related macular degeneration. Eye Disease Case-Control Study Group. JAMA. 1994 Nov 9; 272(18): 1413-20.

52 Thomas J, Mohammad S, Charnigo R, Baffi J, Abdel-Latif A, Ziada KM. Age-Related Macular Degeneration and Coronary Artery Disease in a VA Population. South Med J. 2015: 108(8): 502-6.

53 William S. Yancy Jr., MD, MHS; Maren K Olsen, PhD; John R. Guyton, MD; Ronna P. Bakst, RD; and Eric C. Westman, MD, MHS. A Low-Carbohydrate, Ketogenic Diet versus a Low-Fat Diet To Treat Obesity and Hyperlipidemia. Annals of Internal Medicine. 2004: 140: 769-777.

54 Sharman MJ, Gomez AL, Kraemer WJ, Volek JS. Very low-carbohydrate and low-fat diets affect fasting lipids and postprandial lipemia differently in overweight men. J Nutr. 2004. Apr; 134(4): 880-5.

55 Samaha FF, Foster GD, Makris AP. Low-carbohydrate diets, obesity, and metabolic risk factors for cardiovascular disease. Curr Atheroscler Rep. 2007. Dec: 9(6): 441-7.

56 Stern L, Iqbal N, Seshadri P, Chicano KL, Daily DA, McGrory J, Williams M, Gracely EJ, Samaha FF. The effects of low-carbohydrate versus conventional weight loss diets in severely obese adults: one-year follow-up of a randomized trial.

57 Taubes, Gary. What if It's All Been a Big Fat Lie? The New York Times. July 07, 2002.

58 Mich R, Mozaffarian D, et al., Saturated fat and cardiometabolic risk factors, coronary heart disease, stroke, and diabetes: a fresh look at the evidence. Lipids, 2010 Oct: 45(10): 893-905.

59 Brehm BJ, Seeley RJ, Daniels SR, D'Alessio DA. A randomized trial comparing a very low carbohydrate diet and a calorie-restricted low fat diet on body weight and cardiovascular risk factors in healthy women. J Clin Endocrinol Metab. 2003 Apr; 88(4): 1617-23.

60 Foster GD, Wyatt HR, Hill JO< McGuckin BG, Brill C, Mohammed BS, Szapary PO, Rader DJ, Edman JS, Klein S. A randomized trial of a low-carbohydrate diet for obesity. N Engl J Med. 2003 May 22; 348(21): 2082-90.

61 Meckling KA, O'Sullivan C, Saari D. Comparison of a low-fat diet to a low-carbohydrate diet on weight loss, body composition, and risk factors for diabetes and cardiovascular disease in free-living, overweight men and women. J Clin Endocrinol Metab. 2004 Jun; 89(6): 2717-23.

62 Sharman MJ, Gomez AL, Kraemer WJ, Volek JS. Very low-carbohydrate and low-fat diets affect fasting lipids and postprandial lipemia differently in overweight men. J Nutr. 2004 Apr; 134(4): 880-5.

63 Boden G, Sargrad K, Homko C, Mozzoli M, Stein TP. Effect of a low-carbohydrate diet on appetitie, blood glucose levels, and insulin resistance in obese patients with type 2 diabetes. Ann Intern Med. 2005 Mar 15; 142(6): 403-11.

64 McAuley KA, Hopkins CM, Smith KJ, McLay RT, Williams SM, Taylor RW, Mann JI. Comparison of high-fat and high-protein diets with high-carbohydrate diet in insulin-resistant obese women. Diabetologia. 2005 Jan; 48(1): 8-16.

65 Ravnskov, Uffe. Ignore the Awkward! How the Cholesterol Myths are Kept Alive. 2010. ISBN 1453759409, p. 19.

66 Schulze MB, Manson JE, Ludwig DS, Colditz GA, Stampfer MJ, Willett WC, Hu FB. Sugar-sweetened beverages, weight gain, and incidence of type 2 diabetes in young and middle-aged women. JAMA. 2004 Aug 25; 292(8): 927-34.

67 Bjelakovic G, Nikolova D, et al. Mortality in randomized trials of antioxidant supplements for primary and secondary prevention: systematic review and meta-analysis. JAMA. 2007 Feb 28: 297(8): 842-57/

68 Albert, Daniel M. The History of Ophthalmology. Cambridge, Massachusetts, Blackwell Science, Inc., 1996. p. xvi (Preface).

69 Ibid.

70 Albert, Daniel M. *The History of Ophthalmology.* Blackwell Science, Inc., Cambridge, Massachusetts, 1996, p. 76.

71 Ibid.

72 Keeler CR. A Brief History of the Ophthalmoscope. The Royal College of Ophthalmologists, London, UK, Accepted for publication 16 June 2003. Available at: Optometry in Practice 2003; Vol 4: 137-145.

73 Hirschberg, Julius. The History of Ophthalmology. Vol 10: THE FIRST AND SECOND HALF OF THE NINETEENTH CENTURY (PART NINE TO SEVENTEEN). Originally published in Germany under the title Geschichte der Augenheilkunde. Berlin: Julius Springer, 1914 -1915; (First English edition 1991). P. 293.

74 Albert, Daniel M., Edwards, Diane D. *The History of Ophthalmology.* (Cambridge, Massachusetts, Blackwell Science, 1996) p. 191.

75 Albert, Daniel M., Edwards, Diane D. *The History of Ophthalmology.* Cambridge, Massachusetts, Blackwell Science, 1996. p. 195-196.

76 Keeler CR. A Brief History of the Ophthalmoscope. The Royal College of Ophthalmologists, London, UK, Accepted for publication 16 June 2003. Available at: Optometry in Practice 2003; Vol 4: p. 138.

77 Duke-Elder, WS. *System of Ophthalmology, Volume X.* St. Louis: The C.V. Mosby Company, 1967. p. 535.

78 Hutchinson J, Tay W. Symmetrical central choroido-retinal disease occurring in senile persons. R Lond Ophthalmic Hosp Rep J Ophthalmic Surg. 1874; 8: 231-244.

79 Duke-Elder S, Dobree JH. System of Ophthalmology. Vol. X. Diseases of the retina. London: Kimpton; 1967; p.647.

80 de Jong, Paulus T.V.M. Elusive Ageing Macula Disorder (AMD). Hist Ophthal Intern. 2015; 1: 139-152.

81 Duke-Elder, WS. *Textbook of Ophthalmology - Duke-Elder, Vol. III, Diseases of the Inner Eye.* (St. Louis: The C.V. Mosby Company, 1940) p. 2372.

82 Nagel A. Ueber Chorioiditis areolaris und über Krystalle im Augenhhintergrund. On areolar choroiditis and crystals in the eye fundus. Klin Monbl Augenheilk. 1868; 4: 417-20.

83 Nagel A. Hochgradige Amblyopie, bedingt durch glashäutige Wucherungen und krystallinische Kalkablagerungen an der Innenfläche der Aderhaut. Kl Monatsbl Augenh. 1875; 13:338-51. z

84 Narendran N, Asaria R, Haynes R. Optical coherence tomography of macular crystalline opacities associated with chronic retinal detachment. Nature; Eye (2006) 20, 843-845. Doi:10.1038/sj.eye.6702015; published online 5 August 2005.

85 Pagenstecher: Atlas der pathologischen Anatomie des Augapfels, C. W. Kreidel, Wiesbaden, 1875.

86 Duke-Elder, WS. *Textbook of Ophthalmology - Duke-Elder, Vol. III, Diseases of the Inner Eye.* St. Louis: The C.V. Mosby Company, 1940. p. 2372.

87 Haab, O. Zentralblatt für prakrische Augenheilkunde v. 9, p. 383-4, 1885.

88 Haab O. Atlas und Grundriss der Ophthalmoskopie und ophthalmoskopischen Diagnostik. Atlas and outline of ophthalmoscopy and ophthalmoscopic diagnosis. München, Lehmann; 1895.

89 Haab O. Erkrankungen der Macula Lutea. Diseases of the macula lutea. *Centralblatt für praktische Augenheilkunde.* 1885(9): 383-4.

90 Haab O. Ueber die Erkrankung der Macula lutea. On the disease of the macula lutea. *Siebenter Periodischer Internationaler Ophthalmologen*-Congress Heidelberg. 1888, p. 429.

91 Muller A, McGhee CN. Professor Ernst Fuchs (1851 - 1930): a defining career in ophthalmology. Arch Ophthalmol. 121 (6): 888-91.

92 Fuchs, Ernest. Textbook of Ophthalmology. New York, D. Appleton and Company, 1892. pp. 400 - 419.

93 Fuchs, Ernest. Textbook of Ophthalmology. New York, D. Appleton and Company, 1892. p. 315.

94 Oliver, Charles Augustus, Norris, William Fisher. A Text-Book of Ophthalmology - Primary Source Edition. Philadelphia, Lea Brothers & Co., 1893. p. 496.

95 Oliver, Charles Augustus, Norris, William Fisher. A Text-Book of Ophthalmology - Primary Source Edition (Philadelphia, Lea Brothers & Co., 1893), p. 500.

96 Gradle, Henry. Anomalies of the Retinal Pigment Epithelium and their Clinical Significance. Trans of AAOO. 1913; 332-338.

97 The age of isopter perimetry: Bjerrum and the tangent screen. Imaging and Perimetry Society. Available at: *http://webeye.ophth.uiowa.edu/ips/PerimetryHistory/4-tangentscreen.htm*

98 Hirschberg, Julius. The History of Ophthalmology. Vol 10: THE FIRST AND SECOND HALF OF THE NINETEENTH CENTURY (PART NINE TO SEVENTEEN). Originally published in Germany under the title Geschichte der Augenheilkunde. Berlin: Julius Springer, 1914 -1915; (First English edition 1991). P. 151.

99 Hirschberg, Julius. The History of Ophthalmology. Vol 10: THE FIRST AND SECOND HALF OF THE NINETEENTH CENTURY (PART NINE TO SEVENTEEN). Originally published in Germany under the title Geschichte der Augenheilkunde. Berlin: Julius Springer, 1914 -1915; (First English edition 1991). P. 263.

100 "A Profile of Older Americans: 2014." Department of Health and Human Services, USA. Administration on Aging, 2014. Available at: *http://www.aoa.acl.gov/aging_statistics/profile/2014/docs/2014-Profile.pdf*

101 Klein R, Klein BEK, Cruickshanks KJ. The Prevalence of Age-Related Maculopathy by Geographic Region and Ethnicity. Progress in Retinal and Eye Research. 1999; 18(3): 371-389.

102 Junius P, Kuhnt H. *Die scheibenförmige Entartung der Netzhautmitte.* Degeneratio maculae luteae disciformis. The disciform degeneration of the central retina. Disciform macula lutea degeneration. Berlin: Karger, S.; 1926.

103 de Jong, Paulus. Elusive Ageing Macula Disorder (AMD) - Evolution of Our Understanding and Its Nomenclature. Historia Ophthalmologica Internationalis. 2015; 1: 139-152.

104 Ibid.

105 Duke-Elder, W. Stewart. *Recent Advances in Ophthalmology*. Philadelphia, P. Blakiston's Son & Co., 1927. p. XV.

106 May, Charles H. Manual of the Diseases of the Eye. Thirteenth Edition, Revised. New York. William Wood and Company, 1930, p. 188.

107 Friedenwald, H. The Doyne Memorial Lecture: Pathological changes in the retinal blood-vessels in arterio-sclerosis and hypertension. T.O.S., 1930; 1: 452-531.

108 Verhoeff FH, Grossman HP. The Pathogenesis of Disciform Degeneration of the Macula. Trans Am Ophthalmol Soc. 1937; 35: 262-294.

109 Ibid.

110 Rones, Benjamin. Senile Changes and Degenerations of the Human Eye. American Journal of Ophthalmology. 1938; 21 (3): 239 – 255.

111 Rones, Benjamin. Senile Changes and Degenerations of the Human Eye. American Journal of Ophthalmology. 1938; 21 (3): 239 – 255.

112 Duke-Elder, WS. *Textbook of Ophthalmology – Duke-Elder, Vol. III, Diseases of the Inner Eye*. St. Louis: The C.V. Mosby Company, 1940. p. 2372.

113 Ibid. pp. 2372-2373.

114 Ibid. pp. 2373-2374.

115 Ibid. pp. 2115-2118.

116 Waardenburg, PJ. Some Notes on Publications of Professor Arnold Sorsby and on Aland Eye Disease (Forsius-Eriksson syndrome). Journal of Medical Genetics 1970; 7, 194.

117 Sorsby, Arnold. Systemic Ophthalmology, 2nd Edition. St. Louis: CV Mosby Company, 1958.

118 Kornzweig, AI. Macular Diseases: Pathogenesis. Diseases of the Macula in the Aged. Transactions of the American Academy of Ophthalmology and Otolaryngology. 1965; Jul-Aug: 69: 668-82.

119 Ibid.

120 Ibid.

121 Parsons, John Herbert: *The Pathology of the Eye, Vol. 2*, London, Hodder and Stroughton, 1905, p. 596.

122 Friedenwald, Jonas Stein: *Pathology of the Eye, Ed. 1*, London, Henry Kimpton, 1930, p. 187.

123 Rones, Benjamin: Senile changes and degenerations of the human eye. Amer J Ophthal. 1938; 21: 239-255.

124 Woods, C.G. Russ: Choroidal sclerosis, The Ophthalmoscope. 1915; 13: 374-376.

125 Duke-Elder, WS. *Textbook of Ophthalmology – Duke-Elder, Vol. III, Diseases of the Inner Eye*. St. Louis: The C.V. Mosby Company, 1940. p. 2372.

126 Nagel, A. Hochgradige Amblyopie, bedingt durch gläshautige wucherungen und drystallinische Kalkablagerungen an der innenfläche der Aderhaut, Klin Mbl Augenheilk. 1875; 13: 338-351.

127 Harms, Clemens: Anatomisches über die senile maculaaffektion, Klin Mbl Augenheilk, 1904; 42: 448-461.

128 Behr, Carl. Die Anatomie der "senilen Makula" (der senilen Form der kakularen Heredodegeneration), Klin Mbl Augenheilk, 1921; 67: 551-564.

129 Klein, Bertha A. The heredodegeneration of the macula lutea: diagnostic and differential diagnostic considerations and a histopathologic report. Amer J Ophthal. 1950; 33: 371-379.

130 Klein, Bertha A. Macular lesions of vascular origin, Amer J Ophthal. 1951; 34: 1279-1289.

131 Kornzweig, AI. Macular Diseases: Pathogenesis. Diseases of the Macula in the Aged. Transactions of the American Academy of Ophthalmology and Otolaryngology. 1965; Jul-Aug: 69: 668-82.

132 Duke-Elder, WS. *System of Ophthalmology. Vol IX Diseases of the Uveal Tract*. St. Louis: The C.V. Mosby Company, 1966. pp. 609-614.

133 Kahn HA, Leibowitz HM, Ganley JP, et al: The Framingham Eye Study II. Association of ophthalmic pathology with single variables previously measured in the Framingham Heart Study. Am J Epidemiol 1977; 106: 33.

134 Kahn HA, Leibowitz HM. Ganley JP, et al. The Framingham Eye Study I. Outline and major prevalence findings. Am J Epidemiol. 1977; 106(1): 17-32.

135 Kini MM, Leibowitz HM, Colton T, et al. Prevalence of senile cataract, diabetic retinopathy, senile macular degeneration, and open angle glaucoma in the Framingham Eye Study. Am J Ophthalmol. 1978: 85 (1): 28-34.

136 Vinding T. Age-related macular degeneration. Macular changes, prevalence and sex ratio. An epidemiologic study of 1000 aged individuals. Acta Ophthalmol (Copenh) 1989: 67(6): 609-16.

137 Klein R, Klein BEK, Linton KLP. Prevalence of Age-related Maculopathy. The Beaver Dam Eye Study. Ophthalmology. 1992; 99: 933-43.

138 Mitchell P, Smith W, Attebo K, Wang JJ. Prevalence of age-related maculopathy in Australia. The Blue Mountains Eye Study. Ophthalmology. 1995 Oct; 102(10): 1450-60.

139 Egan KM, Seddon JM. (1994) *Albert & Jakobiec Principles and Practice of Ophthalmology. Basic Sciences* (Philadelphia: W.B. Saunders Co.), p. 1266.

140 1990 Census. United States Census Bureau. Available at: *http://www.census.gov/main/www/cen1990.html*

141 Evans J, Wormald R. Is the incidence of registrable age-related macular degeneration increasing? Br J Ophthalm. 1996; 80: 9-14.

142 Ibid.

143 Rees A, Zekite A, Bunce C, Patel PJ. How many people in England and Wales are registered partially sighted or blind because of age-related macular degeneration? Eye (Lond). 2014; 28(7): 832-7.

144 Penfold, Philip P, Provis, Jan M. Macular Degeneration. Berlin, Heidelberg, New York: Springer, 2005, p. 80.

145 Bird AC. Therapeutic targets in age-related macular disease. J Clin Invest. 2010: 120(9): 3033-3041.

146 Bird, Alan C. "Age Related Macular Disease." National Academy of Sciences, National Academy of Engineering, and Institute of Medicine. *Distinctive Voices* lecture given at the Beckman Center, Irvine, California. 2014. Published online Feb. 6, 2014. Available at: *https://www.youtube.com/watch?v=6ugISIFyxuA*.

147 Search results available at: *http://www.aaojournal.org*.

148 "The History of Nutrition." NaturalHealers. No author listed. ND. Available at: *ww.naturalhealers.com/nutrition-history/*

149 Gradle, Henry. Anomalies of the Retinal Pigment Epithelium and their Clinical Significance. Trans of AAOO. 1913: 332-338.

150 Bedell, Arthur. The Clinical Importance of Pigment in the Fundus. Trans of the American Academy of Ophthalm and Otolaryng. 1936: 446-455.

151 Oliver, Charles Augustus, Norris, William Fisher. A Text-Book of Ophthalmology – Primary Source Edition. Philadelphia, Lea Brothers & Co., 1893. p. 496.

152 Oliver, Charles Augustus, Norris, William Fisher. A Text-Book of Ophthalmology – Primary Source Edition. Philadelphia, Lea Brothers & Co., 1893. p. 449.

153 Rones, Benjamin. Senile Changes and Degenerations of the Human Eye. American Journal of Ophthalmology. 1938; 21 (3): 239 – 255.

154 Ibid.

155 Penfold, Philip L. and Provis, Jan M. *Macular Degeneration.* Berlin, Heidelberg, New York, Springer, 2004, pp. V-VI (preface).

156 Penfold, Philip L. and Provis, Jan M. *Macular Degeneration.* Berlin, Heidelberg, New York, Springer, 2004, p. 26.

157 Thompson, Jennifer Trainer, Seddon, Johanna M. *Eat Right for Your Sight.* New York, The Experiment, LLC, 2015, pp. xxii-xxiii (Introduction).

158 Fritsche LG, Chen W, Schu M, et al. AMD Gene Consortium. Seven new loci associated with age –related macular degeneration. Nat Genet. 2013; 45: 433-439.

159 Davaoudi S and Sobrin L. Genetic Testing for Age-related Macular Degeneration. *Ophthalmology Management.* Dec. 2015, Issue 88.

160 Escher, Jill. "Epigenetics & the Multigenerational Effects of Nutrition, Chemicals and Drugs." Ancestral Health Symposium, 2014. Available at: *https://www.youtube.com/watch?v=k4LezkjN-wnY&list=PLbhWKPDKXIEAhNzG0GiCw7jE59KS6WH5w*

161 Xing C, Sivakumaran TA, Wang JJ, et al. Complement factor H polymorphisms, renal phenotypes and age-related macular degeneration: the Blue Mountains Eye Study. Genes & Immunity 2008; 9, 231-239.

162 Donoso LA, Kim D, Frost A, et al. The role of inflammation in the pathogenesis of age-related macular degeneration. Surv. Ophthalm. 2006; 51: 137-152.

163 Xiao-Feng Hao, Li-Ke Xie, You-Zhi Tang, et al. Associations of complement factor H gene polymorphisms with age-related macular degeneration susceptibility. Int J Clin Exp Pathol. 2015; 8(3): 3186-3191.

164 Thakkinstian A, Han P, McEvoy M, et al. Systematic review and meta-analysis of the association between complement factor H Y402H polymorphisms and age-related macular degeneration. Hum Mol Genet. 2006 Sep 15; 15(18): 2784-90.

165 Schwartz SG, Agarwal A, et al. The ARMS2 A69S Variant and Bilateral Advanced Age-Related Macular Degeneration. Retina. 2012; 32(8): 1486-1491.

166 Bird AC. Therapeutic targets in age-related macular disease. J Clin Invest. 2010: 120(9): 3033-3041.

167 Rivera A, Fisher SA, Fritsche LG, et al. Hypothetical LOC387715 is a second major susceptibility gene for age-related macular degeneration, contributing independently of complement factor H to disease risk. Hum Mol Genet. 2005: 14(21): 3227-3236.

168 Boggs W. Risk Factors Influence Age of Onset of Age-Related Macular Degeneration. Medscape Ophthalmology. March 2, 2015. Available online at *www.medscape.com*.

169 Hyman LG, Lilienfeld AM, Ferris Fl 3rd, Fine AL. Senile macular degeneration: a case control study. Am J Epidemiol. 1983; 118(2): 213-227.

170 Seddon JM, Ajani UA, Mitchell BD. Familial aggregation of age-related maculopathy. Am J Ophthalmol. 1997; 123(2): 199-206.

171 Meyers SM, Greene T, Gutman FA. A Twin Study of Age-related Macular Degeneration. American J Ophthalmol. 1995; 120(6): 757-766.

172 Hammond CJ, Webster AR, Snieder H, et al. Genetic influence on early age-related maculopathy: A twin study. Ophthalmology 2002; 109(4): 730-36.

173 Muehlenbein, Michael P. (Editor) *Human Evolutionary Biology.* Cambridge, New York, Cambridge University Press, 2010, p. 491.

174 Haugen A. Women who smoke: are women more susceptible to tobacco-induced lung cancer? Carcinogenesis. 2002; 23(2): 227-229.

175 Grimes DS. An epidemic of coronary heart disease. QJM: An International Journal of Medicine. 2012; 105(6): 509-18.

176 Meals. The Holocaust Explained. No author listed. ND. Available at: *http://www.theholocaustexplained.org/ks3/the-final-solution/auschwitz-birkenau/meals/#.Vnhb9ek1gXM*

177 Curcio CA, Sloan KR, Kalina RE, Hendrickson AE. Human photoreceptor topography. J Comp Neurol. 1990; 292: 497-523.

178 Penfold, Philip L. and Provis, Jan M. *Macular Degeneration.* Berlin, Heidelberg, New York, Springer, 2004, p. 9.

179 Delori, Francois. "Research Story." Schepens Eye Research Institute, Massachusetss Eye and Ear. 2015. Available online: *http://www.schepens.harvard.edu/restory/francois-delori-phd/research-story.html*

180 Cohen LH, Noell WK. Relationships Between Visual Function and Metabolism. In *Biochemistry of the Retina.* New York: Academic Press; 1965.

181 Strauss O. The Retinal Pigment Epithelium in Visual Function. Physiol Rev 2005;85(3):845-81.

182 Schleicher M, Weikel K, Garber C, Taylor A. Diminishing Risk for Age-Related Macular Degeneration with Nutrition: A Current View. Nutrients. 2013; 5: 2405-2456.

183 Zarbin MA, Current concepts in the pathogenesis of age-related macular degeneration. Arch Ophthalmol 2004;122:598-614.

184 McLeod DS, Grebe R, Bhutto I, et al. Relationships between RPE and choriocapillaris in age-related macular degeneration. Invest Ophthalm Vis Sci 2009;50:4982-4991.

185 Al-Hussaini et al. Mature retinal pigment epithelium cells are retained in the cell cycle and proliferate in vivo. Molecular Vision. 2008: 14: 1784-1791.

186 Xia H, Krebs MP, Kaushal S, Scott EW. Enhanced retinal pigment epithelium regeneration after injury in MRL/MpJ mice. Experimental Eye Research. 2011; 93(6): 862-872.

187 Fuhrmann S, Zou CJ, Levine EM. Retinal pigment epithelium development, plasticity, and tissue homeostasis. Experimental Eye Research. 2014; 123: 141-150.

188 Seagle BLL, Gasyna EM, Mieler WF, Norris JR. Photoprotection of human retinal pigment epithelium cells against blue light-induced apoptosis by melanin free radicals from Sepia officinalis. Proceedings of the National Academy of Sciences of the United States of America. 2006; 103(45): 16644-16648.

189 Zarbin MA. Age-related macular degeneration: review of pathogenesis. Eur J Ophthalmol. 1998: 8(4): 199-206.

190 Chiu, Chung-Jung, Taylor T. Dietary Hyperglycemia, Glycemic Index and Metabolic Retinal Diseases. Prog Retin Eye Res. 2011; 30(1): 18-53.

191 Gonzales-Fernandez F. Interphotoreceptor retinoid-binding protein – an old gene for new eyes. Vision Res. 2003; 43(28): 3021-36.

192 Chong NH, Keonin J, Luthert PJ, et al. Decreased thickness and integrity of the macular elastic layer of Bruch's membrane correspond to the distribution of lesions associated with age-related macular degeneration. Am J Pathol 2005; 166: 241-251.

193 Hogan MJ, Alvarado J. Studies on the human macula. IV. Aging changes in Bruch's membrane. Arch Ophthalmol. 1967; 77(3): 410-420.

194 van der Schaft TL, deBruijn WC, Mooy CM, Ketelaars DA, de Jong PT. Is basal laminar deposit unique for age-related macular degeneration? Arch Ophthalmol 1991; 109: 420-425.

195 Ramrattan RS, van der Schaft TL, Mooy CM, et al. Morphometric analysis of Bruch's membrane, the choriocapillaris, and the choroid in aging. Invest Ophthalmol Vis Sci 1994; 35: 2857-2864.

196 Spraul CW, Lang GE, Grossniklaus HE, Lang GK. Histologic and Morphometric Analysis of the Choroid, Bruch's Membrane, and Retinal Pigment Epithelium in Postmortem Eyes With Age-Related Macular Degeneration and Histologic Examination of Surgically Excised Choroidal Neovascular Membranes. Survey of Ophthalmol. 1999; Vol 44, Supplement 1: S10- S32.

197 Spraul CW, Lang GE, et al. Histologic and Morphometric Analysis of the Choroid, Bruch's Membrane, and Retinal Pigment Epithelium in Postmortem Eyes With Age-Related Macular Degeneration and Histologic Examination of Surgically Excised Choroidal Neovascular Membranes. Survey of Ophthalmol. 1999; Vol 44, Supplement 1: S10- S32.

198 Klein R, Klein BE, et al. The association of cardiovascular disease with the long-term incidence of age-related maculopathy: the Beaver Dam eye study. Ophthalmology. 2003; 110(4): 636-43.

199 Theuwissen E, Smit E, Vermeer C. The Role of Vitamin K in Soft-Tissue Calcification. Advances in Nutrition. 2012; 3: 166-173.

200 Schurgers LJ, Dissel PEP, et al. Role of vitamin K and vitamin K-dependent proteins in vascular calcification. Zeitschrift für Kardiologie. 2001; 90(3): 57-63.

201 Shea MK and Holden RM. Vitamin K Status and Vascular Calcification: Evidence from Observational and Clinical Studies. Advances in Nutrition. 2012; 3: 158-165.

202 Pauleikhoff D, Harper CA, Marshall J, Bird AC. Aging changes in Bruch's membrane. A histochemical and morphologic study. Ophthalmol 1990;97(2):171-8.

203 Sarks S, Cherepanoff S, Killingsworth M, Sarks J. Relationship of basal laminar deposit and membranous debris to the clinical presentation of early age-related macular degeneration. Invest Ophthalmol Vis Sci 2007;48:968-977.

204 Spraul CW, Lang GE, Grossniklaus HE, Lang GK. Histologic and Morphometric Analysis of the Choroid, Bruch's Membrane, and Retinal Pigment Epithelium in Postmortem Eyes With Age-Related Macular Degeneration and Histologic Examination of Surgically Excised Choroidal Neovascular Membranes. Surv Ophthalmol 1999; 44, Supp 1: S10- S32.

205 de Jong Paulus TVM. Age-Related Macular Degeneration. N Engl J Med 2006; 355: 1474 – 1485.

206 Bird, Alan C. "Age Related Macular Disease." National Academy of Sciences, National Academy of Engineering, and Institute of Medicine. *Distinctive Voices* lecture given at the Beckman Center, Irvine, California. 2014. Published online Feb. 6, 2014. Available at: *https://www.youtube.com/watch?v=6ugISIFyxuA*.

207 Alm A, Bill A. Ocular and optic nerve blood flow at normal and increased intraocular pressure in monkeys. Exp Eye Res 1973;15:15-29.

208 Alm A. Ocular Circulation. In: Hart WM, editor. *Adler's Physiology of the Eye.* St. Louis, MO: Mosby-Year Book Inc; 1992:198-227.

209 Spraul CW, Lang GE, Grossniklaus HE, Lang GK. Histologic and Morphometric Analysis of the Choroid, Bruch's Membrane, and Retinal Pigment Epithelium in Postmortem Eyes With Age-Related Macular Degeneration and Histologic Examination of Surgically Excised Choroidal Neovascular Membranes. Survey of Ophthalmol. 1999; 44, Suppl 1: S10- S32.

210 Grunwald JE, Hariprasad SM, DuPont J, et al. Foveolar choroidal blood flow in age-related macular degeneration. Invest Ophthalmol Vis Sci. 1998: 39(2): 385-390.

211 Penfold PL, Killingsworth MC, Sarks SH. Senile macular degeneration. The involvement of giant cells in atrophy of the retinal pigment epithelium. Invest Ophthalmol Vis Sci. 1986: 27(3): 364-71.

212 Curcio CA, Saunders PL, Younger PW, Malek G. Peripapillary chorioretinal atrophy: Bruch's membrane changes and photoreceptor loss. Ophthalmology. 2000; 107 (2): 334-43.

213 Schmetterer, Leopold and Kiel, Jeffrey W. *Ocular Blood Flow.* New York, Springer Heidelberg, 2012. P. 200.

214 Ciulla TA, Harris A, Chung HS, et al. Color Doppler imaging discloses reduced ocular blood flow velocities in nonexudative age-related macular degeneration. Am J Ophthalmol. 1999 Jul; 128(1): 75-80.

215 Snow KK, Seddon JM. Do age-related macular degeneration and cardiovascular disease share common antecedents? Ophthalmic Epidemiol. 1999; 6: 125-143.

216 Johnson LV, Leitner WP, et al. Complement Activation and Inflammatory Process in Drusen Formation and Age Related Macular Degeneration. Exp Eye Res. 2001; 73: 887-896.

217 Anderson DH, Mullins RF, et al. A role for local inflammation in the formation of drusen in the aging eye. Am J Ophthalmol. 2002; 134: 411-431.

218 Mullins RF, Russell SR, et al. Drusen associated with aging and age-related macular degeneration contain proteins common to extracellular deposits associated with atherosclerosis, elastosis, amyloidosis, and dense deposit disease. FASEB J. 2000; 14: 835-846.

219 Ibid.

220 Ibid.

221 Seddon JM, Gensler G, et al. Association Between C-Reactive Protein and Age-Related Macular Degeneration. JAMA. 2004; 291(6): 704-710.

222 Rapin JR, Wiernsperger N. Possible links between intestinal permeability and food processing: A potential therapeutic niche for glutamine. Clinics (Sao Paulo). 2010;65(6):635-43.

223 Schleicher M, Weikel K, Garber C, Taylor A. Diminshing Risk for Age-Related Macular Degeneration with Nutrition: A Current View. Nutrients. 2013; 5: 2405-2456.

224 Penfold, Philip L. and Provis, Jan M. *Macular Degeneration.* Berlin, Heidelberg, New York, Springer, 2004, p. 32.

225 Abugreen S, Muldrew KA, Stevenson MR. CNV subtype in first eyes predicts severity of ARM in fellow eyes. Br J Ophthalmol. 2003; 87(3): 307-11.

226 Adamis AP, Shima DT, Yeo KT, et al. Synthesis and secretion of vascular permeability factor/vascular endothelial growth factor by human retinal pigment epithelial cells. Biochem Biophys Res Commun. 1993; 193: 631-638.

227 Frank RN. Growth factors in age-related macular degeneration: pathogenic and therapeutic implications. Ophthalmic Res. 1997; 29: 341-353.

228 Frank RN, Amin RH, et al. Basic fibroblast growth factor and vascular endothelial growth factor are present in epiretinal and choroidal neovascular membranes. Am J Ophthalmol. 1996; 122: 393-403.

229 Ishibashi T, Hata Y, Yoshikawa H, et al. Expression of vascular endothelial growth factor in experimental choroidal neovascularization. Graefes Arch Clin Exp Ophthalmol. 1997; 235: 159-167.

230 Dawson DW, Volpert OV, Gillis P, et al. Pigment epithelium-derived gactor: a potent inhibitor of angiogenesis. Science. 1999; 285: 245-248.

231 Adamis AP, Shima DT, Yeo KT, et al. Synthesis and secretion of vascular permeability factor/vascular endothelial growth factor by human retinal pigment epithelial cells. Biochem Biophys Res Commun. 1993; 193: 631-638.

232 Lopez PF, Sippy BD, Lambert HM, et al. Transdifferentiated retinal pigment epithelial cells are immunoreactive for vascular endothelial growth factor in surgically excised age-related macular degeneration-related choroidal neovascular membranes. Invest Ophthalmol Vis Sci. 1996; 37: 855-868.

233 Burns MS and Hartz MJ. The retinal pigment epithelium induces fenestration of endothelial cells in vivo. Curr Eye Res. 1992; 11: 863-872.

234 Ford KM, Saint-Geniez M, et al. Expression and role of VEGF in the adult retinal pigment epithelium. Invest Ophthalmol Vis Sci. 2011; 52(13): 9478-87.

235 Kim I, Ryan AM, Rohan R, et al. Constitutive expression of VEFG, VEGFR-1, and VEGFR-2 in normal eyes. Invest Ophthalmol Vis Sci. 2000; 41(2): 368.

236 Robinson GS, Ju M, Shih SC, et al. Nonvascular role for VEGF: VEGFR-1, 2 activity is critical for neural retinal development. FASEB Journal. 2001; 15: 1215-1217.

237 Saint-Geniez M, Maharaj ASR, et al. Endogenous VEGF Is Required for Visual Function: Evidence for a Survival Role on Müller Cells and Photoreceptors. PLOS ONE. 2008, Nov. 8.

238 Grunwald JE, Daniel E, Huang J, et al. Risk of geographic atrophy in the comparison of age-related macular degeneration treatment trials. Ophthalmology. 2014; 121(1): 150-61.

239 Sadda SR. Development of atrophy in neovascular AMD treated with anti-VEGF therapy: Results of the HARBOR Study. Poster presented at: American Academy of Ophthalmology Retina Subspecialty Day. Chicago, IL; Oct. 17, 2014.

240 Jackson GR, Owsley C, McGwin G. Aging and dark adaptation. Vision Research. 1999; 39: 3975-3982.

241 Ibid.

242 Owsley C, Jackson GR, White M, Feist R, Edwards D. Delays in rod-mediated dark adaptation in early age-related maculopathy. Ophthalmology. 2001; 108(7): 1196-1202.

243 Penfold, Philip L. and Provis, Jan M. *Macular Degeneration*. Berlin, Heidelberg, New York, Springer, 2004, p. 54.

244 Owsley C, McGwin G Jr, et al. Delayed Rod-Mediated Dark Adaptation is a Functional Biomarker for Incident Early Age-Related Macular Degeneration. Ophthalmology. 2016; 123(2): 344-51.

245 Ibid.

246 Wang SB, Mitchell P, Chiha J, Liew G, et al. Severity of Coronary Artery Disease Is Independently Associated With the Frequency of Early Age-Related Macular Degeneration. British J Ophthalmol. 2015; 99(3): 365-370.

247 Fallon Morell, Sally. Ancient Dietary Wisdom for Tomorrow's Children. Available at: The Weston A Price Foundation website: *www.westonaprice.org*. Posted January 1, 2000. Available at: *http://www.westonaprice.org/health-topics/ancient-dietary-wisdom-for-tomorrows-children/*

248 Fallon Morell, Sally. "Nourishing Traditional Diets – Sally Fallon" presentation. Published to YouTube on Dec. 23, 2012. Available at: *https://www.youtube.com/watch?v=7ixsBn_lfXE*

249 Price, Weston A. *Nutrition and Physical Degeneration.* 6th Edition. La Mesa, CA, Price-Pottenger Nutrition Foundation, 2003, p. 472.

250 Price, Weston A. Nutrition and Physical Degeneration. 1939, 1945 by Weston A. Price. Lemon Grove, California, The Price-Pottenger Nutrition Foundation, Inc. 1970 – 2008.

251 Ibid, p. 25.

252 Fallon Morell, Sally. "Nourishing Traditional Diets – Sally Fallon" presentation. Published to YouTube on Dec. 23, 2012. Available at: *https://www.youtube.com/watch?v=7ixsBn_lfXE*

253 Price, Weston A. Nutrition and Physical Degeneration. 1939, 1945 by Weston A. Price. Lemon Grove, California, The Price-Pottenger Nutrition Foundation, Inc. 1970 – 2008, p. 120.

254 Ibid, p. 120.

255 Ibid, p. 133.

256 Ibid. p. 124.

257 Ibid. p. 120.

258 Ibid.

259 Fallon-Morell, Sally. "Nourishing Traditional Diets – The Key to Vibrant Health." Published Dec. 23, 2012. Available at: *https://www.youtube.com/watch?v=7ixsBn_lfXE*

260 Cordain S, Eaton SB, Brand-Miller J, Lindeberg S, Jensen C. An evolutionary analysis of the aetiology and pathogenesis of juvenile-onset myopia. Acta Ophthalmologica Scandinavica. 2002; 80: 125-135.

261 Kahl, Kristie L. Concern for myopia progression increases with alarming rise in global prevalence. Ocular Surgery News. March 10, 2016.

262 Ibid.

263 Ogden, CL, Carroll, MD, CDC Division of Health and Nutrition Examination Surveys. Prevalence of overweight, obesity, and extreme obesity among adults: United States, trends 1960-62 through 2007-2008.

264 Ibid.

265 Kahl, Kristie L. Concern for myopia progression increases with alarming rise in global prevalence. Ocular Surgery News. March 10, 2016.

266 Ibid.

267 Price, Weston A. Nutrition and Physical Degeneration. 1939, by Weston A. Price. Lemon Grove, California, The Price-Pottenger Nutrition Foundation, Inc. 1970 – 2008, p. 452.

268 Ibid, p. 452.

269 Ibid, p. 152.

270 Ibid, p. 251-252.

271 Ibid, p. 306.

272 Ibid, p. 309.

273 Ibid, p. 309.

274 Ibid, p. 250.

275 Weston A. Price. *Nutrition and Physical Degeneration.* 6th Edition. La Mesa, CA, Price-Pottenger Nutrition Foundation, 2003, Chapter 18.

276 Price, Weston A. *Nutrition and Physical Degeneration*. Lemon Grove, California, The Price-Pottenger Nutrition Foundation, Inc., 1939, p. xvi.

277 Ibid, p. 452. p. 246-248.

278 Ibid, p. 246-7.

279 "Dr. Weston A. Price Movietone." The Weston A. Price Foundation. Published On-Line Mar 10, 2011. Available at: *http://www.westonaprice.org/about-the-foundation/dr-weston-a-price-movietone/*

280 Masterjohn, Chris. "On the Trail of the Elusive X-Factor: A Sixty-Two-Year-Old Mystery Finally Solved. The Weston A. Price Foundation. Feb 14, 2008. Available at: *http://www.westonaprice.org/health-topics/abcs-of-nutrition/on-the-trail-of-the-elusive-x-factor-a-sixty-two-year-old-mystery-finally-solved/*

281 Ibid. p. 264.

282 Price, Weston A. Nutrition and Physical Degeneration. 1939, 1945 by Weston A. Price. Lemon Grove, California, The Price-Pottenger Nutrition Foundation, Inc. 1970 – 2008.

283 Ibid, p. 246.

284 "Dr. Weston A. Price Movietone." The Weston A. Price Foundation. Published On-Line Mar 10, 2011. Available at: *http://www.westonaprice.org/about-the-foundation/dr-weston-a-price-movietone/*

285 Simmons, Amelia; With an Essay by Mary Tolford Wilson. The First American Cookbook – A Facsimile of "American Cookery," 1796. New York. Oxford University Press, 1958.

286 Ibid. p. xvi.

287 Volo, James M and Dorothy D. The Antebellum Period. (Westport, Connecticut, Greenwood Press, 2004), pp. 169-171.

288 Volo, James M and Dorothy D. The Antebellum Period. (Westport, Connecticut, Greenwood Press, 2004), pp. 169-171.

289 Leslie, Eliza. *Miss Leslie's Directions for Cookery – An Unabridged Reprint of the 1851 Classic.* Introduction by Janice (Jan) Bluestein Longone. Mineola, New York. Dover Publications, 1999.

290 Ibid. p. 209.

291 Ibid. pp. 142, 149, 151.

292 Ibid. p. 128.

293 Ibid. p. 358 -9.

294 Kreidberg, Marjorie. *Food On The Frontier – Minnesota Cooking from 1850 to 1900 With Selected Recipes.* St. Paul. Minnesota Historical Society Press, 1975.

295 Campbell, Grant M. Chapter 7: Roller Milling of Wheat. In: Salman AD, Ghadiri M, Hounslow MJ, ed. *Handbook of Powder Technology*. Vol 12. New York, NY: Elsevier BV; 2007: 383-416.

296 Kreidberg, Marjorie. *Food On The Frontier – Minnesota Cooking from 1850 to 1900 With Selected Recipes.* St. Paul. Minnesota Historical Society Press, 1975, pp. 39-40.

297 Slavin JL, Jacobs D, Marquart L. Grain processing and nutrition. Crit Rev Biotechnol. 2001; 21(1): 49-66.

298 Shewry, PR. Wheat. J Exp Bot. 2009; 60(6): 1537-1553.

299 Steiger Howard, Judy. *1905 Cookbook – Food for Body and Soul.* Oklahoma City, Oklahoma. Dorcas Publishing, 2011.

300 Ibid. p. 73.

301 Ibid. p. 69.

302 Ibid. pp. 1, 3, 4, 27, 49, 60, 66.

303 Ibid. pp. 55, 89, 90.

304 Ibid. p. 104.

305 d'Estries, Michael. "Jack LaLanne: The first fitness superhero." Mother Nature Network. n.d. Available at: *http://www.mnn.com/health/fitness-well-being/blogs/jack-lalanne-the-first-fitness-superhero*

306 Tuttle, Dave. "Jack LaLanne." Life Extension Magazine. August, 2006. Available at: *http://www.lifeextension.com/magazine/2006/8/report_lalanne/Page-01*

307 St. James Encyclopedia of Popular Culture. 2000; Vol 3, pp 81-83.

308 "Fitness guru Jack LaLanne dies at 96." By the CNN Wires Staff. January 24, 2011. Available at: *http://www.cnn.com/2011/SHOWBIZ/celebrity.news.gossip/01/23/obit.jack.lalanne/*

309 "Food processing." Wikipedia. Available at: *https://en.wikipedia.org/wiki/Food_processing*

310 Vergroesen AJ and Gottenbos JJ. "The Role of Fats in Human Nutrition: An Introduction." In *The Role of Fats in Human Nutrition, edited by A.J. Vergroesen.* London, Academic Press. Pp. 1 – 41.

311 Price, Weston A. Nutrition and Physical Degeneration. 1939, 1945 by Weston A. Price. Lemon Grove, California, The Price-Pottenger Nutrition Foundation, Inc. 1970 – 2008.

312 Rosillo-Calle, Frank. A Global Overview of Vegetable Oils, With Reference to Biodiesel. IEA Bioenergy. June, 2009. Available at: *http://www.bioenergytrade.org/downloads/vegetableoilstudyfinaljune18.pdf*

313 O'Brien, Richard D et al. "Cottonseed Oil." Chapter 5 in *Bailey's Industrial Oil and Fat Products.* John Wiley & Sons, Inc. 2005.

314 Proctor & Gamble – A Company History – 1837 – Today. Available online: *https://www.pg.com/translations/history_pdf/english_history.pdf*

315 Siri-Tarino PW, Sun Q, Hu FB, Krauss RM. Meta-analysis of prospective cohort studies evaluating the association of saturated fat with cardiovascular disease. Ameican Journal Clinical Nutrition.

316 "Nutrition and Your Health: Dietary Guidelines for Americans." USDA, Appendix G-5. Brief History of Dietary Guidelines. Available at: *http://health.gov/dietaryguidelines/dga2005/report/html/G5_History.htm*

317 Lustig, Robert H. *Fat Chance – Beating the Odds Against Sugar, Processed Food, Obesity, and Disease.* New York, Hudson Street Press, 2013, p. 169.

318 Fallon, Sally. *Nourishing Traditions – The Cookbook that Challenges Politically Correct Nutrition and the Diet Dictocrats.* Brandywine, Maryland. NewTrends Publishing, Inc., 2001, p. 5.

319 Grimes DS. An epidemic of coronary heart disease. QJM: An International Journal of Medicine. 2012; 105(6): 509-18.

320 Mazzucco, Massimo. *Cancer – The Forbidden Cures.* Buenaonda Films, London, UK. 2013. Available at: *https://www.youtube.com/watch?v=3ncDdqNDcaI*

321 Carter, Nancy Carol. "San Diego Olives: Origins of a California Industry." The Journal of San Diego History. 2008; 54(3): 138-40.

322 Grigg, D. "The European Diet: Regional Variations in Food Consumption in the 1980s." Geoforum. 1993; 24: 277-289.

323 Ibid.

324 "History: Inventor of Advanced Processing Technology." Anderson International Corp. n.d. Available at: *http://www.anderson-intl.net/index_files/History.htm*

325 Nixon, H.C. The Rise of the American Cottonseed Oil Industry. Journal of Political Economy. 1930; 38(1): 73-85.

326 Ibid.

327 Ibid.

328 Cordain L, Eaton SB, et al. Origins and evolution of the Western diet: health implications for the 21st century. Am J Clin Nutr. 2005; 81(2): 341-354.

329 Shurtleff, William, and Aoyagi, Akiko. *History of Soybeans and Soyfoods In The United Kingdom and Ireland (1613 – 2015): Extensively Annotated Bibliography and Sourcebook.* SoyInfo Center, Lafayette, California, 2015, pp. 869-871.

330 Dietary Assessment of Major Trends in U.S. Food Consumption, 1970 – 2005. USDA Economic Research Service. Bulletin Number 33, March 2008.

331 Cordain L, Eaton SB, et al. Origins and evolution of the Western diet: health implications for the 21st century. Am J Clin Nutr. 2005; 81(2): 341-354.

332 Wells, Hodan F., and Jean C. Buzby. Dietary Assessment of Major Trends in U.S. Food Consumption, 1970-2005, Economic Information Bulletin No. 33. Economic Research Service, U.S. Dept of Agriculture. March 2008. Available at: *http://www.ers.usda.gov/media/210681/eib33_1_.pdf*

333 Popkin BM, Gordon-Larsen P. The nutrition transition: worldwide obesity dynamics and their determinants. International Journal of Obesity. 2004; 28: S2-S9.

334 Hawken, Paul and Fred Rohe. "The Dangers of Vegetable Oil Extraction and Processing." *The Mother Earth News.* Nov/December. 1971 Issue 12: 26-27.

335 Fallon, Sally and Mary G. Enig, PhD. "The Skinny on Fats." The Weston A. Price Foundation. Posted January 1, 2000. Available at: *http://www.westonaprice.org/health-topics/the-skinny-on-fats/*

336 Hamm H, Hamilton RJ, Calliauw G. *Edible Oil Processing, Second Edition.* West Sussex, UK: Wiley-Blackwell; 2013.

337 "How its (sic) made Canola Oil." *YouTube.com*. Published May 7, 2013. Available at: *https://www.youtube.com/watch?v=uVe_08TntEU*

338 Ibid.

339 Choe E, Min DB. Mechanisms and Factors for Edible Oil Oxidation. Comprehensive Reviews in Food Science and Food Safety 2006; 5:169-86.

340 Fallon, Sally and Mary G. Enig, PhD. "The Skinny on Fats." The Weston A. Price Foundation. Posted January 1, 2000. Available at: *http://www.westonaprice.org/health-topics/the-skinny-on-fats/*

341 Hawken, Paul and Fred Rohe. "The Dangers of Vegetable Oil Extraction and Procesing." *The Mother Earth News.* Nov/December. 1971 Issue 12: 26-27.

342 Weingarten, Hemi. "What is Expeller Pressed Oil and Why Does it Matter?" *Fooducate.com*. Dec. 8, 2010: Available at: *http://blog.fooducate.com/2010/12/08/what-is-expeller-pressed-oil-and-why-does-it-matter/*

343 Table 6. Food Sources of Alpha-Linolenic Acid. National Cancer Institute, Applied Research Cancer Control and Population Sciences. 18 Oct, 2013. Available at: *http://appliedresearch.cancer.gov/diet/foodsources/fatty_acids/table6.html*

344 Simopoulos AP. Evolutionary aspects of diet, the omega-6/omega-3 ratio and genetic variation: nutritional implications for chronic diseases. Biomedicine & Pharmacotherapy. 2006: 60(9): 502-507.

345 Ibid.

346 Simopoulos Artemis. Human Requirements for N-3 Polyunsaturated Fatty Acids. Article in Poultry Science: August 2000.

347 "Omega-3 Fatty Acids and Health: Fact Sheet for Health Professionals." US National Institutes of Health, Office of Dietary Supplements. 2005. Available at: *https://ods.od.nih.gov/factsheets/Omega3FattyAcidsandHealth-HealthProfessional/*

348 Simopoulos AP. Evolutionary aspects of diet, the omega-6/omega-3 ratio and genetic variation: nutritional implications for chronic diseases. Biomedicine & Pharmacotherapy. 2006; 60(9): 502-507.

349 Simopoulos AP, Childs B. *Genetic Variation and Nutrition.* World Review of Nutrition and Dietetics. Karger and Basel. 1990, Vol. 63.

350 Simopoulos AP, Ordovas J. *Nutrigenetics and Nutrigenomics.* World Review of Nutrition and Dietetics. Karger and Basel. 2004, Vol. 93.

351 Eaton SB, Konner M. Paleolithic nutrition – A consideration of its nature and current implications. N Engl J Med. 1985; 312: 283-289.

352 Simopoulos AP. Omega-3 fatty acids in health and disease and in growth and development. Am J Clin Nutr. 1991; 54: 438-463.

353 Simopoulos AP. *Plants in Human Nutrition.* World Review of Nutrition and Dietetics. 1995, Vol. 77, Karger and Basel.

354 Simopoulos AP. Is insulin resistance influenced by dietary linoleic acid and trans fatty acids? Free Rad Biol Med. 1994; 17(4): 367-372.

355 Simopoulos AP, Robinson J. *The Omega Diet – The Lifesaving Nutritional Program Based On the Diet of the Island of Crete.* New York, Harper Collins, 1999.

356 Simopoulos A. Omega-3 fatty acids in health and disease and in growth and development. American Journal of Clinical Nutrition. 1991; 54: 438-63.

357 Simopoulos AP, Cleland LG. "Omega-6/Omega-3 Essential Fatty Acid Ratio: the Scientific Evidence." World Rev Nutr Diet. Basel and Karger, 2003, Vol 92.

358 de Lorgeril M, Renaud S, et al. Mediterranean a-linolenic acid-rich diet in secondary prevention of coronary heart disease. Lancet. 1994; 343: 1454-1459.

359 Blasbalg TL, Hibbeln JR, Ramsden CE, Majchrzak SF, Rawlings RR. Changes in consumption of omega-3 and omega-6 fatty acids in the United States during the 20th century. Am J Clin Nutr. 2011: 93(5): 950-962.

360 Ibid.

361 Ford ES, Dietz WH. Trends in energy intake among adults in the United States: findings from NHANES. Am J Clin Nutr. 2013; 97(4): 848-53.

362 Dolacek TA. Epidemiological evidence of relationships between dietary polyunsaturated fatty acids and mortality in the multiple risk factor intervention trial. Proc Soc Exp Biol Med. 1992; 200(2): 177-82.

363 Baghurst Kl, Crawford DA, et al. The Victorian Nutrition Survey – intakes and sources of dietary fats and cholesterol in the Victorian population. Med J Aust. 1988; 149(1):12-5, 18-20.

364 Blasbalg TL, Hibbeln JR, Ramsden CE, Majchrzak SF, Rawlings RR. Changes in consumption of omega-3 and omega-6 fatty acids in the United States during the 20th century. Am J Clin Nutr. 2011: 93(5): 950-962.

365 Lands WEM, Libelt B, Morris A, et al. Maintenance of lower proportions of (n-6) eicosanoid precursors in phospholipids of human plasma in response to added dietary (n-3) fatty acids. Biochim Biophys Acta. 1992; 1180: 147-62.

366 Blasbalg TL, Hibbeln JR, Ramsden CE, Majchrzak SF, Rawlings RR. Changes in consumption of omega-3 and omega-6 fatty acids in the United States during the 20th century. Am J Clin Nutr. 2011: 93(5): 950-962.

367 Lands WEM, Libelt B, Morris A, et al. Maintenance of lower proportions of (n-6) eicosanoid precursors in phospholipids of human plasma in response to added dietary (n-3) fatty acids. Biochim Biophys Acta. 1992; 1180: 147-62.

368 Liou YA, King DJ, et al. Decreasing linoleic acid with constant alpha-linolenic acid in dietary fats increases (n-3) eicosapentaenoic acid in plasma phospholipids in healthy men. J Nutr. 2007; 137(4): 945-52.

369 Angela Liou Y, Innis SM. Dietary linoleic acid has no effect on arachidonic acid, but increases n-6 eicosadienoic acid, and lower dihomogamma-linolenic and eicosapentaenoic acid in plasma of adult men. Prostaglandins Leukot Essent Fatty Acids. 2009; 80(4): 201-6.

370 Friesen RW, Innis SM. Linoleic acid is associated with lower long-chain n-6 and n-3 fatty acids in red blood cell lipids of Canadian pregnant women. Am J Clin Nutr. 2010; 91(1): 23-31.

371 Storlien LH, Jenkins AB, et al. Influence of dietary fat composition on development of insulin resistance in rats. Relationship to muscle triglyceride and omega-3 fatty acids in muscle phospholipid. Diabetes. 1991; 40(2): 280-9.

372 Guyenet, Stephan. "My TEDx Talk, "The American Diet: a Historical Perspective." Whole Health Source. 2012 Feb 6. Available at: *http://wholehealthsource.blogspot.com/2012/02/my-tedx-talk-american-diet-historical.html*

373 Witting LA, Lee L. Recommended dietary allowance for vitamin E: relation to dietary, erythrocyte and adipose tissue linoleate. Am J Clin Nutr. 1975; 28(6): 577-83.

374 Berry EM, Hirsch J, et al. The relationship of dietary fat to plasma lipid levels as studied by factor analysis of adipose tissue fatty acid composition in a free-living population of middle-aged American men. Am J Clin Nutr. 1986; 44(2): 220-31.

375 London SJ, Sacks FM, et al. Fatty acid composition of subcutaneous adipose tissue and diet in postmenopausal US women. Am J Clin Nutr. 1991; 54(2): 340-5.

376 Garland M, Sacks FM, et al. The relation between dietary intake and adipose tissue composition of selected fatty acids in US women. Am J Clin Nutr. 1998; 67(1): 25-30.

377 Knutsen SF, Fraser GE, et al. Comparison of adipose tissue fatty acids with dietary fatty acids as measured by 24-hour recall and food frequency questionnaire in Black and White Adventists: the Adventist Health Study. Ann Epidemiol. 2003; 13(2): 119-27.

378 Ren J, Dimitrov I, et al. Composition of adipose tissue and marrow fat in humans by 1H NMR at 7Tesla. J Lipid Res. 2008; 49(9): 2055-2062.

379 Leaf A. Prevention of sudden cardiac death by n-3 polyunsaturated fatty acids. J Cardiovasc Med (Hagerstown) 2007; 8(Suppl 1): S27-9).

380 Rao JS, Lee HJ, et al. Mode of action of mood stabilizers: is the arachidonic acid cascade a common target? Mol Psychiatry. 2008: 13: 585-96.

381 Tjonneland A, Overvad K, et al. Linoleic acid, a dietary n-6 polyunsaturated fatty acid, and the aetiology of ulcerative colitis: a nested case-control study within a European prospective cohort study. Gut. 2009: 58: 1606-11.

382 SanGiovanni JP, Chew EY. The role of omega-3 long-chain polyunsaturated fatty acids in health and disease of the retina. Prog Retin Eye Res. 2005; 24: 87-138.

383 Kishan AU, Modjtahedi BS, et al. Lipids and age-related macular degeneration. Surv Ophthalmol. 2011; 56: 195-213.

384 SanGiovanni JP, Chew EY. The role of omega-3 long-chain polyunsaturated fatty acids in health and disease of the retina. Prog Retin Eye Res. 2005; 24: 87-138.

385 Ibid.

386 Donoso LA, Kim D, Frost A, Callahan A, Hageman G. The role of inflammation in the pathogenesis of age-related macular degeneration. Surv Ophthalmol. 2006; 51: 137-52.

387 Delyfer, Marie-Noëlle, Buaud, Benjamin, et al (Chapter Authors). Omega-3 and Macular Pigment Accumulation: Results from the Pimavosa Study. Preedy, Victor R. *Handbook of Nutrition, Diet, and the Eye.* Amsterdam, Elsevier. 2014, p. 264.

388 Age Related Eye Disease Study Research Group. The Relationship of Dietary Lipid Intake and Age-Related Macular Degeneration in a Case-Control Study. JAMA Ophthalmology. 2007; 125(5): 671-679.

389 Ibid.

390 Guyenet, Stephan. "Cancer Among the Inuit." Whole Health Source. July 4, 2008. Available at: *http://wholehealthsource.blogspot.com/2008/07/cancer-among-inuit.html*

391 Fallon, Sally. *Nourishing Traditions – The Cookbook that Challenges Politically Correct Nutrition and the Diet Dictocrats.* Brandywine, Maryland. NewTrends Publishing, Inc., 2001, p. 10.

392 Fang JL, Vaca CE, Valsta LM, Mutanen M. Determination of DNA adducts of malonaldehyde in humans: effects of dietary fatty acid composition. Carcinogenesis. 1996; 17(5): 1035-40.

393 Turpeinen AM, Basu S, Mutanen M. A high linoleic acid diet increases oxidative stress in vivo and affects nitric oxide metabolism in humans. Prostaglandins Leukot Essent Fatty Acids. 1998; 59(3): 229-33.

394 Ibid.

395 Toborek M, Lee YW, Garrido R, et al. Unsaturated fatty acids selectively induce an inflammatory environment in human endothelial cells. Am J Clin Nutr. 2002; 5(1): 119-125.

396 Endemann DH, Schiffrin EL. Endothelial dysfunction. J Am Soc Nephrol. 2004; 15(8): 1983-92.

397 Fallon, Sally. *Nourishing Traditions – The Cookbook that Challenges Politically Correct Nutrition and the Diet Dictocrats.* Brandywine, Maryland. NewTrends Publishing, Inc., 2001, p. 5.

398 Lichtenstein AH, Ausman LM, et al. Effects of canola, corn, and olive oils on fasting and postprandial plasma lipoproteins in humans as part of a National Cholesterol Education Program Step 2 diet. Arteriosclerosis, Thrombosis, and Vascular Biology. 1993; 13: 1533-1542.

399 Rassias G, Kestin M, Nestel PJ. Linoleic acid lowers LDL cholesterol without a proportionate displacement of saturated fatty acid. Eur. J Clin Nutr. 1991; 45(6): 315-20.

400 Bierenbaum ML, Reichstein RP, et al. Effects of canola oil on serum lipids in humans. J Am Coll Nutr. 1991; 10(3): 228-33.

401 Sacks FM, Katan M. Randomized clinical trials on the effets of dietary fat and carbohydrate on plasma lipoproteins and cardiovascular disease. Amer J Med. 2002; 113(9) Suppl 2: 13-24

402 Toth PP. Cardiology patient page. The "good cholesterol": high-density lipoprotein. Circulation. 2005; 111(5): e89-e91.

403 Kummerow, Fred A. Interaction between sphingomyelin and oxysterols contributes to atherosclerosis and sudden death. Am J Cardiovasc Dis. 2013; 3(1): 17-26.

404 Ravnskov U, DiNicolantonio JJ, Harcombe Z, Kummerow FA, et al. The Questionable Benefits of Exchanging Saturated Fat With Polyunsaturated Fat. Mayo Clinic Proceedings. 2014; 89(4): 451-453.

405 Warner, Melanie. "A Lifelong Fight Against Trans Fats." The New York Times. Dec. 16, 2013. Available at: *www.nytimes.com*.

406 Silaste ML, Rantala M, et al. Changes in Dietary Fat Intake Alter Plasma Levels of Oxidized Low-Density Lipoprotein and Lipoprotein(a). Arterioscler Thromb Vasc Biol. 2004; 24(3): 498-503.

407 Mata P, Alonso R, et al. Effect of dietary fat saturation on LDL oxidation and monocyte adhesion to human endothelial cells in vitro. Arterioscl Thromb Vasc Biol. 1996; 16(11): 1347-55.

408 Ramsden CE, Ringel A, et al. Lowering dietary linoleic acid reduces bioactive oxidized linoleic acid metabolites in humans. Prostaglandins Leukot Essent Fatty Acids. 2012; 87(4-5): 135-41.

409 Reaven P, Parthasarathy S, et al. Effects of oleate-rich and linoleate-rich diets on the susceptibility of low density lipoprotein to oxidative modification in mildly hypercholesterolemic subjects. J Clin Invest. 1993; 91(2): 668-676.

410 Spiteller D, Spitellar G. Oxidation of Linoleic Acid in Low-Density Lipoprotein: An Important Event in Atherogenesis. Angew Chem Int Ed Engl. 2000; 39(3): 585-89.

411 Maingrette F, Renier G. Linoleic acid increases lectin-like oxidized LDL receptor-1 (LOX-1) expression in human aortic endothelial cells. Diabetes. 2005; 54(5): 1506-13.

412 Itabe H, Obama T, Kato R. The Dynamics of Oxidized LDL during Atherogenesis. J Lipids. 2011; 2011: 418313.

413 Ibid.

414 Pohjantähti-Maaroos H, Palomäki A, Kankkunen P, et al. Circulating oxidized low-density lipoproteins and arterial elasticity: comparison between men with metabolic syndrome and physically active counterparts. Cardiovasc Diabetol 2010;9:41.

415 Masterjohn, Chris. "High Cholesterol And Heart Disease – Myth or Truth?" *Cholesterol-and-health.com*. Aug 23, 2008. Available at: *http://www.cholesterol-and-health.com/Does-Cholesterol-Cause-Heart-Disease-Myth.html*

416 Masterjohn, Chris. "Are Animal Fats Good for You?" Lecture at Freedom Law School. Jan 14, 2012 (uploaded). Available at: https://www.youtube.com/watch?v=dkno1A1VpWw

417 Ibid.

418 Itabe H, Takeshima E, at al. A monoclonal antibody against oxidized lipoprotein recognizes foam cells in atherosclerotic lesions. Complex formation of oxidized phosphatidylcholines and polypeptides. Journal of Biological Chemistry. 1994; 269(21): 15274-15279.

419 Ehara S, Ueda M, et al. Elevated levels of oxidized low density lipoprotein show a positive relationship with the severity of acute coronary syndromes. Circulation. 2001; 103(15): 1955-1960.

420 Nishi K, Itabe H, et al. Oxidized LDL in carotid plaques and plasma associates with plaque instability. Arteriosclerosis, Thrombosis, and Vascular Biology. 2002; 22(10): 1649-1654.

421 Palinski W, Hörkkö E, et al. Cloning of monoclonal autoantibodies to epitopes of oxidized lipoproteins from apolipoprotein E-deficient mice: demonstration of epitipes of oxidized low density lipoprotein in human plasma. Journal of Clinical Investigation. 1996; 98(3): 800-814.

422 Itabe H, Obama T, Kato R. The Dynamics of Oxidized LDL during Atherogenesis. J Lipids. 2011; 2011: 418313.

423 Klein R, Peto T, Bird A, Vannewkirk MR. The epidemiology of age-related macular degeneration. Amer J Ophthalmol. 2004; 137(3): 486-495.

424 Gordiyenko N, Campos M, Lee JW, et al. RPE cells internalize low-density lipoprotein (LDL) and oxidized LDL (oxLDL) in large quantities in vitro and in vivo. Invest Ophthalmol Vis Sci 2004;45:2822-2829.

425 Tserentsoodol N, Gordiyenko NV, Pascual I, et al. Intraretinal lipid transport is dependent on high density lipoprotein-like particles and class B scavenger receptors. Mol Vis 2006;12:1319-33.

426 Tserentsoodol N, Sztein J, Campos M, et al. Uptake of cholesterol by the retina occurs primarily via a low density lipoprotein receptor-mediated process. Mol Vis 2006;12:1306-18.

427 Curcio CA, Presley JB, Malek G, et al. Esterified and unesterified cholesterol in drusen and basal deposits of eyes with age-related maculopathy. Exp Eye Res 2005; 81:731-41.

428 Li CM, Chung BH, Presley G, et al. Lipoprotein-like particles and cholesteryl esters in human Bruch's membrane: initial characterization. Invest Ophthalmol Vis Sci 2005;46:2576-86.

429 Bretillon L, Thuret G, et al. Lipid and fatty acid profile of the retina, retinal pigment epithelium/choroid, and the lacrimal gland, and associations with adipose tissue fatty acids in human subjects. Exp Eye Res. 2008; 87(6): 521-8.

430 Kamei M, Yoneda K, Kume N, et al. Scavenger receptors for oxidized lipoprotein in age-related macular degeneration. Invest. Ophthalmol Vis Sci 2007;48: 1801-07.

431 Ates O, Azizi S, Alp HH, et al. Decreased Serum Paraoxonase 1 Activity and Increased Serum Homocysteine and Malondialdehyde Levels in Age-Related Macular Degeneration. Tohoku J Exp Med. 2009;217: 17-22.

432 Grootveld M, Silwood CJL, et al. Health Effects of Oxidized Heated Oils. Foodservice Research International. 2001; 13: 41-55.

433 Friedman E. Pathogenesis: a hemodynamic model. J.W. Berger, S.L. Fine, M.G. Maguire (Eds.), *Age related Macular Degeneration*. Mosby, St. Louis. 1999, pp. 173-178.

434 Potts AM. An hypothesis on macular disease. Trans Am Acad Ophthalmol Otolaryngol. 1966; 70(6): 1058-1062.

435 Bischoff PM, Flower RW. High blood pressure in choroidal arteries as a possible pathogenetic mechanism in senile macular degeneration. Am J Ophthalmol. 1983; 96(3): 398-9.

436 Holz FG, Sheraidah G, Pauleikhoff D, Bird AC. Analysis of lipid deposits extracted from human macular and peripheral Bruch's membrane. Arch Ophthalmol. 1994; 112(3): 402-6.

437 Vingerling JR, Dielemans I, Bots ML, Hofman A, Grobbee DE, and de Jong PTVM. Age-related Macular Degeneration Is Associated with Atherosclerosis. The Rotterdam Study. Am J Epidemiol. 1995; 142(4): 404-409.

438 Ibid.

439 Ibid

440 Wang SB, Mitchell P, Chiha J, Liew G, et al. Severity of Coronary Artery Disease Is Independently Associated With the Frequency of Early Age-Related Macular Degeneration. British J Ophthalmol. 2015; 99(3): 365-370.

441 Klein R, Clegg L, et al. Prevalence of age-related maculopathy in the Atherosclerosis Risk in Communities Study. Arch Ophthalmol. 1999; 117(9): 1203-10.

442 Klein R, Klein BEK, et al. Early age-related maculopathy in the cardiovascular health study. 2003; 110(1): 25-33.

443 Seddon JM, Rosner B, et al. Dietary Fat and Risk for Advanced Age-Related Macular Degeneration. Arch Ophthalmol. 2001; 119(8): 1191-1199.

444 Ibid.

445 Seddon JM, Cote J, Rosner B. Progression of age-related macular degeneration: association with dietary fat, transunsaturaed fat, nuts, and fish intake. Arch Ophthalmol. 2003; 121(12): 1728-37.

446 Tan JS, Wang JJ, et al. Dietary fatty acids and the 10-year incidence of age-related macular degeneration: the Blue Mountains Eye Study. Arch Ophthalmol. 2009; 127(5): 656-65.

447 Chiu CJ, Chang ML, et al. The relationship of major American dietary patterns to age-related macular degeneration. Am J Ophthalmol. 2014; 158(1): 118-127.

448 Seddon JM, George S, Rosner B. Cigarette smoking, fish consumption, omega-e fatty acid intake, and association with age-related macular degeneration: the US Twin Study of Age-Related Macular Degeneration. Arch Ophthalmol. 2006; 124(7): 995-1001.

449 SanGiovanni JP, Chew EY, et al. The relationship of dietary lipid intake and age-related macular degeneration in a case-control study: AREDS Report No. 20. Arch Ophthalmol. 2007; 125(5): 671-9.

450 Chong EW, Robman LD, et al. Fat consumption and its association with age-related macular degeneration. Arch Ophthalmol. 2009; 127(5): 674-80.

451 Parekh N, Voland RP, et al. Association between dietary fat intake and age-related macular degeneration in the Carotenoids in Age-Related Eye Disease Study (CAREDS): an ancillary study of the Women's Health Initiative. Arch Ophthalmol. 2009; 127(11): 1483-93.

452 Chong EW, Robman LD, et al. Fat consumption and its association with age-related macular degeneration. Arch Ophthalmol. 2009; 127(5): 674-80.

453 Ouchi M, Ikeda T, et al. A novel relation of fatty acid with age-related macular degeneration. Ophthalmologica. 2002; 216(5): 363-7.

454 O'Keefe S, Gaskins-Wright S, et al. Levels of Trans-Geometrical Isomers of Essential Fatty Acids In Some Unhydrogenated U.S. Vegetable Oils. Journal of Food Lipids. 1994; 1(3): 165-176.

455 De Greyt W, Radanyl O, et al. Contribution of trans-Fatty Acids from Vegetable Oils and Margarines to the Belgian Diet. European Journal of Lipid Science and Technology. 1996; 98(1): 30-33.

456 Friend, Berta. Nutrients in United States Food Supply – A Review of Trends, 1909-1913 to 1965. Am J Clin Nutr. 1967; 20(8): 907-914.

457 Household USDA Food Facts Sheet. "Oil, Vegetable." USDA. October, 2012. Available at: http://www.fns.usda.gov/sites/default/files/HHFS_OIL_VEGETABLE_100440Oct2012.pdf

458 "Basic Report: 04044, Oil, soybean, salad or cooking." USDA: National Nutrient Database for Standard Reference Release 28. Available at: http://ndb.nal.usda.gov/ndb/foods/show/658?manu=&fgcd=

459 Price, Weston A. Nutrition and Physical Degeneration. 1939, 1945 by Weston A. Price. Lemon Grove, California, The Price-Pottenger Nutrition Foundation, Inc. 1970 – 2008, pp. 386-405.

460 Ibid. p. 405.

461 Geleijnse JM, Vermeer C, et al. Dietary intake of menaquinone is associated with a reduced risk of coronary heart disease: the Rotterdam Study. J Nutr. 2004; 134(11): 3100-5.

462 Beulens JW, Bots ML, et al. High dietary menaquinone intake is associated with reduced coronary calcification. Atherosclerosis. 2009; 203(2): 489-493.

463 Asmar E, Naoum JJ, Arbid EJ. Vitamin k dependent proteins and the role of vitamin k2 in the modulation of vascular calcification: a review. Oman Med J. 2014; 29(3): 172-7.

464 Chiu CJ, Klein R, et al. Does eating particular diets alter the risk of age-related macular degeneration in users of the Age-Related Eye Disease Study supplements? Br J Ophthalmol 2009; 93(9): 1241-6.

465 Sangiovanni JP, Agron E, et al. [omega]-3 Long-chain polyunsaturated fatty acid intake and 12-y incidence of neovascular age-related macular degeneration and central geographic atrophy: AREDS report 30, a prospective cohort study from the Age-Related Eye Disease Study. Am J Clin Nutr. 2009; 90(6): 1601-7.

466 SanGiovanni JP, Chew EY, et al. The relationship of dietary lipid intake and age-related macular degeneration in a case-control study: AREDS Report No. 20. Arch Ophthalmol. 2007; 125(5): 671-9.

467 Sangiovanni JP, Chew EY, et al. The relationship of dietary omega-3 long-chain polyunsaturated fatty acid intake with incident age-related macular degeneration: AREDS report no. 23. Arch Ophthalmol. 2008; 126(9): 1274-9.

468 Cho E, Hung S, et al. Prospective study of dietary fat and the risk of age-related macular degeneration. Am J Clin Nutr. 2001; 73(2): 209-18.

469 Chong EW, Kreis AJ, et al. Dietary omega-3 fatty acid and fish intake in the primary prevention of age-related macular degeneration: a systematic review and meta-analysis. Arch Ophthalmol. 2008; 126(6): 826-33.

470 Chua B, Flood V, et al. Dietary fatty acids and the 5-year incidence of age-related maculopathy. Arch Ophthalmol. 2006; 124(7): 981-6.

471 Smith W, Mitchell P, Leeder SR. Dietary fat and fish intake and age-related maculopathy. Arch Ophthalmol. 2000; 118(3): 401-4.

472 Dietary Guidelines for Americans, 2010. Washington, DC: U.S. Government Printing Office, 2010.

473 Wang T and Wang L. Chemical Modification of Partially Hydrogenated Vegetable Oil to Improve its Functional Properties to Replace Petroleum Waxes. Iowa State University Patents. 2008, Nov. 13. Paper 18.

474 Semma M. Trans Fatty Acids: Properties, Benefits and Risks. Journal of Health Science. 2002; 48(1):7-13.

475 Nixey, Catherine. "Trans Fats/Hydrogenated Oils – The Killer in Non-Organic Processed Foods." Organic Consumers Association. 22 February 2005, Available at : https://www.organicconsumers.org/old_articles/foodsafety/transfat022305.php

476 Proctor & Gamble – A Company History – 1837 – Today. Available online: https://www.pg.com/translations/history_pdf/english_history.pdf

477 Allison DB, Egan SK, Barraj LM, et al. Estimated intakes of trans fatty and other fatty acids in the US population. J Am Diet Assoc 1999; 99(2):166-74.

478 Aro A, Antoine JM, et al. TransFatty Acids in Dairy and Meat Products from 14 European Countries: The TRANSFAIR Study. Journal of Food Composition and Analysis. 1998, 11(2): 150-160.

479 O'Donnell-Megano AM, Barbano DM, Bauman DE. Survey of the fatty acid composition of retail milk in the United States including regional and seasonal variations. J of Dairy Science. 2011; 94(1): 59 – 65.

480 Bendsen NT, Christensen R, et al. Consumption of industrial and ruminant trans fatty acids and risk of coronary heart disease: a systematic review and meta-analysis of cohort studies. European J Clin Nutr. 2011; 65(7): 773-83.

481 Wahle KW, Heys SD, Rotondo D. Conjugated linoleic acids: are they beneficial or detrimental to health? Prog Lipid Res. 2004; 43(6): 553-87.

482 Da Silva MS, Julien P, et al. Natural Rumen-Derived trans Fatty Acids Are Associated with Metabolic Markers of Cardiac Health. Lipids. 2015; 50(9): 873-82.

483 Bhattacharya A, Banu J, Rahman M, et al. Biological effects of conjugated linoleic acids in health and disease. J Nutr Biochem. 2006; 17(2): 789-810.

484 Carlson, Annabeth. "The man behind the trans fat ban." The Daily Illini. 12/4/2013. Available at: http://www.dailyillini.com/article/2013/12/the-man-behind-the-trans-fat-ban

485 Bernhard, Blythe. (2015, October 19). Word's Oldest Working Scientist Is Taking on Alzheimer's. *St. Louis Post-Dispatch*. Retrieved from http://www.vnews.com.

486 Willett WC, Stampfer MJ, Manson JE, et al. Intake of trans fatty acids and risk of coronary heart disease among women. Lancet. 1993; 341: 581-5.

487 Sun Q, Ma J, Campos H, et al. A prospective study of trans fatty acids in erythrocytes and risk of coronary heart disease. Circulation. 2007; 115: 1858-65.

488 Oomen CM, Ocke MC, et al. Association between trans fatty acid intake and 10-year risk of coronary heart disease in the Zutphen Elderly Study: a prospective population-based study. Lancet. 2001; 357: 746-51.

489 Lemaitre RN, King IB, et al. Cell membrane trans-fatty acids and the risk of primary cardiac arrest. Circulation. 2002; 105: 697-701.

490 Ibid.

491 Mozaffarian D, Clarke R. Quantitative effects on cardiovascular risk factors and coronary heart disease risk of replacing partially hydrogenated vegetable oils with other fats and oils. Eur J Clin Nutr. 2009; 63 Suppl 2: S22-33.

492 Kummerow FA, Zhou Q, et al. Trans fatty acids in hydrogenated fat inhibited the synthesis of the polyunsaturated fatty acids in the phospholipid of arterial cells. Life Sciences. 2004; 74(22): 2707-2723.

493 de Souza RJ, Mente A, Maroleanu A, et al. Intake of saturated and trans unsaturated fatty acids and risk of all cause mortality, cardiovascular disease, and type 2 diabetes: systematic review and meta-analysis of observational studies. BMJ. 2015 Aug 11; 351:h3978.

494 Hu FB, Manson JE, et al. Diet, Lifestyle, and the Risk of Type 2 Diabetes Mellitus in Women. N Engl J Med. 2001; 345: 790-797.

495 Gosline A. Why fast foods are bad, even in moderation. New Scientist. 2007-01-09.

496 "Six years of fast-foods supersizes monkeys." New Scientist. (2556): 21. 2006-06-17.

497 Kavanagh K, Jones KL, et al. Trans fat diet induces abdominal obesity and changes in insulin sensitivity in monkeys. Obesity (Silver Spring). 2007; 15(7): 1675-84.

498 Chajes V, et al. Association between serum trans-monounsaturated fatty acids and breast cancer risk in the E3N-EPIC Study. Am J Epidemiol. 2008; 167: 1312-20.

499 Bowman, GL, et al. Nutrient biomarker patterns, cognitive function, and MRI measures of brain aging. Neurology. 2012; 78(4): 241-9.

500 Sanchez-Villegas A, et al. Dietary fat intake and the risk of depression: the SUN Project. PLoS One, 2011. Jan 26;6(1):e16268.

501 Chavarro JE, et al. Dietary fatty acid intakes and the risk of ovulatory infertility. Amer J of Clin Nutr. 2007; 85(1): 231-237.

502 Seddon JM, Cote J, Rosner B. Progression of age-related macular degeneration: association with dietary fat, transunsaturaed fat, nuts, and fish intake. Arch Ophthalmol. 2003; 121(12): 1728-37.

503 Chong EW, Robman LD, et al. Fat consumption and its association with age-related macular degeneration. Arch Ophthalmol. 2009; 127(5): 674-80.

504 Cho E, Hung S, Willett WC, et al. Prospective study of dietary fat and the risk of age-related macular degeneration. Am J Clin Nutr. 2001 73(2): 209-218.

505 Chong EW, Kreis AJ, Wong TY, et al. Dietary omega-3 fatty acid and fish intake in the primary prevention of age-related macular degeneration: a systematic review and meta-analysis. Arch Ophthalmol. 2008; 126(6): 826-33.

506 Seddon JM, Rosner B, Sperduto RD, et al. Dietary fat and risk for advanced age-related macular degeneration. Arch Ophthalmol. 2001; 119(8): 1191-9.

507 Bretillon L, Gilles T, et al. Lipid and fatty acid profile of the retina, retinal pigment epithelium/choroid, and the lacrimal gland, and associations with adipose tissue fatty acids in human subjects. Exp Eye Research. 2008; 87(6): 521-528.

508 Final Determination Regarding Partially Hydrogenated Oils. Federal Register; FDA. 6/17/2015. Available at: *https://www.federalregister.gov/articles/2015/06/17/2015-14883/final-determination-regarding-partially-hydrogenated-oils*

509 Swift, Jennifer. "Trans fats: stealth killers." tfX:: the campaign against trans fats in food. ND. Available at: *http://www.tfx.org.uk*

510 Pitts M, Dorling D, Pattie C. "Oil For Food: The Global Story of Edible Lipids." Journal of World-Systems Research. 2007; Vol. XIII, No 1: pp. 12-32.

511 Davis, William. *Wheat Belly*. Rodale, New York. 2011.

512 Perlmutter, David. Grain Brain. Little Brown and Company, New York. 2013.

513 Colpo, Anthony. Whole Grains Empty Promises. Lulu Publishing, 2014.

514 "Whole Grains 101." Oldways Whole Grains Council. ND. Available at: *http://wholegrainscouncil.org/whole-grains-101*

515 Abdulla G, El-Shourbagy GA, Sitchy MZ. Effect of Pre-drying, Blanching and Citric Acid Treatments on the Quality of Fried Sweet Potato Chips. American Journal of Food Technology. 2014; 9: 39-48.

516 Schuppan D. Current concepts of celiac disease pathogenesis. Gastroenterology. 2000; 119(1): 234-242.

517 Fallon Morell, Sally. "Nourishing Traditional Diets – Sally Fallon" presentation. Published to YouTube on Dec. 23, 2012. Available at: *https://www.youtube.com/watch?v=7ixsBn_lfXE*

518 Pollan, Michael. "What I learned about wheat." 2014 Community Grains Conference. Oakland, California. March 9, 2014. Available at: *YouTube.com*.

519 Wheat: Wheat's Role in the U.S. Diet. USDA Economic Research Service. June 19, 2013. Available at: *http://www.ers.usda.gov/topics/crops/wheat/wheats-role-in-the-us-diet.aspx*

520 Slavin JL, Jacobs D, Marquart L. Grain Processing and Nutrition. Critical Reviews in Biotechnology. 2001; 21(1): 49-66.

521 Campbell, Grant M. "Chapter 7: Roller Milling of Wheat." Handbook of Powder Technology. 2007. Vol 12. Elsevier B.V.

522 Palmer, Marilyn and Neaverson, Peter. Industry In The Landscape, 1700-1900. Routledge, London and New York. 1994, p. 26.

523 Burnett, John. "Brown is Best: the Reform Bread League." History Today. 2005; 55(5). Available at: *www.historytoday.com*.

524 Ibid.

525 Ibid.

526 Thompson, Sir Henry. *Food and Feeding*. F. Warne & Company, London. 1880.

527 Burnett, John. "Brown is Best: the Reform Bread League." History Today. 2005; 55(5). Available at: *www.historytoday.com*.

528 Jacobs DR and Steffen LM. Nutrients, foods, and dietary patterns as exposures in research: a framework for food synergy. Am J Clin Nutr. 2003; 78(3): 5085-5135.

529 Bollet AJ. Politics and pellagra: the epidemic of pellagra in the U.S. in the early twentieth century. Yale J Biol Med. 1992; 65: 211-21.

530 Czapp, Katherine. "Against the Grain." The Weston A Price Foundation. July 16, 2006. Available at: *http://www.westonaprice.org/modern-diseases/against-the-grain/*

531 Ibid.

532 "Wonder Bread." *Wikipedia.org*. ND. Available at: *https://en.wikipedia.org/wiki/Wonder_Bread*

533 Slavin JL, Jacobs D, Marquart L. Grain Processing and Nutrition. Critical Reviews in Biotechnology. 2001; 21(1): 49-66.

534 Hassanein MMM and Abadel-Razek AG. Chromatographic Quantitation of Some Bioactive Minor Components in Oils of Wheat Germ and Grape Seeds Produced as By-Products. Journal of Oleo Science. 2009; 58(5): 227-233.

535 Ibid.

536 Jacobs DR and Steffen LM. Nutrients, foods, and dietary patterns as exposures in research: a framework for food synergy. Am J Clin Nutr. 2003; 78(3): 5085-5135.

537 Brenchley R, Spannagl M, Pfeifer M, et al. Analysis of the bread wheat genome using whole genome shotgun sequencing. Nature 2012; 491: 705-710.

538 Whole Grain Resource for the National School Lunch and School Breakfast Programs. USDA. January, 2014. Available at: *http://www.fns.usda.gov/sites/default/files/WholeGrainResource.pdf*

539 "Government Guidance." Oldways Whole Grains Council. ND. Available at: *http://wholegrainscouncil.org/whole-grain-stamp/government-guidance*

540 Jacobs DR and Steffen LM. Nutrients, foods, and dietary patterns as exposures in research: a framework for food synergy. Am J Clin Nutr. 2003; 78(3): 5085-5135.

541 Cordain L, Eaton SB, et al. Origins and evolution of the Western diet: health implications for the 21st century. Am J Clin Nutr. 2005; 81: 341-54.

542 Camire ME. Chemical changes during extrusion cooking. Recent advances. Adv Exp Med Biol. 1998; 434: 109-21.

543 Stitt, Paul A. *Beating the Food Giants.* Natural Press, Manitowoc, WI. 2007.

544 Fallon-Morell, Sally. "Nourishing Traditional Diets – The Key to Vibrant Health." Presentation published Dec. 23, 2012. Available at: *https://www.youtube.com/watch?v=7ixsBn_lfXE*

545 Stitt, Paul A. *Beating the Food Giants.* Natural Press, Manitowoc, WI. 2007.

546 Minger, Denise. "The China Study: Fact Or Fallacy?" Raw Food SOS. July 7, 2010. Available at: *http://rawfoodsos.com/2010/07/07/the-china-study-fact-or-fallac/*

547 Minger, Denise. "The China Study, Wheat and Heart Disease; Oh My!" Raw Food *SOS.com*. N.D. Available at: *http://rawfoodsos.com/2010/09/02/the-china-study-wheat-and-heart-disease-oh-my/*

548 Jacobs DR and Steffen LM. Nutrients, foods, and dietary patterns as exposures in research: a framework for food synergy. Am J Clin Nutr. 2003; 78(3): 5085-5135.

549 Ibid.

550 Anderson JW. Whole-grains intake and risk for coronary heart disease. In Whole-Grain Foods in Health and Disease, pp. 187-200 [L. Marquart, JL Slavin and RG Fulcher, editors]. St. Paul, MN: Eagan Press, 2002.

551 Morris J, Marr J, and Clayton D. Diet and heart: a postscript. British Medical Journal 1977; 1307-1314.

552 Jacobs DR, Meyer KA, et al. Whole-grain intake may reduce the risk of ischemic heart disease death in postmenopausal women: the Iowa Women's Health Study. Am J Clin Nutr. 1998; 68(2): 248-57.

553 Pietinen P, Rimm EB, et al. Intake of dietary fiber and risk of coronary heart disease in a cohort of Finnish men. The Alpha-Tocopherol, Beta Carotene Cancer Prevention Study. Circulation. 1996; 94: 2720-2727.

554 Rimm EB, Ascherio A, et al. Vegetable, fruit and cereal fiber intake and risk of coronary heart disease among men. Journal of the American Medical Association. 1996; 275: 447-451.

555 Liu SM, Stampfer MJ, Hu FB, et al. Whole-grain consumption and risk of coronary heart disease: results from the Nurse's Health Study. American Journal of Clinical Nutrition. 1999; 78: 920-927.

556 Pereira MA. Whole grain consumption and body weight regulation. In Whole-Grain Foods in Health and Disease, pp. 233-242 [L Marquart, JL Slavin and RG Fulcher, editors]. St. Paul, MN; Eagan Press, 2002.

557 Jacobs DR, Marquart L, Slavin JL, and Kushi LH. Whole-grain intake and cancer: an expanded review and meta-analysis. Nutrition and Cancer. 1998a; 30: 85-96.

558 Pereira MA, Jacobs DR, et al. The association of whole grain intake and fasting insulin in a biracial cohort of young adults: the CARDIA study. CVD Prevention I. 1998; 231-242.

559 Salmeron J, Ascherio A, et al. Dietary fiber, glycemic load, and risk of NIDDM in men. Diabetes Care. 1997a; 20: 545-550.

560 Salmeron J, Manson JE, et al. Dietary fiber, glycemic load, and risk of non-insulin-dependent diabetes mellitus in women. Journal of the American Medical Association. 1997b; 277: 472-477.

561 Jacobs DR, Meyer KA, et al. Is whole-grain intake associated with reduced total and cause-specific death rates in older women? The Iowa Women's Health Study. American Journal of Public Health. 1999; 89: 322-329.

562 van Leeuwen R, Boekhoorn S, Vingerling JR, et al. Dietary Intake of Antioxidants and Risk of Age-Related Macular Degeneration. JAMA. 2005; 294(24): 3101-3107.

563 Weng-Yew W, Selvaduray KR, et al. Suppression of tumor growth by palm tocotrienols via the attenuation of angiogenesis. Nutr Cancer. 2009; 61: 367-373.

564 Shibata A, Nakagawa K, et al. Tocotrienol inhibits secretion of angiogenic factors from human colorectal adenocarcinoma cells by suppressing hypoxia-inducible factor- 1 alpha. J Nutr. 2008; 138: 2136-2142.

565 Miyazawa T, Shibata A, et al. Anti-angiogenic function of tocotrienol. Asia Pac J Clin Nutr. 2008; 17 Suppl 1: 253-256.

566 Nakagawa K, Eitsuka T, et al. DNA chip analysis of comprehensive food function: inhibition of angiogenesis and telomerase activity with unsaturated vitamin E, tocotrienol. Biofactors. 2004; 21: 5-10.

567 Shibata A, Nakagawa K, et al. Delta-Tocotrienol suppresses VEGF induced angiogenesis whereas alpha-tocopherol does not. J. Agric Food Chem. 2009; 57: 8696 – 8704.

568 Cohen, Richard. "Sugar Love (A not so sweet story)." *National Geographic.* August, 2013.

569 Ibid.

570 Guyenet, Stephan. "By 2606, the US Diet will be 100 Percent Sugar." *WholeHealthSource.org*, Feb. 18, 2012. Available at: *http://wholehealthsource.blogspot.com/2012/02/by-2606-us-diet-will-be-100-percent.html*

571 Ibid.

572 Ibid.

573 "Profiling Food Consumption in America." USDA Economic Research Service, Factbook, Chapter 2. ND. Available at: *http://www.usda.gov/factbook/chapter2.pdf*

574 Lustig, Robert. Lecture: "Sugar: The Bitter Truth." University of California Television (UCTV). May 26, 2009. Available at: *https://www.youtube.com/watch?v=dBnniua6-oM*

575 National Cancer Institute. Usual intake of added sugars. In: Usual Dietary Intakes: Food Intakes, US Population 2001-04. November 2008. Available at: *http://riskfactor.cancer.*

576 Putnam, Judy and Gerrior, Shirley. Trends in the U.S Food Supply, 1970-97. USDA Economic Research Service. Available at: *http://www.ers.usda.gov/media/91042/aib750g_1_.pdf*

577 National Institute of Diabetes and Digestive and Kidney Diseases online registration page for "Clinical Research Strategies for Fructose Metabolism," available at: *http://www2.niddk.nih.gov/News/Calendar/FructoseMetab2012.htm*

578 Lustig, Robert. Lecture: "Is a Calorie a Calorie?: Processed Food, Experiment Gone Wrong." Delivered at Stanford Hospital & Clinics, published April 9, 2015. Available at: *https://www.youtube.com/watch?v=nxyxcTZccsE*

579 Lustig, Robert H. *Fat Chance – Beating the Odds Against Sugar, Processed Food, Obesity, and Disease.* Hudson Street Press, New York. 2012, p. 234.

580 Van Horn L, Johnson RK, et al. AHA Conference Proceedings: Translation and Implementation of Added Sugars Consumption Recommendations. Circulation. 2010; 122: 2470-2490.

581 Parnell W, Dodd J, Donnell A. Sugar consumption in New Zealand – with Thornley and McRobbie response. NZMJ 2010; 123 (1325): 102-3; author reply 103-4.

582 Lustig, Robert. Lecture: "Sugar: The Bitter Truth." University of California Television (UCTV). May 26, 2009. Available at: *https://www.youtube.com/watch?v=dBnniua6-oM*

583 Ibid.

584 Cohen, Rich. "Sugar Love (A not so sweet story)." *National Geographic.* August, 2013.

585 Yudkin, John. *Pure, White and Deadly - How Sugar is Killing Us and What We Can Do to Stop It.* Penguin Books, Ltd. London, England. 1972, 1986. Pp. 1 - 2.

586 Ibid.

587 Atkins, Robert C. *Dr. Atkins' Diet Revolution.* David McKay Company. Philadelphia, 1972, p. 63.

588 Lustig, Robert. Lecture: "Sugar: The Bitter Truth." University of California Television (UCTV). May 26, 2009. Available at: *https://www.youtube.com/watch?v=dBnniua6-oM*

589 Ibid.

590 Hellerstein MK, Schwarz JM, Neese, RA. Regulation of Hepatic De Novo Lipogenesis in Humans. Annual Reviews Nutrition. 1996; 16: 523-57.

591 Faeh D, Minehira K, Schwarz JM, et al. Effect of fructose overfeeding and fish oil administration on hepatic de novo lipogenesis and insulin sensitivity in healthy men. Diabetes. 2005; 54(7): 1907-13.

592 Thorburn AW, Storlein LH, Jenkins AB, et al. Fructose-induced in vivo insulin resistance and elevated plasma triglyceride levels in rats. Am J Clin Nutr 1989; 49: 1155-63.

593 Hwang IS, Ho H, et al. Fructose-induced insulin resistance and hypertension in rats. Hypertension. 1987; 10(5): 512-6.

594 Bremer AA, Stanhope KL, et al. Fructose-fed monkeys: a nonhuman primate model of insulin resistance, metabolic syndrome, and type 2 diabetes. Clin Transl Sci. 2011; 4(4): 243-52.

595 Lustig RH, Sen S, Soberman JE, Velasquez-Mieyer PA. Obesity, leptin resistance, and the effects of insulin. Int J Obes Relat Metab Disord. 2004; 28(10): 1344-8.

596 Lirio LM, Forechi L, et al. Chronic fructose intake accelerates non-alcoholic fatty liver disease in the presence of essential hypertension. J Diabetes Complications. 2015 Oct 19. Pii: S1056-8727(15)00398-0. {Epub ahead of print}.

597 Basu S, Yoffe P, Hills N, Lustig RH. The Relationship of Sugar to Population-Level Diabetes Prevalence: An Econometric Analysis of Repeated Cross-Sectional Data. PLOS One. February 27, 2013; 8(2): e57873.

598 EPIC-Interact Consortium. Consumption of sweet beverages and type 2 diabetes incidence in European adults: Results from Epic-Interact. Diabetologia. 2013; 56(7): 1520-30.

599 Basu S, Yoffe P, Hills N, Lustig RH. The Relationship of Sugar to Population-Level Diabetes Prevalence: An Econometric Analysis of Repeated Cross-Sectional Data. PLOS One. February 27, 2013; 8(2): e57873.

600 Yang Q, Zhang Z, et al. Added Sugar Intake and Cardiovascular Diseases Mortality Among US Adults. JAMA Intern Med. 2014; 174(4): 516-524.

601 Thornalley PJ, Langborg A, et al. Formation of glyoxal, methylglyoxal and 3-deoxyglucosone in the glycation of proteins by glucose. Biochem J. 1999; 344: 109-16.

602 Stitt AW. Advanced glycation: an important pathological event in diabetic and age related ocular disease. Br. J Ophthalm. 2001; 85: 746-53.

603 Stitt, Alan W. Advanced glycation: an important pathological event in diabetic and age related ocular disease. Br J Ophthalmol. 2001; 85: 746-753.

604 Hammes HP, Hoerauf H, et al. N(epsiolon)(carboxymethyl) lysine and the AGE receptor RAGE colocalize in age-related macular degeneration. Invest Ophthalmol Vis Sci. 1999; 40(8): 1855-9.

605 Handa JT, Verzijl N, et al. Increase in the advanced glycation end product pentosidine in Bruch's membrane with age. Invest Ophthalmol Vis Sci. 1999; 40: 775-79.

606 Handa JT, Reiser KM, et al. The advanced glycation endproduct pentosidine induces the expression of PDGF-B in human retinal pigment epithelial cells. Exp Eye Res. 1998; 66: 411-419.

607 Farboud B, Aotaki-Keen A, et al. Development of a polyclonal antibody with braod epitope specificity for advanced glycation endproducts and localization of these epitopes in Bruch's membrane of the aging eye. Mol Vis. 1999; 14: 5-11.

608 Hageman GS, Mullins RF, et al. Vitronectin is a constituent of ocular drusen and the vitronectin gene is expressed in human retinal pigmented epithelial cells. FASEB J. 1999; 13: 477-484.

609 Mullins RF, Russell SR, et al. Drusen associated with aging and age-related macular degeneration contain proteins common to extracellular deposits associated with atherosclerosis, elastosis, amyloidosis, and dense deposit disease. FASEB J. 2000; 14: 835-846.

610 Li YM, Dickson DW. Enhanced binding of advanced glycation endproducts (AGE) by the ApoE4 isoform links the mechanism of plaque deposition in Alzheimer's disease. Neurosci Lett. 1997; 226: 155-8.

611 Tabaton M, Perry G, et al. Is amyloid beta-protein glycated in Alzheimer's disease? Neuroreport. 1997; 8: 907-9.

612 Hammes HP, Weiss A, et al. Modification of vitronectin by advanced glycation alters functional properties in vitro and in the diabetic retina. Lab Invest. 1996; 75: 325-38.

613 Moore DJ, Hussain AA, Marshall J. Age-related variation in the hydraulic conductivity of Bruch's membrane. Invest. Ophthalmol Vis Sci. 1995; 36: 1290-7.

614 Okubo A, Rosa RH Jr, et al. The relationship of age changes in retinal pigment epithelium and Bruch's membrane. Invest Ophthalmol Vis Sci. 1999; 40: 443-9.

615 Takagi Y, Kashiwagi A, et al. Significance of fructose-induced protein oxidation and formation of advanced glycation end product. J Diabetes Complications. 1995; 9(2): 87-91.

616 Stitt, Alan W. Advanced glycation: an important pathological event in diabetic and age related ocular disease. Br J Ophthalmol. 2001; 85: 746-53.

617 Lu M, Kuroki M, et al. Advanced Glycation End Products Increase Retinal Vascular Endothelial Growth Factor Expression. J Clin Invest. 1998; 101(6): 1219-1224.

618 Boulton M, McKechnie NM, et al. The formation of autofluorescent granules in cultured human RPE. Invest Ophthalmol Vis Sci. 1989; 30: 82-9.

619 Ghaem Maralani H, Tai BC, et al. Metabolic Syndrome and Risk of Age-Related Macular Degeneration. Retina. 2015; 35(3): 459-66.

620 Thierry M, Pasquis B, Acar N, et al. Metabolic Syndrome Triggered by High-Fructose Diet Favors Choroidal Neovascularization and Impairs Retinal Light Sensitivity in the Rat. PLOS One. 2014; 9(11): e112450.

621 Chiu CJ, Hubbard LD, et al. Dietary glycemic index and carbohydrate in relation to early age-related macular degeneration. Am J Clin Nutr. 2006a; 83: 880-6.

622 Chiu CJ, Milton RC, et al. Association between dietary glycemic index and age-related macular degeneration in the Age-Related Eye Disease Study. Am J Clin Nutr. 2007a; 86: 180-8.

623 Chiu, Chung-Jung, Taylor A. Dietary Hyperglycemia, Glycemic Index and Metabolic Retinal Diseases. Prog Retin Eye Res. 2011; 30(1): 18-53.

624 Guyenet, Stephan. "The Carbohydrate Hypothesis of Obesity: a Critical Examination." *WholeHealthSource.org*. August 13, 2011. Available at: *http://wholehealthsource.blogspot.com/2011/08/carbohydrate-hypothesis-of-obesity.html*

625 Ibid.

626 Miller JB, Pang E, Bramall L. Rice: a high or low glycemic index food? Am J Clin Nutr. 1992; 56: 1034-6.

627 Guyenet, Stephan. "The Carbohydrate Hypothesis of Obesity: a Critical Examination." Whole Health Source.org. August 13, 2011. Available at: *http://wholehealthsource.blogspot.com/2011/08/carbohydrate-hypothesis-of-obesity.html*

628 Lindeberg S, Berntorp E., et al. Age relations of cardiovascular risk factors in a traditional Melanesian society: the Kitava Study. Am J Clin Nutr. 1997; 66(4): 845-52.

629 Lindeberg, Staffan. "Our research." *StaffanLindeberg.com*. ND. Available at: *http://www.staffanlindeberg.com/OurResearch.html*

630 Lindeberg S, Berntorp E., et al. Age relations of cardiovascular risk factors in a traditional Melanesian society: the Kitava Study. Am J Clin Nutr. 1997; 66(4): 845-52.

631 Lindeberg, S. Dietary Shifts and Human Health: Cancer and Cardiovascular Disease in a Sustainable World. J Gastrointest Canc. 2012; 43: 8-12.

632 Ibid.

633 Lindeberg S, Ahren B, et al. Determinants of serum trigylycerides and high-density lipoprotein cholesterol in traditional Trobriand Islanders: the Kitava Study. Scand J Clin Lab Invest. 2003; 63: 175-80.

634 Lindeberg, Staffan. "The Kitava Study." ND. Available at: *http://www.staffanlindeberg.com/TheKitavaStudy.html*

635 Ibid.

636 Lindeberg, Staffan. "Our research." *StaffanLindeberg.com*. ND. Available at: *http://www.staffanlindeberg.com/OurResearch.html*

637 Grundy SM, Vega GL. Two Different Views of the Relationship of Hypertriglyceridemia to Coronary Heart Disease. Arch Intern Med. 1992; 152(1): 28-34.

638 Schulz LO, Bennett PH, Ravussen E, et al. Effects of Traditional and Western Environments on Prevalence of Type 2 Diabetes in Pima Indians in Mexico and the U.S. Diabetes Care. 2006; 29(8): 1866-71.

639 Taubes, Gary. *Good Calories, Bad Calories*. Alfred A. Knopf, New York. 2007. P. 237.

640 Guyenet, Stephan. "Lessons From the Pima Indians." Whole Health Source. May 15, 2008. Available at: *www.wholehealthsource.org*.

641 Taubes, Gary. *Good Calories, Bad Calories*. Alfred A. Knopf. New York. 2007. p. 238-9.

642 Smith CJ, Nelson RG, et al. Survey of the Diet of Pima Indians Using Quantitative Food Frequenty Assessment and 24-Hour Recall. J Amer Diet Assoc. 1996; 96(8): 778-784.

643 Price, Weston A. Nutrition and Physical Degeneration. 1939, 1945 by Weston A. Price. Lemon Grove, California, The Price-Pottenger Nutrition Foundation, Inc. 1970 – 2008.

644 Guyenet, Stephan. "The Kitavans: Wisdom from the Pacific Islands." Whole Health Source. Aug 13, 2008. Available at: *www.wholehealthsource.org*.

645 Writght, JD, et al. Trends in Intake of Energy and Macronutrients - United States, 1971 – 2000, CDC MMWR. Feb 6, 2004; 53(04): 80-82. Data based on the National Health and Nutrition Examination Survey (NHANES 1971 – 2000).

646 Guyenet, Stephan. "Lessons From the Pima Indians." Whole Health Source. May 15, 2008. Available at: *www.wholehealthsource.org*.

647 Lustig, Robert H. "Processed Food: An Experiment That Failed?" Lecture presented at the Stockholm Food Forum 2015. June 1-2, 2015. Stockholm, Sweden.

648 Popkin BM, Hawkes C. Sweetening of the global diet, particularly beverages: patterns, trends, and policy responses. Lancet Diabetes Endocrinol. 2016; 4(2): 174-86.

649 Lustig, Robert H. "Processed Food: An Experiment That Failed?" Lecture presented at the Stockholm Food Forum 2015. June 1-2, 2015. Stockholm, Sweden.

650 Jones NRV, Conklin AI, et al. The Growing Price Gap Between More and Less Healthy Foods: Analysis of a Novel Longitudinal UK Dataset. PLOS One. October 8, 2014. DOI: 10.1371/journal.pone.0109343.

651 "How Much Do Americans Pay for Fruits and Vegetables/ AIB-790." USDA Economic Research Service. 2015. Available at: *http://www.ers.usda.gov/media/303025/aib790d_1_.pdf*

652 Ibid.

653 Klein R, Lee KE, Gangnon RE, Klein BEK. Incidence of Visual Impairment Over a 20-Year Period. Ophthalmology, 2013; 120(6): 1210-1219.

654 Dandona R, Dandona L. Socioeconomic status and blindness. Br J Ophthalmol. 2001; 85: 1484-1488.

655 Yip JL, Khawaja AP, Chan MP, et al. Area deprivation and age related macular degeneration in the EPIC-Norfolk Eye Study. Public Health. 2015; 129(2): 103-9.

656 Tielsch JM, Sommer A, et al. Socioeconomic Status and Visual Impairment Among Urban Americans. Arch Ophthalmol. 1991; 109: 637-641.

657 Klein R, Klein BE, et al. The relation of socioeconomic factors to age-related cataract, maculopathy, and impaired vision. The Beaver Dam Eye Study. Ophthalmology. 1994; 101(12): 1969-1979.

658 Adler NE, Boyce WT, et al. Socioeconomic inequalities in health: no easy solution. JAMA. 1993; 269: 3140-3145.

659 Chiu CJ, Chang ML, et al. The relationship of major American dietary patterns to age-related macular degeneration. Am J Ophthalmol. 2014; 158(1): 118-127.

660 Ibid.

661 Shrank, WH, Patrick AR, Brookhart MA. Healthy User and Related Biases in Observational Studies of Preventive Interventions: A Primer for Physicians. J of Gen Internal Med. 2011; 26(5): 546-550.

662 Brenchley R, Spannagl M, Pfeifer M, et al. Analysis of the bread wheat genome using whole genome shotgun sequencing. Nature 2012; 491: 705-710.

663 Nieto, F. Javier. Cardiovascular Disease and Risk Factor Epidemiology: A Look Back at the Epidemic of the 20th Century. American Journal of Public Health. 1999; 89(3): 292-4.

664 Ibid.

665 Dayton S, Pearce M, et al. A Controlled Clinical Trial of a Diet High in Unsaturated Fat in Preventing Complications of Atherosclerosis. Circulation. 1969; 40:11-1-11-63.

666 Grimes DS. An epidemic of coronary heart disease. QJ Med. 2012; 105: 509-518.

667 Tan JS, Wang JJ, et al. Age-related macular degeneration and mortality from cardiovascular disease or stroke. Br J Ophthalmol. 2008; 92: 509-512.

668 Ogden, CL, Carroll, MD, CDC Division of Health and Nutrition Examination Surveys. Prevalence of overweight, obesity, and extreme obesity among adults: United States, trends 1960-62 through 2007-2008.

669 Hurt RT, Kulisek C, et al. The Obesity Epidemic: Challenges, Health Initiatives, and Implications for Gastroenterologists. Gastroenterol Hepatol (NY). 2010: 6(12): 780-92.

670 CDC Grand Rounds: Childhood Obesity in the United States, Morbidity and Mortality Weekly Report. Jan 21, 2011. 60(02): 42-46.

671 Sclafani A, Springer D. Dietary obesity in adult rats: similarities to hypothalamic and human obesity syndromes. Physiology & Behavior. 1976; 17(3): 461-71.

672 Sclafani A, Gorman A. Effects of age, sex, and prior body weight on the development of dietary obesity in adult rats. Physiology & Behovior. 1977; 18(6): 1021-26.

673 Sampey BP, Vanhoose AM, et al. Cafeteria diet is a robust model of human metabolic syndrome with liver and adipose inflammation: comparison to high-fat diet. Obesity (Silver Spring). 2011; 19(6): 1109-17.

674 Rising R, Alger S, et al. Food intake measured by an automated food-selection system: relationship to energy expenditure. Amer J Clin Nutr. 1992; 55(2): 343-9.

675 Larson DE, Rising R, et al. Spontaneous overfeeding with a 'cafeteria diet' in men: effects on a 24-hour energy expenditure and substrate oxidation. Intl J Obes Relat Metab Disord. 1995; 19(5): 331-7.

676 Larson DE, Tataranni PA, et al. Ad libitum food intake on a "cafeteria diet" in Native American women: relations with body composition and 24-hour expenditure. Amer J Clin Nutr. 1995; 62(5): 911-17.

677 Sampey BP, Vanhoose AM, et al. Cafeteria diet is a robust model of human metabolic syndrome with liver and adipose inflammation: comparison to high-fat diet. Obesity (Silver Spring). 2011: 19(6): 1109-17.

678 Ibid.

679 Howard KP, Klein BE, Lee KE, Klein R. Measures of body shape and adiposity as related to incidence of age-related eye diseases: observations from the Beaver Dam Eye Study. Invest Ophthalmol Vis Sci. 2014; 55(4): 2592-8.

680 Adams MK, Simpson JA, et al. Abdominal obesity and age-related macular degeneration. Am J Epidemiol. 2011; 173(11): 1246-55.

681 Ghaem Maralani H, Tai BC, et al. Metabolic syndrome and risk of age-related macular degeneration. Retina. 2015; 35(3): 459-66.

682 Munch IC, Linneberg A, Larsen M. Precursors of age-related macular degeneration: associations with physical activity, obesity, and serum lipids in the inter99 eye study. Invest Ophthalmol Vis Sci. 2013; 54(6): 3932-40.

683 Cheung LK, Eaton A. Age-related macular degeneration. Pharmacotherapy. 2013; 33(8): 838-55.

684 Cheung N, Wong TY. Obesity and eye diseases. Surv Ophthalmol. 2007; 52(2): 180-95.

685 Sin HP, Liu DT, Lam DS. Lifestyle modification, nutritional and vitamin supplements for age-related macular degeneration. Acta Ophthalmol. 2013; 91(1): 6-11.

686 Peeters A, Magliano DJ, et al. Changes in Abdominal Obesity and Age-Related Macular Degeneration. The Atherosclerosis Risk in Communities Study. Arch Ophthalmol. 2008; 126(11): 1554-1560.

687 Gopinath B, Liew G, et al. Physical activity and the 15-year incidence of age-related macular degeneration. Invest Ophthalmol Vis Sci. 2014; 55(12): 7799-803.

688 McGuinness MB, Karahalios A, et al. Past physical activity and age-related macular degeneration: the Melbourne Collaborative Cohort Study. Br J Ophthalmol. 2016; Jan 19. Pii: bjophthalmol-2015-307633.

689 "Jack LaLanne Biography. *Biography.com*. N.D. Available at: *http://www.biography.com/people/jack-lalanne-273648*

690 Ohkawara K, Tanaka S, Miyachi M, Ishikawa-Takata K, Tabata I. A dose-response relation between aerobic exercise and visceral fat reduction: systematic review of clinical trials. Int J Obes (Lond). 2007; 31(12): 1786-97.

691 Emberts T, Porcari J, et al. Exercise Intensity and Energy Expenditure of a Tabata Workout. Journal of Sports Science and Medicine. 2013; 12: 612-613.

692 2014 National Diabetes Statistics Report. Centers for Disease Control and Prevention. Available at: *http://www.cdc.gov*

693 Choi JK, Lym YL, et al. Diabetes mellitus and early age-related macular degeneration. Arch Ophthalmol. 2011; 129(2): 196-9.

694 Mazzucco, Massimo. *Cancer – The Forbidden Cures.* Buenaonda Films, London, UK. 2013. Available at: *https://www.youtube.com/watch?v=3ncDdqNDcaI*

695 American Cancer Society. "Cancer Facts & Figures 2013." Atlanta: American Cancer Society; 2013. Available at: *http://www.cancer.org/acs/groups/content/@epidemiologysurveilance/documents/document/acspc-036845.pdf*

696 Port AM, Ruth MR, Istfan NW. Fructose consumption and cancer: is there a connection? Curr Opin Endocrinol Diabetes Obes. 2012; 19(5): 367-74.

697 Seely S, Horrobin DF. Diet and breast cancer: the possible connection with sugar consumption.

698 Lustig, Robert H. *Fat Chance – Beating the Odds Against Sugar, Processed Food, Obesity, and Disease.* Hudson Street Press, New York. 2012, p. 96.

699 Beasley JD, Swift JJ. The Kellogg Report. The Institute of Health Policy and Practice, Annandale-on-Hudson, New York. 1989, 129.

700 Enig, Mary, et al. Federation Proceedings. July 1978; 37(9): 2215-2220.

701 Doll, Richard, Armstrong, Bruce. Cancer. In H.C. Trowell and D.P. Burkitt (Eds.), *Western Diseases: their emergence and prevention* (p. 106) Cambridge, Massachusetts, Harvard University Press, 1981.

702 Cordain, Loren. The Paleo Answer. Hoboken, New Jersey: John Wiley and Sons, Inc., 2012.

703 Mandas A, Mereu RM, et al. Cognitive Impairment and Age-Related Vision Disorders: Their Possible Relationship and the Evaluation of the Use of Aspirin and Satins in a 65 Years-And-Over Sardinian Population. Front Agin Neurosci. 2014; 7(6): 309. Epubl 2014 Nov 7.

704 Kaarniranta K, Salminen A, et al. Age-related macular degeneration (AMD): Alzheimer's disease in the eye? J Alzheimers Dis. 2011; 24(4): 615-31.

705 Cleave, T.L. *The Saccharine Disease.* John Wright & Sons Limited, Bristol, Great Britain. 1974, pp. 86-87.

706 Ibid.

707 Nangia V, Jonas JB, et al. Prevalence of age-related macular degeneration in rural central India: the Central India Eye and Medical Study. Retina. 2011; 31(6): 1179-85.

708 Dyer O. First cases of type 2 diabetes found in white UK teenagers. BMJ. 2002; 324(7336): 506.

709 Elder DA, Woo JG, D'Alessio DA. Impaired beta-cell sensitivity to glucose and maximal insulin secretory capacity in adolescents with type 2 diabetes. Pediatr Diabetes. 2010; 11(5): 314-321.

710 Chiu CJ, Milton RC, et al. Association between dietary glycemic index and age-related macular degeneration in nondiabetic participants in the Age-Related Eye Disease Study. Am J Clin Nutr. 2007; 86: 180-8.

711 Kaushik S, Wang JJ, et al. Dietary glycemic index and the risk of age-related macular degeneration. Am J Clin Nutr. 2008; 88: 1104-10.

712 Klein R, Davis MD, et al. The Wisconsin Age-related Maculopathy Grading System. Ophthalmology. 1991; 98: 1128-1134.

713 Bird AC, Bressler SB, Bressler IH, et al. An International Classification and Grading System for Age-related Maculopathy and Age-related Macular Degeneration. The International ARM Epidemiological Study Group. Surv Ophthalmol. 1995; 39: 367-374.

714 Seddon JM, Sharma S, Adelman RA. Evaluation of the Clinical Age-Related Maculopathy Staging System. Ophthalmology. 2006; 113: 260-66.

715 Klein R, Meuer SM, et al. Harmonizing the classification of age-related macular degeneration in the three-continent AMD consortium. Ophthalmic Epidemiol. 2014 21(3): 204-5.

716 Bird, Alan C. "Age Related Macular Disease." National Academy of Sciences, National Academy of Engineering, and Institute of Medicine. *Distinctive Voices* lecture given at the Beckman Center, Irvine, California. 2014. Published online Feb. 6, 2014. Available at: *https://www.youtube.com/watch?v=6ugISIFyxuA*.

717 Mitchell P, Smith W, et al. Prevalence of age-related maculopathy in Australia. The Blue Mountains Eye Study. Ophthalmology. 1995; 102(10): 1450-60.

718 Klein R, Klein BEK, Cruickshanks KJ. The Prevalence of Age-Related Maculopathy by Geographic Region and Ethnicity. Progress in Retinal and Eye Research. 1999; 18(3): 371-389.

719 VanNewkirk MR, Nanjan MB, et al. The Prevalence of Age-related Maculopathy. The Visual Impairment Project. Ophthalmology. 2000; 107: 1593-1600.

720 Schachat AP, Hyman L, et al. Features of Age-Related Macular Degeneration in a Black Population. The Barbados Eye Study Group. Arch Ophthalmol. 1995; 113: 728-35.

721 Li Y, Xu L, et al. Prevalence of age-related maculopathy in the adult population in China: the Beijing eye study. Am J Ophthalmol. 2006; 142(5): 788-93.

722 Li Y., Xu L., Wang Y.X., et al. Prevalence of age-related maculopathy in the adult population in China: the Beijing eye study [letter]. Am J Ophthalmol. 2008; 146: 329.

723 Vinding T. Age-related macular degeneration. Macular changes, prevalence and sex ratio. An epidemiological study of 1000 aged individuals. Acta Ophthalmol (Copenh). 1989; 67(6): 609-16.

724 Korb CA, Kottler UB, et al. Prevalence of age-related macular degeneration in a large European cohort: Results from the population-based Gutenberg Health Study. Graefes Arch Clin Exp Ophthalmol. 2014; 252: 1403-1411.

725 Augood CA, Vingerling JR, de Jong PTVM, et al. Prevalence of Age-Related Maculopathy in Older Europeans. Arch Ophthalmol. 2006; 124: 529-535.

726 Wyatt HT. Abnormalities of cornea, lens and retina survey findings. Can J Ophthalmol. 1973: 8: 291-297.

727 Andersen MVN, Rosenberg T, et al. Prevalence of Age-Related Maculopathy and Age-Related Macular Degeneration among the Inuit in Greenland. The Greenland Inuit Eye Study. Ophthalmology. 2008; 115: 700-707.

728 Jonasson F and Thordarson K. Prevalence of ocular disease and blindness in a rural area in the eastern region of Iceland during 1980 through 1984. Acta Ophthalmol. 1987; 182: 40-43.

729 Jonasson F, Arnarsson A, et al. The Prevalence of Age-Related Maculopathy in Iceland. Arch Ophthalmol. 2003; 121: 379-385.

730 Jain IS, Prasad P, Gupta A, et al. Senile macular degeneration in Northern India. Indian J Ophthalmol. 1984; 32: 343-6.

731 Gupta SK, Murthy GV, et al. Prevalence of early and late age-related macular degeneration in a rural population in northern India: the INDEYE Feasibility Study. Invest Ophthalmol Vis Sci. 2007; 48: 1007-1011.

732 Piermarocchi S, Segato T, et al. The prevalence of age-related macular degeneration in Italy (PAMDI) study: report 1. Ophthalmic Epidemiol. 2011; 18(3): 129-36.

733 Klein R, Klein BEK, Cruickshanks KJ. The Prevalence of Age-Related Maculopathy by Geographic Region and Ethnicity. Progress in Retinal and Eye Research. 1999; 18(3): 371-389.

734 Yasuda M, Kiyohara Y, et al. Nine-year incidence and risk factors for age-related macular degeneration in a defined Japanese population the Hisayama study. Ophthalmol. 2009; 116(11): 2135-40.

735 Mathenge W, Bastawrous A, et al. Prevalence of Age-Related Macular Degeneration in Nakuru, Kenya: A Cross-Sectional Population-Based Study. PLOS. Feb 19, 2013. DOI: 10.1371/journal.pmed.1001393.

736 Yoon KC, Mun GH, et al. Prevalence of eye diseases in South Korea: data from the Korea National Health and Nutrition Examination Survey 2008-2009. Korean J Ophthalmol. 2011; 25(6): 421-33.

737 Cho BJ, Heo JW, et al. Prevalence and Risk Factors of Age-Related Macular Degeneration in Korea: The Korea Natinal Health and Nutrition Examination Survey 2010-2011. Invest Ophthalmol Vis Sci. 2014; 55: 1101-1108.

738 Yitzchak GJ, Mokete M. Survey of Ophthalmic Conditions in Rural Lesotho. Documenta Ophthalmologica. 1980; 49: 285-291.

739 Vingerling JR, Klaver CC, et al. Epidemiology of age-related maculopathy. Epidemiologic Rev. 1995; 17: 347-60.

740 Mann I, Potter D. Geographic Ophthalmology – A Preliminary Study of the Maoris of New Zealand. Am J Ophthalmol. 1969; 67(3): 358-69.

741 Worsley D, Worsley A. Prevalence predictions for age-related macular degeneration in New Zealand have implications for provision of healthcare services. NZ Med J. 2015; 128(1409): 44-56.

742 Nwosu SN. Age-related macular degeneration in Onitsha, Nigeria. Niger J Clin Pract. 2011; 14(3): 327-31.

743 Adegbehingbe BO, Majengbasan TO. Ocular health status of rural dwellers in south-western Nigeria. Aust J Rural Health. 2007; 15: 269-272.

744 Jenchitr W, Ruamviboonsuk P, et al. Prevalence of age-related macular degeneration in Thailand. Ophthalmic Epidemiol. 2011; 18(1): 48-52.

745 Khotcharrat R, Patikulsila D. et al. Epidemiology of Age-Related Macular Degeneration among the Elderly Population of Thailand. J Med Assoc Thai. 2015; 98(8): 790-7.

746 Ngai LY, Stocks N, et al. The prevalence and analysis of risk factors for age-related macular degeneration: 18-year follow-up data from the Speedwell eye study, United Kingdom. Eye (Lond). 2011; 25(6): 784-93.

747 Akuffo KO, Nolan J, et al. Prevalence of age-related macular degeneration in the Republic of Ireland. Br J Ophthalmol. 2015; 99(8): 1037-44.

748 Kahn HA, Leibowitz HM, et al. The Framingham Eye Study. II. Association of ophthalmic pathology with single variables previously measured in the Framingham Heart Study. Amer J Epidemiol. 1977b; 106: 33-41.

749 Klein R, Klein BEK, Cruickshanks KJ. The Prevalence of Age-Related Maculopathy by Geographic Region and Ethnicity. Progress in Retinal and Eye Research. 1999; 18(3): 371-389.

750 Chumbley LC. Impressions of Eye Diseases among Rhodesian Blacks in Mashonaland. S Afr Med J. 1977; 52(8): 316-318.

751 Kahn HA, Leibowitz HM, et al. The Framingham Eye Study. II. Association of ophthalmic pathology with single variables previously measured in the Framingham Heart Study. Amer J Epidemiol. 1977; 106: 33-41.

752 Ibid.

753 Cruickshanks KJ, Hamman RF, Klein R, et al. The prevalence of age-related maculopathy by geographic region and ethnicity. The Colorado-Wisconsin study of age-related maculopathy. Arch Ophthalmol. 1997; 115: 242-250.

754 Klein R, Klein BEK, Cruikshanks KJ. The Prevalence of Age-Related Maculopathy by Geographic Region and Ethnicity. Progress in Retinal and Eye Research. 1999; 18(3): 371-389.

755 Ngai LY, Stocks N, et al. The prevalence and analysis of risk factors for age-related macular degeneration: 18-year follow-up data from the Speedwell eye study, United Kingdom. Eye (Lond). 2011; 25(6): 784-93.

756 Akuffo KO, Nolan J, et al. Prevalence of age-related macular degeneration in the Republic of Ireland. Br J Ophthalmol. 2015; 99(8): 1037-44.

757 Augood CA, Vingerling JR, de Jong, PTVM, et al. Prevalence of Age-Related Maculopathy in Older Europeans. Arch Ophthalmol. 2006; 124: 529-535.

758 Gibson J, Rosenthal A, Lavery J. A study of the prevalence of eye disease in the elderly in an English community. Trans Ophthalmol Soc. 1985; 104: 196-203.

759 Dickinson AJ, Sparrow JM, et al. Prevalence of age-related maculopathy at two points in time in an elderly British population. Eye. 1997; 11: 301-314.

760 Sparrow JM, Dickinson AJ, et al. Seven year follow-up of age-related maculopathy in an elderly British population. Eye. 1997; 11: 315-324.

761 Ghafour IM, Allan D, Foulds WS. Common causes of blindness and visual handicap in the west of Scotland. Br J Ophthalmol. 1983; 67: 209-13.

762 Rees A, Zekite A, et al. How many people in England and Wales are registered partially sighted or blind because of age-related macular degeneration? Eye (Lond). 2014; 28(7): 832-7.

763 Congdon N, O'Colmain B, et al. Causes and prevalence of visual impairment among adults in the United States. Arch Ophthalmol. 2004; 122(4): 477-485.

764 Attebo K, Mitchell P, Smith W. Visual Acuity and the Causes of Visual Loss in Australia. The Blue Mountains Eye Study. Ophthalmology; 1996; 103: 357-364.

765 Mitchell P, Smith W, et al. Prevalence of age-related maculopathy in Australia. The Blue Mountains Eye Study. Ophthalmology. 1995; 102(10): 1450-60.

766 Klein R, Klein BEK, Cruikshanks KJ. The Prevalence of Age-Related Maculopathy by Geographic Region and Ethnicity. Progress in Retinal and Eye Research. 1999; 18(3): 371-389.

767 VanNewkirk MR, Nanjan MB, et al. The Prevalence of Age-related Maculopathy. The Visual Impairment Project. Ophthalmology. 2000; 107: 1593-1600.

768 Vinding T. Age-related macular degeneration. Macular changes, prevalence and sex ratio. An epidemiological study of 1000 aged individuals. Acta Ophthalmol (Copenh). 1989; 67(6): 609-16.

769 la Cour M, Nielsen NV, et al. [Age related macular degeneration. A widespread disease]. Ugeskr Laeger. 2001; 163(46): 6396-6400.

770 Lindekleiv H, Erke MG. Projected prevalence of age-related macular degeneration in Scandinavia 2012-2040. Acta Ophthalmol. 2013; 91(4): 307-11.

771 Vingerling JR, Klaver CC, et al. Epidemiology of age-related maculopathy. Epidemiologic Rev. 1995; 17: 347-60.

772 Bundesausschuβ der Ärzte und Krankenkassen (2001) Photodynamische Therapie (PDT) mit Verteporfin bei altersabhangiger feuchter Makladegeneration mit subfoveolaren Klassischen choriodalen Neovasklarisationen *http://www.kbv.de/hta/hta.htm.*

773 Korb CA, Kottler UB, et al. Prevalence of age-related macular degeneration in a large European cohort: Results from the population-based Gutenberg Health Study. Graefes Arch Clin Exp Ophthalmol. 2014; 252: 1403-1411.

774 Augood CA, Vingerling JR, de Jong PTVM, et al. Prevalence of Age-Related Maculopathy in Older Europeans. The European Eye Study (EUREYE). Arch Ophthalmol. 2006; 124: 529-535.

775 Topouzis F, Coleman AL, et al. Prevalence of age-related macular degeneration in Greece: the Thessaloniki Eye Study. Am J Ophthalmol. 2006; 142(6): 1076-9.

776 Piermarocchi S, Segato T, et al. The prevalence of age-related macula degeneration in Italy (PAMDI) study: report 1. Ophthalmic Epidemiol. 2011; 18(3): 129-36.

777 Ibid.

778 "Culture & History." Greenland Guide. ND. Available at: *http://www.greenland-guide.gl/culture_history.htm*

779 "2006 Census: Aboriginal Peoples in Canada in 2006: Inuit, Metis and First Nations, 2006 Census: Inuit." Statistics Canada. ND. Available at: *https://www12.statcan.gc.ca/census-recensement/2006/as-sa/97-558/p6-eng.cfm*

780 Skydsgaard H. Gronlandske Blinde. Medicinsk oversigt med en socialmedicinsk kommentar. In: Landslaegens arsberetning 1962. Sundhedstilstanden I Gronland. Beretninger vedrorende Gronland 4, 1963.

781 Johnson GJ, Green JS, et al. Survey of ophthalmic conditions in a Labrador community: II. Ocular disease. Can J Ophthalmol. 1984; 19: 224-233.

782 Rosenberg T. Prevalence of Blindness Caused by Senile Macular Degeneration in Greenland." Arct Med Res. 1987; 46(2): 64-70.

783 Ibid.

784 Ibid.

785 Rosenberg T. Prevalence of blindness caused by senile macular degeneration in Greenland. Arctic Med Res. 1987; 46:64-70.

786 Alsbirk PH. Eye health service in Greenland. Acta Ophthalmol Scand. 2002; 80(Suppl. 234): 39-43.

787 Wyatt HT. Abnormalities of cornea, lens and retina survey findings. Can J Ophthalmol. 1973: 8: 291-297.

788 Johnson, GJ, Green JS, et al. Survey of ophthalmic conditions in a Labrador community: II. Ocular disease. Can J Ophthalmol. 1984; 19: 224-233.

789 Zammit MP, Torres A, et al. The prevalence and patterns of dental caries in Labrador Inuit youth. J Public Health Dent. 1994; 54(3): 132-8.

790 Andersen MVN, Rosenberg T, et al. Prevalence of Age-Related Maculopathy and Age-Related Macular Degeneration among the Inuit in Greenland. The Greenland Inuit Eye Study. Ophthalmology. 2008; 115: 700-707.

791 Rens van GHMB. Ophthalmologic findings among Alaskan Eskimos of the Norton Sound and Bering Straits region. Thesis. Department of Ophthalmology of the Catholic University of Nijmegen, The Netherlands.

792 Gadsby, Patricia and Steele, Leon. "The Inuit Paradox – How can people who gorge on fat and rarely see a vegetable be healthier than we are?" Discover. October, 2004 Issue. Available: *http://discovermagazine.com/2004/oct/inuit-paradox*

793 Ibid.

794 Bjerregaard P, Jeppesen C. Inuit Dietary Patterns In Modern Greenland. Int J Circumpolar Health 2010; 69(1):13-24.

795 Bang HO, Dyerberg J, Nielsen AB, et al. Plasma lipid and lipoprotein pattern in Greenland West-coast Eskimos. Lancet 1971(June);5:1134-1146.

796 Dyerberg J, Ban HO, Hjorne N. Fatty acid composition of the plasma lipids in Greenland Eskimos. Am J Clin Nutr 1975;28:958-66.

797 Dyerberg J, Ban HO, Hjorne N. Plasma cholesterol concentration in Caucasian Danes and Greenland West-coast Eskimos. Dan Med Bull 1977;24:52-5.

798 Dyerberg J, Bang HO, Stoffersen E. Eicosapentaenoic acid and prevention of thrombosis and atherosclerosis. Lancet 1978 (july);15:117-9.

799 Bang HO, Dyerberg J. The lipid metabolism in Greenlanders. Meddelelser om Gronland. Man & Soc. 1981;2:3-18.

800 Bang HO, Dyerberg J, Sinclair HM. The composition of the Eskimo food in northwestern Greenland. Am J Clin Nutr 1980;30:2657-2661.

801 Deutch B, Dyerberg J, Pedersen HS, et al. Dietary composition and contaminants in north Greenland, in the 1970s and 2004. Sci Total Environ 2006;370(2-3):372-81.

802 Ibid.

803 Deutch B, Dyerberg J, Pedersen HS, et al. Traditional and modern Greenlandic food – Dietary composition, nutrients and contaminants. Sci Total Environ 2007;384(1-3):106-119.

804 Deutch B, Pedersen HS, Hansen JC. Increasing Overweight in Greenland: Social, Demographic, Dietary and Other Life-Style Factors. Int J Circumpolar Health 2005;64(1):86-98.

805 Andersen S, Mulvad G, Pedersen HS, Laurberg P. Gender diversity in developing overweight over 35 years of Westernization in an Inuit hunter cohort and ethno-specific body mass index for evaluation of body-weight abnormalities. Eur J Endocrinol 2004;151:735-740.

806 Jonasson F, Thordarson K. Prevalence of Ocular Disease and Blindness in a Rural Area in the Eastern Region of Iceland during 1980 through 1984. Acta Ophthalmol. 1987; 182: 40-43.

807 Ibid.

808 Jonasson F, Arnarsson A, et al. The Prevalence of Age-Related Maculopathy in Iceland. Arch Ophthalmol. 2003; 121: 379-385.

809 FOA Fisheries Statistics 1986: Commodities 63. Rome, Italy: Food and Agriculture Organization of the United Nations; 1988.

810 Jonasson F, Arnarsson A, et al. The Prevalence of Age-Related Maculopathy in Iceland. Arch Ophthalmol. 2003; 121: 379-385.

811 Leske MC. Wu SY, et al. Nine-Year Incidence of Age-Related Macular Degeneration in the Barbados Eye Studies." Ophthalmology. 2006; 113: 29-35.

812 Schachat AP, Hyman L, et al, The Barbados Eye Study Group. Features of Age-Related Macular Degeneration in a Black Population. Arch Ophthalmol. 1995; 113: 728-735.

813 Leske, MC. Wu SY, et al. Nine Year Incidence of Age-Related Macular Degeneration in the Barbados Eye Studies. The Barbados Eye Studies Group. Ophthalmol. 2006; 113: 29-35.

814 "Food production zones coming." *Barbados Today.* August 7, 2013. Available at: *http://www.barbadostoday.bb/2013/08/07/food-production-zones-coming/*

815 Ibid.

816 Sharma S., Cao X. et al. Assessing dietary patterns in Barbados highlights the need for nutritional intervention to reduce risk of chronic disease. J Hum Nutr Diet. 2008; 21(2): 150-158.

817 Ibid.

818 Gaskin PS, Lai P, Guy D, et al. Diet, Physical Activity, Weight Status, and Culture in a Sample of Children from the Developing World. J Nutr Metab 2012; 2012:242875.

819 Foster C, Rotimi C, Fraser H, et al. Hypertension, diabetes, and obesity in Barbados: findings from a recent population-based survey. Ethn Dis 1993; 3(4): 404-12.

820 Gaskin PS, Broome H, Alert C, Fraser H. Misperceptions, inactivity and maternal factors may drive obesity among Barbadian adolescents. Public Health Nutr 2008; 11(1):41-8.

821 Klein R, Klein BEK, Cruickshanks KJ. The Prevalence of Age-Related Maculopathy by Geographic Region and Ethnicity. Progress in Retinal and Eye Research. 1999; 18(3): 371-389.

822 Li Y, Xu L, Jonas JB, Yang H, Ma Y, Li J. Prevalence of age-related maculopathy in the adult population in China: the Beijing eye study. Am J Ophthalmol. 2006; 142(5): 788-93.

823 Li Y, Xu L, Wang YX, et al. Prevalence of Age-Related Maculopathy in the Adult Population in China: The Beijing Eye Study [letter]. Am J Ophthalmol. 2008; 146: 329.

824 Popkin, Barry. "The World Is Fat: New Dynamic Shifts in Patterns of the Nutrition Transition." Lecture at the International Congress of Nutrition, Oct 4-9, 2009, Bangkok, Thailand. Available from: University of North Carolina, Chapel Hill.

825 Wells, Hodan F., and Jean C. Buzby. Dietary Assessment of Major Trends in U.S. Food Consumption, 1970-2005, Economic Information Bulletin No. 33. Economic Research Service, U.S. Dept of Agriculture. March 2008. Available at: *http://www.ers.usda.gov/media/210681/eib33_1_.pdf*

826 Avisar R, Frilling R, et al. Estimation of prevalence and incidence rates and causes of blindness in Israel, 1998-2003. Isr Med Assoc J. 2006; 8(12): 880-1.

827 Mathenge, Wanjiku. "The Nakuru Eye Disease Study." E-mail. October, 2015.

828 Mathenge W, Bastawrous A, et al. Prevalence of Age-Related Macular Degeneration in Nakuru, Kenya: A Cross-Sectional Population-Based Study. PLOS. Feb 19, 2013. DOI: 10.1371/journal.pmed.1001393.

829 "The Kikuyu Tribe." Kenya-Information-Guide.com. 19 Feb, 2013. Available at: *http://www.kenya-information-guide.com/kikuyu-tribe.html*

830 Mathenge W, Bastawrous A, et al. Prevalence of Age-Related Macular Degeneration in Nakuru, Kenya: A Cross-Sectional Population-Based Study. PLOS. Feb 19, 2013. DOI: 10.1371/journal.pmed.1001393.

831 "The Kikuyu Tribe." *Kenya-Information-Guide.com*. 19 Feb, 2013. Available at: *http://www.kenya-information-guide.com/kikuyu-tribe.html*

832 Lowe, L. Nakuru – a study in urbanization. Intermediate Technology Development Group. 2001. Available at: *http://www.ucl.ac.uk/dpu-projects/drivers_urb_change/urb_infrastructure/pdf_appropriate_technology/ITDG_lowe_Nakuru.pdf*

833 Mungati, J.K. "Food Industry In Kenya." Presentation held at the Industrialization Week conference at KICC Nairobi, Nov. 19, 2013. Available online at *Slideshare.net*, Slide #5: *http://www.slideshare.net/KenyaVision2030/food-industry-in-kenya-november-2013*

834 "Vegetable Oil Industry In Kenya 2005." Export Processing Zones Authority. 2005. Available at: *http://www.epzakenya.com/UserFiles/files/kenyaVegetableOil.pdf*

835 Rischke R, Kimenju SC, et al. Supermarkets and food consumption patterns: The case of small towns in Kenya. Food Policy. 2015; 52: 9-21.

836 Yoon KC, Mun GH, et al. Prevalence of eye diseases in South Korea: data from the Korea National Health and Nutrition Examination Survey 2008-2009. Korean J Ophthalmol. 2011; 25(6): 421-433.

837 Cho BJ, Heo JW, et al. Prevalence and Risk Factors of Age-Related Macular Degeneration in Korea: The Korea National Health and Nutrition Examination Survey 2010-2011. Invest Ophthalmol Vis Sci. 2014; 55: 1101-1108.

838 Jenchitr W, Ruamviboonsuk P, et al. Prevalence of age-related macular degeneration in Thailand. Ophthalmic Epidemiol. 2011; 18(1): 48-52.

839 Khotcharrat R, Patikulsila D, et al. Epidemiology of Age-Related Macular Degeneration among the Elderly Population in Thailand. J Med Assoc Thai. 2015; 98(8): 790-7.

840 Bird, Alan C. Age-Related Macular Disease: Aetiology and Clinical Management. Community Eye Health. 1999; 12(29): 8-9.

841 Bird, Alan C. "Age Related Macular Disease." National Academy of Sciences, National Academy of Engineering, and Institute of Medicine. *Distinctive Voices* lecture given at the Beckman Center, Irvine, California. 2014. Published online Feb. 6, 2014. Available at: *https://www.youtube.com/watch?v=6ugISIFyxuA*.

842 Klein R, Klein BEK, Cruickshanks KJ. The Prevalence of Age-Related Maculopathy by Geographic Region and Ethnicity. Progress in Retinal and Eye Research. 1999; 18(3): 371-389.

843 Ichikawa H: The visual functions and aging, Rinsho Ganka. Japanese J Clinic Ophthalmol. 1981: 35: 9-26.

844 Hoshino M, Mizuno K, Ichikawa H. Aging Alterations of Retina and Choroid of Japanese: Light Microscopic Study of Macular Region of 176 Eyes. Japanese J of Ophthalmology. 1984; 28(1): 89-102.

845 Maruo T, Ikebukuro N, et al. Changes in Causes of Visual Handicaps in Tokyo. Jpn J Ophthalmol. 1991; 35: 268-272.

846 Yamada M, Hiratsuka Y, et al. Prevalence of visual impairment in the adult Japanese population by cause and severity and future projections. Ophthalmic Epidemiol. 2010; 17(1): 50-7.

847 Yuzawa M, Tamakoshi A, et al. Report on the nationwide epidemiological survey of exudative age-related macular degeneration in Japan. Int Ophthalmol. 1997; 21(1): 1-3.

848 Ibid.

849 Oshima Y, Ishibashi T, et al. Prevalence of age related maculopathy in a representative Japanese population: the Hisayama study. Br J Ophthalmol. 2001; 85(10): 1153-7.

850 Klein R, Klein BEK, Linton KLP. Prevalence of Age-related Maculopathy. The Beaver Dam Eye Study. Ophthalmology. 1992; 99: 933-43.

851 Miyazaki M, Nakamura H, et al. Risk factors for age related maculopathy in a Japanese population: the Hisayama study. Br J Ophthalmol. 2003; 87(4): 469-72.

852 Miyazaki M, Kiyohara Y, et al. The 5-year incidence and risk factors for age-related maculopathy in a general Japanese population: the Hisayama study. Invest Ophthalmol Vis Sci. 2005; 46(6): 1907-10.

853 Yasuda M, Kiyohara Y, et al. Nine-year incidence and risk factors for age-related macular degeneration in a defined Japanese population the Hisayama study. Ophthalmol. 2009; 116(11): 2135-40.

854 Nakata I, Yamashiro K, et al. Prevalence and characteristics of age-related macular degeneration in the Japanese population: the Nagahama study. Am J Ophthalmol. 2013; 156(5): 1002-1009.

855 Popkin, Barry M. Global nutrition dynamics: the world is shifting rapidly toward a diet linked with noncommunicable diseases. Am J Clin Nutr. 2006; 84(2): 289-298.

856 Ferreira SRG, Lerario DDG, et al. Obesity and Central Adiposity in Japanese Immigrants: Role of the Western Dietary Pattern. J Epidemiol. 2002; 12: 431-438.

857 Ibid.

858 Oguido AP, Casella AM, et al. Prevalence of age-related macular degeneration in Japanese immigrants and their descendents living in Londrina (PR) - Brazil. Arq Bras Oftalmol. 2008; 71(3): 375-80.

859 Medina NH. Epidemiologia do envelhecimento: estudo oftalmologico populacional de idosos [tese]. São Paulo: Universidade Federal de São Paulo; 1997.

860 Stein JD, VanderBeek BL, et al. Rates of Nonexudative and Exudative Age-Related Macular Degeneration among Asian American Ethnic Groups. 2011; 52(9): 6842-6848.

861 "Trading In Agricultural Products - Edible Oil." PEC Ltd. - A Premier Indian International Trading Company. 2004. Available at: *http://www.peclimited.com/agricultural_edibleoil.htm*

862 Jain IS, Prasad P, Gupta A, et al. Senile macular degeneration in Northern India. Indian J Ophthalmol. 1984; 32: 343-6.

863 Dandona L, Dandona R, et al. Blindness in the Indian state of Andhra Pradesh. Invest Ophthalmol Vis Sci. 2001; 42(5): 908-16.

864 Evans J, Wormald R. Is the incidence of registrable age-related macular degeneration increasing? Br J Ophthalm. 1996; 80: 9-14.

865 Krishnaiah S, Das T, et al. Risk factors for age-related macular degeneration: findings from the Andhra Pradesh Eye Disease Study in South India. Invest Ophthalmol Vis Sci. 2005; 46: 4442-4449.

866 Nirmalan PK, Katz J, et al. Prevalence of vitreoretinal disorders in a rural population of southern India: the Aravind Comprehensive Eye Study. Arch Ophthalmol. 2004; 122: 581-586.

867 Gupta SK, Murthy GV, et al. Prevalence of early and late age-related macular degeneration in a rural population in northern India: the INDEYE Feasibility Study. Invest Ophthalmol Vis Sci. 2007; 48: 1007-1011.

868 Nangia V, Jonas JB, et al. Prevalence of age-related macular degeneration in rural central India: the Central India Eye and Medical Study. Retina. 2011; 31(6): 1179-85.

869 Rauf A, Malik R, Bunce C, Wormald R. The British Asian community eye study: outline of results on the prevalence of eye disease in British Asians with origins from the Indian subcontinent. Indian J Ophthalmol. 2013; 61(2): 53-8.

870 Ibid.

871 Mann I, Potter D. Geographic Ophthalmology - A Preliminary Study of the Maoris of New Zealand. Am J Ophthalmol. 1969; 67(3): 358-69.

872 Ibid.

873 Martinez GS, Campbell AJ, et al. Prevalence of Ocular Disease in a Population Study of Subjects 65 Years Old and Older. Am J Ophthalmol. 1982; 94: 181-189.

874 Worsley D, Worsley A. Prevalence predictions for age-related macular degeneration in New Zealand have implications for provision of healthcare services. NZ Med J. 2015; 128(1409): 44-55.

875 Chumbley LC. Impressions of Eye Diseases among Rhodesian Blacks in Mashonaland. S Afr Med J. 1977; 52(8): 316-318.

876 Ibid.

877 Mann, Ida. *Culture, Race, Climate and Eye Disease.* Charles C. Thomas, Springfield, Ill. 1966.

878 Chumbley LC. Impressions of Eye Diseases among Rhodesian Blacks in Mashonaland. S Afr Med J. 1977; 52(8): 316-318.

879 Yitzchak GJ, Mokete M. Survey of Ophthalmic Conditions in Rural Lesotho. Documenta Ophthalmologica. 1980; 49: 285-291.

880 Ibid.

881 Leete M, Damen B, Rossi A. "Lesotho – BEFS Country Brief. BEFS – Bioenergy and Food Security Projects. FAO.org. 2013. Available at: http://www.fao.org/energy/36343-0c514e6a60af9b-94495f8420c451a105b.pdf

882 "Nutrition Country Profile Kingdom of Lesotho – 2010." FAOSTAT. 2010. Avaialbe at: http://www.fao.org/3/a-ap839e.pdf

883 Oluleye TS. Is age-related macular degeneration a problem in Ibadan, Sub-Saharan Africa? Clin Ophthalmol. 2012; 6: 561-564.

884 Adegbehingbe BO, Majengbasan TO. Ocular health status of rural dwellers in south-western Nigeria. Aust J Rural Health. 2007; 15: 269-272.

885 "Onitsha, Nigeria." Encyclopedia Britannica. ND. Available at: http://www.britannica.com/place/Onitsha-Nigeria

886 Nwosu SN. Age-related macular degeneration in Onitsha, Nigeria. Niger J Clin Pract. 2011; 14(3): 327-31.

887 Rural Poverty in Nigeria. Rural Poverty Portal Website: http://www.ruralpovertyportal.org/country/home/tags/nigeria. No published date. Accessed May 4, 2016.

888 Pagliarini S, Moramarco A, Wormald RPL, et al. Age-related Macular Disease in Rural Southern Italy. Arch Ophthalmol. 1997; 115: 616-622.

889 Ibid.

890 Ibid.

891 Ibid.

892 Pagliarini, Sergio. "AMD in Southern Italy." E-mail, Jan 14, 2016.

893 Moramarco, Antonietta. "Questions Regarding Salandra Study, Please!" E-mail, Jan 22, 2016, and Jan 25, 2016.

894 Keeffe, Jill. "Prevalence of AMD in Pacific Islands – Help With Research?" E-mail, Jan 04, 2016.

895 Cama, Ana. ""Prevalence Question Regarding AMD in South Pacific, Please!" E-mail, Jan 29, 2016.

896 Sikivou Biu. "Prevalence Question Regarding AMD in South Pacific, Please!" E-mail, Jan 30, 2016.

897 Rakabu-Hicks, Tarai. "Help With AMD Study, Please!" E-mail, Feb 2, 2016.

898 Ibid. Mar 2, 2016.

899 Mallam, Patricia. "Record Year for Tourism." Tourism Fiji. Feb 20, 2015. Available at: http://www.fiji.travel/us/news/record-year-tourism

900 Ibid.

901 Posala, Claude. "Need Help With AMD Study, Please – Referred by Dr Ana Cama." E-mail, Jan 31, 2016.

902 Ah Ching, Lucilla. "Help With AMD Research, Please! Referred by Dr Ana Cama." E-mail. Jan 31, 2016.

903 Ramke J, Franzco GB, et al. Eye disease and care at hospital clinics in Cook Islands, Fiji, Samoa and Tonga. Clinical and Experimental Ophthalmology. 2007; 35: 627-634.

904 Seiden A, Hawley NL, et al. Long-Term Trends in Food Availability, Food Prices, and Obesity in Samoa. American J Human Biology. 2012; 24: 286-295.

905 "Kiribati." Wikitravel. ND. Available at: http://wikitravel.org/en/Kiribati

906 Tekeraoi, Rabebe. "Help with AMD Study Please! Referred by Dr Ana Cama, in Fiji." E-mail. Jan 31, Feb 4, 2016.

907 Plauche, William and Bossen, Andrew. "AMD Practice Volume Assessment." E-mail. May 19, 2016.

908 Anand, Rajiv. "Quote on AMD Patient Volume." E-mail, May 25, 2016.

909 Keeffe, J, Taylor HR, et al. Prevalence and causes of vision loss in Southeast Asia and Oceania: 1990-2010. Br J Ophthalmol. 2014; 98: 586-591.

910 Ibid.

911 World Health Organization. World Health Statistics 2013. Geneva: World Health Organization, 2013.

912 Keeffe, J, Taylor HR, et al. Prevalence and causes of vision loss in Southeast Asia and Oceania: 1990-2010. Br J Ophthalmol. 2014; 98: 586-591.

913 Teicholz, Nina. "What if Bad Fat is Actually Good for You?" Men's Health. October 10, 2007. Available at: http://www.menshealth.com/health/saturated-fat

914 Ibid.

915 Price, Weston A. Nutrition and Physical Degeneration. 1939, 1945 by Weston A. Price. Lemon Grove, California, The Price-Pottenger Nutrition Foundation, Inc. 1970 – 2008.

916 British Medical Journal. No authors listed. The Masai's cholesterol. 1971; 3(5769): 262-3.

917 Shaper AG, Leonard PJ, et al. Environmental effects on the body build, blood pressure and blood chemistry of nomadic warriors serving in the army of Kenya. East Afr Med J. 1969; 46(5): 282-9.

918 British Medical Journal. No authors listed. The Masai's cholesterol. 1971; 3(5769): 262-3.

919 Fallon, Sally. *Nourishing Traditions.* New Trends Publishing, Inc. Brandywine, MD, 1999, 2001, p. 7.

920 Burr ML. Explaining the French paradox. J R Soc Health. 1995; 115(4): 217-9.

921 López-Miranda V, Soto-Mntenegro ML, et al. Resveratrol: a neuroprotective polyphenol in the Mediterranean diet. Rev Neurol. 2012; 54(6): 349-356.

922 Parodi PW. The French paradox unmasked: the role of folate. Med Hypotheses. 1997; 49(4): 313-8.

923 Petyaev IM, Bashmakov YK. Could cheese be the missing piece in the French paradox puzzle? Med Hypotheses. 2012; 79(6): 746-9.

924 Rozin P, Kabnick K, et al. The ecology of eating: smaller portion sizes in France Than in the United States help explain the French paradox. Psychol Sci. 2003; 14(5): 450-4.

925 Rozin P, Fischler C, et al. Attitudes to food and the role of food in life in the U.S.A., Japan, Flemish Belgiu and France: possible implications for the diet-health debate. Appetite. 1999; 33(2): 163-80.

926 Gadsby, Patricia and Steele, Leon. "The Inuit Paradox." Discover. October, 2004. Available: http://discovermagazine.com/2004/oct/inuit-paradox

927 Guyenet, Stephan. "The Tokelau Island Migrant Study: Background and Overview." WholeHealthSource.org, Jan 4, 2009.

928 Wessen, Albert F. Migration and Health in a Small Society: the Case of Tokelau. Clarenton Press, the University of Michigan, 1992.

929 Guyenet, Stephan. "The Tokelau Island Migrant Study: The Final Word." WholeHealthSource.org, Jan 25, 2009.

930 Ministry of Agriculture, Fisheries and Food, Annual Report of the National Food Survey Committee, London, HMSO, 1966.

931 Department of Health and Social Security, Prevention and Health, p. 63. London, HMSO, 1976.

932 Michaels L. Aetiology of coronary artery disease: an historical approach. British Heart Journal, 1966; 28(2): 258-264.

933 Guyenet, Stephan. "The American Diet: A Historical Perspective." A TEDx Presentation given at Harvard Law, Oct. 21, 2011. Available at: https://www.youtube.com/watch?v=HC20OoIgG_Y

934 Antar MA, Ohlson MA, Hodges RE. Changes in Retail Market Food Supplies in the United States in the Last Seventy Years in Relation to the Incidence of Coronary Heart Disease, With Special Reference to Dietary Carbohydrates and Essential Fatty Acids. Am J Clin Nutr. 1964; 14: 169-78.

935 Ibid.

936 Minger, Denise. *Death by Food Pyramid.* Primal Blueprint Publishing, Malibu, CA, 2013, p.89.

937 Taubes, Gary. *Why We Get Fat.* Alfred A. Knopf, New York, 2011, p. 25.

938 Keys A. Atherosclerosis: a problem in newer public health. J Mt Sinai Hosp N Y. 1953; 20(2): 118-39.

939 Yerushalmy J, Hilleboe HE. Fat in the diet and mortality from heart disease; a methodological note. N Y State Med. 1957; 57: 2343-2354.

940 Keys A. Coronary heart disease in seven countries. Circulation. 1970; 41(suppl 1): 1-211.

941 Brody, Jane. Jane Brody's Nutrition Book. W.W. Norton & Company, New York, pp. 9-11.

942 Siri-Tarino PW, Sun Q, et al. Meta-analysis of prospective cohort studies evaluating the association of saturated fat with cardiovascular disease. Am J Clin Nutr. 2010; 91(3): 535-46.

943 Micha, R, Mozaffarian D. Saturated fat and cardiometabolic risk factors, coronary heart disease, stroke, and diabetes: a fresh look at the evidence. Lipids. 2010 Oct: 45(10): 893-905.

944 Masterjohn, Christopher. "Understanding the Essential Fatty Acids." The Weston A. Price Foundation. Sep 22, 2010. Available at: *http://www.westonaprice.org/know-your-fats/precious-yet-perilous/*

945 Ibid.

946 Mares-Perlman JA, Brady WE, et al. Dietary fat and age-related maculopathy. Arch Ophthalmol. 1995; 113(6): 743-8.

947 Seddon JM, Cote J, Rosner B. Progression of Age-Related Macular Degeneration Associated With Dietary Fat, Transunsaturated Fat, Nuts, and Fish Intake. Arch Ophthalmol. 2003; 121(12): 1728-1737.

948 Piermarocchi S, Segato T, et al. The PAMDI Study Group. The Prevalence of Age-Related Macular Degeneration in Italy (PAMDI) Study: Report 1. Ophthalmic Epidemiology. 2011; 18(3): 129-136.

949 Drewnowski A. Sensory Properties of Fats and Fat Replacements. Nutrition Reviews. 1992; 50(4): 17-20.

950 Kramsch DM, Franzblau C, Hollander W. The Protein and Lipid Composition of Arterial Elastin and Its Relationship to Lipid Accumulation in the Atherosclerotic Plaque. J Clin Invest. 1971; 50(8): 1666-1677.

951 Gown AM, Tsukada T, Ross R. Human atherosclerosis. II. Immunocytochemical analysis of the cellular composition of human atherosclerotic lesions. Am J Pathol. 1986; 125(1): 191-207.

952 Fitzpatrick LA, Severson A, et al. Diffuse calcification in human coronary arteries. Association of osteopontin with atherosclerosis. J Clin Invest. 1994; 94(4): 1597-1604.

953 Pletcher MJ, Tice JA, et al. Using the Coronary Artery Calcium Score to Predict Coronary Heart Disease Events. Arch Intern Med. 2004; 164(12): 1285-1292.

954 Ravnskov, Uffe. Ignore the Awkward! How the Cholesterol Myths are Kept Alive. 2010. ISBN 1453759409, p. 19.

955 Ravnskov, Uffe. Ignore the Awkward! How the Cholesterol Myths are Kept Alive. 2010. ISBN 1453759409, p. 35.

956 Sachdeva A, Cannon C, Deedwania P, LaBresh K, Smith S, Dai D, Hernandez A, Fonarow G. Lipid levels in patients hospitalized with coronary artery disease: An analysis of 136,905 hospitalizations in Get With The Guidelines. American Heart Journal. Jan 2009. 157(1): 111-17.

957 Jacobs D, Blackburn H, Higgins M, Reed D, Iso H, McMillan G, Neaton J, Nelson J, Potter J, and Rifkind B. Report of the Conference on Low Blood Cholesterol: Mortality Associations. Circulation 1992; 86: 1046-1060.

958 Ravnskov, Uffe. Ignore the Awkward! How the Cholesterol Myths are Kept Alive. 2010. ISBN 1453759409, p. xi.

959 Komachi Y, Iida M, Shimamoto T, Chikayama Y, Takahashi H, Konishi M, Tominaga S. Geographic and occupational comparisons of risk factors in cardiovascular diseases in Japan. Jpn Circ J 1971; 35: 189-207.

960 Komachi Y, Iida M, Ozawa H, Shimamoto T, Ueshima, Tanigaki M, Tsujioka K. Risk factors of stroke (in Japanese). Saishin Igaku 1977; 32: 2264-2269.

961 Ueshima H, Iida M, Shimamoto T, Konishi M, Tsujioka K, Tanigaki M, Nakanishi N, Ozawa H, Kojima S, Komachi Y. Multivariate analysis of risk factors for stroke: Eight-year followup study of farming villages in Akita, Japan. Prev Med 1980; 9:722-740.

962 Tanaka H, Ueda Y, Hayashi M, Date C, Baba T, Yamshita H, Shoji H, Tanaka Y, Owada K, Detels R. Risk factors for cerebral hemorrhage and cerebral infarction in a Japanese rural community. Stroke 1982; 13: 62-73.

963 Konishi M, Komachi Y, Iso H, Iida M, Naito Y, Sato S, Kiyama M, Shimamoto T, Kitamura A, Doi M, Ito M. Secular trends in atherosclerosis of the coronary arteries and basal cerebral arteries in Japan. The Akita Pathology Study. Arteriosclerosis 1990; 10: 535-540.

964 Yano K, Reed DM, Maclean CJ. Serum cholesterol and hemorrhagic stroke in the Honolulu Heart Program. Stroke 1989; 20:1460-1465.

965 Kagan A, Popper JS, Rhoads GG, Yano K. Factors related to stroke incidence in Hawaii Japanese men. The Honolulu Heart Study. Stroke 1980; 11: 14-21.

966 Iso H, Jacobs DR, Wentworth D, Neaton JD, Cohen. Serum cholesterol levels and six-year mortality from stroke in 350,977 men screened for the Multiple Risk Factor Intervention Trial. N Engl J Med 1989; 320: 904-910.

967 Authors not listed. Cholesterol, diastolic blood pressure, and stroke: 13,000 strokes in 450,000 people in 45 prospective cohorts. Prospective studies collaboration. Lancet 1995 Dec 23-30; 346(8991-8992): 1647-53.

968 Ravnskov, Uffe. Ignore the Awkward! How the Cholesterol Myths are Kept Alive. 2010. ISBN 1453759409, p. 37.

969 Ravnskov, Uffe. Ignore the Awkward! How the Cholesterol Myths are Kept Alive. 2010. ISBN 1453759409, p. 20,

970 Mann GV, Shaffer RD, Anderson RS, Sandstead HH. Cardiovascular disease in the masai. Journal of Atherosclerosis Research. July 8, 1964, 4(4): 289-312.

971 Ravnskov U. The questionable role of saturated and polyunsaturated fatty acids in cardiovascular disease. J Clin Epidemiol. 1998 Jun; 51(6): 443-60.

972 Ravnskov, Uffe. Ignore the Awkward! How the Cholesterol Myths are Kept Alive. 2010. ISBN 1453759409, p. 30.

973 Neil HAW, Hawkins MM, Durrington PN, Betteridge DJ, Capps NE, Humphries SE. Non-coronary heart disease mortality and risk of fatal cancer in patients with treated heterozygous familial hypercholesterolemia: a prospective registry study. Atherosclerosis. April 2005, 179(2): 293-297.

974 Ravnskov, Uffe. Is atherosclerosis caused by high cholesterol? QJ Med. 2002; 95: 397-403.

975 Bruschke AVG, Kramer JR Jr, et al. The dynamics of progression of coronary atherosclerosis studied in 168 medically treated patients who underwent coronary arteriography three times. Am Heart J. 1989; 117: 296-305.

976 Bisset JK, Wyeth RP, et al. Plasma lipid concentrations and subsequent coronary occlusion after a first myocardial infarction. The POSCH group. Am J Med Sci. 1993; 305: 139-44.

977 Bemis CE, Gorlin R, et al. Progression of coronary artery disease: a clinical arteriographic study. Circulation. 1973: 47: 455-64.

978 Shub C, Vlietstra RE, et al. The unpredictable progression of symptomatic coronary artery disease: a serial clinical-angiographic analysis. May Clin Proc. 1981; 56: 155-60.

979 Krauss RM, Lindgren FT, et al. Intermediate-density lipoproteins and progression of coronary artery disease in hypercholesterolaemic men. Lancet. 1987; 2: 62-66.

980 Masterjohn, Chris. Foods High in Cholesterol Could Save Your Health! *Cholesterol-and-health.com*. Available at: http://www.cholesterol-and-health.com/Foods-High-In-Cholesterol.html#1

981 Fernandez ML. Dietary cholesterol provided by eggs and plasma lipoproteins in healthy populations. Curr Opin Clin Nutr Metab Care. 2006; 9(1): 8-12.

982 Taylor F, Huffman MD, Macedo A, Moore THM, Burke M, Davey Smith G, Ward K, Ebrahim S. Statins for the primary prevention of cardiovascular disease. Published online: Cochrane Summaries. Jan 20, 2014. Available at: *http://summaries.cochrane.org/CD004816/statins-for-the-primary-prevention-of-cardiovascular-disease*

983 Ray KK, Cannon CP. The Potential Relevance of the Multiple Lipid-Independent (Pleiotropic) Effects of Statins in the Management of Acute Coronary Syndromes. Journal of the American College of Cardiology. 2005, 46(8): 1425-33.

984 Cassels A. Eminence vs. evidence. Posted to *Cochrane.org* on 2012, Nov 30. Available at: *http://www.cochrane.org/news/blog/eminence-vs-evidence*

985 Lerche Davis, Jeanie. Baycol Removed From Market – Cholesterol Drug Linked to 31 Deaths. WebMD Health News. August, 2001. Available at: *http://www.webmd.com/cholesterol-management/news/20050322/baycol-removed-from-market*

986 Sultan S, Hynes N. The Ugly Side of Statins. Systemic Appraisal of the Contemporary Unkown Unknowns. Open Journal of Endocrine and Metabolic Diseases. 2013 Vol. 3, No. 3. Article ID: 34065, 7 pages.

987 Muldoon MF, Ryan CM, Sereika SM, Flory JD, Manuck SB. Randomized trial of the effects of simvastatin on cognitive functioning in hypercholesterolemic adults. Am J Med. 2004 Dec 1; 117(11): 823-9.

988 Muldoon MF, Barger SD, Ryan CM, Flory JD, Lehoczky JP< Matthews KA, Manuck SB. Effects of lovastatin on cognitive function and psychological well-being. Am J Med. 2000 May; 108(7): 538-46.

989 Bang CN, Okin PM. Statin treatment, new-onset diabetes, and other adverse effects: a systematic review. Curr Cardiol Rep. 2014; 16(3): 461.

990 Ibid.

991 Klinefelter GR, Laskey JW, Amann RP. Statin drugs markedly inhibit testosterone production by rat Leydig cells in vitro: Implications for men. Reprod Toxicol. 2014 Jan 22; 45C: 52-58.

992 Lipitor (Atorvastatin calcium). Pfizer. Available at: *http://www.lipitor.com/aboutlipitor.aspx*

993 Stout, Hilary. Viagra: The Thrill That Was. The New York Times. June 3, 2011. Available at: *http://www.nytimes.com/2011/06/05/fashion/viagra-the-thrill-that-was-cultural-studies.html?pagewanted=all&_r=0*

994 Fernandez AB, Karas RH, Alsheikh-Ali AA, Thompson PD. Statins and Interstitial Lung Disease. A Systematic Review of the Literature and of Food and Drug Administration Adverse Event Reports. Chest. 2008; 134(4): 824-830.

995 Huang X, Chen H, Miller WC, Mailman RB, Woodard JL, Chen PC, Xiang D, Murrow RW, Wang Y, Poole C. Lower Low-Density Lipoprotein Cholesterol Levels Are Associated With Parkinson's Disease. Movement Disorders. 2007; 22(3): 377-381.

996 Nakazato R, Gransar H, Berman DS, et al. Statins Use and Coronary Artery Plaque Composition: Results from the International Multicenter Confirm Registry. Atherosclerosis. 2012; 225(1): 148-53.

997 Raggi P, Davidson M, Callister TQ, et al. Aggressive versus Moderate Lipid-Lowering Therapy in Hypercholesterolemic Postmenopausal Women: Beyond Endorsed Lipid Lowering with EBT Scanning (BELLES). Circulation. 2005; Vol. 112, 563-571.

998 Schmermund A, Achenback S, Budde T, et al. Effect of Intensive versus Standard Lipid-Lowering Treatment with Atorvastatin on the Progression of Calcified Coronary Atherosclerosis over 12 Months: A Multicenter, Randomized, Double-Blind Trial. Circulation. 2006; Vol. 113, 427-437.

999 Bang CN, Okin PM. Statin treatment, new-onset diabetes, and other adverse effects: a systematic review. Curr Cardiol Rep. 2014 Mar; 16(3): 461.

1000 Statin Adverse Effects. University of California – San Diego online, available at: *https://www.statineffects.com/info/*

1001 Kaiserman N, Vinker S, Kaiserman I. Statins do not decrease the risk for wet age-related macular degeneration. Curr Eye Res. 2009; 34(4): 304-10.

1002 Masterjohn, Chris. "On the Trail of the Elusive X-Factor: A Sixty-Two Year-Old Mystery Finally Solved." The Weston A. Price Foundation." Feb 14, 2008. Available at: *http://www.westonaprice.org/health-topics/abcs-of-nutrition/on-the-trail-of-the-elusive-x-factor-a-sixty-two-year-old-mystery-finally-solved/*

1003 "Vitamin D In-Depth Report." The New York Times. ND. Available at: *http://www.nytimes.com/health/guides/nutrition/vitamin-d/print.html*

1004 Fulgoni VL, Keast DR, et al. Foods, Fortificants, and Supplements: Where Do Americans Get Their Nutrients? J Nutr. 2011; 141: 1847-1854.

1005 Ibid.

1006 Food and Nutrition Board. Recommended Dietary Allowances: 10th Edition. 1989. Available at: *http://www.nap.edu/catalog/1349.html*

1007 Moshfegh, Alanna; Goldman, Joseph; and Cleveland, Linda. 2005. *What We Eat in America*, NHANES 2001-2002: Usual Nutrient Intakes from Food Compared to Dietary Reference Intakes. U.S.D.A., Agricultural Research Service. Available at: *http://www.ars.usda.gov/SP2UserFiles/Place/80400530/pdf/0102/usualintaketables2001-02.pdf*

1008 Age-Related Eye Disease Study Research Group. The Relationship of Dietary Carotenoid and Vitamin A, E, and C Intake With Age-Related Macular Degeneration in a Case-Control Study. AREDS Report No. 22. Arch Ophthalmol. 2007; 125(9): 1225-1232.

1009 Seddon JM, Ajani UA, et al. Dietary carotenoids, vitamins A, C, and E, and advanced age-related macular degeneration. JAMA. 1994; 272(18): 1413-20.

1010 Snellen EL, Verbeek AL, et al. Neovascular age-related macular degeneration and its relationship to antioxidant intake. Acta Ophthalmol Scand. 2002; 80(4): 368-371.

1011 Snodderly DM, Brown PK, et al. The macular pigment. I. Absorbance spectra, localization, and discrimination from other yellow pigments in primate retinas. Invest Ophthalmol Vis Sci. 1984: 25: 660-673.

1012 Khachik F, Beecher GR, et al. Separation and identification of carotenoids and their oxidation products in the extracts of human plasma. Anal Chem. 1992; 64: 2111-2122.

1013 Sabour-Pickett S, Nolan JM, et al. A review of the evidence germane to the putative protective role of the macular carotenoids for age-related macular degeneration. Mol Nutr Food Res. 2012; 56(2): 270-87.

1014 Landrum JT, Bone RA. Lutein, zeaxanthin, and the macular pigment. Arch Biochem Biophys. 2001; 385(1): 28-40.

1015 Nolan JM, Stack J, et al. Risk factors for age-related maculopathy are associated with a relative lack of macular pigment. Exp Eye Res. 2007; 84(1): 61-74.

1016 Kirby ML, Beatty S, et al. A Central Dip in the Macular Pigment Spatial Profile Is Associated with Age and Smoking. Invest Ophthalmol Vis Sci. 2010; 51: 6722-6728.

1017 Sabour-Pickett S, Nolan JM, et al. A review of the evidence germane to the putative protective role of the macular carotenoids for age-related macular degeneration. Mol Nutr Food Res. 2012; 56: 270-286.

1018 Müller H. {Daily intake of carotenoids (carotenes and xanthophylls) from total diet and the carotenoid content of selected vegetables and fruit}. Article in German. Z Ernahrungswiss. 1996; 35(1): 45-50.

1019 Sommerburg O, Keunen JE, Bird AC, van Kuijk FJ. Fruits and vegetables that are sources for lutein and zeaxanthin: the macular pigment in human eyes. Br J Ophthalmol. 1998; 82(8): 907-10.

1020 Gunnars, Kris. "Pastured vs Omega-3 vs Conventional Eggs – What's The Difference?" Authority Nutrition. January, 2016. Available at: *http://authoritynutrition.com/pastured-vs-omega-3-vs-conventional-eggs/*

1021 Spronk HM, Soute BA, et al. Tissue-specific utilization of menaquinone-4 results in the prevention of arterial calcification in warfarin-treated rats. J Vasc Res. 2003; 40(6): 531-7.

1022 Shea MK, Holden RM. Vitamin K Status and Vascular Calcification: Evidence from Observational and Clinical Studies. Adv. Nutr. 2012; 3:158-165.

1023 Age-Related Eye Disease Study Research Group. The Relationship of Dietary Carotenoid and Vitamin A, E, and C Intake With Age-Related Macular Degeneration in a Case-Control Study. AREDS Report No. 22. Arch Ophthalmol. 2007; 125(9): 1225-1232.

1024 Price, Weston A. *Nutrition and Physical Degeneration.* The Price-Pottenger Nutrition Foundation. Lemon Grove, CA, USA, 1939, p. xvi.

1025 Millen AE, Meyers KJ, et al. Association Between Vitamin D Status and Age-Related Macular Degeneration by Genetic Risk. JAMA Ophthalmol. 2015: 133(10): 1171-79.

1026 Ibid.

1027 Alsalem JA, Patel D, et al. Characterization of vitamin D production by human ocular barrier cells. Invest Ophthalmol Vis Sci. 2014; 55(4): 2140-47.

1028 Parekh N, Chappell RJ, et al. Association between vitamin D and age-related macular degeneration in the Third National Health and Nutrition Examination Survey. 1988 through 1994. Arch Ophthalmol. 2007; 125(5): 661-69.

1029 Millen AE, Voland R, et al. CAREDS Study Group. Vitamin D status and early age-related macular degeneration in postmenopausal women. Arch Ophthalmol. 2011; 129(4): 481-489.

1030 Graffe A, Milea D, et al. Association between hypovitaminosis D and late stages of age-related macular degeneration: a case-control study. J Am Geriatr Soc. 2012; 60(7): 1367-1369.

1031 Kim EC, Han K, Jee D. Inverse relationship between high blood 25-hydroxyvitamin D and late stage of age-related macular degeneration in a representative Korean population. Invest Ophthalmol Vis Sci. 2014; 55(8): 4823-31.

1032 Lee V, Rekhi E, et al. Vitamin D rejuvenates aging eyes by reducing inflammation, clearing amyloid beta and improving vision. Neurobiology of Aging. 2012; 33(10): 2382-2389.

1033 Ibid.

1034 Lipner, Maxine. "On the AMD plate – Eyeing vitamin D levels in connection with disease development." EyeWorld. March 2016; 21(3): 114-117.

1035 Calvo MS, Babu US, et al. Vitamin D2 from light-exposed edible mushrooms is safe, bioavailable and effectively supports bone growth in rats. Osteoporos Int. 2013; 24: 197-207.

1036 Jäpelt RB, Jakobsen J. Vitamin D in plants: a review of occurrence, analysis, and biosynthesis. Front Plant Sci. 2013; 4:136

1037 Fallon, Sally. "Cod Liver Oil Basics and Recommendations." *WestonAPrice.org*. Nov 23 2015. Available at: *http://www.westonaprice.org/health-topics/cod-liver-oil-basics-and-recommendations/*

1038 Price, Weston A. *Nutrition and Physical Degeneration.* The Price-Pottenger Nutrition Foundation, Inc. Lemon Grove, CA, USA. 1939, pp. 367-8.

1039 Jäpelt RB, Jakobsen J. Vitamin D in plants: a review of occurrence, analysis, and biosynthesis. Front Plant Sci. 2013; 4:136

1040 Dietary Reference Intakes (DRIs): Estimated Average Requirements. Food and Nutrition Board, Institute of Medicine, National Academies. 2001. Available at: *https://iom.nationalacademies.org/~/media/Files/Activity%20Files/Nutrition/DRIs/5_Summary%20Table%20Tables%201-4.pdf*

1041 Robert Forbes & Associates Pty Ltd. RFA Vitamin Conversion Chart. 2008. Available at: *http://www.robert-forbes.com/images/pdfs/vitamin_conversion.pdf*

1042 Fairfield KM, Fletcher RH. Vitamins for Chronic Disease Prevention in Adults. JAMA. 2002; 287(23): 3116-3126.

1043 Masterjohn, Chris. "Vitamin A: The Forgotten Bodybuilding Nutrient." The Weston A. Price Foundation. Dec 14, 2004. Available at: *http://www.westonaprice.org/health-topics/vitamin-a-the-forgotten-bodybuilding-nutrient/*

1044 Geubel AP, De Galocsy C, et al. Liver damage caused by therapeutic vitamin A administration: estimate of dose-related toxicity in 41 cases. Gastroenterology. 1991; 100(6): 1701-9.

1045 Ibid.

1046 Price, Catherine. *Vitamania.* Penguin Press, New York, NY, p. 102.

1047 Ibid.

1048 Price, Catherine. *Vitamania.* Penguin Press, New York, NY. Pp. 102-3.

1049 Ibid, p. 103.

1050 Dietary Reference Intakes (DRIs): Estimated Average Requirements. Food and Nutrition Board, Institute of Medicine, National Academies. 2001. Available at: *https://iom.nationalacademies.org/~/media/Files/Activity%20Files/Nutrition/DRIs/5_Summary%20Table%20Tables%201-4.pdf*

1051 Sharma S, Sheehy T, and Kolonel L. Sources of vegetables, fruits and vitamins A, C and E among five ethnic groups: Results from a multiethnic cohort study. Eur J Clin Nutr. 2014; 68: 384-391.

1052 Fallon, Sally. "Vitamin A Saga." The Weston A. Price Foundation. Mar 30, 2002. Available at: *http://www.westonaprice.org/health-topics/abcs-of-nutrition/vitamin-a-saga/*

1053 Ibid.

1054 Gomboeva SB, Shumaev KB, et al. The Mechanism of Oxidation of β-Carotene and Polyunsaturated Fatty Acids. Doklady Biochemistry and Biophysics. 2001; 377: 98-101.

1055 Dietary Assessment of Major Trends in U.S. Food Consumption, 1970 – 2005. USDA Economic Research Service. Bulletin Number 33, March 2008.

1056 Owsley C, Jackson GR, White M, Feist R, Edwards D. Delays in rod-mediated dark adaptation in early age-related maculopathy. Ophthalmology. 2001; 108(7): 1196-1202.

1057 Owsley C, McGwin G Jr, et al. Delayed Rod-Mediated Dark Adaptation is a Functional Biomarker for Incident Early Age-Related Macular Degeneration. Ophthalmology. 2016; 123(2): 344-51.

1058 Ibid.

1059 Haskell MJ, Handelman GJ, et al. Assessment of vitamin A status by the deuterated-retinol-dilution technique and comparison with hepatic vitamin A concentration in Bangladeshi surgical patients. Am J Clin Nutr. 1997; 66(1): 67-74.

1060 Tanumihardjo SA. Assessing Vitamin A Status: Past, Present and Future. J Nutr. 2004;134(1): 290S-293S.

1061 Dogru M, Tsubota K. Pharmacotherapy of dry eye. Expert Opin Pharmacother. 2011; 12(3): 325-34.

1062 Schilling H, Koch JM, et al. [Treatment of the dry eye with vitamin A acid—an impression cytology controlled study]. Fortschr Ophthalmol. 1989; 86(5): 530-4.

1063 Faustino, JF, Ribeiro-Silva A, et al. Vitamin A and the eye: an old tale for modern times. Arquivos Brasileiros de Oftalmologia. 2016; 79(1): 56-61.

1064 Cui X, Xiang J, et al. Vitamin A Palmitate and Carbomer Gel Protects the Conjunctiva of Patients With Long-term Prostaglandin Analogs Application. J Glaucoma. 2015 Aug 27 [Epub ahead of print]

1065 Kojima T, Higuchi A, et al. Autologous serum eye drops for the treatment of dry eye diseases. Cornea. 2008; Suppl 1: S25-30.

1066 Kim EC, Choi JS, Joo CK. A comparison of vitamin A and cyclosporine a 0.05% eye drops for treatment of dry eye syndrome. Am J Ophthalmol. 2009; 147(2): 206-213.

1067 Dorey CK, Wu G, et al. Cell loss in the aging retina. Relationship to lipofuscin accumulation and macular degeneration. Invest Ophthalmol Vis Sci. 1989; 30:1691-99.

1068 Mata N, Lichter JB, et al. Investigation of Oral Fenretinide For Treatment of Geographic Atrophy in Age-Related Macular Degeneration. Retina. 2013; 33(3): 498-507.

1069 Quadro L, Blaner WS, et al. The role of extrahepatic retinol binding protein in the mobilization of retinoid stores. J Lipid Res. 2004; 45: 1975-1982.

1070 Formelli F, Clerici M, et al. Five-year administration of fenretinide: pharmocokinetics and effects on plasma retinol concentrations. J Clin Oncol. 1993; 11: 2036-2042.

1071 Mata N, Lichter JB, et al. Investigation of Oral Fenretinide For Treatment of Geographic Atrophy in Age-Related Macular Degeneration. Retina. 2013; 33(3): 498-507.

1072 Ibid.

1073 Van Duyn MA, Pivonka E. Overview of the health benefits of fruit and vegetable consumption for th dietetics professional: selected literature. J Am Diet Assoc. 2000; 100: 1511-1521.

1074 Sharma S, Sheehy T, Kolonel L. Sources of vegetables, fruits and vitamins A, C and E among five ethnic groups: Results from a multiethnic cohort study. Eur J Clin Nutr. 2014; 68: 384-391.

1075 Genkinger JM, Plats EA, et al. Fruit, vegetable, and antioxidant intake and all-cause, cancer, and cardiovascular disease mortality in a community-dwelling population in Washington County, Maryland. Am J Epidemiol. 2004; 160(12): 1223-33.

1076 Dauchet L, Ferrieres J, et al. Frequency of fruit and vegetable consumption and coronary heart disease in France and Northern Ireland: the PRIME study. Br J Nutr. 2004; 92: 963-972.

1077 Dauchet L, Amouyel P, et al. Fruit and vegetable consumption and risk of coronary heart disease: a meta-analysis of cohort studies. J Nutr. 2006; 136: 2588-2593.

1078 He FJ, Nowson CA, et al. Fruit and vegetable consumption and stroke: meta-analysis of cohort studies. Lancet. 2006; 367: 320-326.

1079 Denmark-Wahnefried W, Rock CL, et al. Lifestyle interventions to reduce cancer risk and improve outcomes. Am Fam Physician. 2008; 77: 1573-1578.

1080 Anand P, Kunnumakkara AB, et al. Cancer is a preventable disease that requires major lifestyle changes. Pharm Res. 2008; 25: 2097-2116.

1081 Galimanis A, Mono ML, et al. Lifestyle and stroke risk: a review. Curr Opin Neurol. 2009; 22: 60-68.

1082 Nagura J, Iso H, et al. Fruit, vegetable and bean intake and mortality from cardiovascular disease among Japanese men and women: the JACC Study. Br J Nutr. 2009; 102: 285-292.

1083 Lane JS, Magno CP, et al. Nutrition impacts the prevalence of peripheral arterial disease in the United States. J Vasc Surg. 2008; 48: 897-904.

1084 Roy JN. The Eyesight of the Negroes of Africa. Can Med Assoc J. 1919; 9(2): 144-54.

1085 Ibid.

1086 Ibid.

1087 Wolchover, Natalie. "What If Humans Had Eagle Vison?" LiveScience. Feb 24, 2012. Available at: *http://www.livescience.com/18658-humans-eagle-vision.html*

1088 Roy JN. The Eyesight of the Negroes of Africa. Can Med Assoc J. 1919; 9(2): 144-54.

1089 Ibid.

1090 Price, Weston A. *Nutrition and Physical Degeneration.* The Price-Pottenger Nutrition Foundation. Lemon Grove, CA, USA, 1939, p. xvi.

1091 DiNicolantonio JJ, Bhutani J, O'Keefe, JH. The health benefits of vitamin K. Open Heart. 2015; Oct 6; 2(1): e000300.

1092 Ibid.

1093 Cockayne S, Adamson J, et al. Vitamin K and the prevention of fractures: systematic review and meta-analysis of randomized controlled trials. Arch Intern Med. 2006; 166: 1256-61.

1094 Spronk HMH, Soute BAM, et al. Tissue-Specific Utilization of Menaquinone-4 Results in the Prevention of Arterial Calcification in Warfarin-Treated Rats. J Vasc Res. 2003; 40: 531-537.

1095 Theuwissen E, Smit E, Cees V. The Role of Vitamin K in Soft-Tissue Calcification. Adv. Nutr. 2012; 3: 166-173.

1096 Geleijnse JM, Vermeer C, et al. Dietary Intake of Menaquinone Is Associated with a Reduced Risk of Coronary Heart Disease: The Rotterdam Study. J Nutr. 2004; 134(11): 3100-3105.

1097 Theuwissen E, Smit E, Cees V. The Role of Vitamin K in Soft-Tissue Calcification. Adv. Nutr. 2012; 3: 166-173.

1098 Bolland MJ, Grey A, et al. Calcium supplements with or without vitamin D and risk of cardiovascular events: reanalysis of the

Women's Health Initiative limited acess dataset and meta-analysis. The British Medical Journal. 2011; 342

1099 Ibid.

1100 Spraul CW, Lang GE, et al. [Characteristics of drusen and changes in Bruch's membrane in eyes with age-related macular degeneration. Histological study]. Ophthalmologe. 1998; 95(2): 73-9.

1101 Biswas J, Raman R. Age-related changes in the macula. A histopathological study of fifty Indian donor eyes. Indian J Ophthalmol. 2002; 50(3): 201-4.

1102 Booji JC, Baas DC, et al. The dynamic nature of Bruch's membrane. Prog Retin Res. 2010; 29(1): 1-18.

1103 Spraul CW, Grossniklaus HE. Characteristics of Drusen and Bruch's Membrane in Postmortem Eyes With Age-Related Macular Degeneration. Arch Ophthalmol. 1997; 115: 267-73.

1104 Spraul CW, Lang GE, et al. Histologic and Morphometric Analysis of the Choroid, Bruch's Membrane, and Retinal Pigment Epithelium in Postmortem Eyes With Age-Related Macular Degeneration and Histologic Examination of Surgically Excised Choroidal Neovascular Membranes. Surv of Ophthalmol. 1999; 44 (Suppl 1): S10-S32.

1105 Davis WL, Jones RG, Hagler HK. An electron microscopic histochemical and analytical X-ray microprobe study of calcification in Bruch's membrane from human eyes. J Histochem Cytochem. 1981; 29(5): 601-8.

1106 van der Schaft TL, Moov CM et al. Histologic features of the early stages of age-related macular degeneration. A statistical analysis. Ophthalmology. 1992; 99(2): 278-86.

1107 Moore, DJ, Hussain AA, Marshall J. Age-Related Variations in the Hydraulic Conductivity of Bruch's Membrane. Invest Ophthalmol Vis Sci. 1995: 36: 1290-1297.

1108 Feeney-Burns L, Ellersieck M. Age-related changes in the ultrastructure of Bruch's membrane. Am J Ophthalmol. 1985; 100: 686-97.

1109 Hogan MJ. Role of the RPE in macular disease. Am Acad Ophthalmol. 1972; 76: 64-80.

1110 Ishibashi T, Sorgente N, et al. Aging changes in Bruch's membrane of monkeys: An electron microscopic study. Ophthalmologica. 1986; 192: 179-90.

1111 Jonczyk-Skorka K, et al. [Does acetylsalicylic acid and vitamin K antagonists are risk factors of macular degeneration related with age?] Pol Merkur Lekarski. 2015; 38(225): 144-9.

1112 Sivaprasad S, Bailey TA, Chong VN. Bruch's membrane and the vascular intima: is there a common basis for age-related changes and disease? Clin Experiment Ophthalmol. 2005; 33(5): 518-23.

1113 Donoso LA, Kim D, et al. The Role of Inflammation in the Pathogenesis of Age-related Macular Degeneration. Survey of Ophthalmology. 2006; 51(2): 137-152.

1114 Grunwald JE, Hariprasad SM, DuPont J, et al. Foveolar choroidal blood flow in age-related macular degeneration. Invest Ophthalmol Vis Sci. 1998: 39(2): 385-390.

1115 Theuwissen E, Smit E, Cees V. The Role of Vitamin K in Soft-Tissue Calcification. Adv. Nutr. 2012; 3: 166-173.

1116 Schurgers LJ, Cranenburg EC, Vermeer C. Matrix Gla-protein: the calcification inhibitor in need of vitamin K. Thromb Haemost. 2008; 100(4): 593-603.

1117 Shanahan CM, Proudfoot D, et al. The role of Gla proteins in vascular calcification. Crit Rev Eykaryot Gene Expr. 1998; 8(3-4): 357-75.

1118 Theuwissen E, Smit E, Cees V. The Role of Vitamin K in Soft-Tissue Calcification. Adv. Nutr. 2012; 3: 166-173.

1119 Schurgers LJ, Cranenburg EC, Vermeer C. Matrix Gla-protein: the calcification inhibitor in need of vitamin K. Thromb Haemost. 2008; 100(4): 593-603.

1120 Trost A, Schroedl F, et al. Neural crest origin of retinal and choroidal pericytes. Invest Ophthalmol Vis Sci. 2013; 54(13): 7910-21.

1121 Shanahan CM, Proudfoot D, et al. The role of Gla proteins in vascular calcification. Crit Rev Eykaryot Gene Expr. 1998; 8(3-4): 357-75.

1122 Proudfoot D, Shanahan CM. Molecular mechanisms mediating fascular calcification: role of matrix Gla protein. Nephrology (Carlton). 2006; 11(55): 455-61.

1123 Ravnskov U. Is atherosclerosis caused by high cholesterol? QJ Med. 2002; 95: 397-403.

1124 Masterjohn, Chris. "On the Trail of the Elusive X-Factor: A Sixty-Two-Year-Old Mystery Finally Solved." The Weston A. Price Foundation. Feb 14, 2008. Available at: *http://www.westonaprice.org/health-topics/abcs-of-nutrition/on-the-trail-of-the-elusive-x-factor-a-sixty-two-year-old-mystery-finally-solved/#article*

1125 Duke-Elder, WS. *Textbook of Ophthalmology – Duke-Elder, Vol. III, Diseases of the Inner Eye*. St. Louis: The C.V. Mosby Company, 1940, p. 2373.

1126 Klein R, Knudtson MD, Klein BE, et al. Inflammation, complement factor h, and age-related macular degeneration: the Multi-ethnic Study of Atherosclerosis. Ophthalmology. 2008; 115(10): 1742-9.

1127 Wagley S, Marra KV, et al. Periodontal Disease and Age-Related Macular Degeneration: Results From the National Health and Nutrition Examination Survey III. Retina. 2015; 35(5): 982-8.

1128 Kalayoglu MV, Bula D, et al. Identification of Chlamydia pneumoniae within human choroidal neovascular membranes secondary to age-related macular degeneration. Graefes Arch Clin Exp Ophthalmol. 2005; 243: 1080-1090.

1129 Robman L, Mahdi OS, et al. Exposure to Chlamydia pneumoniae infection and age-related macular degeneration: the Blue Mountains Eye Study. Invest Ophthalmol Vis Sci. 2007; 48: 4007-4011.

1130 Kalayoglu MV, Bula D, et al. Identification of Chlamydia pneumoniae within human choroidal neovascular membranes secondary to age-related macular degeneration. Graefes Arch Clin Exp Ophthalmol. 2005; 243: 1080-1090.

1131 Ibid.

1132 Lockhart PB, Bolger AF, et al. Periodontal disease and atherosclerotic vascular disease: does the evidence support an independent association?: a scientific statement from the American Heart Association. Circulation. 2012; 125(20): 252044.

1133 Ibid.

1134 Bird AC, Marshall J. Retinal pigment epithelial detachments in the elderly. Trans Ophthalmol Soc UK. 1986; 105: (Pt 6): 674-82.

1135 "A brief history of tobacco." No author. ND. CNN.com. Available at: *http://edition.cnn.com/US/9705/tobacco/history/*

1136 Goodman, J. Webs of Drug Dependence: Towards a Political History of Tobacco. In: Lock S, Reynolds LA, and Tansey, EM, ed. *Ashes to Ashes: The History of Smoking and Health*. Amsterdam – Atlanta, Editions Rodopi B.V., 1998: 16-28.

1137 Piermarocchi S, Tognetto D, et al. Risk Factors and Age-Related Macular Degeneration in a Mediterranean-Basin Population: the PAMDI (Prevalence of Age-Related Macular Degeneration in Italy) Study – Report 2. Ophthalmic Res. 2016; 55(3): 111-8.

1138 Rasoulinejad SA, Zarghami A, et al. Prevalence of age-related macular degeneration among the elderly. Caspian J Intern Med. 2015; 6(3): 141-7.

1139 Velilla S, Garcia-Medina JJ, et al. Smoking and Age-Related Macular Degeneration: Review and Update. J of Ophthalmol. 2013; 2013:895147.

1140 Chakravarthy U, Wong TY, Fletcher A, et al. Clinical risk factors for age-related macular degeneration: a systematic review and meta-analysis. BMC Ophthalmology. 2010: Dec 13;10: 31.

1141 Tomany SC, Wang JJ, Van Leeuwen R, et al. Risk factors for incident age-related macular degeneration: pooled findings from 3 continents. Ophthalmology. 2004; 111(7): 1280-7.

1142 Seddon JM, Sobrin L. "Epidemiology of age-related macular degeneration." In Albert and Jakobiec's Principles and Practice of Ophthalmology, D. Albert, J. Miller, et al. Vol. 1, pp. 413-422, Saunders, Philadelphia, PA, USA, 3rd Edition, 2008.

1143 de Jong, PTVM. Age-related macular degeneration. New England Journal of Medicine. 2006; 355(14): 1474-1485.

1144 Seddon JM, Ajani UA, et al. Dietary carotenoids, vitamins A, C, and E, and advanced age-related macular degeneration. JAMA; 1994; 272(18): 1413-20.

1145 Seddon JM, Willett WC, et al. A prospective study of cigarette smoking and age-related macular degeneration in women. JAMA. 1996; 276(14): 1141-46.

1146 Seddon JM, Cote J, et al. Progression of age-related macular degeneration: association with body mass index, waist circumference, and waist-hip ratio. Archives of Ophthalmol. 2003; 121(6): 785-792.

1147 Seddon JM, Cote J, Rosner B. Progression of age-related macular degeneration: association with dietary fat, transunsaturated fat, nuts, and fish intake. Arch of Ophthalmol. 2003; 121(12): 1728-37.

1148 Seddon JM Rosner B, et al. Dietary fat and risk for advanced age-related macular degeneration. Arch of Ophthalmol. 2001; 119(8): 1191-99.

1149 Fowles J, Dybing E. Application of toxicological risk assessment principles to the chemical constituents of cigarette smoke. Tobacco Control. 2003; 12(4): 424-430.

1150 "Smoking & Tobacco Use." Centers for Disease Control and Prevention. ND. Available at: *http://www.cdc.gov/tobacco/data_statistics/sgr/2010/consumer_booklet/chemicals_smoke/*

1151 Roth F, Bindewald A, et al. Key pathophysiologic pathways in age-related macular disease. Graefe's Archive for Clinical and Experimental Ophthalmology. 2004; 242(8): 710-716.

1152 "Learn about Dioxin." EPA. United States Environmental Protection Agency. Available at: *http://www.epa.gov/dioxin/learn-about-dioxin*

1153 Hoffman EC, Reyes H, et al. Cloning of a factor required for activity of the Ah (dioxin) receptor. Science. 1991; 252(5008): 954-958.

1154 Takeuchi A, Takeuchi K, et al. Effects of dioxin on vascular endothelial growth factor (VEGF) production in the retina associated with choroidal neovascularization. Investigative Ophthalmology and visual Science. 2009; 50(7): 3410-3416.

1155 Yang YM, Huang DY, et al. Effects of 2,3,7,8-tetrachlorodibenzo-p-dioxin on vitamin A metabolism in mice. J Biochem Mol Toxicol. 2005; 19(5): 327-35.

1156 Yang YM, Huang DY, et al. Inhibitory effects of vitamin A on TCDD-induced cytochrome P-450 1A1 enzyme activity and expression. Toxicol Sci. 2005; 85(1): 727-34.

1157 Woodside JV, Young IS, et al. Factors associated with serum/plasma concentrations of vitamins A, C, E, and carotenoids in older people throughout Europe: the EUREYE study. Eur J Nutr 2013; 52: 1493-1501.

1158 Snodderly DM. Evidence for protection against age-related macular degeneration by carotenoids and antioxidant vitamins. Am J Clin Nutr 1995; 62: 1448S-1461S.

1159 Woodside JV, Young IS, et al. Factors associated with serum/plasma concentrations of vitamins A, C, E, and carotenoids in older people throughout Europe: the EUREYE study. Eur J Nutr 2013; 52: 1493-1501.

1160 Baybutt RC, Hu L, Molteni A. Vitamin A deficiency injures lung and liver parenchyma and impairs function of rat type II pneumocytes. J Nutr. 2000; 130(5): 1159-65.

1161 Li T, Molteni A, et al. Vitamin A depletion induced by cigarette smoke is associated with the development of emphysema in rats. J Nutr. 2003; 133(8): 2629-34.

1162 Ibid.

1163 Ibid.

1164 Titova OE, Ayvazova EA, et al. The influence of active and passive smoking during pregnancy on umbilical cord blood levels of vitamins A and E and neonatal anthropometric indices. Br J Nutr. 2012; 108(8): 1341-5.

1165 Ibid.

1166 Morabia A, Sorenson A, et al. Vitamin A, Cigarette Smoking, and Airway Obstruction. American Review of Respiratory Disease. 1989; 140(5): 1312-1316.

1167 Hirayama F, Lee AH, et al. Do vegetables and fruits reduce the risk of chronic obstructive pulmonary disease? A case-control study in Japan. Prev Med. 2009; 49(2-3): 184-9.

1168 Brot C, Jorgensen NR, Sorensen OH. The influence of smoking on vitamin D status and calcium metabolism. Eur J Clin Nutr. 1999; 53(12): 920-926.

1169 Schectman G, Byrd JC, Gruchow HW. The influence of smoking on vitamin C status in adults. American Journal of Public Health. 1989; 79(2): 158-162.

1170 Preston AM. Cigarette smoking-nutritional implications. Progress in Food & Nutrition Science. 1991; 15(4): 183-217.

1171 Klein R, Klein BEK, Linton KLP. Prevalence of Age-related Maculopathy. The Beaver Dam Eye Study. Ophthalmology. 1992; 99: 933-943.

1172 Wolf PA, D'Agostino RB, et al. Cigarette Smoking as a Risk Factor for Stroke. The Framingham Study. JAMA. 1988; 259: 1025-1029.

1173 Mendez D, Warner KE, Courant PN. Has Smoking Cessation Ceased? Expected Trends in the Prevalence of Smoking in the United States. Am J Epidemiol. 1998; 148: 249-58.

1174 Kessaram T, McKenzie J, et al. Tobacco Smoking in Islands of the Pacific Region, 2001-2013. Prev Chronic Dis. 2015; 12:150155. DOI: *http://dx.doi.org/10.5888/ped12.15055.*

1175 Tuomilehto J, Zimmet P, et al. Smoking rates in Pacific islands. Bulletin of World Health Organization. 1986; 64(3): 447-456.

1176 Rasanathan K, Tukuitonga CF. Tobacco smoking prevalence in Pacific Island countries and territories: a review. The New Zealand Medical Journal. 2007; 120(1263): U2742. Review.

1177 Cama, Dr Ana. AMD Prevalence in Fiji. 2016. E-mail.

1178 Sikivou, Dr Biu. AMD Prevalence in Fiji. 2016. E-mail.

1179 Rakabu-Hicks, Dr Tarai. AMD Prevalence in Western Fiji. 2016. E-mail.

1180 Tuomilehto J, Zimmet P, et al. Smoking rates in Pacific islands. Bulletin of World Health Organization. 1986; 64(3): 447-456.

1181 Rasanathan K, Tukuitonga CF. Tobacco smoking prevalence in Pacific Island countries and territories: a review. The New Zealand Medical Journal. 2007; 120(1263): U2742. Review.

1182 Tekeraoi, Dr Rabebe. AMD Prevalence in Kiribati. 2016. E-mail.

1183 Tuomilehto J, Zimmet P, et al. Smoking rates in Pacific islands. Bulletin of World Health Organization. 1986; 64(3): 447-456.

1184 Rasanathan K, Tukuitonga CF. Tobacco smoking prevalence in Pacific Island countries and territories: a review. The New Zealand Medical Journal. 2007; 120(1263): U2742. Review.

1185 Ah Ching, Dr Lucilla. AMD Prevalence in Samoa. 2016. E-mail.

1186 Rasanathan K, Tukuitonga CF. Tobacco smoking prevalence in Pacific Island countries and territories: a review. The New Zealand Medical Journal. 2007; 120(1263): U2742. Review.

1187 Kessaram T, McKenzie J, et al. Tobacco Smoking in Islands of the Pacific Region, 2001-2013. Prev Chronic Dis. 2015; 12:150155. DOI: *http://dx.doi.org/10.5888/ped12.15055*.

1188 Posala, Dr Claude. Prevalence of AMD in the Solomon Islands. 2016. E-mail.

1189 Stoffel, Tim. "Lion Facts." Lionlamb. Feb 15, 2004. Available at: *http://foodbabe.com/2014/02/24/healthiest-bread-on-the-market/, http://www.lionlamb.us/lion/lionfact.html*

1190 Offit, Paul. "The Vitamin Myth: Why We Think We Need Supplements." *The Atlantic.* Jul 19, 2013. Available at: *http://www.theatlantic.com/health/archive/2013/07/the-vitamin-myth-why-we-think-we-need-supplements/277947/*

1191 Ibid.

1192 Ibid.

1193 Price, Catherine. *Vitamania - Our Obsessive Quest For Nutritional Perfection.* Penguin Press, New York, 2015, pp. 1-11.

1194 Svirbely JL, Szent-Gyorgyi A. The chemical nature of vitamin C. Biochem J. 1932: 26865-870.

1195 Waugh WA, King CG. Isolation and identification of vitamin C. J Biol Chem. 1932, 97: 325-331.

1196 Frankenburg, Frances Rachel. *Vitamin Discoveries And Disasters.* Praeger, Santa Barbara, CA, 2009, pp. 15-32.

1197 Price, Catherine. *Vitamania - Our Obsessive Quest For Nutritional Perfection.* Penguin Press, New York, 2015, pp. 27-46.

1198 Kamminga, Harmke and Andrew Cunningham (Editors). *The Science And Culture of Nutrition, 1840 - 1940.* Amsterdam - Atlanta, GA, Editions Rodopi B.V., 1995.

1199 Price, Catherine. *Vitamania - Our Obsessive Quest For Nutritional Perfection.* Penguin Press, New York, 2015, pp. 27-46.

1200 Fulgoni VL, Keast DR, et al. Foods, Fortificants, and Supplements: Where Do Americans Get Their Nutrients? J Nutr. 2011; 141: 1847-1854.

1201 Price, Catherine. *Vitamania - Our Obsessive Quest For Nutritional Perfection.* Penguin Press, New York, 2015, p. 26.

1202 Evans JR, Lawrenson JG. Antioxidant vitamin and mineral supplements for preventing age-related macular degeneration (Review). The Cochrane Collaboration. The Cochrane Library, 2012, Issue 6.

1203 Age-Related Eye Disease Study Research Group. A randomized, placebo-controlled, clinical trial of high-dose supplementation with vitamins C and E, beta carotene, and zinc for age-related macular degeneration and vision loss: AREDS report no. 8. Arch Ophthalmol. 2001; 119(10): 1417-36.

1204 Bressler NM, Bressler SB, et al. Potential public health impact of Age-Related Eye Disease Study results: AREDS report no. 11. Arch Ophthalmol. 2003; 121: 1621-1624.

1205 Age-Related Eye Disease Study 2 Research Group. Lutein + zeaxanthin and omega-3 fatty acids for age-related macular degeneration: the Age-Related Eye Disease Study 2 (AREDS2) randomized clinical trial. JAMA. 2013; 309(19): 2005-15.

1206 Ibid.

1207 Evans JR, Lawrenson JG. Antioxidant vitamins and mineral supplements to slow the progression of age-related macular degeneration. Cochrane. 14 Nov. 2012.

1208 The Alpha-Tocopherol, Beta Carotene Cancer Prevention Study Group. The effect of vitamin E and beta carotene on the incidence of lung cancer and other cancers in male smokers. N Engl J Med. 1994; 330: 1029-35.

1209 Lonn E, Bosch J, et al. Effects of long-term vitamin E supplementation on cardiovascular events and cancer: a randomized controlled trial. JAMA. 2005; 293(11): 1338-47.

1210 Harrison, Laird. "Supplements to Slow Macular Degeneration May Backfire." Medscape. August 13, 2014.

1211 Awh CC, Lane AM, Hawken S, et al. CFH and ARMS2 genetic polymorphisms predict response to antioxidants and zinc in patients with age-related macular degeneration. Ophthalmol. 2013; 120(11): 2317-23.

1212 Harrison, Laird. "Supplements to Slow Macular Degeneration May Backfire." Medscape. August 13, 2014.

1213 Yong JJ, Scott IU, Greenberg PB. Ocular nutritional supplements: are their ingredients and manufacturers' claims evidence based? Ophthalmology. 2015; 122(3): 595-9.

1214 Bjelakovic G, Nikolova D, et al. Antioxidant supplements for prevention of mortality in healthy participants and patients with various diseases. Cochrane. 14 March, 2012. Available at: *http://www.cochrane.org/CD007176/LIVER_antioxidant-supplements-for-prevention-of-mortality-in-healthy-participants-and-patients-with-various-diseases*

1215 Mazzucco, Massimo. *Cancer - The Forbidden Cures.* Buenaonda Films, London, UK. 2013. Available at: *https://www.youtube.com/watch?v=3ncDdqNDcaI*

1216 Price, Weston A. Nutrition and Physical Degeneration. 1939, 1945 by Weston A. Price. Lemon Grove, California, The Price-Pottenger Nutrition Foundation, Inc. 1970 – 2008.

1217 Wilcox, Christie. "Are lower pesticide residues a good reason to buy organic? Probably not." Scientific American. Sep 24, 2012. Available at: *http://blogs.scientificamerican.com/science-sushi/pesticides-food-fears/*

1218 Smith-Spangler C, Brandeau ML, et al. Are organic foods safer or healthier than conventional alternatives? A systemic review. Ann Intern Med. 2012; 157(5): 348-66.

1219 Ibid.

1220 Ibid.

1221 Velimirov A, Lindenthal T. Opinion on the publication of the Stanford University Medical School study: "Are Organic Foods Safer or Healthier than Conventional Alternatives? A Systematic Review. Annals of Internal Medicine. 2012; 157: 348-366.

1222 Ibid.

1223 Benbrook, Charles. Initial Reflections on the Annals of Internal Medicine Paper "Are Organic Foods Safer and Healthier Than Conventional Alternatives? A Systematic Review." Center for Sustaining Agriculture and Natural Resources, Washington State University. Sep 4, 2012. Available at: *http://www.tfrec.wsu.edu/pdfs/P2566.pdf*

1224 Ibid.

1225 Ibid.

1226 Ibid.

1227 Arbuckle, TE, Lin ZQ, & Mery LS. An exploratory analysis of the effect of pesticide exposure on the risk of spontaneous abortion in an Ontario farm population. Environmental Health Perspectives. 2001; 109: 851-857.

1228 Bellinger D. A Strategy for Comparing the Contributions of Environmental Chemicals and Other Risk Factors to Neurodevelopment of Children." Environmental Health Perspectives. 2012: 20(4): 501-507.

1229 Bouchard ME, et al. Prenatal Exposure to OP Pesticides and IQ in 7-Year Old Children. Environmental Health Perspectives. April 21, 2011. Available at: http://ehp.niehs.nih.gov/1003185

1230 Engel SM, et al. Prenatal Exposure to Ops, Paraoxonase 1, and Cognitive Development in Children. Environmental Health Perspectives. April 21, 2011. Available at: http://ehp.niehs.nih.gov/1003183

1231 Garry VF, Harkins ME, et al. Birth defects, season of conception, and sex of children born to pesticide applicators living in the red river valley of Minnesota, USA. Environmental Health Perspectives. 2002; 110: 441-449.

1232 Rauh V, et al. 7-Year Neurodevelopmental Scores and Prenatal Exposure to Chlorpyrifos, a Common Agricultural Insecticide. Environmental Health Perspectives. April 21, 2011. Available at: http://ehp.niehs.nih.gov/1003160

1233 Schreinemachers D. Birth malformations and other adverse perinatal outcomes in four U.S. wheat-producing states. Environmental Health Perspectives. 2003; 111: 1259-1264. Available at: http://www.ncbi.nlm.nih.gov/pmc/articles/PMC1241584

1234 "How to Decipher Egg Carton Labels." The Humane Society of the United States. ND. Available at: http://www.humanesociety.org/issues/confinement_farm/facts/guide_egg_labels.html?credit=web_id95843339

1235 "Egg, whole, cooked, hard-boiled." SELFNutritionData.com. ND. Available at: http://nutritiondata.self.com/facts/dairy-and-egg-products/117/2

1236 Karsten HD, Patterson PH, et al. Vitamins A, E and fatty acid composition of the eggs of caged hens and pastured hens. Renewable Agriculture and Food Systems. 2010; 25: 45-54.

1237 "Home: The Facts About Real Raw Milk." Real Milk.com. A Campaign for Real Milk. Dec 10, 2015. Available at: http://www.realmilk.com

1238 Fallon, Sally. *Nourishing Traditions.* New Trends Publishing, Brandywine, MD, 1999, 2001, pp. 34-35.

1239 "State Updates." Real Milk.com. A Campaign for Real Milk. Jan 23, 2016. Available at: http://www.realmilk.com/state-updates/

1240 Taubes, G. Why We Get Fat and What To Do About It. New York. Alfred A. Knopf. 2011. pp. 175-6.

1241 Price, Weston A. *Nutrition and Physical Degeneration.* The Price-Pottenger Nutrition Foundation, Lemon Grove, CA. 1939, p. 69.

1242 Daley CA, Abbott A, et al. A review of fatty acid profiles and antioxidant content in grass-fed and grain-fed beef. Nutrition Journal. 2010 Mar 10;9:10. Doi: 10.1186/1475-2891-9-10.

1243 Ponnampalam EN, Mann NJ, Sinclair AJ. Effect of feeding systems on omega-3 fatty acids, conjugated linoleic acid and trans fatty acids in Australian beef cuts: potential impact on human health. Asia Pac J Clin Nutr. 2006; 15(1): 21-29.

1244 Daley CA, Abbott A, et al. A review of fatty acid profiles and antioxidant content in grass-fed and grain-fed beef. Nutrition Journal. 2010 Mar 10;9:10. Doi: 10.1186/1475-2891-9-10.

1245 Leheska JM, Thompson LD, et al. Effects of conventional and grass-feeding systems on the nutrient composition of beef. J Anim Sci. 2008; 86(12): 3575-85.

1246 Ponnampalam EN, Mann NJ, Sinclair AJ. Effect of feeding systems on omega-3 fatty acids, conjugated linoleic acid and trans fatty acids in Australian beef cuts: potential impact on human health. Asia Pac J Clin Nutr. 2006; 15(1): 21-29.

1247 Ponnampalam EN, Mann NJ, Sinclair AJ. Effect of feeding systems on omega-3 fatty acids, conjugated linoleic acid and trans fatty acids in Australian beef cuts: potential impact on human health. Asia Pac J Clin Nutr. 2006; 15(1): 21-29.

1248 Whisnant, Patricia. "Frequently Asked Questions of American Grass Fed Beef." American Grass Fed Beef. ND. Available at: http://www.americangrassfedbeef.com/faq-grass-fed-beef.asp

1249 Hossain MA. Fish as Source of n-3 Polyunsaturated Fatty Acids (PUFAs), Which One is Better – Farmed or Wild? Advance Journal of Food Science and Technology. 2011; 3(6): 455-466.

1250 Mozaffarian D, Rimm EB. Fish Intake, Contaminants, and Human Health. JAMA. 2006; 296(15): 1885-1899.

1251 "Cage-Free vs. Battery-Cage Eggs – Comparison of animal welfare in both methods." The Human Society of the United States. ND. http://www.humanesociety.org/issues/confinement_farm/facts/cage-free_vs_battery-cage.html

1252 "Scientists and Experts on Gestation Crates and Sow Welfare. The Humane Society of the United States. October, 2012. Available at: http://www.humanesociety.org/assets/pdfs/farm/HSUS-Synopsis-of-Expert-Opinions-on-Gestation-Crates-and-Sow-Welfare.pdf

1253 Cordain, Loren. *The Paleo Answer.* John Wiley & Sons, Inc. Hoboken, New Jersey, 2012.

1254 Guyenet, Stephan. "Book Review: Dangerous Grains." Whole Health Source. Nov 1, 2008. Available at: http://wholehealthsource.blogspot.com/2008/11/book-review-dangerous-grains.html

1255 Holm FA, Johnson EN. "The history of herbicide use for weed management on the prairies." *Prairie Soils and Crops,* 2009: 2:1 Available Online: http://prairiesoilsandcrops.ca/articles/volume-2-1-print.pdf

1256 Schreinemachers DM. Birth malformations and other adverse perinatal outcomes in four U.S. Wheat-producing states. Environ Health Perspect. 2003; 111(9): 1259-1264.

1257 Czapp, Katherine. "Our Daily Bread." The Weston A. Price Foundation. July 12, 2003. Available at: http://www.westonaprice.org/health-topics/our-daily-bread/

1258 Luo Y, Xie W, Luo F. Effect of several germination treatments on phosphatases activities and degradation of phytate in faba bean (Vicia faba L.) and azuki bean (Vigna angularis L.). J Food Sci. 2012; 77(10): C1023-9.

1259 Centeno C, Viveros A, et al. Effect of several germination conditions on total P, phytate P, phytase, and acid phosphatase activities and inositol phosphate esters in rye and barley. J Agric Food Chem. 2001; 49(7): 3208-15.

1260 Chitra U, Singh U, Rao PV. Phytic acid, in vitro protein digestibility, dietary fiber, and minerals of pulses as influenced by processing methods. Plant Foods Hum Nutr. 1996; 49(4): 307-16.

1261 Bjarnadottir, Adda. "10 Healthy Ways to Replace Conventional Wheat Bread." Authority Nutrition.com. Aug, 1015.

1262 Hari, Vani. "Before You Ever Buy Bread Again… Read This! (And Find the Healthiest Bread On the Markt." FoodBabe.com, ND. Available at: https://authoritynutrition.com/10-ways-to-replace-bread/

1263 Hari, Vani. "If You Eat, You Need Us." FoodBabe.com. ND. Available at: http://foodbabe.com/subscribe

1264 Schlemmer U, Frolich W, et al. Phytate in foods and significance for humans: food sources, intake, processing, bioavailability, protective role and analysis. Mol Nutr Food Res. 2009; 53 Suppl 2: S330-75.

1265 Ibid.

1266 Tabekhia MM, Luh BS. Effect of germination, cooking, and canning on phosphorus and phytate retention in dry beans. J Food Sci. 1980; 45: 406-408.

1267 Arnarson, Atli. "Phytic Acid 101: Everything You Need to Know." Authority Nutrition.com, July, 2015. Available at: *https://authoritynutrition.com/phytic-acid-101/*

1268 Fallon, Sally. *Nourishing Traditions*. New Trends Publishing, Brandywine, Maryland, 1999, 2001, pp. 452-510.

1269 Price, Weston A. *Nutrition and Physical Degeneration*. Price-Pottenger Nutrition Foundation, Lemon Grove, California, pp. 229- 238.

1270 Price, Weston A. *Nutrition and Physical Degeneration*. Price-Pottenger Nutrition Foundation, Lemon Grove, California, p. 238.

1271 Ibid, p. 241.

1272 Geleijnse JM, Vermeer C, et al. Dietary intake of menaquinone is associated with a reduced risk of coronary heart disease: the Rotterdam Study. J Nutr. 204; 134(11): 3100-5.

1273 Schurgers LJ, Spronk HMH, Soute BAM, et al. Regression of warfarin-induced medial elastocalcinosis by high intake of vitamin K in rats. Blood. 2007;109(7):2823-2831.

1274 Allbritton, Jen. "Sacred Foods for Exceptionally Healthy Babies… and parents, too!" The Weston A. Price Foundation. Sep 28, 2010. Available at: *http://www.westonaprice.org/childrens-health/sacred-foods-for-exceptionally-healthy-babies-and-parents-too/*

1275 Lentjes MAH, Welch AA, et al. Cod Liver Oil Supplement Consumption and Health: Cross-sectional Results from the EPIC-Norfolk Cohort Study. Nutrients. 2014; 6(10): 4320-4337.

1276 Fallon Morell, Sally. "Questions and Answers About Fermented Cod Liver Oil (FCLO)." The Weston A. Price Foundation. Aug 28, 2015. Available at: *http://www.westonaprice.org/uncategorized/questions-and-answers-about-fermented-cod-liver-oil-fclo/*

1277 Wetzel, David. "Cod Liver Oil Manufacturing." The Weston A. Price Foundation. Feb 28, 2006. Available at: *https://web.archive.org/web/20120311195548/*; *http://www.westonaprice.org/cod-liver-oil/clo-manufacturing*

1278 Möller, F. Peckel. *Cod Liver Oil and Chemistry*. W.H. Schieffelin & Co., New York, 1895, p. xliv-xlv.

1279 Ibid, p. lv.

1280 Price, Weston A. *Nutrition and Physical Degeneration*. Price-Pottenger Foundation, Lemon Grove, California, 1939, p. 390-392.

1281 Fallon, Sally. "Cod Liver Oil Basics and Recommendations." The Weston A. Price Foundation. Feb 9, 2015, Updated, Nov 23, 2015. Available at: *http://www.westonaprice.org/health-topics/cod-liver-oil-basics-and-recommendations/*

1282 Lopez Alonso, M, Benedito JL, et al. Arsenic, cadmium, lead, copper and zinc in cattle from Galicia, NW Spain. Science of The Total Environment. 2000; 246(2-3): 237-248.

1283 Peralta-Videa JR, Lopez ML, et al. The biochemistry of environmental heavy metal uptake by plants: Implications for the food chain. The International Journal of Biochemistry & Cell Biology. 2009; 41(8-9): 1665-1677.

1284 Tchounwou PB, Yedjou CG, et al. Heavy Metals Toxicity and the Environment. EXS. 2012; 101: 133-164.

1285 Geubel AP, De Galocsy C, et al. Liver damage caused by therapeutic vitamin A administration: estimate of dose-related toxicity in 41 cases. Gastroenterology. 1991; 100: 1701-1709.

1286 Masterjohn, Chris. "The Benefits of Liver, Cod Liver Oil, and Dessicated Liver." Cholesterol and Health. Aug, 2005. Available at: *http://www.cholesterol-and-health.com/Benefit-Of-Cod-Liver-Oil.html*

1287 Razaltis, Lynn. "The Liver Files." The Weston A. Price Foundation. July 29, 2005. Available at: *http://www.westonaprice.org/health-topics/the-liver-files/*

1288 Deutch B, Dyerberg J, Pedersen HS, Ashlund E, Hansen JC. Traditional and modern Greenlandic food – Dietary composition, nutrients and contaminants. Sci Tot Environ. 2007; 384: 106-119.

1289 Lavinder CH: The prevalence and geographic distribution of pellagra in the United States. Public Heal Rep. 1912; 27: 2076-2088.

1290 Goldberger J, Waring CH, Willets DG. The prevention of pellagra: a test of diet among institutionalized inmates. Public Health Rep. 1915: 30: 3117-3131.

1291 Goldberger J, Wheeler GA: Experimental pellagra in the human subject brought about by a restricted diet. Public Health Rep. 1915; 30: 3336-3339.

1292 Terris M: Human experiments. Goldberger on Pellagra. (Reprint of Goldberger J, Wheeler GA: The experimental production of pellagra in human subjects by means of diet. Hyg Lab Bull. 1920; 120: 7-116.) Baton Rouge, Louisiana State University Press, 1964, pp. 54-94.

1293 Frankenburg, Frances Rachel. *Vitamin Discoveries and Disasters – History, Science, and Controversies. Santa Barbara, California. Praeger. 2009, p. 41.*

1294 Elvehjem CA, Madden RJ, Strong FM, et al. Relation of nicotinic acid and nicotinic acid amide to canine black tongue. J Am Chem Soc. 1937; 59: 1767-1768.

1295 Sydenstricker VP: The history of pellagra, its recognition as a disorder of nutrition and its conquest. Am J Clin Nutr. 1958; 6: 409-414.

1296 Stoppler, Melissa Conrad. "Smoker's Lung Pathology Photo Essay. *MedicineNet.com*. May 09, 2013. Available at: *MedicineNet.com*.

1297 "Smoking and lung cancer." Netdoctor (*Netdoctor.co.uk*.) Jan 12, 2010. Available at: *http://www.netdoctor.co.uk/conditions/cancer/a10467/smoking-and-lung-cancer/*

1298 Duke-Elder, WS. *Textbook of Ophthalmology – Duke-Elder, Vol. III, Diseases of the Inner Eye*. St. Louis: The C.V. Mosby Company, 1940. pp. 2372-2373.

1299 Ibid. pp. 2373-2374.

1300 Ibid. p. 3193, 3328, 3285.

1301 The Eye Disease Prevalence Research Group. Prevalence of Age-Related Macular Degeneration in the United States. Arch Ophthalmol. 2004; 122(4): 564-572.

1302 Gillies MC, Campain A, et al. Long-Term Outcomes of Treatment of Neovascular Age-Related Macular Degeneration: Data from an Observational Study. Ophthalmology. 2015; 122(9): 1837-45.

1303 Gass, J Donald M. Drusen and Disciform Macular Detachment and Degeneration. Arch Ophthalmol. 1973; 90: 206-217.

1304 Smith, R T, Sohrab, MA, et al. Dynamic soft drusen remodeling in age-related macular degeneration. Br J Ophthalmol. 2010; 94(12): 1618-1623.

1305 Bressler NM, Munoz B, et al. Five-year incidence and disappearance of drusen and retinal pigment epithelial abnormalities. Waterman study. Arch Ophthalmol. 1995; 113(3): 301-8.

1306 Guyenet, Stephan. "The American Diet: A Historical Perspective." TEDx Harvard Law Lecture. October 21, 2011. Available at: *https://www.youtube.com/watch?v=HC20OoIgG_Y*

1307 Smith, Jeffrey M. *Seeds of Deception*. Yes! Books, Fairfield, Iowa, 2003.

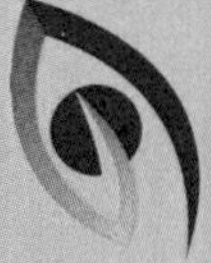

Index

Numbers

A

B

J

K

L

M

N

O